ANNALS OF THE NEW YORK ACADEMY OF SCIENCES

VOLUME 149, ART. 1 PAGES 1-583

March 29, 1968

Editor-in-Chief
EDWARD M. WEYER

Managing Editor
MARC KRAUSS

ERYTHROPOIETIN*

Consulting Editor
JAMES W. FISHER

Conference Cochairmen
JAMES W. FISHER AND ALBERT S. GORDON

CONTENTS

Dedication to Paul Carnot .... Frontispiece

Opening Remarks. *By* KARL H. BEYER, JR. 7

Introduction. *By* JAMES W. FISHER 9

Part I. Assay and Standardization of Erythropoietin

Quantitative Estimation of Erythropoietin. *By* P. MARY COTES 12

Further Experiences with Assays, Units, and Standards of Erythropoietin. *By* GEOFFREY KEIGHLEY 18

Studies on the Erythropoietic Effects of Hyperbaric Hyperoxia. *By* JAMES W. LINMAN AND ROBERT V. PIERRE 25

Use of Silicone Rubber Membrane Enclosures for Preparation of Erythropoietin Assay Mice. *By* R. D. LANGE, M. L. SIMMONS AND T. P. MCDONALD 34

Comparative Assay of Erythropoietin Standards. *By* JAMES F. CAMISCOLI, ARTHUR H. WEINTRAUB AND ALBERT S. GORDON 40

Quantitative Estimation of Erythropoietin. *By* NOMIE A. SHORE, NASSER MOVASSAGHI AND DENMAN HAMMOND 46

Part II. Chemistry and Purification of Erythropoietin

Progress in the Purification of Erythropoietin. *By* EUGENE GOLDWASSER AND CHARLES K. H. KUNG 49

The Fractionation of Erythropoietin from Anemic and Normal Human Urine. *By* PETER H. LOWY AND GEOFFREY KEIGHLEY 54

Preliminary Purification of Sheep and Mouse Erythropoietin by Vertical Flat Bed Discontinuous Electrophoresis in Acrylamide Gel. *By* ROBERT C. ALLEN, DOROTHY J. MOORE AND JAMES W. FISHER 63

The Commercial Production of Erythropoietin from Anemic Sheep Plasma. *By* R. H. PAINTER, W. R. BRUCE AND E. GOLDWASSER 71

* This series of papers is the result of a conference entitled Erythropoietin, held by The New York Academy of Sciences on June 1, 2 and 3, 1966.

Part III. Sites of Erythropoietin Production and Appearance in Tissue Fluids and Extracts

Effects of Testosterone, Cobalt and Hypoxia on Erythropoietin Production in the Isolated Perfused Dog Kidney. *By* James W. Fisher and J. W. Langston 75

Effects of Hypothalamic Stimulation on Erythropoiesis and on the Production of Erythropoiesis-Stimulating Factors in Intact and Nephrectomized Rabbits. *By* Sverre Halvorsen 88

Extra-Renal and Renal Control of Erythropoietin Production. *By* E. A. Mirand 94

Erythrocytosis, Juxtaglomerular Apparatus (JGA), and Erythropoietin in the Course of Experimental Unilateral Hydronephrosis in Rabbits. *By* W. J. Mitus, Keisuke Toyama and Mark J. Brauer 107

The Renal Erythropoietic Factor. I. Studies on Its Purification and Properties. *By* Joseph F. Contrera and Albert S. Gordon 114

Studies on the Site of Production of Erythropoietin. *By* Robert Katz, George W. Cooper, Albert S. Gordon and Esmail D. Zanjani 120

The Renal Mechanism of the Formation and Inactivation of Erythropoietin. *By* Z. Kuratowska 128

Renal Transplantation and Extracts and Erythropoiesis. *By* E. E. Muirhead, B. E. Leach, J. W. Fisher and Mary Kosinski 135

Erythropoiesis in Renal Insufficiency and in Anephric Man. *By* J. P. Naets, M. Wittek, C. Toussaint and J. Van Geertruyden 143

Part IV. Kinetics of Erythropoiesis and Sites of Action of Erythropoietin

Restoration of Stem Cell Function after Irradiation. *By* D. D. Porteous and L. G. Lajtha 151

Regulation of Erythropoiesis. XX. Kinetics of Red Cell Production. *By* Frederick Stohlman, Jr., Shirley Ebbe, Bernard Morse, Donald Howard and Janet Donovan 156

Effect of Polycythemic Serum on the Rate of Red Cell Production. *By* A. J. Erslev and E. B. Thorling 173

Studies on Hypoxia. VI. Changes in Lymphocytes and Transitional Cells in the Marrow during the Intensification of Primary Hypoxia and Rebound. *By* J. M. Yoffey, R. V. Jeffreys, D. G. Osmond, M. S. Turner, S. C. Tahsin and P. A. R. Niven 179

Selective Inhibition of Erythroid Cell Differentiation in the Mouse by Low Doses of Actinomycin D. *By* Kurt R. Reissmann and Kenjiro Ito 193

Ultrastructural and Autoradiographic Studies of Erythropoietin-Induced Red Cell Production. *By* Donald Orlic, Albert S. Gordon and Johannes A. G. Rhodin 198

The Increased Dose-Response of ESF after ESF Stimulation. *By* Jan Fogh 217

Enzymatic Studies on Erythroid Differentiation and Proliferation. *By* Kiku Nakao, Shigeru Sassa, Osamu Wada and Fumimaro Takaku 224

The Participation of Spleen and Bone Marrow in the Recovery of Mice after Suppression of Erythropoiesis by Actinomycin D. *By* José L. Scaro 229

Changes in the Erythropoietin-Responsive Cell after Exposure to Irradiation. *By* George Hodgson and Irma Eskuche 230

Humoral Effects on Marrow Cell Differentiation. *By* Donald R. Korst and Janet Quirk 236

Effect of Erythropoietin on Reticulocyte Release from the Isolated Perfused Rat Spleen. *By* Burton S. Dornfest, George W. Cooper and Albert S. Gordon 249

Erythropoietin and Erythropoiesis in Isolated Perfused Hind Legs of Rats: A Preliminary Study. *By* Joseph LoBue, Francis C. Monette, James F. Camiscoli, Albert S. Gordon and Po-Chuen Chan 257

Part V. Immunological Studies on Erythropoietin

A Summary of Some Studies on Erythropoiesis Using Anti-Erythropoietin Immune Serum. *By* JOHN C. SCHOOLEY, JOSEPH F. GARCIA, LINDA N. CANTOR AND VIRGINIA W. HAVENS 266

Application of Erythropoietin Antisera to Studies of Erythropoiesis. *By* ROBERT D. LANGE, LOIS F. O'GRADY, JERRY P. LEWIS AND FRANK E. TROBAUGH, JR. 281

Some Observations on the Localization of Erythropoietin. *By* EUGENE P. FRENKEL, WADI SUKI AND JOHN BAUM 292

Investigations on an Immunoassay of Erythropoietin. *By* P. G. L. C. KRUGERS DAGNEAUX, R. GOUDSMIT AND H. W. KRIJNEN 294

Part VI. Endocrine and Drug Influences on Erythropoiesis

Further Observations on the Mechanism by which Androgens and Growth Hormone Influence Erythropoiesis. *By* HOWARD A. MEINEKE AND ROGER C. CRAFTS 298

Effects of Angiotensin, Norepinephrine and Renal Artery Constriction on Erythropoietin Production. *By* JAMES W. FISHER, ALAN SAMUELS AND JAMES LANGSTON 308

Androgen Actions on Erythropoiesis. *By* ALBERT S. GORDON, EDWIN A. MIRAND, JEFFREY WENIG, ROBERT KATZ AND ESMAIL D. ZANJANI 318

The Interrelationships of the Endocrine and Erythropoietic Systems in the Rat with Special Reference to the Mechanism of Action of Estradiol and Testosterone. *By* SAM J. PILIERO, PAUL T. MEDICI AND CLARA HABER 336

The Erythropoietic-Stimulating Effects of Androgens. *By* W. FRIED AND C. W. GURNEY 356

The Mechanism of Action of Androgens on Erythropoiesis. *By* J. P. NAETS AND M. WITTEK 366

Hemolysis and Erythropoiesis. III. The Effect of Hemolysis and Hemolysates on Erythropoiesis. *By* L. SÁNCHEZ-MEDAL AND JUAN LABARDINI 377

Observations on the Effect of Testosterone and Hydrocortisone on Erythropoiesis. *By* BERTIL E. GLADER, WALTER A. RAMBACH AND HOWARD L. ALT 383

The Effect of Testosterone on the Uptake of Tritiated Thymidine by the Bone Marrow of Children. *By* W. JACOBSON, R. L. SIDMAN AND L. K. DIAMOND 389

Effects of Acetylcholinesterase on Erythropoiesis in Polycythemic and Mildly Plethoric Mice. *By* ALAN I. SAMUELS, LOTTE MOLLER AND JAMES W. FISHER 406

Discussion. *By* T. P. MCDONALD 409

Part VII. In Vitro Studies on Erythropoietin

Studies on the Control of Hemoglobin Formation in Marrow Cells. *By* MICHAEL E. HRINDA AND EUGENE GOLDWASSER 412

The Change of Hemoglobin Synthesis from Minor to Major in the Course of Erythroblast Maturation. *By* HENRY BORSOOK 416

Effect of Erythropoietin upon Hemoglobin Biosynthesis. *By* LORRAINE M. KRAUS, IWAO IUCHI AND BROTHER THOMAS KRAUS, F.S.C. 423

Application of the In Vitro Erythropoietin System to the Study of Human Bone Marrow Disease: Polycythemia Vera. *By* SANFORD B. KRANTZ 430

In Vitro Studies on DNA Synthesis of Bone Marrow Cells Stimulated by Erythropoietin. *By* PETER P. DUKES 437

Studies on Mitotic Activity In Vitro and Kinetics of Proliferation of Erythroid Cells from Splenic Colonies in Irradiated, Marrow-Transfused Mice. *By* Y. MATOTH 445

Studies on the Control of Hemoglobin Synthesis: Nucleic Acid Synthesis and Normoblast Proliferation in the Presence of Erythropoietin. *By* THOMAS F. NECHELES, RICHARD G. SHEEHAN AND HEIDI J. MEYER 449

Part VIII. Subjects Related to the Physiology of Erythropoietin

The Effect of Carbon Dioxide on Erythropoiesis. *By* José Faura, Clifford W. Gurney and Walter Fried 456

The Physiological Significance of an Erythropoietic Inhibitor Factor Appearing in Plasma Subsequent to Hypertransfusion. *By* Walter H. Whitcomb and Margaret Moore 462

Humoral Regulation of the Erythropoietic Depression of High Altitude Polycythemic Subjects after Return to Sea Level. *By* César Reynafarje 472

Two Hereditary Mouse Anemias (Sl/Sl^d and W/W^v) Deficient in Response to Erythropoietin. *By* Seldon E. Bernstein, Elizabeth S. Russell and Geoffrey Keighley 475

Murine Viral-Induced Polycythemia. *By* E. A. Mirand 486

Part IX. Clinical and Pathological Conditions Related to Erythropoietin Production

Erythropoietin Production in Fetal Hypoxia and in Anemic Uremic Patients. *By* Per Haavardsholm Finne 497

Human Erythropoiesis Following Kidney Transplantation. *By* George C. Hoffman..... 504

The Erythropoiesis-Stimulating Factors Produced by Tumors. *By* Thomas A. Waldmann, Wendell F. Rosse and Richard L. Swarm 509

Production, Utilization and Excretion of Erythropoietin: I. Chronic Anemias. II. Aplastic Crisis. III. Erythropoietic Effects of Normal Plasma. *By* Denman Hammond, Nomie Shore and Nasser Movassaghi 516

Inappropriate Erythropoietin Elaboration. *By* Neil I. Gallagher and Robert M. Donati 528

Erythrocyte Production and Metabolism in Anephric and Uremic Men. *By* David G. Nathan, Laurence H. Beck, Constantine L. Hampers and John P. Merrill..... 539

Fetal and Neonatal Erythropoiesis. *By* G. Lucarelli, A. Porcellini, C. Carnevali, A. Carmena and F. Stohlman, Jr. 544

Erythropoietin and the Polycythemias. *By* John W. Adamson and Clement A. Finch..... 560

Collection of Erythropoietin from Urine of Patients with Anemia Secondary to Hookworm. *By* Abraham Gutnisky, Luis Malgor, Mary Lou Nohr and Donald Van Dyke 564

High Hematocrit in Hypertension and Its Relationship with Renal Arterial Disease. *By* Edward D. Frohlich and Robert C. Tarazi 569

Renal Erythropoietin Excretion as a Function of Acid Base Balance. *By* Diana Marver and Clifford W. Gurney 570

Erythropoietin Production in the Human Fetus and Newborn. *By* Sverre Halvorsen and Per Haavardsholm Finne 576

Summary of Conference on Erythropoietin. *By* Leon O. Jacobson and Sanford B. Krantz 578

Dedicated to

PAUL CARNOT

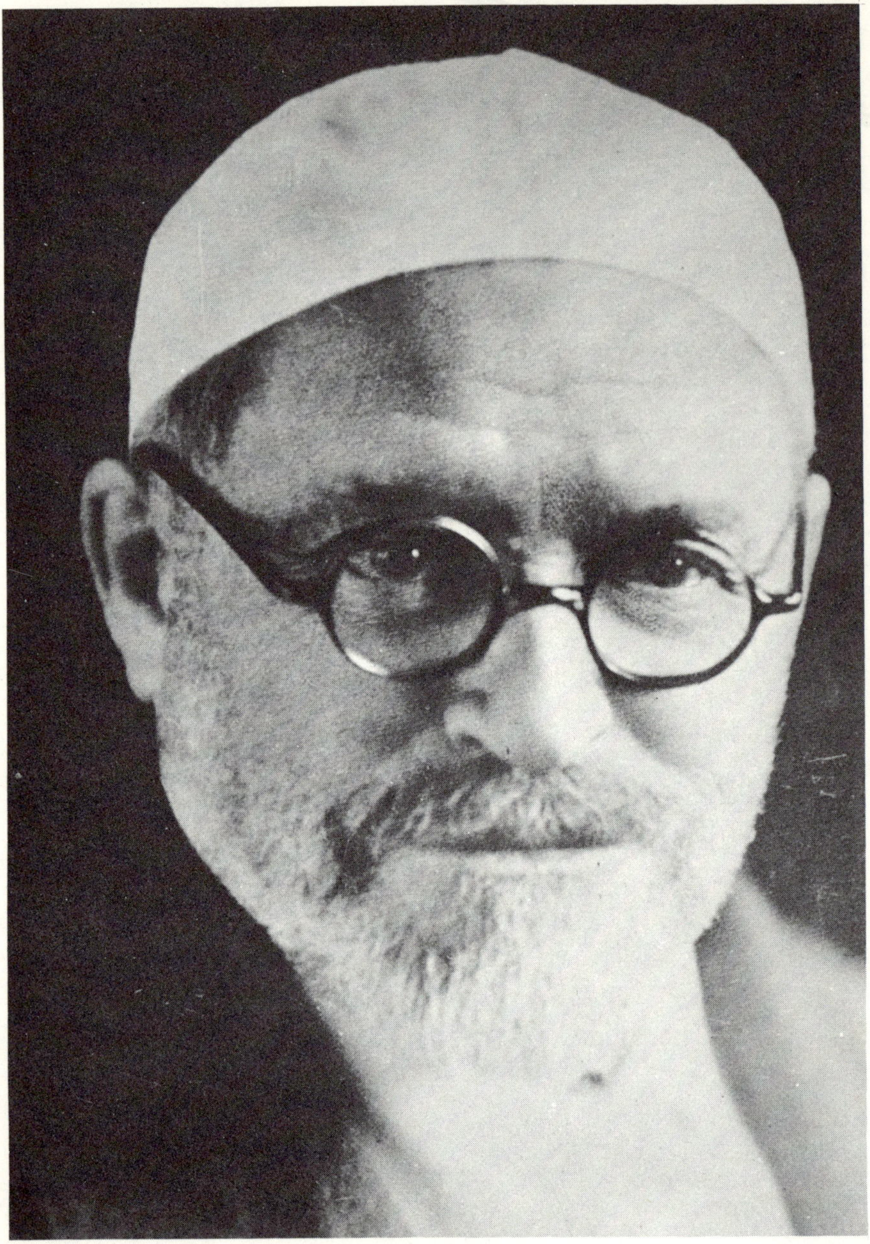

PAUL CARNOT

1869–1957

First to propose that red cell production is regulated by a humoral factor.

"We have observed with Mlle. Déflandre that regeneration of blood after blood letting is under the influence of a humoral process . . . we give this substance the generic name Hémopoïétine."

OPENING REMARKS

Karl H. Beyer, Jr.
Merck, Sharp & Dohme Research Laboratories
West Point, Pa.

I find myself neither greeting you for the Academy, of which I have been a member for perhaps 20 years, nor reciting the aims of the Conference which Dr. Fisher and Dr. Gordon are better qualified to do. Then, too, I note that Dr. Jacobson has drawn the assignment to summarize the Conference. What can I do to be helpful, even though my associates and I have not been particularly active in this field?

I have been interested in erythropoietin for about 20 years, so, for me, this is not some brand new fad in medical research that has just come to the fore for its day in the sun. All aspects of its research have been tediously worked over and the present structure of knowledge in this field seems reasonably based on experimental evidence. As one reviews the literature, this includes substantial symposia by responsible groups and reviews in the best journals by thoughtful investigators over a period of years.

It seems certain that erythropoietin is secreted by the kidney and that its elaboration responds especially to reduction in oxygen tension. Presumably, it is elaborated by the juxtaglomerular apparatus, but I should like to hear more about this for I do not know that the sulfhydryl-inhibiting diuretics influence this mechanism except by the induction of hypovolemia, in which case the effects of potent diuretic agents should be more general across categories. Even the association of renal disease with anemia suggests a more general source within the kidney. The fact that there may be extra renal sources of erythropoietic-stimulating factors does not seem remarkable.

I shall be interested in hearing about the current status of assay for erythropoietin, for on this factor rests the further characterization of such a natural substance. Is it too much to ask for a still sharper, more rapid, sensitive, specific assay? This is what the chemists have needed to break through problems equally difficult.

I am impressed by what the immunologic technics have done to sharpen up the initial part that erythropoietin plays in erythropoiesis, and that it does not appear to be needed for subsequent maturation of cells. If this is so, this knowledge is helpful and reassuring as one tries to group the essential features of this homeostatic mechanism.

The program for this Conference on erythropoietin contains a wealth of detail regarding seemingly every aspect of research in this field, from the standardization of erythropoietin and its kinetics to clinical and pathological conditions related to erythropoietin production. Drs. Fisher and Gordon are to be congratulated on this good effort and the New York Academy of Sciences should be complimented for scheduling such an important conference.

My final comments relate to my own personal attitude toward research at this stage of investigation. Each of these presentations covering three days hopefully will be important as a contribution to knowledge in this and tangential fields. This alone would be a worthy objective for such a conference. Personally, when I moved from physiology to pharmacology I carried an interest in function, such as we are to discuss, to the modulation of function for the advancement of therapy.

It is clear that erythropoietin is a potent factor in the homeostasis of erythropoiesis. In turn, erythropoiesis, certain anemias and (to a lesser extent) polycythemias, are the facts of life with which the physician must deal on a daily basis throughout his career.

I am hopeful that some day we may better handle the practical problems of medicine to which this research relates. We need not know all about a biological phenomenon to control it. This is certain. But we do need to know enough about it to manipulate that phenomenon at will and in a quantitative way. Have we arrived at that point in erythropoiesis? Is erythropoietin sufficiently dominant in this homeostasis to serve our purpose of controlling this overall process? A practical, conceptual knowledge of this field will be needed for systematic advancement in therapy.

INTRODUCTION

James W. Fisher
University of Tennessee Medical Units, Memphis, Tenn.

We are very grateful to the New York Academy of Sciences for making it possible for a group of scientists from all parts of the world interested in erythropoietin to meet together for presentation and discussion of their research work. I should also like to thank each of the participants for his interest and cooperation in helping us make this Conference possible, especially those who have traveled such long distances and at great expense to come to the Conference. I believe we may have at least 14 countries outside of the United States represented here. Investigators from Argentina, Belgium, Canada, Chile, Denmark, England, Germany, Holland, Israel, Italy, Japan, Mexico, Norway and Peru are participating in this Conference. Regrettably, other investigators in the field of erythropoietin and control of erythropoiesis were unable to attend.

I wonder what Doctors Carnot and Déflandre might have thought had they been present at this Conference. Although their techniques may have been crude in the year 1906, they must be given credit for being first to postulate the existence of an erythropoietic-stimulating factor in plasma which they called "Hémopoïétine." We now generally refer to this substance as erythropoietin. We all know very well the oft-referred-to experiments of Carnot and Déflandre in which they demonstrated an increase in peripheral red cell counts in normal rabbits injected with plasma from rabbits made anemic by bleeding.[1,2] Of course we know today that the conclusions drawn from these data could have been invalid because it is possible that the effects seen may have been due to hemoconcentration or splenic contraction. The important point is that they were right in hypothesizing a humoral control of erythropoiesis. In a listing of his most important research works in 1918, Paul Carnot discussed regeneration of blood after blood-letting.[3] He said, "We have observed with Mlle. Déflandre that this repair is under the influence of a humoral process and that an animal's blood or serum, extracted during a period of active hematic regeneration and injected into a second animal, induces in the latter a hematopoietic flare-up. This is evidenced by increased bone marrow activity and by hematic proliferation. We have given this substance the generic name 'Hémopoïétine'." We are very pleased to dedicate this conference to Doctor Carnot. We were very fortunate in being able to locate the daughter of Dr. Carnot, Mme. Coquoin Carnot, who herself is a research scientist in the Laboratory of Histology on the Faculty of Medicine, University of Paris. I also wish to thank Dr. Marcel Bessis in Paris, for assisting me in this search. Mme. Carnot has generously supplied me with some 679 publications of her father, Dr. Paul Carnot, published during the years 1894 and 1949, as well as his picture, which is included in the monograph.

Paul Carnot was born on January 16, 1896 in Limoges, France and died in Paris, April 1, 1957. He was the father of nine children and belonged to an illustrious French family. His greatgrandfather was Minister of Armies in the time of Napoleon Bonaparte. Other ancestors include Sadi Carnot who enunciated the second law of thermodynamics. He held doctorate degrees in physics (Sorbonne, Faculté des Sciences) and medicine (Faculté de Médicine) from The University of Paris. His research works cover a broad area and extend from physiological aspects of the digestive system to humoral control of hematopoiesis. He also studied cytopoietins and extracted substances from the blood of unilaterally nephrectomized animals which stimulated renal regeneration. He called these substances "nephropoietins." He was a teacher, researcher and clinician. He was Professor of the Faculty of Medicine of The University of Paris (1903) and Professor and Head of the Medical Clinic at the Hôtel-Dieu Hospital (1927). He was also a member of the National Academy of Medicine and Commandeur de la Légion d'Honneur.

Even though much credit is due Carnot for being the first, I believe most of the credit for the rapid progress in this field should go to workers who have made major contributions during the last 10–15 years. We owe much thanks to Erslev[4] for having the courage to inject large quantities of serum from bled rabbits into recipient animals to demonstrate an erythropoietic effect. Stohlman's[5] observations on a patient with regional hypoxia and polycythemia secondary to a patent ductus arteriosus was also a landmark in helping to establish a humoral control of erythropoiesis. Borsook's[6] demonstration that the erythropoietic-stimulating substance is present in acidified boiled plasma added much to our understanding of the physicochemical properties of this substance. The findings by Hodgson and coworkers[7] of erythropoietic activity in urine and plasma of bled rabbits also helped to establish erythropoietin as a specific substance. Other experiments confirming a humoral control of erythropoiesis were those of Reissmann[8] who exposed one member of a pair of parabiotic rats to air at lowered oxygen tension while the other partner breathed normal air. Erythropoietic stimulation occurred in both animals, indicating the passage of a humoral erythropoietic substance from one partner to the other. Jacobson and colleagues[9] markedly advanced our knowledge in this field with their concept of a relation between oxygen tension of the blood and oxygen demand by the tissues as well as their work implicating the kidney as the site of production of erythropoietin. Their initiative in developing more sensitive and quantitative assay methods has also been of great value in advancing this field. Much credit must also go to Gordon and coworkers[10] for their contributions to endocrine influences on erythropoiesis as well as their studies on clinical sources, physicochemical properties, biogenesis and assay of erythropoietin.

These are only a few of the workers who have made important contributions to the field of erythropoietin and control of erythropoiesis. There are many more of us who have only recently come on the scene in this extremely interesting field and time does not allow us to mention other important contributors to our knowledge of sites of production, mechanism of action and chemistry of erythropoietin. However, I do believe that the time has passed when some of my friends in physiology will ask me the question, "Do you really think there is such a substance as erythropoietin?"

Since our last meeting on erythropoiesis in San Francisco, California in 1962, many new and important developments in this field have occurred. We hope that this Conference will help to clarify some of the vexing problems on the chemistry and purification of erythropoietin, sites of production (renal and extrarenal), sites and mechanisms of action on erythroid cells, clinical implications of erythropoietin, more sensitive assay techniques for this substance, advances in the immunology of erythropoietin and the significance of erythropoietin and the kidney in the normal physiological control of erythropoiesis.

References

1. CARNOT, P. & G. DEFLANDRE. 1906. Sur l'activité hémopoïétique du sérum au cours de la régénération du sang. Compt. rend. Acad. Science. **143:** 384–386.

2. Carnot, P. & C. Deflandre. 1906. Sur l'activité hémopoïétique des différents organes au cours de la régénération du sang. Compt. rend. Acad. Sci. **143**: 432–435.
3. Carnot, P. 1918. Exposé de Titres et Travaux. : 58.
4. Erslev, A. J. 1953. Blood **8**: 349.
5. Stohlman, F., Jr., C. E. Roth & J. C. Rose. 1954. Blood **9**: 721.
6. Borsook, H. A., A. Grayfield, G. Keighley & E. Windsor. 1954. Blood **9**: 734.
7. Hodgson, G. & J. Toha. 1954. Blood **9**: 299.
8. Reissman, K. R. 1950. Blood **5**: 372.
9. Jacobson, L. O., E. Goldwasser, W. Fried & L. Plzak. 1957. Nature **179**: 633.
10. Gordon, A. S., S. J. Piliero, W. Kleinberg, H. H. Freedman. 1964. Proc. Soc. Exp. Biol. Med. **86**: 255.

PART I. ASSAY AND STANDARDIZATION OF ERYTHROPOIETIN

QUANTITATIVE ESTIMATION OF ERYTHROPOIETIN

P. Mary Cotes

Division of Biological Standards, National Institute for Medical Research, Mill Hill, London, England

I should like to discuss the importance of selection of suitable test animals for bioassay, to comment on some problems involved in quantitation of bioassay results, and to draw attention to the availability of the International Reference Preparation of Erythropoietin for use as a standard for bioassay purposes.

Erythropoietin-like activity in samples of biological materials can be demonstrated by a range of in vivo and in vitro techniques, but definitive demonstration of erythropoietin, at least according to our present concepts, depends upon the ability of the preparation under test to induce an increase in the total red cell mass of a normal animal. Thus, for quantitative estimation of erythropoietin, we must use some variant of a bioassay system in which red cell formation, induced by known amounts of a standard preparation of erythropoietin, is compared with that induced by the sample whose activity is to be estimated. In the normal animal, the effect of a small dose of exogenous erythropoietin may be masked by the effect of endogenous erythropoietin; therefore, for most assays the system is made more sensitive by suppression of endogenous red cell formation in the test animals by starvation (in rats) (Fried *et al.*, 1957; Hodgson *et al.*, 1958) or by polycythemia from transfusion (Fried *et al.*, 1957; Jacobson *et al.*, 1960) or hypoxia (in mice) (Cotes & Bangham, 1961). Small increments in red cell formation, which need not cause a significant increase in the total red cell mass, are demonstrated by measurement of appearance of tracer amounts of injected Fe-59 iron into circulating red cells. Sensitivity and precision of assays are affected by the nature of the dose-response relationship, animal to animal variability, assay design including appropriateness of standard, relative doses of standard and unknown, and the number of animals used. If estimates of potency obtained on different occasions are to be compared, it is axiomatic that the reference standard should be stable.

In some assays we wish to find out not the minimum amount of erythropoietin detectable (which depends upon the sensitivity of the assay system), but the precision of an estimate of potency of a particular sample. The precision obtainable is limited in practice by the cost of the assay in terms of the total amount of erythropoietin used and the number of test animals needed to achieve given statistical fiducial limits for the estimate of potency. On the other hand, for assay of erythropoietin in clinical or experimental samples available in only limited quantities, it may be of more concern to measure very small amounts of erythropoietin and to use a small number of animals.

Selection of Animals

Since both the precision of the assay and the smallest dose of erythropoietin detectable in the system are influenced by the form of the dose-response relationship and by variability of responses, the choice and preparation of suitable test animals are extremely important. After selection of schedules for the assay using animals of different species and strain (1) amount and frequency of transfusions or level and duration of hypoxia or period of starvation in pretreatment; (2) route, number of doses and time of erythropoietin administration; (3) time and route of administration of Fe-59 iron; and (4) interval before blood sampling), it is still found that various strains of mice and rats differ in the reproducibility of responses and in the slope and dose range of the linear portion of the log-dose response (or log-dose log-response) regression.

Using essentially similar assay regimes in polycythemic mice of different strains, concurrent estimates of the relative potency of two preparations of erythropoietin were carried out in two laboratories (my own and Dr. Sephton Smith's). The results of these estimates are summarized in TABLE 1. For estimates of potency with comparable fiducial limits, five times as many mice and three times as much erythropoietin were used in one laboratory compared with the other. This difference was largely attributable to differences between the two strains of mice used. A_2G mice transferred to my laboratory gave better assay performance (index of precision $\lambda = 0.20$) than the M.R.C. TO mice which we had used previously (range of $\lambda = 0.31–0.52$). This improved performance was not maintained when the A_2G mice were bred in our laboratory and after trial of mice from five strains (M.R.C. TO, Parkes, Schneider (a virus-susceptible minimal disease stock), A_2G and CBA), we now use inbred CBA mice (females of 22 g weight).

Similarly, in the starved rat assay it is worthwhile to choose a suitable strain of rat. Hodgson (personal communication) found that one hooded strain of outbred rats gave very variable responses, whereas A × C rats were consistently satisfactory. Results from two laboratories which show the reproducibility of repeated estimates of the relative potency of two preparations of erythropoietin in different assays using the starved rat are shown in TABLE 2. The results of assays of the International Reference Preparation (Standard B) in terms of Standard A using as test animal the starved rat (TABLE 2, assays 26 and 27) may be compared with those obtained using as test animal the polycythemic mouse (TABLE 1). It can be seen from these assays that when similar numbers of animals and comparable dose levels are used, the starved rat gives assays which are comparable in precision with those obtained in the polycythemic mouse. The index of precision (λ) in 11 assays from four laboratories using the starved rat as test animal ranged from 0.092–0.204 (Cotes & Bangham, 1966) and in other results from seven laboratories from 0.128–0.467 (Gordon & Weintraub, 1962).

For detection of small amounts of erythropoietin, the polycythemic mouse is usually more sensitive than the starved rat (Gordon & Weintraub, 1962). In our laboratory, and using the hypoxia-induced polycythemic mouse, the response to a dose of 0.05 units of erythropoietin is usually detectable and in the linear range of the log-dose log-response curve, whereas in the starved rat a dose of about 0.5 units is required to give a response in or just below the linear range of the curve. Thus, if we are not limited by the amounts of erythropoietin (both standard and unknown) used in the assay, the starved rat and polycythemic mouse may be regarded as equally satisfactory assay animals with the reservation that nonspecific stimulation of red cell formation can probably be induced more easily in the starved rat than in the polycythemic mouse.

Specificity of Assay

Specificity of the assay depends upon the assumption that stimulation of incorporation of Fe-59 iron into red cells is induced only by exogenous ery-

TABLE 1

CONFIDENCE LIMITS OF ESTIMATES OF THE RELATIVE POTENCY OF TWO PREPARATIONS OF ERYTHROPOIETIN FROM TWO LABORATORIES USING SIMILAR ASSAY METHODS BUT DIFFERENT STRAINS OF MICE

Laboratory	Test Mice			Potency of IRP (B) in Units of Standard A per Ampoule	Confidence Limits ($p = 0.95$) as % of Potency Ratio	No. of Mice Used	Total Quantity of EPTN Used (Units of IRP)		λ
	Strain	Sex	Weight				Preparation 1 Standard A	Preparation 2 IRP (Standard B)	
P.M.C.	M.R.C. TO	♀	20–22 g	9.9	78.2–127.7*	253*	73.5	66.8	0.31–0.52
R.S.S.	A_2G	♀	30–32 g	10.1	79.9–125.1	48	27.7	27.7	0.167

Note: λ = Index of precision = s/b where s^2 is error variance for that assay and where b is common slope of the log-dose log-response lines for that assay.

* Based on combined results from six assays. In one assay polycythaemia from hypoxia was supplemented by transfusion and in another polycythaemia was induced by transfusion alone.

TABLE 2

REPRODUCIBILITY OF REPEATED ESTIMATES OF THE RELATIVE POTENCY OF PREPARATIONS OF ERYTHROPOIETIN USING THE STARVED RAT ASSAY

Lab. No.*	Assay No.*	Preparations Compared		Total Quantity of Erythropoietin Used in Units of IRP(B) and, in Parenthesis, no. of Animals Used		Estimate of Potency of Test Substance	Fiducial Limits of Estimate of Potency (p = 0.95)	λ	Weighted Mean Potency	Confidence Limits as % of Potency (p = 0.95)	Total No. of Animals Used
		Standard	Test	Standard	Test						
7	13	IRP (B)	Rabbit Plasma (Batch 1)	16(8)	84(8)	10.34 units per ml plasma	6.29–24.32	0.137	10.51 units per ml plasma	83.9–119.8	52
	14	IRP (B)	"	16(8)	16.3(8)	11.65 units per ml plasma	9.23–14.93	0.092			
	15	IRP (B)	"	20(10)	68(15)	7.76 units per ml plasma	5.29–11.82	0.195			
16	26	Standard A	IRP (B)	35(15)	35(15)	10.2 units Standard A per ampoule B	7.35–13.86	0.176	10.1 units Standard A per ampoule B	80.2–124.7	60
	27	A	IRP (B)	44(15)	44(15)	10.1 units Standard A per ampoule B	7.25–14.05	0.190			

* Laboratory and assay number from Cotes and Bangham, 1966.

thropoietin administered to the test animal. Thus, it is assumed that the test substance neither stimulates endogenous erythropoietin secretion nor activates erythropoietin precursors present in the test animal. Quantitation of the assay is achieved by comparison of the response induced by the test material with that induced by the standard administered simultaneously to other animals. (Despite the use of inbred strains of test animal, maintained under controlled environmental conditions, and random distribution between groups treated with test and standard preparations, elimination of variation in animal responsiveness from one time to another can never be relied upon. Thus, for quantitative assays it is necessary to test the two or more preparations under consideration simultaneously.) Test substances which differ from the standard in their mode of action, in rate of absorption, in species of origin, in degree of purification or nature of contaminants may give invalid assays. There may also be significant nonparallelism of log-dose (log-) response lines which would lead to difficulties in the estimation of the relative potency.

The International Reference Preparation of Erythropoietin

Estimates of potency of different preparations made on different occasions or in different laboratories can only be correlated if a stable and common standard has been used. There is no practicable way of detecting small losses of potency in a standard (Bangham, 1962; Jerne & Perry, 1956). The usual measures taken to safeguard the stability of other international standards of various biological materials were taken in the case of Standard B which has since become the International Reference Preparation of Erythropoietin. This preparation (fully described by Cotes and Bangham, 1966) was freeze-dried and sealed in nitrogen-filled ampoules after extensive secondary desiccation and it has been stored in the dark at −10° C. In accelerated degradation tests the activity of material from ampoules stored at 20° C was compared with that from ampoules stored at −10° C. After two years at +20° C there was no evidence of any change in activity (Cotes & Bangham, 1966), and after nearly three years at 20° C there was possibly some loss in activity (TABLE 3). This represents a high order of stability in the International Reference Preparation since this is kept at −10° C.

The World Health Organization has now established Standard B as the First International Reference Preparation of Erythropoietin (Cotes & Bangham, 1966) and ampoules of this material, which each contain 10 units of erythropoietin (based on bioassay against Standard A), are distributed on behalf of the World Health Organization by the Division of Biological Standards at the National Institute for Medical Research, London, England. This material is available on request as a standard for bioassay purposes only and is intended for the calibration of laboratory working standards.

TABLE 3

STABILITY OF THE INTERNATIONAL REFERENCE PREPARATION OF ERYTHROPOIETIN (STANDARD B)

Storage at +20° C for Period: (Days)	Potency Ratio*	Confidence Limits (p = 0.95)
724	1.021	0.82–1.27
1016	0.75	0.49–1.10

* Comparison of Standard stored at +20°C with Standard stored at −10°C.

Acknowledgments

I am very grateful to Miss M. V. Mussett and to Miss P. M. Woodward who carried out the statistical analysis and helped with its evaluation.

References

BANGHAM, D. R. 1962. Biological assay and a standard for erythropoietin. *In* Erythropoiesis. L. O. Jacobson and M. Doyle, Eds. : 23–28. Grune and Stratton. New York, N. Y.

COTES, P. M. & D. R. BANGHAM. 1961, Bio-assay of erythropoietin in mice made polycythaemic by exposure to air at a reduced pressure. Nature **191:** 1065.

COTES, P. M. & D. R. BANGHAM. 1966. An international reference preparation for bioassay of erythropoietin. Bull. Wld. Hlth. Org. **35:** 751.

FRIED, W. L., F. PLZAK, L. O. JACOBSON & E. GOLDWASSER. 1957. Studies on erythropoietin. III. Factors controlling erythropoietin production. Proc. Soc. Exp. Biol. **94:** 237.

GORDON, A. S. & A. H. WEINTRAUB. 1962. Assay of the erythropoietin simulating factor (ESF). *In* Erythropoiesis. L. O. Jacobson and M. Doyle, Eds. : 1–16. Grune and Stratton. New York, N. Y.

HODGSON, G., M. PERRETA, D. YUDILEVICH & I. ESKUCHE. 1958. Assay of "hémopoïétine" in starved animals; Properties of urinary hemopoïétine. Proc. Soc. Exp. Biol. **99:** 137.

JACOBSON, L. O., E. GOLDWASSER & C. W. GURNEY. 1960. Transfusion-induced polycythaemia as a model for studying factors influencing erythropoiesis. *In* Haemopoiesis, Cell Production and Its Regulation. G. E. W. Wolstenholme & M. O'Connor, Eds. : 423–445. Ciba Foundation Symposium. Churchill, London.

JERNE, N. K. & W. L. M. PERRY. 1956. The stability of biological standards. Bull. Wld. Hlth. Org. **14:** 167.

FURTHER EXPERIENCES WITH ASSAYS, UNITS, AND STANDARDS OF ERYTHROPOIETIN*

Geoffrey Keighley

Division of Biology, California Institute of Technology, Pasadena, Calif.

In this paper I shall offer some results from our assays of erythropoietin. They are extensions of those presented four years ago.[1] At that time we used a fasted-rat assay. Now we use a polycythemic mouse assay with incorporation of ^{59}Fe into red cells.

Our method, a modification of that of Cotes and Bangham,[2] is summarized in TABLE 1. Mice of the kind and size described were made polycythemic by a stay of 10 days in a chamber at reduced air pressure, approximately 340 mm Hg. During the 10 days the tank was opened twice to provide clean cages, fresh food, and water. On the 10th day (day zero in TABLE 1) the mice were removed from the tank. On the third day the rest of the schedule was started. A substance to be tested was injected subcutaneously (s.c.) in equally divided doses on the third and fourth days. On the fifth day ^{59}Fe was injected intravenously (i.v.). On the seventh day 43 hours later, blood samples were taken. Mice with hematocrits of less than 52% were not used. The radioactivity of an aliquot of the blood was measured. Blood volumes of the mice were taken as 7.5% of the body weight. The results are expressed as percent of the injected ^{59}Fe which has been incorporated into the red cells. With this schedule erythropoiesis is suppressed (the suppression lasts beyond the seventh day) incorporation in negative controls is low, and small doses of erythropoietin will raise it. Saline was used as a negative control, and pools of frozen plasma from anemic rabbits were used as positive controls and as a working reference standard.

FIGURE 1 is a plot of ^{59}Fe incorporation vs. dose of erythropoietin given to polycythemic, ex-reduced pressure mice. The points and vertical bars show the mean ($\pm$ SE) ^{59}Fe incorporations after six different doses of a batch of Step 2 human urinary material.[3] The dose range is almost 1000:1. We do not as a rule run assays at some of these larger and wasteful doses. We were led to them in attempts to get increased incorporations in anemic mice[4] and at the same time, for control purposes, gave the same large doses to hematologically normal mice. The high uptakes have a certain amount of interest in themselves. The upper limit of iron incorporation of course is 100%. Up to 2 mg dose the log dose response curve is roughly a straight line, but it appears that beyond 2 mg with this material in this assay, higher incorporations are unlikely.

There are two assays of standard B, the large open circles, at doses of 0.1 and 0.5 units.† The dose response is similar to that of the Step 2 material.

FIGURE 2 is of an assay of a pool of plasma from anemic rabbits which had been injected with phenylhydrazine. The bars show the SE's; the numbers below are the total numbers of mice injected with each dose; the numbers in parentheses are the numbers of mice which died. The shape of the dose response curve is similar to that with Step 2 material (FIGURE 1). However, the upper limit appears to be at a dose of about 1.0 ml at an ^{59}Fe incorporation of about 50%; beyond

* This work was supported by research grant HE 07683 from the United States Public Health Service.

† Supplied through D. R. Bangham, Department of Biological Standards, National Institute for Medical Research, London, England.

TABLE 1

ERYTHROPOIETIN ASSAY IN POLYCYTHEMIC MICE*

Days after Return to Normal Pressure			
0	3 and 4	5	7
Mice returned to normal pressure	Substance to be tested injected s.c. in equal doses each day at 8 AM	^{59}Fe injected i.v. at 1 PM	Blood samples taken at ^{59}Fe measured at 8 AM
	<-------- 53 hr ----->	<----- 43 hr --->	

B6D2F$_1$ female mice, 18–20 g Hcts 42–45%, polycythemia induced by 10 days continuous exposure to an ambient pressure of 340 mm Hg.

Mice with Hcts less than 52% on day 7 not used. Results expressed as percent of injected ^{59}Fe which has been incorporated into the red cells.

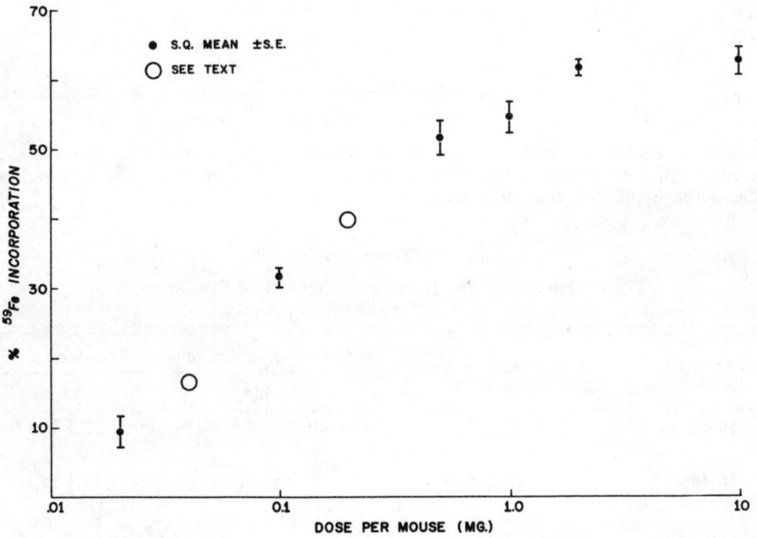

FIGURE 1. ^{59}Fe incorporation in ex-reduced pressure polycythemic mice injected subcutaneously (s.c.) with human urinary erythropoietin, Step 2 material, at the doses shown. The large circles show the mean incorporations, eight mice per point, after the injection of standard B at the levels of 0.1 and 0.5 units per mouse.

this there is only a doubtful increase, and some mice died. We know that this is not the limit of the assay (see FIGURE 1); something in this batch of plasma is interfering at the high doses. Other batches of plasma with higher specific activities have produced higher incorporations. In each particular circumstance it would be well to be certain that this region of a dose response curve is not entered.

TABLE 2 shows assays of the same pool of anemic rabbit plasma, as in FIGURE 2, at doses of 0.08 and 0.8 ml. The ^{59}Fe incorporations are listed for three sets of polycythemic mice which had been exposed to the low pressure for the usual ten-day period, for 16 days, and for 22 days. There is some increase of the hematocrits with longer exposures and the changes in incorporation are small.

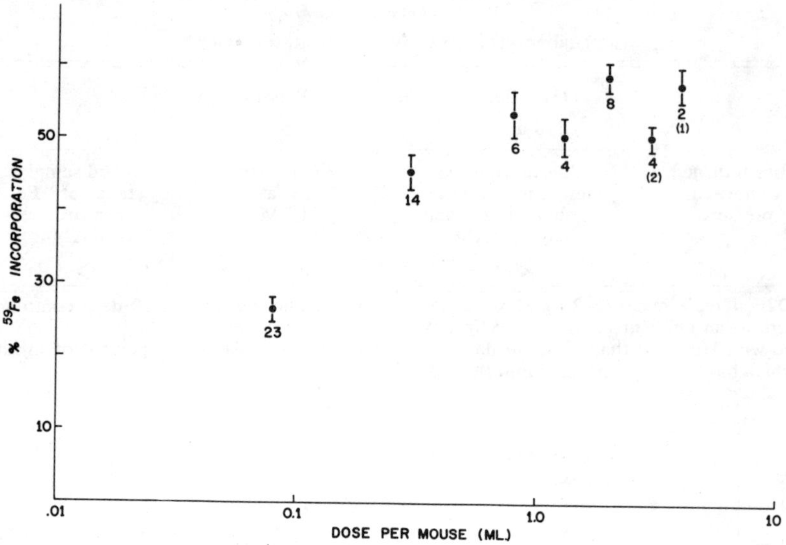

FIGURE 2. ^{59}Fe incorporation in ex-reduced pressure polycythemic mice injected s.c. with anemic rabbit plasma. The total number of mice in the assay at each dose is given, and in parentheses the number of mice that died.

TABLE 2

POLYCYTHEMIC MICE: EFFECT OF LENGTH OF EXPOSURE TO REDUCED PRESSURE ON THE ASSAY

Length of Exposure	Hcts at End of Assay Mean ± SE	^{59}Fe Incorporation, Mean ± SE after a dose of:	
		0.08 ml*	0.8 ml
10 days	54.3 ± 4.7	26.2 ± 1.5 (23)**	53.5 ± 3.0 (6)
16 days	57.7 ± 4.2 P < .01†	25.3 ± 1.5 (18) NS	59.1 ± 1.2 (18) P < .05
22 days	57.5 ± 3.6 P < .01	22.0 ± 1.0 (19) P < .05	58.5 ± 1.2 (19) P < .01

* Pool of plasma from anemic rabbits.
** No. of mice in assay.
† Probability values (compared to means at 10 days) from t-test (Snedecor, '40).

From these figures and others like them we came to the conclusion that a ten-day exposure was adequate. There are some obvious advantages in conducting the assay in as short a time as possible.

FIGURE 3 shows three sets of assays of Step 2 material. The four incorporations shown by plain dots are repeated from FIGURE 1 for comparison; the material was injected s.c. The two incorporations with vertical bars for the SE's are from the same Step 2 material injected intraperitoneally (i.p.); there is no difference. The third set of incorporations, lower in the Figure, was obtained with the same doses injected s.c. in hypertransfused mice.[6] The mice had been injected i.p.

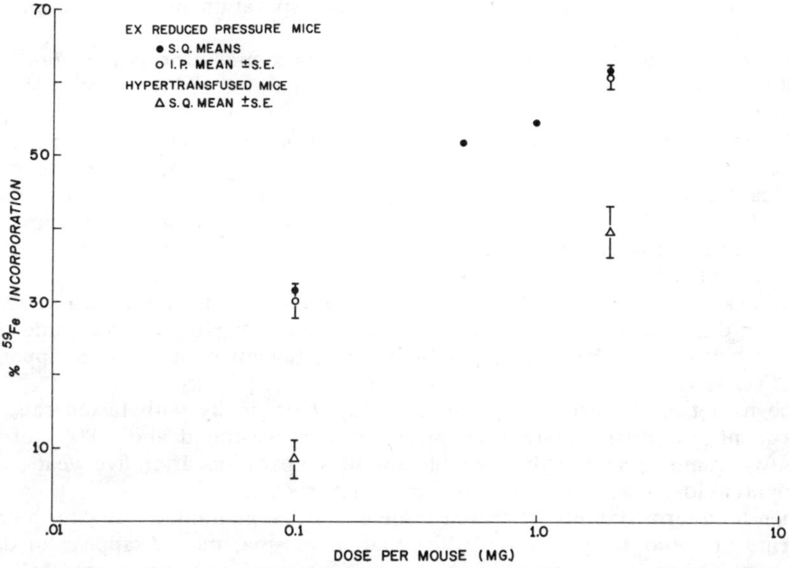

FIGURE 3. ^{59}Fe incorporation in mice injected with Step 2 material. Solid points, ex-reduced pressure polycythemic mice injected s.c. Open circles, the means and SE's of similar mice injected i.p. Triangles, the means and SE's of hypertransfused mice injected s.c.

with 1 ml of washed, packed red cells on the first and second days, with the material to be assayed on the seventh day, with ^{59}Fe on the ninth day, and bled on the 12th day. Their hematocrits had a mean of 64.3 ± 0.7%, the ex-reduced pressure mice had mean hematocrit of 55.4 ± 0.4%. Polycythemic ex-reduced pressure mice have an erythropoietic apparatus which was hyperactive and is now suppressed, and which responds more vigorously to the stimulus of erythropoietin than that of hypertransfused mice which was in a normal state before suppression.

In TABLE 3 we see the incorporation of ^{59}Fe into ten-day ex-reduced pressure mice, injected with a standard dose of erythropoietin. When the dose is divided in two and given on succeeding days, there is a slight advantage over the same amount as a single dose. When we injected it i.v. instead of s.c., there was no

TABLE 3

INCORPORATION OF ^{59}FE IN EX-REDUCED PRESSURE POLYCYTHEMIC MICE*

		^{59}Fe Incorporation, Mean + SE
42 mice, erythropoietin divided into two doses on two days		27.1 ± 0.9
38 mice, erythropoietin given in one dose		23.5 ± 1.07
	P > .01	
Seven mice, erythropoietin injected s.c. in two doses		24.2 ± 2.2
Eight mice, erythropoietin injected i.v. in two doses difference is not significant		22.0 ± 3.5
25 saline controls		0.97 ± 0.07

* One preparation of erythropoietin at one-dose level.

clear benefit. Added at the bottom are the incorporation in 25 saline-injected control mice.

As we did four years ago, we are presenting some information about the stability of preparations which we have had frozen and stored for varying lengths of time.

The first set of assays in TABLE 4 is of a pool of frozen plasma from anemic rabbits which we used for some time as our working standard. There is no significant difference between the assays made with 68 mice and those made with 20 mice two years later. In 1963 the plasma was already two years old. Soon after the last assays the pool began to lose activity. We have put it away for future reference.

The next assays are of a dried soluble preparation from rabbit plasma which had been dissolved in saline and kept frozen, in solution, for two years and four and one-half months. Based on assays with only a few mice there was no apparent loss of activity.

The next two preparations had been assayed originally with fasted rats. By subsequent assays with ex-reduced pressure mice, we found about 80% of the activity remaining in the dry, soluble rabbit preparation after five years, and no apparent loss in a sample of frozen urine after six years.

Such long-term stability of frozen urine cannot be guaranteed. Erythropoietin in urine at room temperature, unlike that in plasma, may disappear in days or hours. Others have reported loss of activity in frozen urine in weeks or months,[7] and we have experienced it occasionally. However, on the basis of hundreds of samples from different patients kept at deep-freeze temperatures, I think it reasonable to expect such frozen samples to be stable for at least three to six months.

TABLE 5 lists the effects of several substances on the assay, and on erythropoiesis. In the third column is a number which we call a dose ratio. It is the ratio between the dose we have given to mice to doses of the same material which others have found to be effective in one way or another in similar or different situations. In some cases we have had to compare on a body weight basis doses given to large animals, e.g. men, to doses for a 20-gram mouse, and in some cases the route of administration has been quite different. Nevertheless, these ratios do have some meaning and their range is large.

The last columns of the Table summarize the effects. Blank spaces mean

TABLE 4

STABILITY OF ERYTHROPOIETIN PREPARATIONS, FROZEN AND STORED FOR SOME TIME

Date	Kind of Sample	Dose	No. of Mice	^{59}Fe Incorporation Mean ± SE
4-19-63	anemic rabbit plasma	0.08 ml	68	22.7 ± 0.8
4-9-65	anemic rabbit plasma	0.08 ml	20	19.7 ± 1.9
	difference not significant			
12-30-65	A soluble preparation from rabbits dissolved in saline, had been stored frozen for two years, 4½ months. By mouse assays.			no apparent loss
4-29-66	A soluble dried preparation from rabbits. Had been assayed in fasted rats five years earlier. By a mouse assay remaining activity found to be			83%
4-29-66	Frozen human urine. Had been assayed in rats six years earlier. By mouse assay			no apparent loss

TABLE 5

EFFECT OF VARIOUS SUBSTANCES

Substance	Dose per Mouse	Dose Ratio*	Effect** on ^{59}Fe Incorporation in Assay Mice: When Given with Erythropoietin	Effect** on ^{59}Fe Incorporation in Assay Mice: When Given without Erythropoietin	Effect on Production of Erythropoietin in Hypoxic Mice
Testosterone	5 mg s.c.	1	+	+	
Polyuridylic acid	1–4 mg s.c.	1–4	0	0	
Puromycin	5 mg i.p.	1	—		0
Hydroxyurea	10 mg s.c.	10	—		
Glucosamine	300 mg s.c.	1	— ?		—
Hydrochlorothiazide	8 mg s.c.	15	0	0	
Lead acetate	5 mg s.c.	250	0 ?		
Sodium fluoride	2 mg s.c.	25	—		
Dimethyl sulfoxide	150 mg s.c.	1	— ?		
Actinomycin D	4 μg i.p.	1	—		0

* Dose ratio: Estimate of ratio of this dose to doses found effective under other circumstances. See text.

** Effect: + shows enhancement, — shows suppression, 0 shows no effect, blank shows not tested.

that the test was not made, a zero, that the substance had no discernible effect, a minus sign, that the course of the assay was suppressed and a plus sign, that the assay was enhanced. The substances were tried in the normal 10-day ex-reduced pressure mouse assay together with a standard stimulating dose of erythropoietin (4th column); tested in an assay without erythropoietin (5th column); and tested for their effect on the production of erythropoietin in hypoxic mice (last column). For the latter test otherwise unmanipulated normal mice were injected with doses of the various substances and placed in a chamber through which a mixture of air and nitrogen at a pO_2 of 58 mm Hg was circulated. After 12 hr the mice were removed and bled immediately. Pools of the plasma were assayed for their erythropoietin content. Control plasmas from hypoxic mice at doses of 0.4 ml regularly produce ^{59}Fe incorporations of 10–15% in recipient assay mice.

The first substance on the list is testosterone. It has been included to show that its effects in our system are similar to those reported by others.[8] It stimulates ^{59}Fe incorporation when given alone or with erythropoietin. Next is polyuridylic acid, which in some systems has been shown to stimulate the incorporation of amino acids into protein.[9] In our assay system, at doses which might be expected to have some effect, we found none. Puromycin, which can inhibit hemoglobin synthesis,[10] did have a suppressive effect on the incorporation of ^{59}Fe in our assay system following the injection of erythropoietin. It did not prevent the production of erythropoietin in hypoxic mice. Hydroxyurea, a substance which has been studied as a chemotherapeutic agent,[11] also had a depressing effect on the influence of erythropoietin in our assay. Glucosamine has been reported to suppress hypoxic erythropoietin formation in rats.[12] We have confirmed this inhibition of erythropoietin production in mice. We were also able to get some suppression of the effect of exogenous erythropoietin in our assay mice, but only with larger doses not far from the lethal range. Hydrochlorothiazide–a diuretic and antihypertensive drug–had no effect on the assay when given either with or without erythropoietin. With lead acetate, at what seem like relatively enormous doses, over 100 times greater than doses which cause objective symptoms of poisoning in men, we were able to get a small, perhaps doubtful, suppression of the effect of erythropoietin. With sodium fluoride, again with rather large doses, we were able to get suppression of the effect of erythropoietin. Dimethyl sulfoxide, which is reported to have many effects, and can cause a reduction of tissue pO_2,[13] had at most a doubtful effect on the incorporation following a stimulating dose of erythropoietin. Actinomycin D in small microgram doses can suppress entirely the effect of erythropoietin but the same or larger doses have no effect on the production of erythropoietin in hypoxic mice.[14]

The figures suggest that agents which in small amounts affect erythropoiesis, and therefore the assays, are specific, and interference with the assays by accidental contamination is not a great danger.

Summary

An assay for erythropoietin, using mice made polycythemic by exposure to hypoxia and the incorporation of ^{59}Fe into the blood, has been examined when some changes are made in the period of hypoxia, and in the route or timing of the injection of material to be tested. Satisfactory responses are possible over a wide range of doses up to high incorporations. Samples of erythropoietin of different origin and preparation have been assayed after storage for some years; most have lost no activity. Although Actinomycin D and testosterone affect erythropoiesis and the assay, some substances which might be suspected of having some influence have little or none.

References

1. KEIGHLEY, G. 1962. *In* Erythropoiesis. L. O. Jacobson and M. Doyle, Eds. : 17. Grune and Stratton. New York, N. Y.
2. COTES, P. M. & D. R. BANGHAM. 1961. Nature **191**: 1065.
3. LOWY, P. H. & H. BORSOOK. 1962. *In* Erythropoiesis. L. O. Jacobson and M. Doyle, Eds. : 33. Grune and Stratton. New York, N. Y.
4. KEIGHLEY, G., P. LOWY, E. S. RUSSELL & M. W. THOMPSON. 1966. Brit. J. Haematol. In press.
6. FILMANOWICZ, E. & C. W. GURNEY. 1961. J. Lab. Clin. Med. **57**: 65.
7. MIRAND, E. A. & T. C. PRENTICE. Private communication.
8. GORDON, A. S. & H. A. CHARIPPER. 1947. Ann. N. Y. Acad. Sci. **48**: 615.
9. RAMPERSAD, O. R. & I. J. WOOL. 1965. Science **149**: 1102.
10. MORRIS, A., S. FAVELUKES, R. ARLINGHAUS & R. SCHWEET. 1962. Biochem. Biophys. Res. Comm. **7**: 326.
11. GALE, G. R. 1964. Biochem. Pharmacol. **13**: 1377.
12. SCHMAUS, J. W. & K. R. REISSMANN. 1965. Fed. Proc. **24**: 402 (abstract).
13. VAN DER MEER, C., P. W. VALKENBURG & M. REMMELTS. 1963. Int. J. Rad. Biol. **6**: 151.
14. KEIGHLEY, G. & P. H. LOWY. 1966. Blood **27**: 637.

STUDIES ON THE ERYTHROPOIETIC EFFECTS OF HYPERBARIC HYPEROXIA*

James W. Linman

Mayo Clinic and the Mayo Graduate School of Medicine, Rochester, Minn.

and

Robert V. Pierre†

Veterans Administration Research Hospital and Northwestern University Medical School, Chicago, Ill.

The past 15 years have seen significant advances in the understanding of the physiologic and pathophysiologic control of erythropoiesis. Although the complete solution to this complex problem is not yet at hand, the existence of a humoral erythropoietic regulatory mechanism can no longer be denied.[1–4] Future experimentation may necessitate changes in current concepts; however, it is reasonable to conclude from studies to date that humoral factors exert homeostatic control over erythropoiesis. Hypoxia resulting from changes in the dynamic relationship between tissue oxygen tension and cellular metabolic requirements is generally accepted as the fundamental erythropoietic stimulus. Abundant clinical and experimental data provide compelling support for the thesis that the hypoxic stimulus is mediated by the humoral regulatory mechanism.

Any disorder that decreases arterial oxygen saturation or the oxygen-carrying capacity of the blood will sequentially reduce the oxygen content of the blood, produce tissue hypoxia, enhance humoral erythropoietic factor activity, stimulate the bone marrow, and augment red cell mass; in this manner the balance between oxygen supply and cellular needs is restored. Anemia due to acute blood loss acts in this way to enhance marrow erythropoiesis. A decrease in the oxygen tension of inspired air also imparts a potent erythropoietic stimulus, as do other causes of hypoxic hypoxia such as hypoventilation, an alveolar-capillary block, or an admixture of venous and arterial blood. If the resultant increase in oxygen-carrying capacity is adequate to correct the tissue oxygen deficit, erythrocytic equilibrium is reestablished at a higher level. Otherwise, the humoral physiologic corrective mechanism continues to operate and an unphysiologic secondary polycythemia ensues.

The erythropoietic stimulatory effects of hypoxic and anemic hypoxia appear to be transmitted to the marrow by the humoral regulatory mechanism. Therefore, it is logical to surmise that pulmonary hyperoxia or an augmented red cell mass might curtail endogenous erythropoietic factor elaboration which, in turn, would lead to decreased erythropoiesis and a reduction in the oxygen-carrying capacity of the blood. At normal atmospheric pressure an increase in the oxygen tension of inspired air suppresses erythrocyte production,[5–9] and transfusion-induced polycythemia causes an almost complete cessation of erythropoiesis.[10–15] The supposition that these suppressive effects are also mediated by the humoral erythropoietic regulatory mechanism possesses strong indirect and teleologic support. However, technical difficulties concerned with the quantification of less than

* This investigation was supported in part by Research grants AM–01991, AM–10079 and AM–0954 from the National Institute of Arthritis and Metabolic Diseases, Public Health Service.

† Present address: Mayo Clinic, Rochester, Minn.

normal levels of erythropoietin activity have precluded direct documentation. Recent studies in our laboratories on the erythropoietic effects of hyperbaric oxygenation deal with this problem.

Materials and Methods

Adult Swiss-Webster mice weighing about 25 to 30 g have been maintained for varying periods at four absolute atmospheres of air, that is, normal barometric pressure plus a gauge pressure equivalent to three atmospheres (atm); pressure within the chamber was 3,040 mm Hg or 60 pounds per square inch absolute (psia). The steel chamber used in these experiments measures 136 by 76 cm and has a volume of 580 l. Hyperbarism was achieved with a three-fourths horsepower, electric, single-stage, oil-less compressor. Pressure and ventilation were regulated by a spring-loaded control valve that permits an exhaust flow at 4 atm of 12.75 l/min and a complete change of air within the chamber every 45 min. The chamber temperature was essentially that of the ambient room air (about 75 F). At 4 atm (absolute) of air, the partial pressure of oxygen in the chamber was 640 mm Hg. The chamber was decompressed for servicing once daily without staging; exposure to normal atmospheric pressure never exceeded 20 min/day, and the entire process of decompression, servicing, and recompression required less than 90 min. Mice were maintained on a normal laboratory diet containing adequate amounts of all nutrients including vitamin E; they were permitted water ad libitum.

Uptake of ^{59}Fe by the erythrocytes, reticulocyte counts, and peripheral erythroid values were used to assess rates of erythropoiesis. In addition, Wright-stained splenic imprints and marrow preparations provided morphologic confirmation of changes in erythropoiesis. At varying intervals of time the mice were injected with ^{59}Fe (0.5 ml containing 0.5 μc of ^{59}ferrous citrate) and then returned to the hyperbaric chamber. Erythrocyte uptake of ^{59}Fe was measured 48 hr later; blood volume was assumed to be 6% of the animal's final body weight. Blood samples were obtained by cardiac puncture or from the retro-orbital plexus; radioactivity was quantified in a well-type scintillation counter and expressed as percent of injected counts. The erythroid measurements included microhematocrit readings, hemacytometer erythrocyte counts, and determinations of hemoglobin concentration by the cyanmethemoglobin technique; reticulocytes were counted on brilliant cresyl blue coverslip films counterstained with Wright's stain.

In some groups of mice, exogenous erythropoietin was given intraperitoneally in the form of erythropoietin standard B prepared from anemic human urine and kindly supplied by the National Institute for Medical Research, Mill Hill, London. An injection of 0.5 unit was given after residence in the hyperbaric chamber for 120 and again at 144 hr; the animals were returned to the chamber, and ^{59}Fe was given 24 hr later. For the purpose of comparing responses to erythropoietin in hyperoxic mice with those in animals conditioned in other ways, mice were hypertransfused (1 ml of packed red cells daily times two with a final hematocrit value of 65 to 70%) or made polycythemic by exposure to simulated high altitude (0.4 atm for 12 hr/day for 20 days). The latter animals were given comparable amounts of erythropoietin standard B in the form of two injections 24 hr apart; ^{59}Fe was given 24 hr later, and erythrocyte uptake was determined 48 hr thereafter.

Results

The effect of residence in a hyperbaric environment (4 atm absolute or 60 psia of air) on ^{59}Fe incorporation in hemoglobin is shown in FIGURE 1. During the

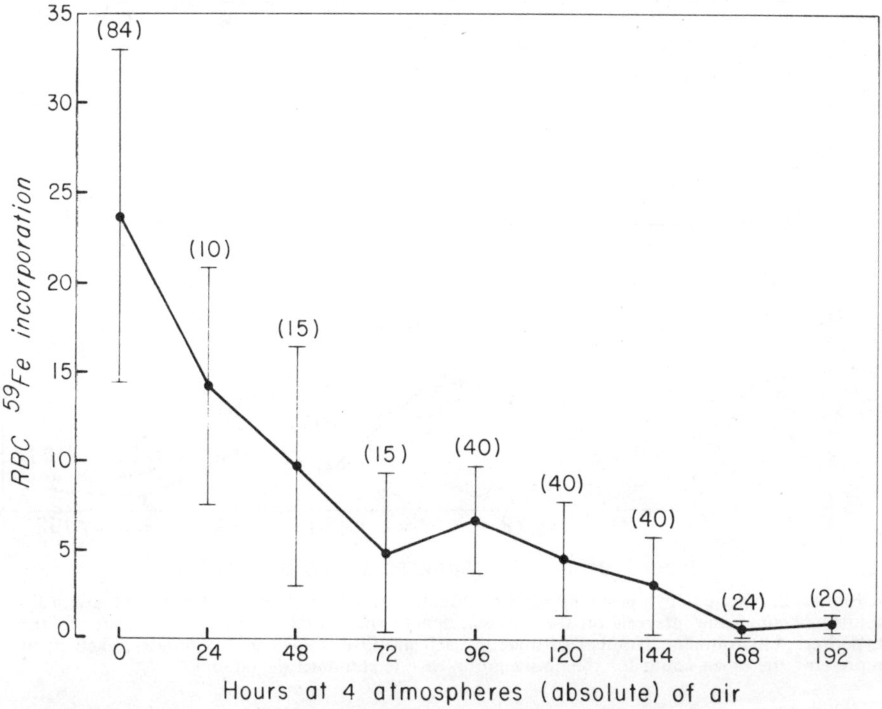

FIGURE 1. Erythrocytic uptake of ^{59}Fe in mice maintained in a hyperbaric chamber at 4 atm (absolute) of air. Time intervals on the abscissa mark the duration of hyperbarism at the time the ^{59}Fe was given. Number of mice in each group is indicated in parentheses; each point indicates the mean for the entire group, with one standard deviation shown to indicate the scatter about the mean.

first 72 hr, ^{59} Fe uptake fell to about 5%. Continued hyperbarism resulted in a slower, progressive decline to less than 1% in mice exposed for 168 to 192 hr. Preliminary observations on the effects of more prolonged hyperbaric hyperoxia are difficult to evaluate and require further study. Some mice have remained depressed for 240 to 264 hr; however, other animals have exhibited a progressive increase in ^{59}Fe uptake beginning about 216 hr after the onset of hyperbaric oxygenation.

The number of hours per day of exposure to hyperbaric hyperoxia appears to be of fundamental importance as does the magnitude of the hyperbarism. In the experiments depicted in FIGURE 1, mice were exposed to 4 atm (absolute) of air (60 psia) for at least 22.5 hr/day; when the exposure time was reduced to 20 hr/day, variable and less marked suppression ensued. When the animals were maintained at 4 atm (absolute) of air for only 16 hr daily, erythrocytic uptake of ^{59}Fe at 120 hr did not differ significantly from that in control animals not placed in the hyperbaric chamber. In mice exposed to only 3 atm of air (45 psia) for 22.5 hr/day, ^{59}Fe uptake fell to about 5%; however, even prolonged exposure failed to inhibit erythropoiesis to the degree shown in FIGURE 1.

The sharp diminution in erythrocytic uptake of ^{59}Fe in mice exposed to 4 atm (absolute) of air was accompanied by reticulocytopenia (FIGURE 2). No signif-

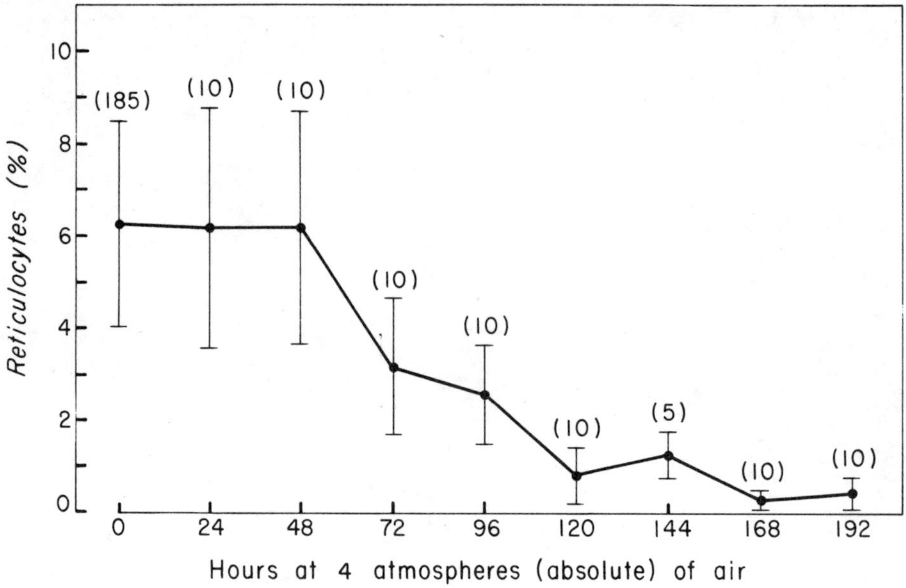

FIGURE 2. Reticulocytopenia in mice maintained in a hyperbaric chamber at 4 atm (absolute) of air. Time intervals on the abscissa denote the actual duration of exposure to the hyperbaric environment. Number of mice in each group is shown in parentheses; each point represents the mean count for the entire group ± one standard deviation.

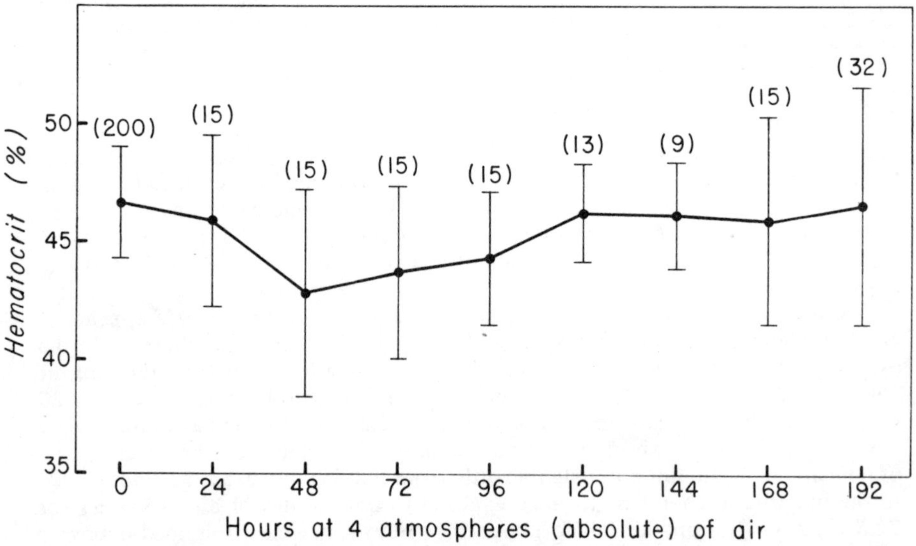

FIGURE 3. Hematocrit values in mice maintained at 4 atm (absolute) of air. Number of mice in each group is indicated in parentheses; each point represents the mean for all animals in the group ± one standard deviation.

icant changes were detected in the hematocrit levels (FIGURE 3) or other peripheral erythroid values in these relatively short-term experiments. In view of the clear-cut evidence of erythropoietic suppression, more lengthy exposure should be reflected by a decrement in red cell mass. A relatively high mortality rate encountered in animals subjected to prolonged hyperbarism has precluded a definitive solution to this problem; however, preliminary observations in a few animals indicate that mice maintained at 4 atm of air for 10 to 14 days or longer do manifest significant reductions in hemoglobin level, hematocrit and erythrocyte count.

Alterations in splenic and marrow cytology provided corroborative evidence that hyperbaric hyperoxia depresses erythropoiesis. In the mouse the spleen constitutes an important site of erythrocytogenesis. Wright-stained imprints of spleens from normal mice reveal numerous foci of active erythropoiesis; erythrocytic precursors were virtually absent in the spleens as well as in the bone marrows of mice subjected to hyperbarism (60 psia of air) for 192 hr.

Mice with depressed erythropoiesis consequent to hyperbaric hyperoxia exhibited unequivocal responses to exogenous erythropoietin (FIGURE 4) and appear to be suitable recipients for the bioassay of erythropoietin. In an attempt to assess the relative "sensitivity" of mice prepared in this manner, their responses to

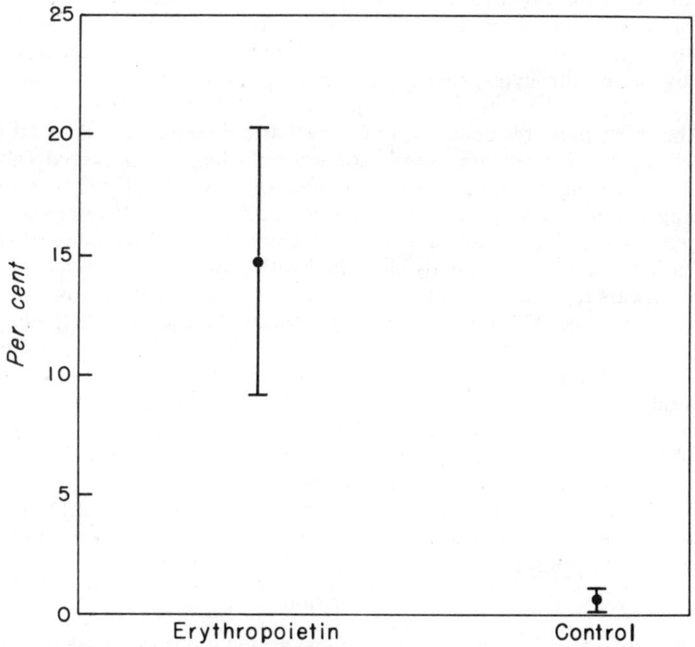

FIGURE 4. Erythrocytic uptake of ^{59}Fe in mice exposed to hyperbaric hyperoxia. One group of animals received 0.5 unit of erythropoietin standard B at 120 and again at 144 hr; a second group received equivalent quantities of saline and served as controls. ^{59}Fe was given 24 hr after the second injection of erythropoietin or saline; incorporation in hemoglobin was determined 48 hr later. Each point represents the average uptake of 16 animals, with one standard deviation shown to indicate the scatter about the mean.

TABLE 1

ERYTHROCYTIC INCORPORATION OF ^{59}Fe IN MICE (EIGHT ANIMALS IN EACH GROUP) CONDITIONED BY HYPEROXIA, HYPOXIA, AND TRANSFUSION-INDUCED POLYCYTHEMIA

Type of Recipients	Test Material	^{59}Fe Uptake (%)	
		Mean	SD
Hyperoxic (4 atm of air for 168 hr)	saline	0.56	0.40
	erythropoietin (standard B)	14.87	5.70
Hypoxic (0.4 atm 12 hr/day for 20 days)	saline	0.52	0.12
	erythropoietin (standard B)	25.97	4.28
Polycythemic (transfusion-induced)	saline	0.26	0.12
	erythropoietin (standard B)	16.88	4.04

erythropoietin standard B were compared with similar observations in groups of mice conditioned by hypoxic hypoxia or transfusion-induced polycythemia. The results of this experiment are shown in TABLE 1. The degree of erythropoietic suppression was similar in all three groups. The hyperoxic and polycythemic recipients of erythropoietin standard B exhibited comparable increments in ^{59}Fe uptake by the erythrocytes; the hypoxic mice manifested a considerably greater response.

For the most part, residence in the hyperbaric chamber for 8 to 10 days has been well tolerated, although usually some weight loss has occurred (about 5 to 10% of initial weight). Under the conditions of these experiments, no evidence of decompression sickness has been encountered, and manifestations attributable to oxygen toxicity have been unusual.[16–19] Convulsions have been observed on rare occasions, and a few animals have died with a fibrinous pneumonitis. A critical time appears to occur about five days after onset of hyperbarism, when certain animals begin to die with pulmonary complications; those mice that survive seem to be able to tolerate even prolonged hyperbarism without serious untoward effects. To date, no evidence of hemolysis has been uncovered in our studies on the erythropoietic effects of breathing air under increased pressure. It should be noted, however, that the response to this type of hyperbarism is somewhat variable, and further observations are needed to clarify its toxicity; for example, some animals display no adverse effects to residence in a hyperbaric environment, whereas others react poorly with high mortality rates. Additional factors such as the temperature and humidity within the chamber may contribute significantly to these variable responses.

Discussion

Despite widespread interest in the clinical applications of hyperbaric oxygenation,[19] the hematologic manifestations of hyperbarism have received relatively little investigative attention. Most of the published observations on the erythropoietic effects of hyperoxia have involved exposure to high concentrations of oxygen at normal atmospheric pressure; the majority of investigators have reported evidence of erythropoietic suppression,[5–9] but some have observed no effect.[20]

The oxygen content of the blood depends on the concentration of hemoglobin (each gram of hemoglobin can carry 1.34 ml of oxygen) and on the amount of hemoglobin present as oxyhemoglobin, that is, the percent oxygen saturation. When hemoglobin is fully saturated with oxygen, any further increase in the oxygen content of the blood is limited to the amount of gas that can be carried in physical solution. For each 100 mm Hg oxygen tension, 0.3 ml of oxygen will dissolve in 100 ml of blood. The pO_2 of the chamber air in our experiments was 640 mm Hg or four times that of ambient air. Because of the constant pressure in the lungs of water vapor (47 mm Hg) and carbon dioxide (40 mm Hg), the pO_2 of the alveolar air in mice maintained at 60 psia of air was approximately 620 mm Hg or the equivalent of breathing about 92% oxygen at normal atmospheric pressure. If a close correlation between alveolar and arterial pO_2 at high oxygen tensions exists, the oxygen content of the arterial blood in the mice exposed to the hyperbaric environment should have been increased by about 1.8 volumes percent (oxygen in the form of physically dissolved gas). However, further studies, for example, determinations of arterial blood gas, are needed to clarify this point, since data exist indicating a progressive decrease in the diffusing capacity of the pulmonary membrane in the face of a rising oxygen tension.[21] Such a difference in alveolar-arterial oxygen tension could have an important effect on the increase in oxygen content of the blood evoked by pulmonary hyperoxia. It is also noteworthy that it would be necessary to raise arterial pO_2 by about 450 mm Hg to equal the increase in oxygen-carrying capacity that would be provided by 1 g of additional hemoglobin per 100 ml of blood.

The demonstration in mice maintained under hyperbaric conditions of decreased ^{59}Fe incorporation in hemoglobin together with reticulocytopenia and a paucity of erythrocytic precursors in their spleens and bone marrow indicates that breathing air under increased pressure depresses erythropoiesis. These observations are in accord with the thesis that tissue oxygen tension exerts homeostatic control over erythrocyte production and contributes to the maintenance of the normal erythroid steady state. It is suggested that the erythropoietic suppressive effect of hyperbaric hyperoxia is mediated by the humoral erythropoietic regulatory mechanism. It should be emphasized, however, that proof of this hypothesis must await the development of assay techniques sufficiently sensitive to demonstrate unequivocally less than normal levels of plasma erythropoietic factor activity. In addition, it has been suggested that an erythropoietic inhibitor may contribute to the depressed erythropoiesis brought about by hypertransfusion.[22,23] If future studies confirm the presence of such an inhibitor, a similar factor might be "activated" by hyperoxia.

Hyperbarism provides another experimental tool for the investigation of the physiologic and pathophysiologic control of erythropoiesis. It also provides a means to condition animals as recipients for the bioassay of erythropoietin. The range of ^{59} Fe uptake by the erythrocytes in normal animals is so great (see FIGURE 1) that it is difficult to demonstrate clear-cut differences between control animals and recipients of erythropoietically active test materials. When erythropoiesis is suppressed prior to the administration of an erythropoietic stimulant, augmentation in ^{59}Fe uptake becomes more evident. For example, a 15% increase in ^{59}Fe incorporation in hemoglobin is much more apparent in a group of mice with a control of $0.5 \pm 0.2\%$ than in a group with base-line values of $24 \pm 10\%$. Several techniques have been used to suppress erythropoiesis in recipient animals; hypertransfused mice[11,12] or mice with erythrocytosis brought about by exposure to simulated high altitude[13,14] have proved most reliable.

It was hoped that hyperbaric hyperoxia would provide a quick and relatively simple way to condition mice for erythropoietin assay. Such animals are suitable recipients and do exhibit clear-cut responses to exogenous erythropoietin; however, the variable incidence of adverse reactions encountered in mice maintained in the hyperbaric chamber constitutes a serious obstacle. Pending further adaptation of the chamber to permit more precise control of such factors as temperature and humidity, hyperbaric hyperoxia remains more of an experimental tool to study mechanisms controlling erythropoiesis rather than a means to condition recipients for erythropoietin assay.

Summary

From the studies described herein the following observations are made:

1. Normal mice exposed to a hyperbaric environment (four absolute atmospheres or 60 psia of air) exhibit erythropoietic depression manifested by a sharp curtailment in erythrocytic ^{59}Fe uptake, reticulocytopenia, and morphologic evidence of decreased erythropoiesis.

2. The erythropoietic effects of hyperbaric hyperoxia are in accord with the concept that tissue oxygen tension exerts homeostatic control over erythropoiesis; it is suggested (but not proved) that this suppressive effect is transmitted to the marrow by the humoral regulatory mechanism.

3. Exogenous erythropoietin evokes a clear-cut increase in the incorporation of ^{59}Fe in hemoglobin of mice conditioned by breathing air under pressure. However, certain adverse effects associated with residence in a hyperbaric chamber must be eliminated before hyperbarism can be recommended as a completely acceptable method to prepare animals for erythropoietin assay.

References

1. GORDON, A. S. 1959. Hémopoïétine. Physiol. Rev. **39:** 1–40.
2. LINMAN, J. W. & F. H. BETHEL. 1960. Factors Controlling Erythropoiesis. Charles C Thomas. Springfield, Illinois. 208 pp.
3. JACOBSON, L. O. & M. DOYLE, Eds. 1962. Erythropoiesis. Grune & Stratton, Inc. New York, N. Y. 399 pp.
4. STOHLMAN, F., JR. 1962. Erythropoiesis. New England J. Med. **267:** 342–348; 392–399.
5. REINHARD, E. H., C. V. MOORE, R. DUBACH & L. J. WADE. 1944. Depressant effects of high concentrations of inspired oxygen on erythrocytogenesis: Observations on patients with sickle cell anemia with a description of the observed toxic manifestations of oxygen. J. Clin. Invest. **23:** 682–698.
6. TINSLEY, J. C., JR., C. V. MOORE, R. DUBACH, V. MINNICH & M. GRINSTEIN. 1949. The role of oxygen in the regulation of erythropoiesis: Depression of the rate of delivery of new red cells to the blood by high concentrations of inspired oxygen. J. Clin. Invest. **28:** 1544–1564.
7. COOPERBERG, A. & K. SINGER. 1951. The reaction of the bone marrow to high oxygen tension in normal and anemic guinea pigs. J. Lab. Clin. Med. **37:** 936–947.
8. FRIED, W., L. F. PLZAK, L. O. JACOBSON & E. GOLDWASSER. 1957. Studies on erythropoiesis. **III.** Factors controlling erythropoietin production. Proc. Soc. Exper. Biol. Med. **94:** 237–241.
9. GYLLENSTEN, L. & G. SWANBECK. 1959. Influence of concentrated oxygen on the circulating erythrocytes in growing mice. Acta path. microbiol. scandinav. **45:** 229–236.
10. BIRKHILL, F. R., M. A. MALONEY & S. M. LEVENSON. 1951. Effect of transfusion polycythemia upon bone marrow activity and erythrocyte survival in man. Blood **6:** 1021–1033.
11. GURNEY, C. W. & C. PAN. 1958. Studies on erythropoiesis. **IX.** Mechanism of decreased erythropoiesis in experimental polycythemia. Proc. Soc. Exper. Biol. Med. **98:** 789–793.
12. JACOBSON, L. O., E. GOLDWASSER & C. W. GURNEY. 1960. Transfusion-induced polycythaemia as a model for studying factors influencing erythropoiesis. *In* Ciba Foundation Symposium on Haemopoiesis: Cell Production and Its Regulation. G. E. W. Wolstenholme & M. O'Connor, Eds. : 423–445. Little, Brown & Company. Boston, Mass.

13. DeGowin, R. L., D. Hofstra & C. W. Gurney. 1962. The mouse with hypoxia-induced erythremia, an erythropoietin bioassay animal. J. Lab. Clin. Med. **60:** 846–852.
14. Weintraub, A. H., A. S. Gordon & J. F. Camiscoli. 1963. Use of the hypoxia-induced polycythemic mouse in the assay and standardization of erythropoietin. J. Lab. Clin. Med. **62:** 743–752.
15. Monette, F. C., J. LoBue, A. S. Gordon & P. Chan. 1965. Erythropoiesis in transfusion-induced polycythemic rats studied with H^3-thymidine autoradiography. Proc. Soc. Exper. Biol. Med. **119:** 445–449.
16. Mengel, C. E., H. E. Kann, W. W. Smith & B. D. Horton. 1964. Effects of *in vivo* hyperoxia on erythrocytes. 1. Hemolysis in mice exposed to hyperbaric oxygenation. Proc. Soc. Exper. Biol. Med. **116:** 259–261.
17. Mengel, C. E., H. E. Kann, Jr., A. Heyman & E. Metz. 1965. Effects of in vivo hyperoxia on erythrocytes. II. Hemolysis in a human after exposure to oxygen under high pressure. Blood **25:** 822-829.
18. Fuson, R. L., H. A. Saltzman, W. W. Smith, R. E. Whalen, S. Osterhout & R. T. Parker. 1965. Clinical hyperbaric oxygenation with severe oxygen toxicity: Report of a case. New England J. Med. **273:** 415–419.
19. Pittinger, C. B. 1966. Hyperbaric Oxygenation. Charles C Thomas. Springfield, Illinois. 113 pp.
20. Zalusky, R., F. Ulvedal, J. E. Herlocher & B. E. Welch. 1964. Physiologic response to increased oxygen partial pressure. **III.** Hematopoiesis. Aerospace Med. **35:** 622–626.
21. Nairn, J. R., G. G. Power, R. W. Hyde, R. E. Forster, C. J. Labertsen & J. Dickson. 1965. Diffusing capacity and pulmonary capillary blood flow at hyperbaric pressures. J. Clin. Invest. **44:** 1591–1599.
22. Krzymowski, T. & H. Krzymowska. 1962. Studies on the erythropoiesis inhibiting factor in the plasma of animals with transfusion polycythemia. Blood **19:** 38–44.
23. Whitcomb, W. H. & M. Z. Moore. 1965. The inhibitory effect of plasma from hypertransfused animals on erythrocyte iron incorporation in mice. J. Lab. Clin. Med. **66:** 641–651.

USE OF SILICONE RUBBER MEMBRANE ENCLOSURES FOR PREPARATION OF ERYTHROPOIETIN ASSAY MICE*

R. D. Lange, M. L. Simmons and T. P. McDonald

University of Tennessee Memorial Research Center, Knoxville, Tenn.

Bioassays utilizing polycythemic mice are currently in general use for the indirect determination of erythropoietin.[1–3] Assay animals are usually prepared either by transfusion or by exposure to reduced oxygen tension in specially constructed chambers, or by a combination of the two methods.[4–6] Recently we described the use of cage enclosures covered with a dimethyl silicone rubber membrane to produce hypoxic erythrocythemia in mice.[7] Because of the permeability properties of the membranes, the oxygen concentration within the enclosure is inversely proportional to the number of mice housed. It is the purpose of this paper to extend earlier observations and to report experiments designed to develop an assay procedure utilizing animals which had been housed for varying lengths of time in the membrane enclosures.

Methods and Materials

The membrane enclosures were hand fabricated in the laboratories of the General Electric Company utilizing standard laboratory cages (FIGURE 1). One hundred forty-three square inches of the dimethyl silicone rubber membrane, bonded on both sides with "Dacron" mats, were used for each enclosure. In earlier experiments the enclosures were flushed with 10% O_2 after being opened. Based on results of subsequent experiments, it was found that this was not necessary; therefore, currently, after the cages are opened for cleaning, they are resealed with plastic tape and equilibrium is established in approximately eight hours.

A/Jax mice were used in all of the experiments described herein. Oxygen content was measured by a Beckman oxygen analyzer. The CO_2 partial pressure was measured in an Instrumentation Laboratory Inc. meter. Hematocrits were determined by the micro method and the radioiron incorporation in red blood cells was measured 48 hr after an intraperitoneal injection of 0.5 μc of ^{59}Fe, utilizing a well-type scintillation counter. The data were analyzed in all cases by the one-way classification analysis of variance method and Duncan's Multiple Range test.[8]

Results

The effect of enclosing different numbers of mice on the oxygen content within the enclosure and the hematocrit and iron incorporation of the mice is shown in FIGURE 2. It should be noted that with increasing numbers of enclosed mice, the oxygen content decreased from 18% with one mouse enclosed to 6.5% with 11 mice enclosed in the cage. By increasing the degree of hypoxia by enclosing more mice, the hematocrit of 11 mice enclosed for three weeks and measured seven days post enclosure was increased to 58%. Similarly, the red blood cell iron incorporation, measured seven days post enclosure, decreased to less than 0.75% when 9, 10, or 11 mice were enclosed. Statistically the ^{59}Fe incorporations in red blood cells are not different when 9, 10, or 11 mice are enclosed per cage ($P < 0.01$).

* Supported in part by grant no. GB–4818 from the National Science Foundation and U.S.P.H.S. grant no. HE–10567–01.

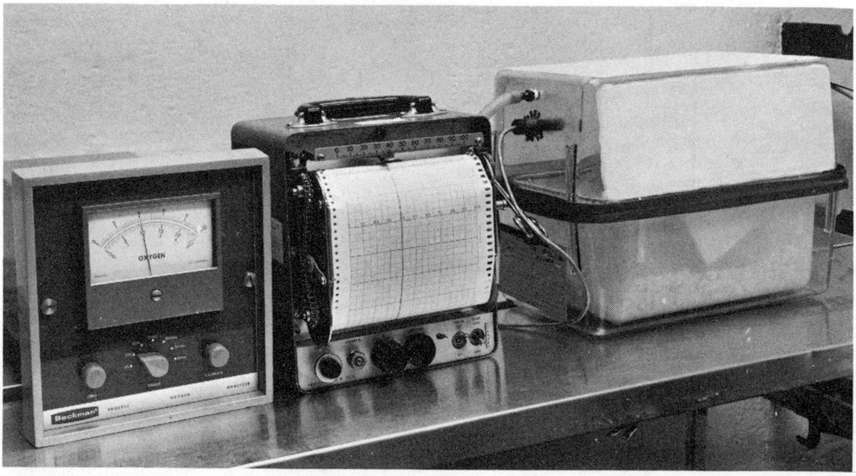

FIGURE 1. A mouse cage covered with a silicone rubber membrane with O_2 analyzer attached.

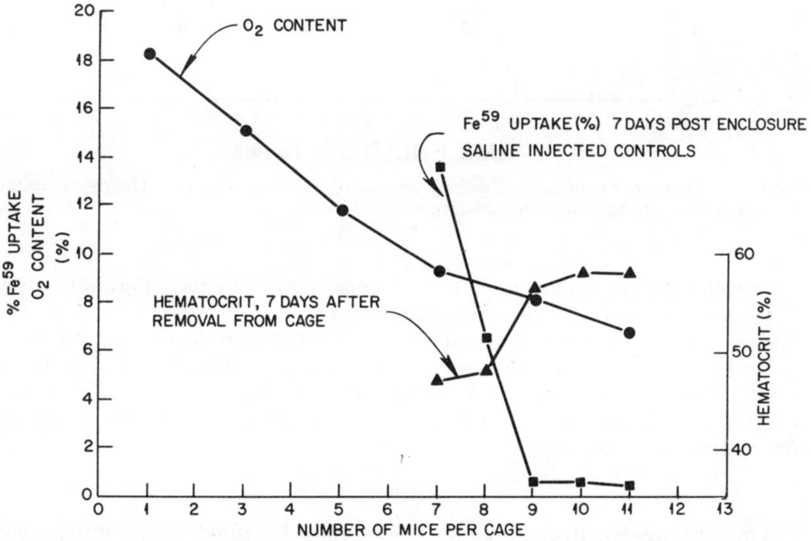

FIGURE 2. The effects of enclosing different numbers of mice on the oxygen content within the cage, hematocrits and percent ^{59}Fe red blood cell incorporation in mice.

With 11 mice enclosed, the mean hematocrit, measured at weekly intervals, increased from 48% to 73% (FIGURE 3). Significantly higher hematocrits were obtained at 3 weeks over 2 weeks; 2 weeks $>$ 1 week $>$ 0 week at the 5% level.

The 48-hour percentage of radioiron incorporated into red blood cells was measured at timed intervals following removal from the enclosure. The results are graphically portrayed in FIGURE 4. As shown, minimal iron incorporations were recorded during the period of 6 to 12 days post enclosure and by 14 days

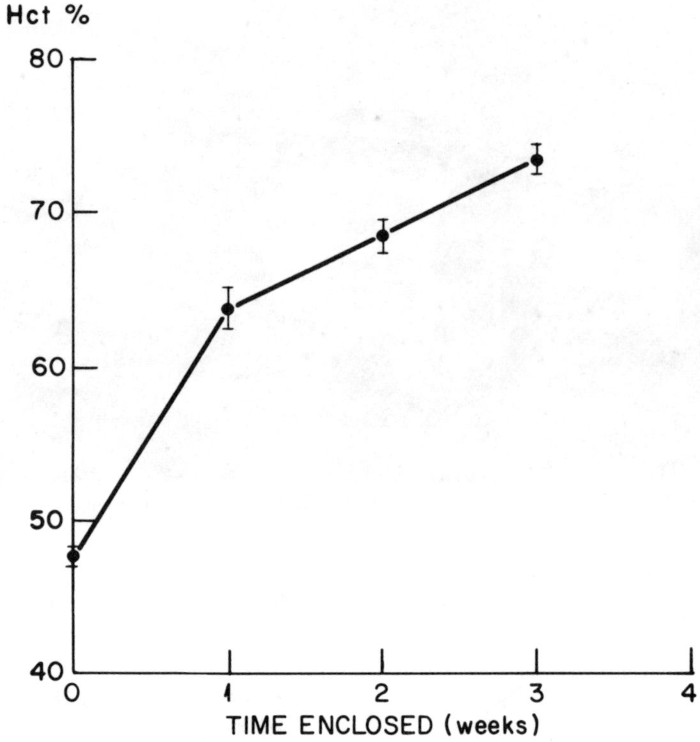

FIGURE 3. Hematocrits of mice at weekly intervals following enclosure. The cages contained 11 mice each. Verticle bars indicate standard error of mean.

an increased iron incorporation was noted once more. ^{59}Fe incorporations on days 6–12 were not statistically different at the 1% level.

The results of a dose response experiment are recorded in FIGURE 5. For these experiments 11 mice were enclosed for a three-week period and 0.05 to 0.4 unit of erythropoietin was injected. A statistically significant response ($P < 0.01$) was found to 0.05 unit of erythropoietin and increasing the dose led to increased incorporations of radioiron.

Discussion

The membranes which enclosed the cages utilize the nineteenth century concept of using semipermeable membranes for the separation of gases and vapors. As shown schematically in FIGURE 6, permselective membranes differ from ordinary porous membranes in that the permeability depends on the solubility and rate of diffusion and as a consequence gas A will permeate the membrane faster than gas B and gas B faster than gas C. The membrane used in the present experiments, a dimethyl silicone rubber film, was 0.001 inch in thickness. Some of the properties of this membrane have been published.[9,10] In the enclosure described in this report, as the animals consumed oxygen, the partial pressure of oxygen inside the cage was lowered below ambient air and produced a partial pressure difference across the membrane. Because of the difference in permeability, the partial pres-

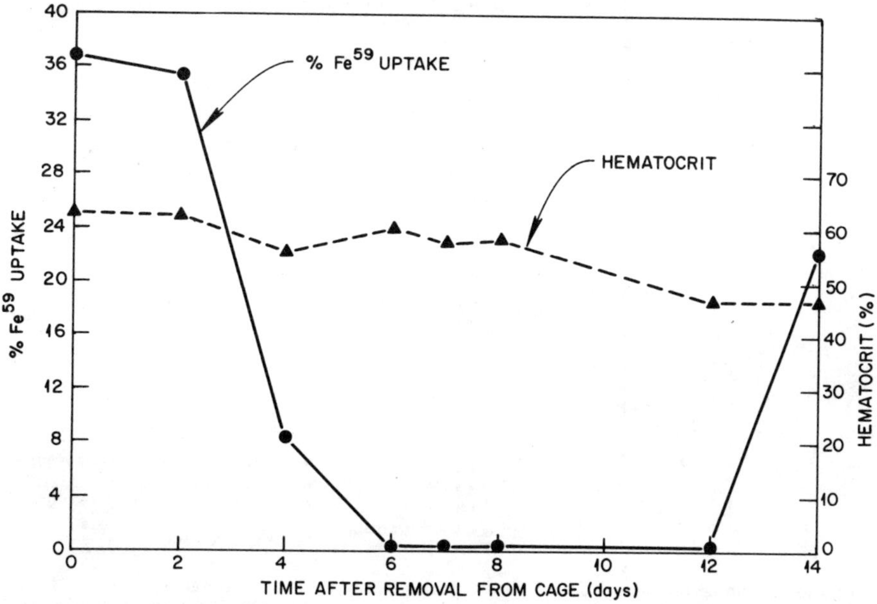

FIGURE 4. The percent ^{59}Fe incorporation and hematocrits of mice measured at timed intervals following removal from the enclosure. The cages contained 11 mice each.

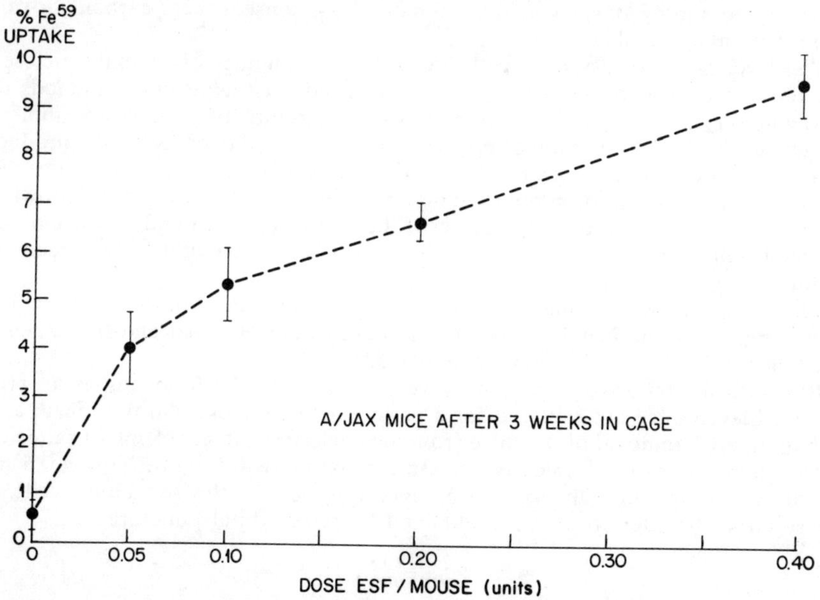

FIGURE 5. The percent ^{59}Fe incorporation of mouse red blood cells after enclosure for three weeks utilizing different doses of erythropoietin. Verticle bars indicate standard error of mean.

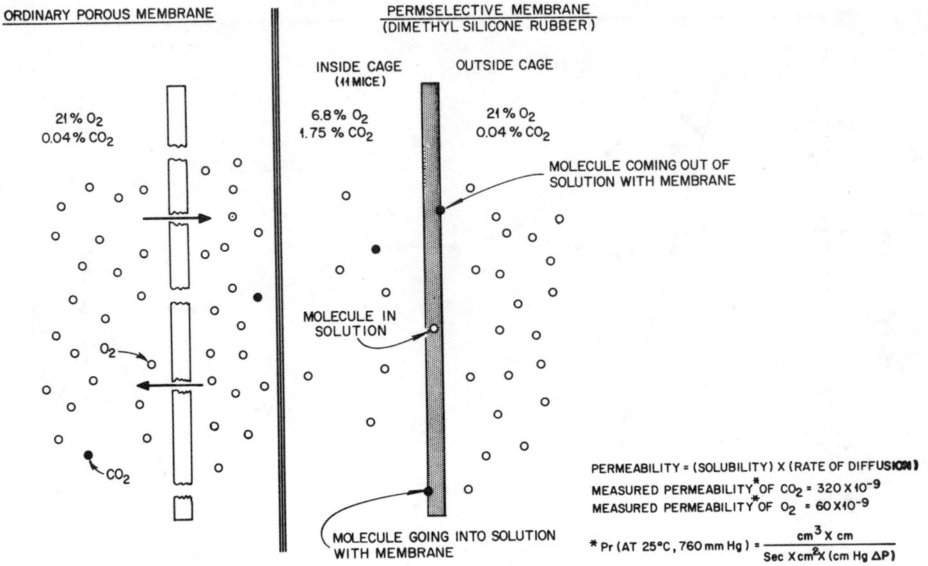

FIGURE 6. Some characteristics of porous versus permselective membranes. Modified from Esmond and Dibelius, Trans. Am. Soc. Artif. Intern. Organs **11:** 325, 1965, and published by consent of the authors and publisher.

sure difference to drive carbon dioxide out of the cage is less than one-fifth that necessary to supply oxygen to the animals. As a consequence, carbon dioxide levels were in a tolerable range.

The level of hypoxia was directly related to the number of animals enclosed and the expected increase in hematocrits occurred. Just as in other methods of producing erythropoietin assay animals, with the return of animals to ambient oxygen levels after production of polycythemia, a marked decrease in the production of new erythrocytes occurred. This was shown by the decrease in the red blood cell iron incorporation reported herein. Also, as in other methods, following a period of suppression of erythropoiesis, the hematocrits fell and erythropoiesis resumed. This is apparently related to suppression and production of endogenous erythropoietin.[11]

The use of the membrane cages represents a simple and safe method of producing polycythemia in mice. Mechanical failures are obviated and the expense and time involved in transfusions are avoided.

Based on the reported experiments we have adapted the following assay procedure. Eleven mice are enclosed for a period of three weeks. On the fourth and fifth days, after removal of the mice from the enclosure, either 0.5 ml. of saline or test substance in saline is injected i.p. On the sixth day, 0.5 μc of ^{59}Fe in 0.5 ml of saline is given i.p.; the radio-iron incorporation in the red blood cells is measured 48 hr later from blood obtained by retro-orbital puncture.

Summary

1. The use of silicone rubber membrane enclosures for the preparation of erythropoietin assay mice is reported.

2. The method represents a safe, simple method for producing hypoxia.
3. The results of hematocrit elevation, iron incorporation and response to erythropoietin parallel established assay methods.

References

1. GORDON, A. S. & A. H. WEINTRAUB. 1962. Assay of the erythropoietic stimulating factor (ESF). *In* Erythropoiesis. L. O. Jacobson & M. Doyle, Eds. : 1–16. Grune & Stratton. New York.
2. DEGOWIN, R. L., D. HOFSTRA & C. W. GURNEY. 1962. A comparison of erythropoietin bioassays. Proc. Soc. Exp. Biol. Med. **110:** 48–51.
3. LANGE, R. D. & V. PAVLOVIC-KENTERA. 1964. Erythropoietin. *In* Progress in Hematology. IV. C. V. Moore & E. B. Brown, Eds. : 72. Grune & Stratton. New York.
4. COTES, P. M. & D. R. BANGHAM. 1961. Bioassay of erythropoietin in mice made polycythemic by exposure to air at a reduced pressure. Nature **191:** 1065–1067.
5. DEGOWIN, R. L., D. HOFSTRA & C. W. GURNEY. 1962. The mouse with hypoxia-induced erythremia, an erythropoietic bioassay animal. J. Lab. Clin. Med. **60:** 846-852.
6. WEINTRAUB, A. H., A. S. GORDON & J. F. CAMISCOLI. 1963. Use of the hypoxia-induced polycythemic mouse in the assay and standardization of erythropoietin. J. Lab. Clin. Med. **62:** 743–752.
7. LANGE, R. D., M. L. SIMMONS & N. R. DIBELIUS. 1966. Polycythemic mice produced by hypoxia in silicone rubber membrane enclosures: a new technique. Proc. Soc. Exp. Biol. Med. **122:** 761–764.
8. LECLERG, E. L. 1957. Mean separation by the functional analysis of variance and multiple comparisons. U.S. Dept. Agr. Agriculture Research Service. : 20–3.
9. ROBB, W. L. 1965. Preliminary report entitled "Air ecology using thin silicone membranes in an aqueous environment," Prepared by the General Electric Company and presented before the 159th Annual Medical Society of the State of New York.
10. ESMOND, W. G. & N. R. DIBELIUS. 1965. Permselective ultra-thin disposable silicone rubber membrane blood oxygenator: Preliminary report. Trans. Amer. Soc. Artif. Intern. Organs **11:** 325–329.
11. GURNEY, C. W., N. WACKMAN & E. FILMANOWICZ. 1961. Studies on erythropoiesis. XVII. Some quantitative aspects of the erythropoietic response to erythropoietin. Blood **17:** 531–546.

COMPARATIVE ASSAY OF ERYTHROPOIETIN STANDARDS*

James F. Camiscoli, Arthur H. Weintraub and Albert S. Gordon
Department of Biology, Graduate School of Arts and Science, New York University, New York, N. Y.

In a previous review of this subject in 1962[1] we summarized the numerous assay methods used for the detection of erythropoietic activity and emphasized the advantages of the polycythemic mouse as a test animal. We further suggested that erythropoietin activity be reported in terms of the then available sheep plasma standard, erythropoietin standard A (ESA). In the four years since that time there has been widespread acceptance of radioiron uptake in the blood of the transfused or hypoxia-induced plethoric mouse as the method of choice for the estimation of erythropoietin activity. Furthermore, supplies of ESA were being rapidly exhausted, necessitating the preparation of a new standard, erythropoietin standard B (ESB), derived from human urinary sources. With a view toward its establishment as an international reference preparation, ESB was subjected to an international collaborative assay, with the participation of seventeen different laboratories under the direction of Dr. P. Mary Cotes of the Division of Biological Standards, National Institute for Medical Research, Mill Hill, London, England. The detailed results of this collaborative study are now in press.[2] Recently, the 17th session of the World Health Organization Expert Committee on Biological Standardization has declared ESB as the International Reference Preparation for Erythropoietin (IRPE) and defined an international unit of erythropoietin as the activity contained in 1.48 mg of IRPE.

At this point, with the availability of an international reference standard and considering the many new investigators entering the field of erythropoietin research, it seems appropriate to reemphasize certain technical aspects of the routine bioassay of erythropoietin preparations:

1) Each laboratory should prepare sufficient quantities of a working standard and calibrate it against the international preparation. Both preparations should be stored under conditions minimizing rapid loss of activity preferably in the dry state at $-10°$ C or lower. The working standard should be rechecked against the international standard at regular intervals, preferably at three dose levels (six-point assay) so that both linearity and parallelism may be assessed. The choice of a particular working standard will be largely dictated by the nature of the studies being conducted and by the availability of materials in a given laboratory. However, the storage of standard at several convenient dose levels provides flexibility in the assay of unknown substances of widely divergent potencies.

2) Measurement of test substances and standard should be carried out simultaneously, preferably in a balanced four-point assay. It is imperative that doses be selected within the linear range of the dose-response curve if valid results are to be obtained.

3) Appropriate statistical methods (i.e., variance analysis) should be employed in all assays to insure both significant regression and parallelism of standard and test preparations. If statistical confirmation of these parameters is not obtainable, the results must be regarded as invalid.

4) Expression of erythropoietin activity should be in terms of the international

* Supported by Grant 5–R01–HE03357–09 from the National Heart Institute of the National Institutes of Health, U.S.P.H.S.

standard as units of IRPE. Some estimate of error, either the standard error of the potency and/or the 95 percent confidence limits, should be included with estimates of potency. Methods for the calculation of the above values are found in standard texts.[3,4]

It should be noted that "pilot assays" of unknowns are frequently helpful in reducing error by allowing closer matching of unknown and standard doses. Finally, the careful selection of animals cannot be overemphasized. We have noted that randomized groups of homogeneous mice consistently give the best results, i.e., the lowest indices of precision.

It is obvious from the above considerations that a working standard must show parallel regression against the international standard and that its usefulness is in large part determined by its parallelism with erythropoietically active substances from a broad spectrum of sources. This is particularly true in our laboratory where routine assays of active material from a variety of animal and human sources are conducted. From time to time we have encountered erythropoietin preparations, usually samples of raw human urine, which showed regressions markedly different from those of the simultaneously assayed sheep plasma standard.[5,6] Others have reported similar findings.[2] It is perhaps not surprising that crude preparations may contain inhibitors or hemolysins which could have a profound influence on the regression of the active substance. On the other hand, the mere addition of plasma or urine to partially purified erythropoietin does not appear to influence its potency or regression.[5]

This report presents data obtained from comparative assays of seven different erythropoietin preparations employed in our laboratory. These substances have been used as standards for investigational purposes and provide a reasonably representative sample of erythropoietically active substances. Our objectives in conducting this comparative study were: 1) to assay ESB (now IRPE) in terms of ESA, largely as our contribution to the international collaborative assay mentioned above; 2) to compare the relative regressions and to test the parallelism of erythropoietin preparations from various sources and of different potencies and states of purification; 3) and to obtain some information regarding the loss of activity of two partially purified preparations (ELS-3 and ELS-4) that had been stored under defined conditions for several years.

Materials and Methods

Assay Procedures

A modification of the method described by Weintraub *et al.* was employed.[5] CF-1 female mice with initial weights of 22–25 g were exposed to a simulated altitude of 23,000 feet, 19 hr per day for two weeks. Erythropoietin preparations were administered i.p. in divided doses on the third and fourth days posthypoxia; 0.5 μc $^{59}Fe\ Cl_3$ in 0.2 ml 0.9% saline was given i.v. on the fifth day, and animals were killed by removal of blood via cardiac puncture under light ether anesthesia on the seventh day. The radioactivity of 0.5 ml samples of cardiac blood was determined in a well-type scintillation counter and expressed as percent RBC ^{59}Fe incorporation. Microhematocrits were done in duplicate and mice with values less than 57% were discarded. Four assays were carried out at three dose levels (six-point design), with a minimum of five mice per dose, and ESA was used as the primary reference standard. Due to the limited quantities of ESA, fewer animals were employed per dose level for this material and the results obtained in the four assays were pooled. Potencies and error calculations were done by standard methods.[4] Protein determinations were made on each erythropoietin preparation by the Biuret method, employing a Beckman DU spectrophotometer, and erythropoietin activities were expressed as units of ESF per mg protein.

Erythropoietin Preparations

1) *Erythropoietin Standard A* (ESA), sheep plasma erythropoietin prepared by the Armour Pharmaceutical Co. in cooperation with the University of Chicago for distribution by the U.S.P.H.S. under research grant H-5393. Batch AL-0336, Lot K 103-124 was distributed in ampoules containing 10 units of activity which were prepared under the direction of Drs. D. R. Bangham and P. M. Cotes, Dept. of Biological Standards, National Institute for Medical Research, Mill Hill, London, England.

2) *Erythropoietin Standard B* (ESB), human urinary erythropoietin prepared by pooling partially fractionated batches from anemic patients. Ampoules containing approximately 10 units of activity relative to ESA were prepared under the direction of Drs. D. R. Bangham and P. M. Cotes, Dept. of Biological Standards, National Institute for Medical Research, Mill Hill, London, England. Details of the individual fractions and preparation of the standard are published elsewhere.[2]

3) *Erythropoietin Laboratory Standard 3* (ELS-3), Step III sheep plasma erythropoietin, Armour Lot K 147-137, originally assaying at 7.3 units per mg protein. Preparation supplied by the Hematology Study Section, National Institutes of Health, U.S.P.H.S.

4) *Erythropoietin Laboratory Standard 4* (ELS-4), Step IV sheep plasma erythropoietin, Armour Lot K 103-124, originally assaying at 23 units per mg protein. Preparation supplied by the Hematology Study Section, National Institutes of Health, U.S.P.H.S.

5) *Human Urinary Erythropoietin (HUE Hammond)*, fractionated material from the urine of patients with anemia due to hookworm infestation. Kindly supplied by Dr. G. Denman Hammond.

6) *Human Urinary Erythropoietin (HUE Stohlman)*, material fractionated from the urine of patients with hypoplastic anemia. Kindly supplied by Dr. F. Stohlman, Jr.

7) *Hypoxic Rat Plasma (HRP 18-hour)*, plasma collected and pooled from male, 180-190 g Long-Evans rats immediately after 18 hr continuous exposure to a simulated altitude of 23,000 feet.

8) *Erythropoietin Laboratory Standard-Phenylhydrazinized Rat Plasma-Fraction 1 (ELS-PRP-F_1)*, the dialyzed, 40–80-percent ammonium sulfate fraction of plasma obtained from male, 280-300 g Long-Evans rats treated with 35 mg neutralized phenylhydrazine per rat in divided doses over four days.

All preparations except ELS-3 and ELS-4 were stored in the freezer at −10° C until just before use. ELS-3 and ELS-4 have been stored dry in injection bottles at 10° C for about five years.

Results and Discussion

The relative potencies, slopes, and error data for the seven preparations studied are presented in Table 1. The potencies ranged from a low for hypoxic rat plasma of 0.005 units per mg protein to 24.6 units per mg protein for Stohlman's highly active urinary fraction or about a 5,000-fold increment of specific activities. The activity of ESB was found to be about 1/20 of this range, 1.17 units per mg protein, and approximately 5% potency relative to ESA on a units per

TABLE 1

COMPARISON OF ASSAY REFERENCE STANDARDS WITH ESA

ESF Preparation*	Slope ± S.E.**	Relative Potency (R.P.) (units ESA/mg. prot.)	S.E. of R.P.† (percent)	95 percent Confidence Limits (percent)	Index of Precision (s/b)
HRP (18-hr)	24.3 ± 4.25	0.005	13.9	49.7–201.2	0.18
ELS-PRP-F_1	29.2 ± 7.21	0.044	12.5	62.9–158.8	0.21
ESB	29.8 ± 10.23	1.17	14.4	47.1–217.2	0.27
ELS-3	30.0 ± 7.18	3.04	12.4	63.8–156.6	0.20
HUE (Hammond)	30.2 ± 3.58	6.60	11.7	72.1–138.6	0.15
ELS-4	31.6 ± 5.65	16.3	11.5	75.0–134.0	0.13
HUE (Stohlman)	29.4 ± 4.32	24.6	11.4	75.6–132.1	0.11
ESA	30.0 ± 5.48	—	—	—	—

* For explanation, see text.
** S.E. = standard error.
† R.P. = relative potency.

mg basis. Highly purified fractions of sheep plasma erythropoietin with activities ranging up to 6,500 units per mg protein or higher have been reported.[7] Such highly active material, although very unstable and available only in very small quantities, serves to emphasize the relatively low specific activity of the currently available standard. The low activity has been attributed to the presence of inactive pigment and protein, largely derived from patients with paroxysmal nocturnal hemoglobinuria.[2] While low activity per se is not objectionable, it may prove to be undesirable in the assay of highly active preparations since it is obviously easier to dilute a standard of known activity than an unknown. However, careful calibration of working laboratory standards should alleviate this difficulty.

The individual regression lines of radioiron uptake on log dose for the seven preparations and ESA are plotted in FIGURE 1 and the values of the respective slopes (± standard errors) are listed in TABLE 1. All slopes were highly significant ($P < 0.001$) and despite the wide range of potencies and the heterogeneity of sources, there was no significant difference between the slope of any preparation and that of ESA (dash line in FIGURE 1). Furthermore, all slope values were homogeneous, with $\chi^2 = 13.1$ and 7 d.f. at $p > 0.05$. Only the slope of the crudest material, the hypoxic rat plasma, showed any tendency toward deviation from the other values and this was not significant. Such a surprising degree of parallelism among these preparations was unexpected in view of our prior experience and lends confidence to the expression of comparative activities.

Since all of the above preparations have parallel regressions, theoretically any of them could serve as a satisfactory standard. Selection of one or two may then be based on 1) activity appropriate to that of the unknown and 2) statistical considerations. It should be noted (TABLE 1) that the two urinary preparations (HUE Hammond; HUE Stohlman) and ELS-4 showed lower indices of precision (λ) and narrower 95-percent confidence intervals than the other substances and hence might be expected to provide more precise results. While not included in the present study, we have prior evidence that erythropoietic activity extracted from the kidneys of hypoxic rats[8] or produced by in vitro incubations of a subcellular fraction[9,10] is also parallel when assayed against preparations evaluated here.

The degradation of active material in stored standard preparations has fre-

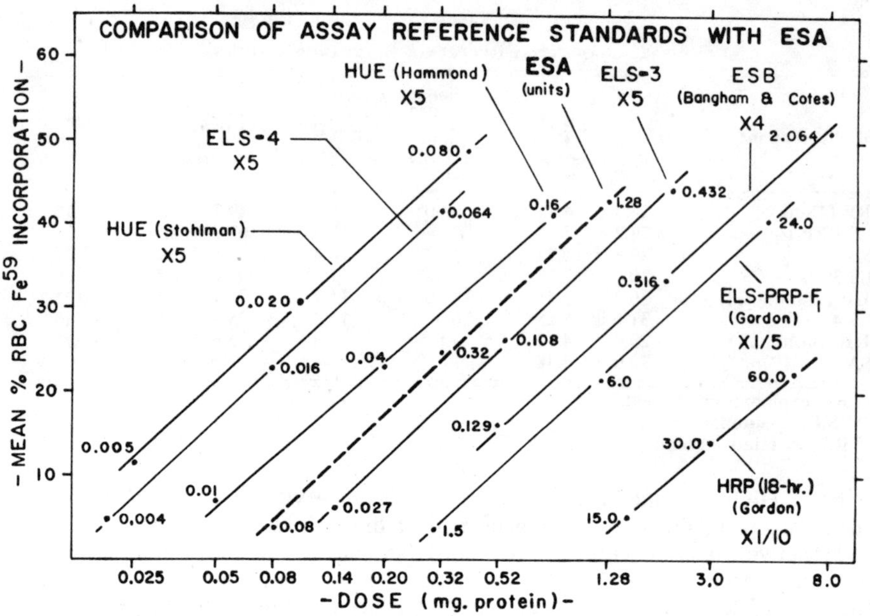

FIGURE 1. Comparison of assay reference standards with ESA. In order to facilitate comparison of preparations with widely divergent activities on a reasonable scale, original doses have been multiplied by appropriate factors. The factors are listed next to the individual regression lines and the original doses in mg protein are listed adjacent to each point. For identification of individual preparations, see text.

quently been pointed to as a possible source of error,[1,5,11] but little actual data concerning this important point have been available. In the current study we have had the opportunity to re-assay two partially purified fractions of sheep plasma erythropoietin (ELS-3 and ELS-4) which were stored in their original containers at 10° C since 1961. Assay of these fractions against ESA in 1962 and 1963 revealed no significant change from the original potency estimates of 7.3 (ELS-3) and 23 (ELS-4) units per mg protein.[5] The current assays reveal a value for ELS-3 of 3.0 units per mg protein or about 40 percent of its original activity; and a potency for ELS-4 of 16.3 units per mg protein, about 70 percent of its original value. These findings are of interest because they indicate that at this general range of activity, the more purified preparation had significantly greater stability. This is in contradistinction to the established lability of very highly purified material with activities in the range of thousands of units per mg protein.[7] It should be noted that ELS-4 and ESA were derived from the same original lot (K 103-124) of Step IV sheep plasma erythropoietin, the major difference between the two being the addition of lactose and buffer in the preparation of ESA and its subsequent storage in vacuo at −10° C. Hence the current study may be interpreted as an accelerated degradation test of sheep plasma erythropoietin by exposure to higher temperature and air. The preparation, ELS-4, stored at 10° C lost 30 percent of its activity compared with the preparation stored at −10° C over a period of five years. No difference in activity was found at the end of two years. These data should be compared with those reported by Cotes and Bangham on the effects of heat on the current urinary standard

ESB (IRPE).[2] They found no loss of activity after storage at 37° C for one year or at 20° C for about two years, but noted an approximate 50-percent decrement in activity of material stored at 37° C for about two years. These findings indicate that the loss of activity from erythropoietin standards is slow but definite and that storage at −10° C or lower (in vacuo) will retard decay.

Summary

Assays of seven different erythropoietin preparations, of various sources, potencies and states of purification, were conducted employing Erythropoietin Standard A as the primary reference standard. Despite a 5,000-fold range of activities among the preparations, all showed parallel regressions with that of Standard A and the slopes of all were found to be homogeneous. Data are presented indicating that the loss of activity from sheep erythropoietin standards is slow and is related to the method of storage, degree of purity, and storage temperature. Technical aspects of the routine bioassay of erythropoietin are discussed and procedural details are outlined.

References

1. Gordon, A. S. & A. H. Weintraub. 1962. Assay of the erythropoietic stimulating factor (ESF). *In* Erythropoiesis. L. O. Jacobson & M. Doyle, Eds. : 1–16. Grune & Stratton. New York, N. Y.
2. Cotes, P. M. & D. R. Bangham. 1966. The international reference preparation of erythropoietin. Bull. WHO **35**: 751–760.
3. Bliss, C. L. 1952. The Statistics of Bioassay. Academic Press. New York, N. Y.
4. Finney, D. J. 1964. Statistical Method in Biological Assay. Second Edition. Hafner Publishing Co. New York, N. Y.
5. Weintraub, A. H., A. S. Gordon & J. F. Camiscoli. 1963. Use of the hypoxia-induced polycythemic mouse in the assay and standardization of erythropoietin. J. Lab. Clin. Med. **62**: 743–752.
6. Gordon, A. S., A. H. Weintraub, J. F. Camiscoli & J. F. Contrera. 1964. Plasma and urinary levels of erythropoietin in Cooley's anemia. Ann. N. Y. Acad. Sci. **119**: 561–577.
7. Goldwasser, E. & C. Kung. 1967. On the purification and properties of sheep plasma erythropoietin. Ann. N. Y. Acad. Sci. This Annal.
8. Contrera, J. F., J. F. Camiscoli, A. H. Weintraub & A. S. Gordon. 1965. Extraction of erythropoietin from kidneys of hypoxic and phenylhydrazine-treated rats. Blood **25**: 809–816.
9. Contrera, J. F. & A. S. Gordon. 1966. Erythropoietin: Production by a particulate fraction of rat kidney. Science **152**: 653–654.
10. Contrera, J. F., A. S. Gordon & A. H. Weintraub. 1966. Extraction of an erythropoietin-producing factor from a particulate fraction of rat kidney. Blood **28**: 330–343.
11. Bangham, D. R. 1962. Biological assay and a standard for erythropoietin. *In* Erythropoiesis. L. O. Jacobson and M. Doyle, Eds. : 23–28. Grune & Stratton. New York, N. Y.

QUANTITATIVE ESTIMATION OF ERYTHROPOIETIN*

Nomie A. Shore, Nasser Movassaghi and Denman Hammond
Division of Hematology, The Children's Hospital of Los Angeles and
The Department of Pediatrics, University of Southern California School of Medicine

Assays for erythropoietin have enabled investigators to measure erythropoietin activity in terms of its biological effect. However, a standard was needed that could be exchanged among workers to permit the results of the assays run in different laboratories to be expressed in comparable quantitative terms.

Several reference materials have been proposed as interlaboratory standards. Although it is not the intent of this discussion to review the history of erythropoietin standards, such material as cobalt,[1] a dried filtrate of boiled anemic rabbit plasma,[2,3] and anemic sheep plasma[4] have been proposed and used. For a variety of reasons, no one substance has been in general use for assays of erythropoietin.

The need for the development of a material which would satisfy the definition of a biological standard and at the same time be relatively abundant and easy to obtain has been widely recognized. Cotes and Bangham prepared a material derived from urine from anemic humans which was extracted by three different methods. The three extracts were pooled and freeze-dried in ampules. Assay of this material in terms of anemic sheep plasma (Standard A) by three laboratories, using either polycythemic mice (hypoxia- or transfusion-induced) or starved rats, gave a potency estimate of 10.1 units per ampule, with a 95% confidence interval of 8.8 to 11.4 units per ampule.[5] The slope of the log-dose-log-response curve of Standard A was slightly steeper than that of the pooled urinary extract. However, there was no statistically significant nonparallelism between the slopes. This material was assigned a value of 10 units per ampule and designated Standard B. It has since been recognized by the World Health Organization as the International Reference Preparation of Erythropoietin.[5]

Our desire to quantitate erythropoietin in samples of biological material led us to use Standard B, kindly provided by Drs. Cotes and Bangham. We have used Standard B to quantitate a secondary standard for routine use in this laboratory and for estimation of the potency of crude erythropoietin-containing materials. The laboratory standard consists of a single pool of plasma from rabbits made anemic by administration of phenylhydrazine.

In recent years we have utilized the exhypoxic polycythemic mouse for assay of erythropoietin by measuring the incorporation of ^{59}Fe into the circulating red blood cells. The assay is described in detail elsewhere in this Annal.[6]

Between July, 1964, and April, 1966, dose-response slopes have been constructed from data obtained from assays using Standard B on eight separate occasions. Log-dose response curves were obtained using Standard B at three to five dose levels between 0.01 and 5 units per mouse. The curves were linear between doses of 0.1 unit and 2.0 units per mouse. Slopes of the best fit lines, as calculated by the method of least squares, varied from $b = 21.6$ to $b = 12.0$ (FIGURE 1). Despite the range of b values obtained, analysis of variance between the slopes with the highest and lowest b values, utilizing the Student t test, showed no significant difference ($.90 < P < .95$).

* Supported by U.S.P.H.S. funds from research grant AM 04048, postgraduate training grant 2T1 HD 48, Clinical Research Center grant FR-86 and funds from the Medical Research Committee of Delta Delta Delta.

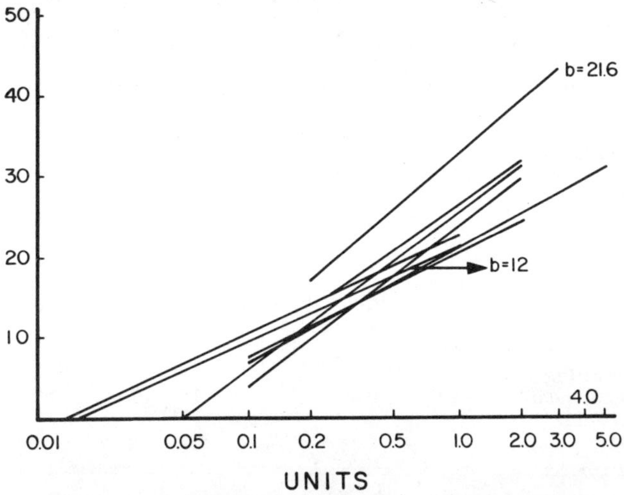

FIGURE 1. Log-Dose Response for ESF Standard B Slopes (7/9/64-4/22/66) calculated by least squares method from curves obtained by exhypoxic polycythemic mouse assay. Each point of curve is the mean value from five mice. Regression analysis comparison of slopes shows they are not significantly different (Student t test $0.90 < P < 0.95$).

Ampules of Standard B received in 1964 and stored in this laboratory at −20° C for a period of 21 months showed no apparent loss of potency when compared to ampules received in 1966. These were assayed concurrently and gave slopes of best fit lines of b = 12.0 and b = 12.2. From this experience we conclude that Standard B has maintained its potency within the confidence limits determined by Cotes and Bangham.

Currently erythropoietin is assayed by a number of different techniques in which the type of animal, the preparation of the animal, the dose and time of administration of the sample, and the method of measurement of erythropoiesis varies widely between laboratories. The variability of current erythropoietin bioassays is likely to give quantitatively divergent results among laboratories.

Examples from our laboratory illustrate this point. At the time each of the Standard B dose-response slopes was determined, the erythropoietin activity of our laboratory standard was simultaneously assayed. The mean ^{59}Fe RBC uptake was 27 ± 2.9%. The 95% confidence interval was 24.9% to 29.0% (TABLE 1).

Calculating the potency of the laboratory standard on eight separate occasions from the Standard B dose-response slope determined concurrently, the "concentration of erythropoietin" appeared to vary from 2.15 to 8.75 units per ml (mean 4.70 ± 2.32). Thus, the unit potency of this pool appeared to vary over a threefold range.

There was no nonparallelism between the eight separate dose-response slopes of Standard B. Also, the range of variability in ^{59}Fe RBC uptake produced by the laboratory standard was small. Therefore, the threefold difference in unit potency assigned to the laboratory standard in terms of Standard B must mean that their variability was independent. We believe the variability demonstrated is a characteristic of biological assay systems since the standards are presumed not to show such variability.

TABLE 1

ASSAY OF LABORATORY STANDARD IN TERMS OF STANDARD B

	Dates of Assays	7/19/64	8/7/64	12/3/65	2/4/66	2/4/66	2/25/66	4/22/66	4/22/66
Standard B	Slopes of Log-Dose Response Curves (b value)	21.6	17.6	14.4	12.0	12.2	20.0	13.4	20.1
Laboratory Standard	RBC ^{59}Fe Uptake (%)	31.0	25.0	24.0	26.0	26.0	32.0	28.0	26.0
Laboratory Standard	Potency of Laboratory Standard (Units Std B/ml)	0.9	0.86	1.7	2.7	2.0	2.2	3.5	1.2

If this be true for a single assay system in one laboratory, it is reasonable to expect greater variability when results are compared from different types of assays in use in different laboratories. Investigators using a standard reference material for quantitation of erythropoietin in biological materials should be aware of the variability of dose-response slopes using the standard by the technique they employ in their own laboratory.

Although a useful standard reference preparation of erythropoietin is available, a valid bioassay, as defined by Bangham,[7] has not yet been proposed. Even when identical assay systems are used in different laboratories, there is no general agreement on the dose or activity level at which an unknown specimen should be quantitated against a standard curve. Until isolation of a pure erythropoietin is achieved and a precise means of quantitation is available, the usefulness of the available standard would be improved by adoption of a standard assay methodology.

References

1. GOLDWASSER, E. & W. F. WHITE. 1959. Purification of sheep erythropoietin. Fed. Proc. **18:** 236.
2. KEIGHLEY, G. 1962. Experiences with assays, units and standards of erythropoietin. *In* Erythropoiesis. L. O. Jacobson & M. Doyle, Eds. : 17. Grune & Stratton, New York, N.Y.
3. KEIGHLEY, G., P. H. LOWY, H. BORSOOK, E. GOLDWASSER, A. S. GORDON, T. C. PRENTICE, W. A. RAMBACH, F. STOHLMAN, JR. & D. C. VAN DYKE. 1960. A cooperative assay of a sample with erythropoietic stimulating activity. Blood **16:** 1424.
4. JACOBSON, L. O., E. GOLDWASSER, & C. W. GURNEY. 1960. Transfusion induced polycythemia as a model for studying factors influencing erythropoiesis. *In* CIBA Foundation Symposium on Haemopoiesis. G. E. W. Wolstenholme & M. O'Connor, Eds. : 423. Little Brown & Co. Boston, Mass.
5. COTES, M. & D. R. BANGHAM. An International Reference Preparation for bioassay of erythropoietin. In press.
6. HAMMOND, G. D., N. A. SHORE & N. MOVASSAGHI. 1966. Production, utilization, and excretion of erythropoietin. This Annal.
7. BANGHAM, D. R. 1962. Biological assay and a standard for "erythropoietin." *In* Erythropoiesis. L. O. Jacobson & M. Doyle, Eds. : 23. Grune & Stratton. New York, N. Y.

PART II. CHEMISTRY AND PURIFICATION OF ERYTHROPOIETIN

PROGRESS IN THE PURIFICATION OF ERYTHROPOIETIN

Eugene Goldwasser and Charles K. H. Kung

Argonne Cancer Research Hospital and the Department of Biochemistry, University of Chicago, Chicago, Ill.*

In our last publication[1] on the purification of sheep plasma erythropoietin (EPO), we reported a potency of about 450 units/mg of protein; since that time we have purified the hormone by another factor of about 13.

The material used for the earlier purification was a side fraction (0.67 saturated ammonium sulfate supernate) from the sheep plasma erythropoietin produced in the large scale program undertaken by the United States Public Health Service in collaboration with the University of Chicago and Armour and Company. Experiments with that fraction indicated that potencies in the range of 400–500 could be achieved, but quantities of the best fraction were insufficient to carry the fractionation any further. In part, this was due to the extensive losses of activity in the calcium phosphate gel adsorption step. More recently, we have developed methods for reproducibly obtaining fractions of anemic sheep plasma with potencies of about 6,500 units/mg protein; this communication presents some of our results.

Materials and Methods

The starting erythropoietin fraction was the Step III material provided by the Hematology Study Section of the United States Public Health Service. Except where otherwise stated, assays were done by the fasted rat method.[2] The standard used in each assay was anemic sheep plasma (6.8 units/ml) that had been standardized with reference to both cobaltous chloride and Standard A. Protein concentrations were usually determined by the absorbancy at 278 mμ in a Zeiss PMQII spectrophotometer. At that wave length, the absorbancy of a one percent solution of mixed plasma glycoproteins is approximately 10, so that for rough analysis we used one absorbancy unit as equivalent to a concentration of 1 mg/ml. When protein concentrations were very low, they were calculated from the absorbancy at 194 mμ determined with a Perkin-Elmer model 202 spectrophotometer. Because of the inherent danger of stray light artefacts at the short wave length, determinations of A_{194} at various concentrations of protein (both crystalline beef serum albumin and highly purified sheep orosomucoid) were carried out. The data in FIGURE 1 show that the curve goes through the origin, indicating that there is no stray light problem, that the A_{194} is proportional to the protein concentration, that the nature of the protein is not important, and that a few μg per ml of protein can be determined by this method.

Calcium phosphate gel was prepared by the method of Tsuboi and Hudson[3] as previously reported, and the other reagents used were the best possible commercial grades.

Results and Discussion

One of the major disadvantages in our earlier fractionation method involved the calcium phosphate gel adsorption step. Although the purification effected by this method was appreciable, the yield was small, and we found that if too much gel were used, the erythropoietin activity was adsorbed and in many cases

* Operated by the University of Chicago for the United States Atomic Energy Commission.

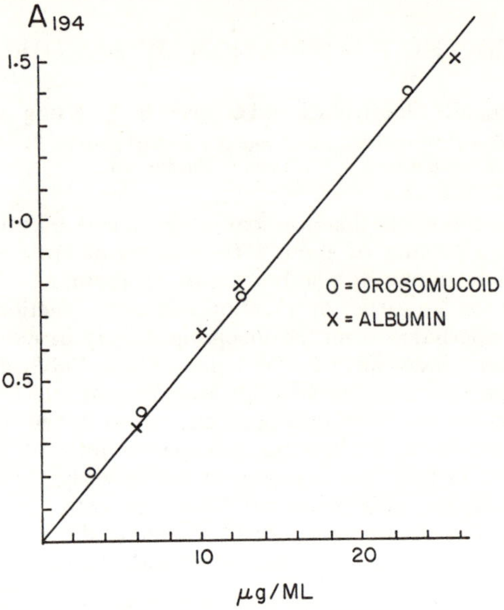

FIGURE 1. Absorbency of orosomucoid and bovine plasma albumin at 194 mμ.

little or no activity could be eluted.[1] This loss of activity was, in fact, more apparent than real. Data in TABLE 1 demonstrate that addition of serum albumin to the assay aliquots prevents the loss of an appreciable amount of activity. This protection of the erythropoietin activity appears to be the result of diminished surface denaturation of the hormone in very dilute solution, since orosomucoid and gelatin also had the same effect. This expedient enabled us to recover substantial amounts of activity from calcium phosphate gels at very high potency.

Step III erythropoietin (2.7 μ/mg) prepared by DEAE-cellulose and Amberlite XE-97 adsorption was further fractionated with ammonium sulfate to yield a Step IV fraction in 57-percent yield with a potency of 15. The dialyzed Step IV fraction was dissolved in 0.005 *M* acetate buffer, pH 4.5, and chromatographed on a sulfoethyl Sephadex (SES) column (2.2 cm × 34.4 cm) equilibrated with the same buffer. Elution was done in a stepwise fashion as indicated in TABLE 2. The major portion of the activity was located in fraction SES-5 eluted with the 0.015 *M* acetate, pH 5.0 buffer. The potency of this fraction was about 130 and recovery at this step was 52% making the yield from Step III 30%.

The SES-5 fraction was dialyzed against de-ionized water until the conductivity was < 100 μ mho cm^{-1} before adsorption on gel. During the handling of this fraction there was an appreciable decline in potency. In TABLE 3, data from a typical gel adsorption experiment are collected; it can be seen that the calcium phosphate gel eluate 2B (CaP-2B) eluted with 0.0005 *M* phosphate buffer at pH 7.4 had the highest potency—about 6,500 units per mg protein. The recovery of activity from Step III was 6.3%, and the yield from the original anemic plasma was about 2.2%. Since the original plasma had a potency of about 0.007, the overall purification factor to the CaP-2B fraction is approximately 930,000. A summary of the purification processes is presented in TABLE 4.

TABLE 1

PROTECTION OF ERYTHROPOIETIN ACTIVITY BY PROTEIN

Addition	Units Recovered
None	6.9
Albumin, 5 mg/ml	18.0
Orosomucoid, 5 mg/ml	18.6
Gelatin, 1 mg/ml	18.0

TABLE 2

CHROMATOGRAPHY OF STEP IV ERYTHROPOIETIN ON SULFOETHYL-SEPHADEX

Fraction	Buffer	Units/mg	Percent Recovery
Step IV	0.005 *M* acetate, pH 4.5	19.2	100
SES–1	0.005 *M* acetate, pH 4.5	4.5	7.8
SES–2	0.005 *M* acetate, pH 4.5	12.8	7.8
SES–3	0.01 *M* acetate, pH 4.5	0	0
SES–4	0.015 *M* acetate, pH 5.0	23.5	3.1
SES–5	0.015 *M* acetate, pH 5.0	133	52
SES–6	0.02 *M* acetate, pH 5.6	18.4	8

TABLE 3

CALCIUM PHOSPHATE GEL PURIFICATION OF ERYTHROPOIETIN

Fraction	Buffer	Units/mg	Percent Recovery
SES–5	—	79	100
Sup–2	—	435	28.6
CaP–1A	0.0005 *M* phosphate, pH 7.4	1,430	17.8
CaP–2B	0.0005 *M* phosphate, pH 7.4	6,500	37.5

TABLE 4

SUMMARY OF PURIFICATION OF ERYTHROPOIETIN

Fraction	Units/mg	Percent Recovery	Purification Factor
Anemic plasma	0.007	100	—
Step III	2.7	35	388
Step IV	19	20	2,700
SES–5	133	10.4	19,000
CaP–2B	6,500	2.2	930,000

Because of inadequate supplies of starting material (anemic sheep plasma and/or Step III), we have not yet been able to accumulate enough of the CaP-2B fraction to do any tests for heterogeneity. During the gel phosphate procedure, however, we have occasionally obtained fractions with potencies in the region of 8,000 units/mg. If this can be confirmed, we must conclude that the CaP-2B fraction is not pure erythropoietin. The heterogeneity may be due either to the presence of some erythropoietin that had been inactivated during the purification processes or to the presence of a protein unrelated to erythropoietin. Until more material becomes available this uncertainty will, unfortunately, remain.

Because of the severely limited supplies of active sheep plasma we have also been attempting to purify human urinary erythropoietin, but with much less success in obtaining very high potency fractions. As starting material we have used material precipitated from urine of anemic patients by addition of three volumes of acetone. The dried precipitate was extracted with 0.14 *M* NaCl, dialyzed, lyophilized and then fractionated by a reverse ammonium sulfate gradient dissolution method. The active fraction from the ammonium sulfate technique was then further fractionated with CaP gel to yield a fraction with a potency of about 300 units/mg protein. It is evident that this material is, at best, only about 5% pure.

Because of the minute amount of plasma fraction CaP-2B obtained, it is impossible to do any direct determinations of its chemical and physical properties. We have been forced, therefore, to rely on biological assay as a means of studying the nature of the hormone. What meager information exists from other laboratories and our own can be summarized at follows:

1) Erythropoietin is a sialic acid containing protein.
2) Serine and/or threonine hydroxyls do not seem to be required for biological activity.
3) Sulfhydryl groups do not seem to be required for biological activity.
4) Phenolic hydroxyls and/or free amino groups may be required for biological activity.
5) It probably has a molecular weight in the region 50,000–60,000.

The data in support of points (2) and (4) have come, in the main, from the work of Lowy and Borsook.[4] We have confirmed the inactivation of erythropoietin by fluoresceinisothiocyanate, and have found that p-chloromercuribenzoate[5] does not inactivate it (point 3).

The question of molecular size has been studied by Rosse *et al.*,[6] using inactivation by ionizing radiation. They concluded that erythropoietin was an elongated (axial ratio 10:1) molecule of molecular weight 27,000. Hodgson, on the other hand, found a target size of 68,000 by γ-ray inactivation.[7] We have measured the sedimentation coefficient of erythropoietin by bioassay, using the moving-partition separation cell[8] in the analytical ultracentrifuge, and found a value of 5–6 S. A sedimentation coefficient this large is not compatible with a molecular weight of 27,000, but is compatible with a molecular weight of 60–70,000. The elution volume for erythropoietin activity using gel filtration on Sephadex G-200 is also suggestive of the larger molecular size. It is clear that much work remains to be done before this relatively simple problem is solved.

Several laboratories have presented data showing that removal of sialic acid by either sialidase[9] or dilute acid[10] results in the complete loss of erythropoietin activity determined by bioassay. If the desialated erythropoietin is assayed by a marrow cell culture method,[11] however, there is no loss of activity (TABLE 5).[12] We consider the difference between the two groups assayed in vitro to be of

TABLE 5

EFFECT OF SIALIDASE ON ERYTHROPOIETIN ACTIVITY

		Units Recovered
Assayed in vivo	Control	11.4
	Sialidase-treated	0
Assayed in vitro	Control	0.04
	Sialidase-treated	0.05

doubtful significance. We do not yet understand this phenomenon but think it may relate to the binding of erythropoietin by a carrier substance. Attempts to restore activity to desialated erythropoietin by adding suspected carrier glycoproteins have been uniformly without success, leading us to our current idea that sialic acid is an intrinsic part of the erythropoietin molecule but is not required either for interaction with the target cells in the marrow or for action within the cell. Sialic acid may be required in the whole animal for binding to a carrier, or may serve to protect erythropoietin from degradation in, or excretion by, the assay animal. If this is the case, we should not expect the desialated erythropoietin to be active (except perhaps in massive amounts) in whole animals, but to be effective in cell cultures. It would also be impossible to restore in vivo activity to desialated erythropoietin, short of reforming the specific covalent bonds that had been broken.

Conclusion

The obvious need at present is a supply of starting material large enough to yield an adequate quantity of erythropoietin at the highest purity obtainable for further study. If we want, for example, 10 mg of material with a potency of 6,500, we should need about 3,250,000 units as anemic plasma. Present methods in use at the Connaught Laboratories of the University of Toronto (see the paper by Painter *et al.*, this Annal) yield about 10,000 units per sheep so that the plasma from a herd of 325 sheep must be processed to produce the desired amount. While these figures do not make the problem impossible of solution, they do indicate that it will be some time before what may be considered the final purification and characterization are achieved. It may be that urine from anemic patients will prove to be the only feasible large scale source despite what, in our experience, appears to be a lower stability for the hormone found in urine. Using the same end point and assuming a two-percent yield, we calculate that 3,250 l of urine would be required, assuming that 1 unit per ml could be obtained. This would represent about three years' daily collection from a single patient, or one month's collection from 36 patients, which does not seem to be an impossible goal. Whatever the source, it is abundantly clear that much work needs to be done before we can begin to study the chemical and structural properties of this hormone and the relationship of these properties to its striking role in red cell development.

References

1. Goldwasser, E., W. F. White & K. B. Taylor. 1962. Biochim. Biophys. Acta **64:** 487.
2. Fried, W., L. F. Plzak, L. O. Jacobson & E. Goldwasser. 1957. Proc. Soc. Exp. Biol. Med. **92:** 203.
3. Tsuboi, K. K. & P. B. Hudson. 1957. J. Biol. Chem. **224:** 879.
4. Lowy, P. H. & H. Borsook. 1962. *In* Erythropoiesis. L. O. Jacobson & M. Doyle, Eds. : 33–42. Grune and Stratton. New York, N. Y.
5. Goldwasser, E. & C. Kung. Unpublished data.
6. Rosse, W. F., R. J. Berry & T. A. Waldman. 1963. J. Clin. Invest. **42:** 124.
7. Hodgson, G. Personal communication.
8. Yphantis, D. A. & D. F. Waugh. 1956. J. Phys. Chem. **60:** 623.
9. Lowy, P. H., G. Keighly & H. Borsook. 1960. Nature **185:** 102.
10. Rambach, W. A., R. A. Shaw, J. A. D. Cooper & H. A. Alt. 1958. Proc. Soc. Exp. Biol. Med. **99:** 482.
11. Krantz, S. B., O. Gallien-Lartigue & E. Goldwasser. 1963. J. Biol. Chem. **238:** 4085.
12. Dukes, P. P., C. Kung & E. Goldwasser. Unpublished data.

THE FRACTIONATION OF ERYTHROPOIETIN FROM ANEMIC AND NORMAL HUMAN URINE*

Peter H. Lowy and Geoffrey Keighley

Division of Biology, California Institute of Technology, Pasadena, Calif.

Since the discovery of erythropoietin (EP) in the urine of bled rabbits by Hodgson,[1] urine of human anemic patients has become one of its prime sources[2–6] for experimentation. Our present fractionation scheme is shown in TABLE 1. We have previously described the procedures leading to Step 2 and recently, those leading to Step 4-A and 4-B material.[6] We now report on the presence of erythropoietin in a normal preparation. We also compare normal and anemic Step 4-A material chemically and immunologically.

By our extraction method we have obtained good yields of EP from all the urines we have examined. An advantage is that small and very large batches can be handled in a similar manner. We have reduced with relatively little labor as much as 100 l of urine to a few hundred grams of dry powder (Step 1). The urines from anemic patients were obtained with the kind cooperation of Dr. Denman Hammond, Children's Hospital of Los Angeles, California. They were kept frozen after voiding until the start of a fractionation.

Previous fractionations of Step 2 material by ethanol precipitations and DEAE cellulose chromatography had been only partially successful because preparations from different human subjects showed different distributions of activity when identical methods were applied.[4] More recently, we reported further steps giving consistent improvement of specific activities with all urines examined.[6]

The development of more sensitive assay methods is beginning to facilitate the demonstration of erythropoietin in normal plasmas and urines.[7–11] The specific activity obtainable with our Step 3 and Step 4 materials is great enough to show the presence of erythropoietin in the urine of a hematologically normal male. We were able to raise the ^{59}Fe incorporation in the assay animals from the control level of 1% to over 40%, while keeping moderate the weight of material injected.

Methods and Results

TABLE 2 shows assays of normal Step 3 material in ex-hypoxic B6D2F$_1$ female mice, according to a modification[6] of the technique of Cotes and Bangham.[12] The slope of the dose response curve over an 18-fold dose range is the same as that of preparations from anemic urine or rabbit plasma (FIGURE 1). Rabbit anti-human urinary erythropoietin serum abolishes the biological effect of erythropoietin.[13] When such serum** was injected simultaneously with the normal preparation, the ^{59}Fe incorporation was reduced to the saline control level. TABLE 3 shows a comparison of specific activities of Step 3 and Step 4-A materials from a normal and an anemic subject.

By our definition erythropoietin, when administered in sufficient amounts, stimulates erythropoiesis in a normal animal to a point where above normal blood volumes and circulating hemoglobin can be demonstrated.[6,14] Since EP is usually determined by measuring ^{59}Fe incorporation in erythropoietically suppressed animals, it is desirable to test substances derived in new ways and assayed by ^{59}Fe incorporation for their ability to produce erythrocytosis in normal animals. Daily doses of 40 μg of Step 4-A material given to normal mice for 25 to 27 days did

* This work was supported by a research grant, HE–07683, from the U.S. Public Health Service.

** Kindly supplied by Dr. John C. Schooley.

TABLE 1

FRACTIONATION OF ERYTHROPOIETIN FROM HUMAN URINE*

	Material Isolated	Weight of best fraction mg
1 l urine + 1 g phenol + 4 l ethanol		
Sup (discarded)		
ppt dialyzed	Step 1 (contains salt)	1500–3500
Insoluble ppt and dialyzate (discarded)		
Dialyzand, freeze-dried	Step 2	100–200
dissolved in 3 *M* NaCl, + 2 vol. ethanol		
0–67 ppt (dialyzed, freeze-dried)		
67–Sup, dialyzed, freeze-dried	Step 3	4–20
← A or B →		
+ sat. $(NH_4)_2SO_4$		
a. 0–50 ppt, dialyzed, freeze-dried		
b. *50–75 ppt, dialyzed, freeze-dried*	Step 4–A	1–6
c. 75–Sup (discarded)		
Acrylamide gel chromatography (Ref. 6) (water as eluent)		
Fractions 1–4, 6 and 7, freeze-dried		
Fraction 5, freeze-dried	Step 4–B	1–2

* Best fractions italicized.

indeed raise the hematocrit from 45 to 69%, and the blood volume from 6.2 to 8.1 ml/100 g body weight.[6]

Step 4-A material from normal and anemic human urines besides being assayed for erythropoietic activity was also examined for androgenic activity by disc electrophoresis, immunoelectrophoresis, and chemical determinations of sialic acid and hexose content.

In view of the known enhancement of erythropoiesis by testosterone and related compounds[15–17] it seemed of interest to examine potent Step 4-A preparations for androgenic activity. Because of the preparation method it is unlikely that low-

TABLE 2

ASSAYS OF STEP 3 MATERIAL FROM A NORMAL URINE*

	Step 3 Material Total Dose mg	^{59}Fe Percent
	3.6	4.0
	13.1	22.1
	13.1	17.3
	13.1	19.0
	65.9	38.9
	65.9	42.6
	66.0	45.5
+ anti-EP serum	13.1	0.77
	66.0	0.90
Saline control	—	0.83
Recovered: Recovered: 1.1 A u/l of urine.		

* Each value is the mean of 4–6 exhypoxic mice.

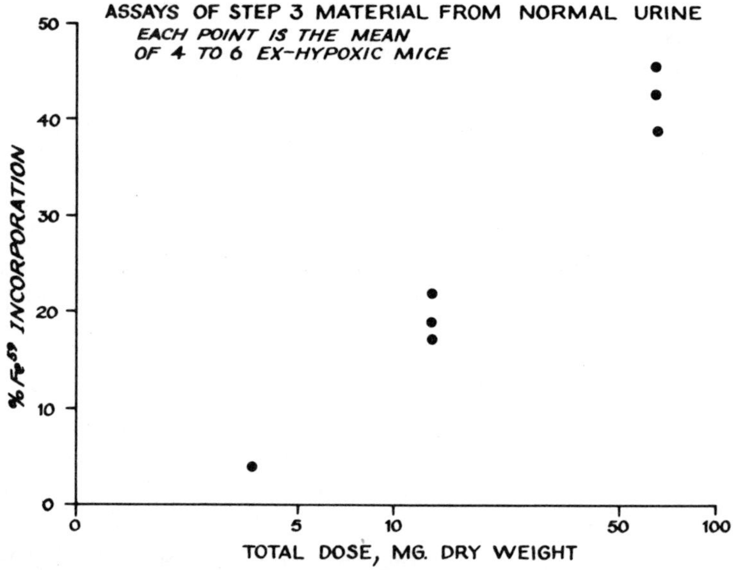

FIGURE 1. Dose response of exhypoxic B6D2F$_1$ female mice to Step 3 material from a normal human urine.

molecular compounds like androgens could be present in free form. But the question of an androgen-like molecule bound or associated to a protein, thereby conferring erythropoietic specificity, could be raised. Materials from one normal subject (0.14 u/mg) and from three anemic subjects (50–180 u/mg) were tested by the chick androgen assay method of Dorfman.[18] No androgenic activity was found and if present, it could not have exceeded 10 μg equivalents of testosterone per mg of Step 4-A material.*

* We are greatly indebted to Dr. Ralph I. Dorfman, Syntex Research, Palo Alto, California, for performing these assays.

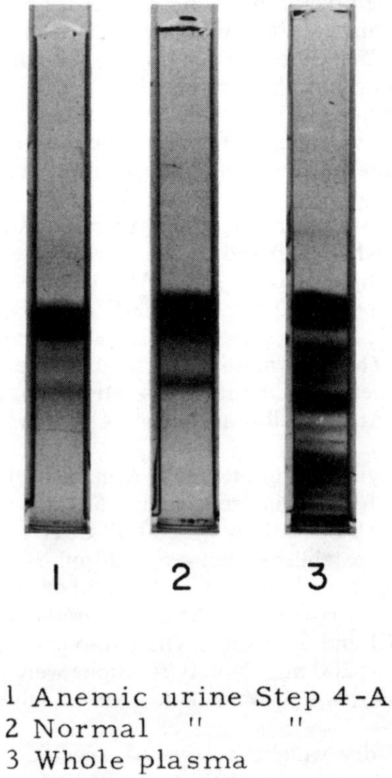

FIGURE 2. Acrylamide gel column disc electrophoresis. 128 μg (180 A units per mg) of anemic, 144 μg (0.14 u/mg) of normal and 0.002 ml of plasma, respectively, were applied to 7% gels in Tris buffer, pH 8.3. "Canalco" disc electrophoresis apparatus, Canal Industrial Corporation, Bethesda, Maryland.

TABLE 3

SPECIFIC ACTIVITIES OF PREPARATIONS FROM A NORMAL AND A POTENT ANEMIC URINE (A u/mg)

Materials	Step 3	Step 4-A
Normal	0.03	0.14
Anemic	88.0	254.0

FIGURE 2 shows acrylamide gel disc electrophoresis patterns of normal and anemic Step 4-A materials, with human plasma as a reference. Similar patterns were obtained with Step 4-A materials from other anemic patients. The bulk component of Step 4-A material appears to be albumin.

Further verification was made by positive precipitin reactions (ring-test)[19] with rabbit anti-human albumin (Hyland Laboratories, prepared with Human Fraction V as the antigen). Immunoelectrophoresis[20] of 80 μg each of normal and anemic Step 4-A materials (specific activities 0.14 and 50 units per mg, respectively) was carried out on agar gel in 0.05 *M* barbital buffer, pH 8.6, for two hr at 70 volts and 10 ma per slide. The precipitin reactions against goat anti-human serum and rabbit anti-human albumin are shown in FIGURE 3. There is a prominent reaction in the albumin zone. Two additional faint lines in the potent preparation and one in the normal preparation are also present.

Determinations of sialic acid[21] and total neutral hexose (orcinol-H_2SO_4 method)[22] for a normal and two anemic Step 4-A preparations are shown in TABLE 4. These values indicate the presence of a considerable amount of material other than albumin.

One of the attempts to further fractionate the albumin-rich Step 4-A material is the following Step 5, which is based on the work of Rejnek *et al.*[23] with human albumin by use of a diethylaminoethyl (DEAE) cellulose column.[24] In a manner similar to theirs we suspended 2.5 g of DEAE cellulose ("Selectacel" reagent, Schleicher & Schuell Co., Keene, New Hampshire) in several changes of buffer A which was 0.04 *M* Tris (hydroxymethyl) aminomethane (Tris) ("Trizma" Base, reagent grade, Sigma Chemical Co., St. Louis, Missouri), adjusted to pH 8.5 with 85% phosphoric acid. After equilibration for 24 hr it was poured into a column (1 × 23 cm).

One hundred and fifty-eight mg of Step 4-A material (36 units/mg) were dissolved in 3.5 ml of buffer A, dialyzed against 500 ml of the same buffer, and applied to the column. All operations were at 5° C. After washing with 30 ml of buffer A, a gradient was established between 120 ml of buffer B which was 0.35 *M* Tris, 0.35 *M* phosphoric acid, pH 4.0, and 120 ml of buffer A. Effluent fractions were collected at a rate of 6.4 ml/hr. After the gradient the column was eluted stepwise with 3 *M* NaCl and 8 *M* LiCl. The elution was monitored by measurement of optical density at 280 mμ. Ninety fractions were collected and combined into 12 pools (FIGURE 4), which were then freed of salts by dialysis and freeze-dried.

TABLE 5 is a list of dry weights recovered, specific activities and sialic acid contents of the pools. One hundred thirty mg (82%) of dry weight were recovered, containing 88% of the erythropoietic activity.

The Step 5 DEAE pools were tested by immunodiffusion against goat anti-human serum and against two rabbit anti-human albumin sera, including one prepared against crystallized human serum albumin, obtained from Mann Research Laboratories, Inc., New York, N. Y.

All the pools, ranging from 12 to 106 units per mg in specific activity, and from 0.6 to 11.7% in sialic acid content, showed identical single precipitin arcs of fusion. The patterns obtained with five of the pools are shown in FIGURE 5. The only detectable antigenicity is that of human albumin. One can assume that the fractions with very little sialic acid contain the purer albumin, while the others are high in glycoprotein. It remains to be seen, however, whether high potency erythropoietin, free of the albumin antigenicity, can be obtained from Step 4-A urinary material. The Step 5 DEAE fractionation has given similar elution pat-

TABLE 4
SIALIC ACID AND HEXOSE DETERMINATIONS OF ONE NORMAL AND TWO ANEMIC STEP 4-A PREPARATIONS

Step 4-A Material	Spec. Activity A u/mg	Sialic Acid Percent	Hexose Percent
Normal	0.14	4.2	5.3
Anemic A	30.0	4.2	6.4
Anemic B	134.0	6.4	6.4

TABLE 5

STEP 5: DEAE COLUMN CHROMATOGRAPHY

	mg	Sialic Acid Percent	Sp. Activity A u/mg	Total Units
Starting Material (4–A)	158	4.2	36.0	5700
Pool 1	0.3		0	
2	3.1		0	
3	3.6	8.1	0	
4	18.5	3.1	13.4	248
5	23.0	0.6	12.1	278
6	19.0	1.4	24.2	460
7	10.4	3.2	51.5	535
8	19.7	4.0	106.8	2100
9	3.1	3.8	29.5	92
10	4.8	7.4	61.4	294
11	18.1	11.7	50.4	914
12	6.5	1.3	10.4	67
Recovered	130.1 (82%)			4988 (88%)

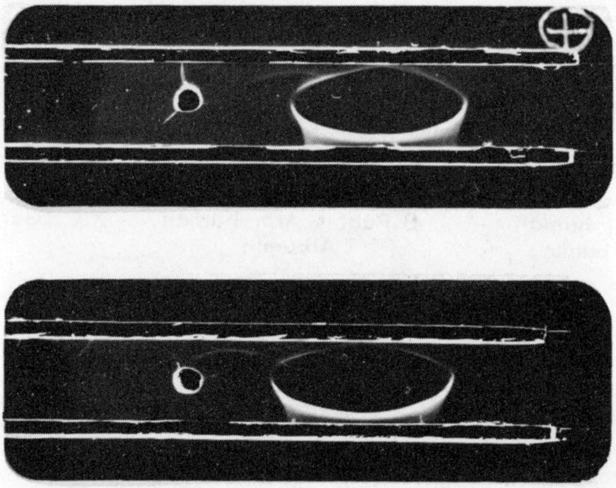

FIGURE 3. Immunoelectrophoresis (microslide method).[20] Eighty μg of sample, 10 ma constant current per slide, 70 volts, two hr.
Top: Normal urine Step 4-A.
Bottom: Anemic urine Step 4-A.
Upper troughs: Anti-human serum.
Lower troughs: Anti-human albumin.

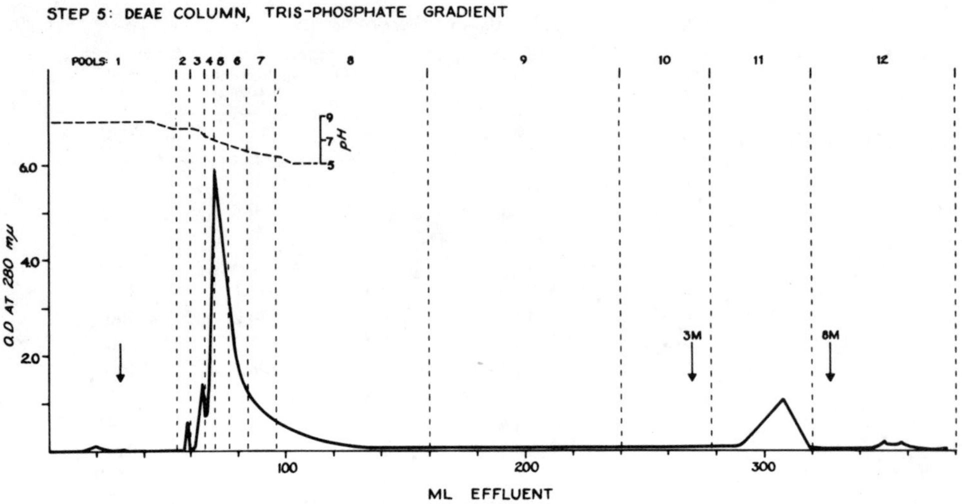

FIGURE 4. DEAE-cellulose column (1 × 23 cm). Applied: 158 mg Step 4-A material derived from 24 l of anemic urine. Arrows (from left) indicate start of gradient, and stepwise elutions with 3 *M* NaCl and 8 *M* LiCl. Ninety fractions were collected and combined in 12 pools, as shown.

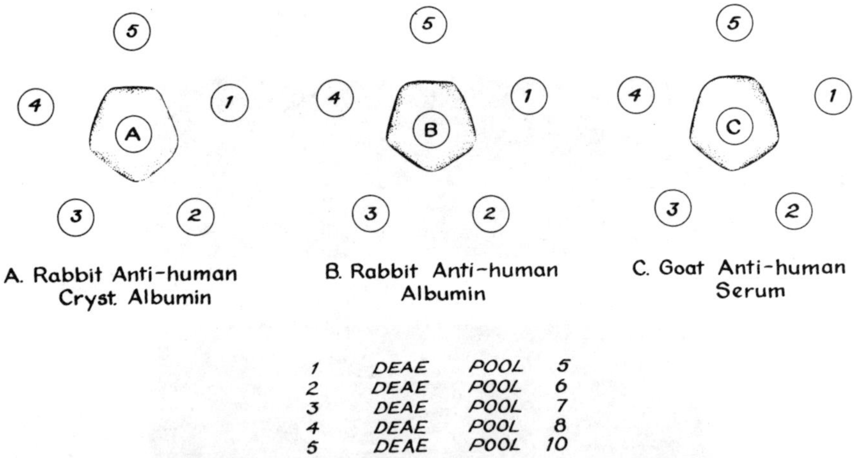

FIGURE 5. Immunodiffusion precipitin patterns of freeze-dried pools from Step 5 DEAE-cellulose chromatography. Antisera were in the center wells, samples of DEAE pools in the numbered outside wells. Specific activities and sialic acid content of the pools are listed in TABLE 5.

terns, albumin antigenicity and sialic acid distribution, when carried out with one normal and two anemic Step 4-A preparations. Here again a physicochemical difference between biologically very potent and very weak material has not yet been shown.

Discussion

Among the problems to be met in preparing erythropoietin concentrates from urine are these:

1. Water and low-molecular substances such as salts and urea must be removed.
2. The inactivation of erythropoietin by enzymes and extreme pH (approximately below 5 and above 9)[3,4] should be minimized.

The effectiveness of ethanol throughout the first three steps may be partly due to denaturation of enzymes which inactivate erythropoietin. The four consecutive steps of our scheme have given consistent improvements at each step with all urines.

One can carry the procedure to any given step and store the dry product. There may be short cuts, omitting or combining some of the steps. So far we have mostly used the given sequence. (The sequence may matter.)

With a substance sensitive to enzymes one must expect some loss during various operations, particularly when aqueous solutions are being handled for prolonged periods. Enzymes may be present in the original urines and in fractions prepared from them, but they can also arise from subsequent bacterial contamination. We had noted losses in DEAE column chromatography of a Step 2-type material, and were able to avoid them by use of phenol.[25] A drop in specific activity has been observed[5] in column chromatography of urinary material which had been isolated by procedures using entirely aqueous media.

A step which fails to produce at least one fraction whose specific activity is increased over the starting material cannot be considered useful. On the other hand any step which raises specific activity may be better than it looks for three reasons:

1) Almost any step will destroy some activity (due to enzymes, etc.).
2) No enhancing effect has yet been observed between two active fractions or an active and inactive fraction.
3) Assay solutions containing very small amounts might be assumed to be less stable (more subject to enzymatic destruction).

In fractionations the activity often becomes distributed over a number of fractions. The fraction with the highest specific activity (and hopefully with the greatest total activity) is assumed to be the best for further purification attempts.

Two of our side fractions, the 0–67 ethanol precipitate of Step 3 and the 0–50 ammonium sulfate precipitate of Step 4-A, contain considerable amounts of erythropoietin but their specific activity is low compared to the main fraction of the same step.

Reextractions of side fractions in attempts to transfer all the activity into a fraction corresponding to the main fraction have not been successful.[6] This failure together with the distribution of active material over different fractions in column chromatography[4–6] could mean:

1. Formation of artifacts.
   a) EP attaching to different macromolecules.
   b) EP-macromolecule complex being partially hydrolyzed, thereby acquiring different physicochemical properties, while remaining biologically active.
2. Natural binding to or association with various macromolecules.

Our present isolation scheme leading to Step 4-A is probably biased towards the isolation of albumin components from urine. But in view of the high specific activities obtained, this seems to be where the most potent EP is found.

We will continue the attempt to separate high-activity erythropoietin from "albumin" or any other inert protein components which we may encounter. One should, however, keep in mind that their presence in potent erythropoietin may be related to the binding and transport of the active moiety in the living organism.

To date it has not been possible to demonstrate a physicochemical difference between preparations which have been carried to the same state in a fractionation scheme, but whose erythropoietic activities range from near-zero to hundreds of A units per mg.

References

1. Hodgson, G. & J. Tohá. 1954. Blood **9**: 299–309.
2. Van Dyke, D. C., J. F. Garcia & J. H. Lawrence. 1957. Proc. Soc. Exp. Biol. Med. **96**: 541–544.
3. Winkert, J. W. & A. S. Gordon. 1960. Biochim. Biophys. Acta **42**: 170–171.
4. Lowy, P. H. & H. Borsook. 1962. *In* Erythropoiesis. L. O. Jacobson and M. Doyle, Eds. : 33–42. Grune and Stratton. New York, N. Y.
5. Lewis, J. P., N. I. Gallagher, S. E. Carmody & R. D. Lange. 1965. Biochim. Biophys. Acta **104**: 218–228.
6. Lowy, P. H. & G. Keighley. 1966. Clin. Chim. Acta **13**: 491–497.
7. Mirand, E. A., A. H. Weintraub, A. S. Gordon, T. C. Prentice & J. T. Grace, Jr. 1965. Proc. Soc. Exp. Biol. Med. **118**: 823–826.
8. Finne, P. H. 1965. Brit. Med. J. **1**: 697–699.
9. Alexanian, R. 1966. Blood **27**: 581 (Author's summary).
10. Van Dyke, D. C. Private communication.
11. Finch, C. A. Private communication.
12. Cotes, P. M. & D. R. Bangham. 1961. Nature **191**: 1065–1067.
13. Schooley, J. C. & J. F. Garcia. 1965. Blood **25**: 204–217.
14. Borsook, H., A. Graybiel, G. Keighley & E. Windsor. 1954. Blood **9**: 734–742.
15. Gordon, A. S. & H. A. Charipper. 1947. Ann. N. Y. Acad. Sci. **48**: 615–641.
16. Mirand, E. A., A. S. Gordon & J. Wenig. 1965. Nature **206**: 270–272.
17. Naets, J. P. & M. Wittek. 1966. Am. J. Physiol. **210**: 315–320.
18. Dorfman, R. I. & A. S. Dorfman. 1963. Acta Endocrinol. **42**(suppl. 74): 3–22.
19. Campbell, D. H., J. S. Garvey, N. E. Cremer & D. H. Sussdorf. 1963. Methods in Immunology. W. A. Benjamin, Inc. New York, N. Y.
20. Scheidegger, J. J. 1955. Intern. Arch. Allergy Appl. Immunol. **7**: 103–110.
21. Warren, L. 1959. J. Biol. Chem. **234**: 1971–1975.
22. Winzler, R. J. 1955. *In* Methods of Biochemical Analysis. D. Glick, Ed. **2**: 290–292. Interscience Publishers, Inc. New York, N. Y.
23. Rejnek, J., T. Bednarík & J. Kocí. 1963. Clin. Chim. Acta **8**: 116–126.
24. Peterson, E. A., M. M. Wyckoff & H. A. Sober. 1961. Arch. Biochem. Biophys. **93**: 428–434.
25. Lowy, P. H. & G. Keighley. 1961. Nature **192**: 75.

PRELIMINARY PURIFICATION OF SHEEP AND MOUSE ERYTHROPOIETIN BY VERTICAL FLAT BED DISCONTINUOUS ELECTROPHORESIS IN ACRYLAMIDE GEL*

Robert C. Allen and Dorothy J. Moore
Biology Division, Oak Ridge National Laboratory, Oak Ridge, Tenn.

and

James W. Fisher
Department of Pharmacology, University of Tennessee Medical Units, Memphis, Tenn.

Introduction

Some investigators have been able to accomplish partial purification of plasma and urinary erythropoietin by combining ion exchange, precipitation, and absorption methods.[1,2] However, the erythropoietin available for experimental studies still contains contaminating proteins. In order to study the direct effects of erythropoietin on erythroid cells, it is of the utmost importance to purify erythropoietin completely. It should be possible to have this substance isotopically labeled for the study of its metabolic distribution and sites of localization and to have it available as a pure protein for immunologic and structural studies. The work described in this report is the result of a two step purification of sheep and mouse plasma erythropoietin with the use of a discontinuous vertical flat bed acrylamide gel electrophoresis technique.[3]

Materials and Methods

The discontinuous gel system was cast in modified Tiselius cells with interior dimensions of 3 mm in depth by 25 mm wide by 75 mm long. From the top or cathodal end of the cell to the bottom of anodal end, the gel was cast in the following manner: a 0.8 ml cap of 5% acrylamide spacer gel, pH 6.9, 2.95 mg protein sample in 0.2 ml of 50% sucrose buffered to pH 6.9 with 0.12 *M* tris-phosphate, 1 ml of 3.3% acrylamide spacer gel similarly buffered and a separating or lower gel consisting of 4.8 ml of 6.5% acrylamide concentration buffered at pH 8.9 with 0.36 *M* tris-chloride. All molarities are in respect to the tris; sufficient anion was added to give the desired pH at 25° C. Cells were cast upside down in the order stated and then inverted and placed in the electrophoresis tanks containing 0.05 *M* tris-glycine buffer, pH 8.9 at 8° C. Separations were carried out at 8 ma per gel, until the bromophenol blue tracking dye had traversed the length of the lower gel. Protein zones were located by one of three techniques: (1) a longitudinal strip of gel was removed from the slab following separation and stained with Amido Schwartz. The bands were then located by Rf measurements to the tracking dye front. (2) One: one schlieren optical pattern polaroid photos were taken following electrophoresis and prior to removing the gel slab from the cell. The slabs were overlayed on the photos and the protein zones excised with a razor blade. (3) Esterase zymograms were used to locate mouse plasma protein zones. A three-minute reaction time with alpha-naphthyl-butyrate and Fast blue RR as the diazonium salt was employed. The individual protein zones located by these procedures were excised from the gel slabs, finely minced, and placed in modified Tiselius cells in 50% sucrose buffered at pH 6.9

* Research sponsored by the United States Atomic Energy Commission under contract with the Union Carbide Corporation and USPHS grant AM–02973–07.

with tris-phosphate buffer. One ml of spacer gel was cast on sucrose-gel mixture and then a dialysis bag containing 3 ml of tris-glycine buffer, pH 8.9, was attached to the anodal end of the cell. The cell was then placed in an electrophoresis tank and the protein eluted electrophoretically into the buffer in the dialysis bag. Quantitative esterase studies were performed as previously described,[4,8] employing a high resolution microspectrophotometer coupled to an electronic integrating system[5] and quantitative protein determinations were carried out after the method of Warburg and Christian.[6]

The various protein fractions obtained from the electrophoretic separation of Step III sheep erythropoietin (Armour and Co.) and from mouse plasma were assayed in mice made polycythemic by a modification of the method of DeGowin *et al.*[7] Male Swiss-Webster mice were placed in a low pressure tank at 0.5 atmosphere for three weeks. Then on the day they were removed from the tank they were injected intraperitoneally with 1 ml of blood obtained from isologous donors with a hematocrit of 70. On the fifth day out of the tank, the mice were injected subcutaneously with various protein fractions. Each mouse was injected intraperitoneally with 0.5 mc of ^{59}Fe citrate two days later and exsanguinated 72 hr after injection of the iron. The hematocrit and ^{59}Fe incorporated in RBC were determined on each blood sample. Mice with hematocrits of less than 55% on the final day of the study were discarded from the assay.

Results

The schlieren pattern, electropherogram, and optical density trace (FIGURE 1) indicated that some 13 protein bands were separated by this procedure in Step III sheep erythropoietin.** Excision of bands into five regions as indicated in FIGURE 1, and their subsequent assay for erythropoietic activity by direct injection of the homogenized gel regions in saline indicated that the erythropoietin activity was found in band E only.

The results of the assay of 10.4 mg of electrophoretically eluted band E are shown in TABLE 1. A 20 percent recovery of the initial activity was effected, giving a specific activity of 2.5 units of erythropoietin per mg of protein. The results of reelectrophoresis of the eluate, shown in FIGURE 2, indicated that it migrated as a single protein band with some slight tailing, while the schlieren pattern (FIGURE 1) suggests two possibly overlapping bands. As may also be seen in FIGURE 2, band E is a glycoprotein, by virtue of a positive Schiff stain, and showed some esterase activity with alpha-naphthyl-butrate as a substrate. This latter finding, however, was not consistent in different lots of the Step III material. Sedimentation velocity studies on the eluted band indicated a single component which had a sedimentation coefficient of 3.4. However, molecular weight studies, based on the meniscus depletion method run at 29,500 rpm for 24 hr at a concentration of 1 mg per ml and an assumed partial specific volume of 0.75, indicated that possibly two proteins were present, one with a molecular weight of 40,000 and the other with a molecular weight on the order of magnitude of 100,000.

The low recovery of activity in the band E eluate and the evidence that it might not be adequately separated with this technique prompted us to turn to another source from which to isolate erythropoietin.

A pool of plasma obtained from C57B1/6 mice made anemic by phenylhydrazine, containing 2.4 units of erythropoietin activity per ml of plasma, was employed for the electrophoretic isolation and purification of erythropoietin. Ery-

** Supplied by the U.S.P.H.S. Hematology Study Section.

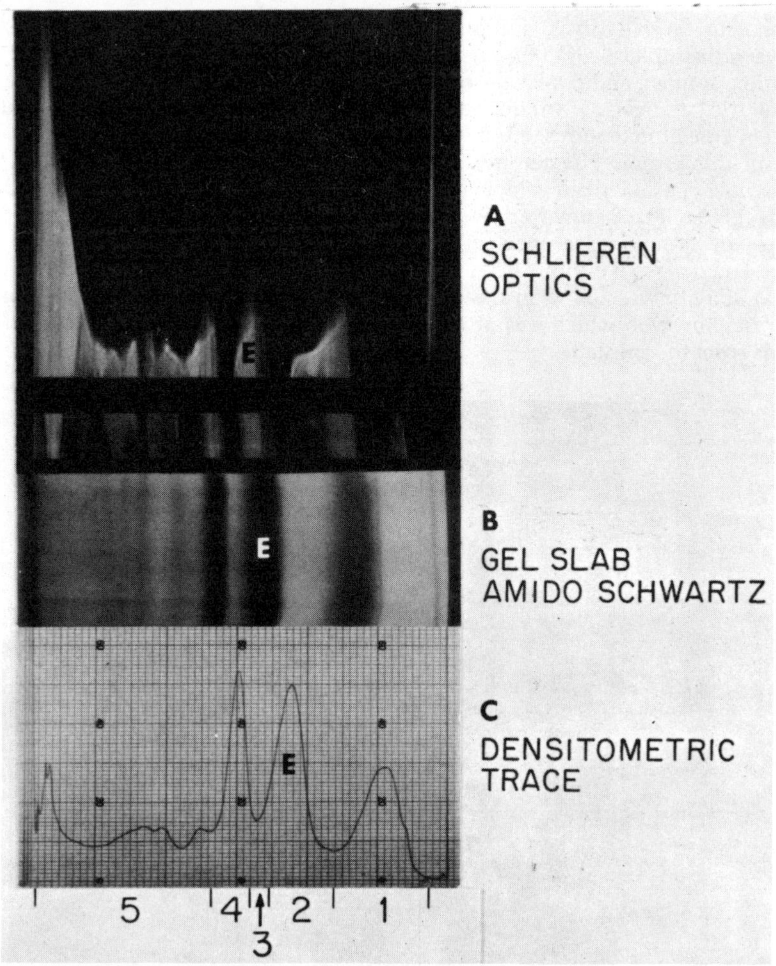

FIGURE 1. (A) Schlieren pattern of electrophoretic separation in the flat-bed system of sheep plasma erythropoietin purified to Step III (Armour Co., Chicago) prior to removal of the gel slab from the cell. (B) Gel slab A above with protein stained with Amido Schwartz. (C) Densitometric trace of gel slab B. Erythropoietin activity was found in band E only.

TABLE 1

ERYTHROPOIETIN ASSAY OF BAND-E ELUATE OF STEP III SHEEP ERYTHROPOIETIN SEPARATED BY ACRYLAMIDE GEL ELECTROPHORESIS

Treatment	No. Mice	Percent ^{59}Fe Incorporation in RBC of Polycythemic Mice	Total Dose of Protein Injected Per Mouse in μg
Saline	7	.44 ± .11	
Standard B (1.0 unit)*	5	7.43 ± 2.0	
Band E Eluate	6	2.84 ± 1.1	160 μg

thropoietin activity was predominantly located in a protein band migrating between the alpha 1 globulin region and the albumin region, and was in the same location as the band 6 plasma esterase isozyme. (FIGURE 3). Quantitative densitometric studies of Amido Schwartz-stained pherograms indicated that this protein constituted about 0.34% of the total plasma protein. Electrophoretic elution of this protein effected a 102% recovery of the amount initially present in the whole plasma from which it was separated. The eluted protein (band E) from this zone contained an average of 0.4 units of erythropoietin activity per 51 μg of protein or a specific activity of 7.9 units per mg (TABLE 2). This represented a recovery of 64.5% of the initial activity. An additional 11% of the initial activity was found in the adjoining protein zone corresponding to band 7 esterase, however, which was probably due to a slicing error in separating the two bands from the gel slab.

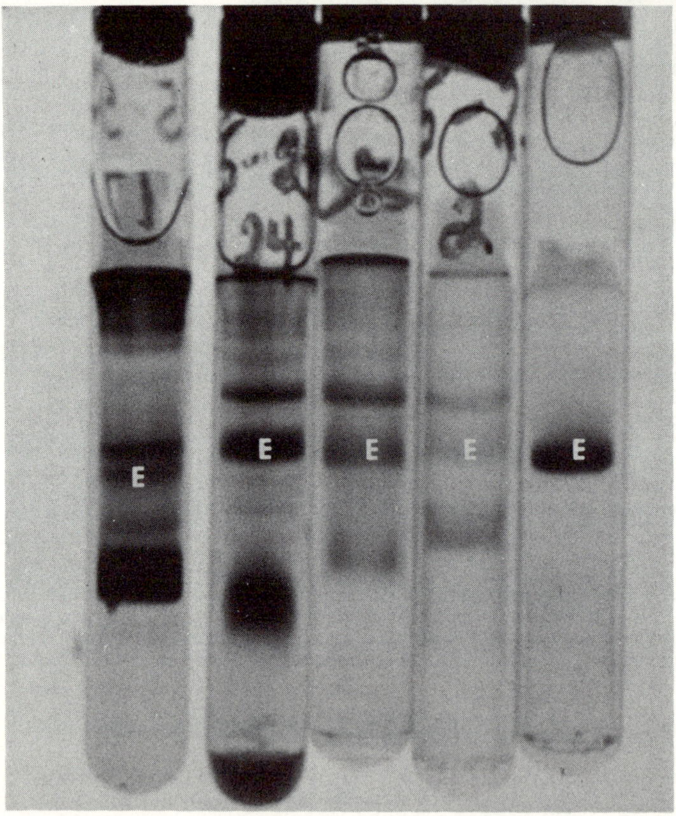

A B C D E

FIGURE 2. Electrophoretic separations of sheep plasma and sheep plasma erythropoietin Step III. (A) Sheep plasma protein stained with Amido Schwartz. (B) Step III erythropoietin stained with Amido Schwartz. (C) Step III erythropoietin stained with Schiff reagent. (D) Step III erythropoietin esterase zymogram α-naphthyl butyrate as substrate. (E) Reelectrophoresis of the eluate from Band E-E stained with Amido Schwartz.

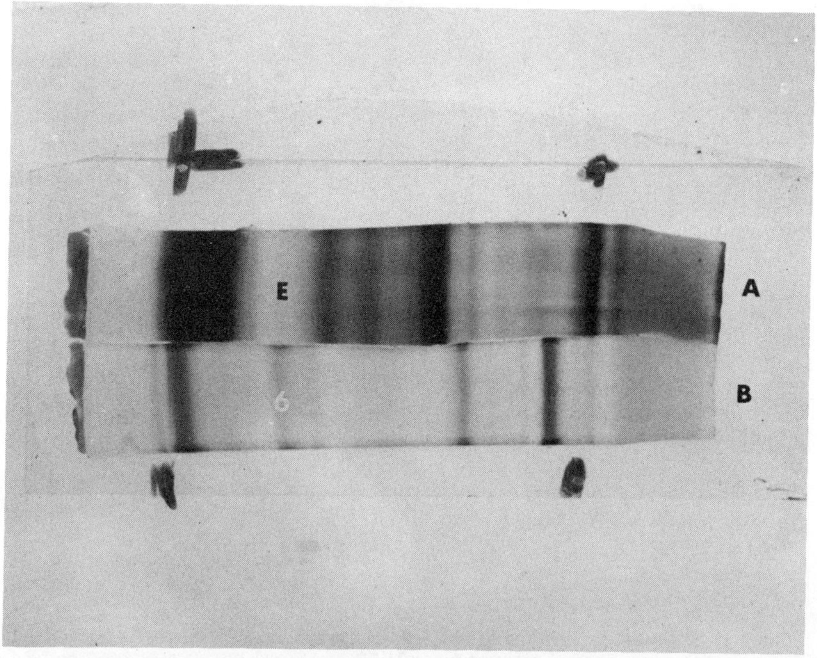

FIGURE 3. Localization of erythropoietin activity in anemic mouse plasma activity was found in protein band marked E. (A) Protein stained with Amido Schwartz. (B) Esterase zymogram with α-naphthyl butyrate as substrate. The gel concentration of lower gel was 6.5.

TABLE 2
ERYTHROPOIETIC ACTIVITY OF ANEMIC MOUSE PLASMA AND PROTEIN FRACTIONS SEPARATED BY ACRYLAMIDE GEL ELECTROPHORESIS

Treatment	No. Mice	Percent ^{59}Fe Incorporation in RBC	Total Dose Protein Injected per Mouse	Specific Activity
Saline	13	.34 ± .10	—	
Standard B (1.0 unit)	10	8.84 ± 1.8	—	
Anemic mouse whole plasma	6	17.87 ± 2.6	56.8 mg	0.36 U/mg
Band E	5	3.41 ± 1.3	51 μg	7.55 U/mg
Band 7 esterase	6	.93 ± .96	0.34 mg	0.21 U/mg

Following 10-fold concentration of the eluted mouse protein band E by vacuum dialysis in the cold, it was again submitted to electrophoretic separation; six protein bands, three of which were esterases, were apparent. (FIGURE 4). Which of these bands have erythropoietic activity has not yet been determined, and nor have their molecular weights been determined.

Since the protein zone containing erythropoietin activity also contained esterase activity, we initiated quantitative studies on the esterase activity of this band prior to and following phenylhydrazine treatment on the assumption that if the esterase was also the erythropoietin, its activity might increase. However, sufficient treatment to reduce the hematocrit to levels of 6–18 produced a marked decrease in the esterase activity (TABLE 3).

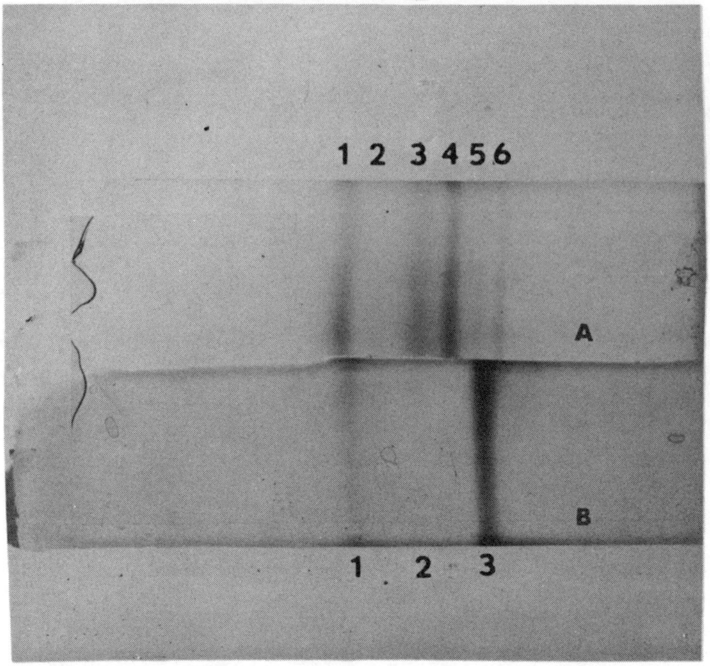

FIGURE 4. Pherogram of 440 μg of concentrated mouse band E eluate. (A) protein stained with Amido Schwartz. Bands 1 through 6 are 21.8%, 5.1%, 22.3%, 35.4%, 8.0% and 7.4% of the total protein concentration, respectively. (B) Esterase zymogram of second half of gel with α-naphthyl butyrate as substrate. The major esterase band corresponds with Band 5 protein. The lower gel concentration was 6.5%.

TABLE 3
ESTERASE CONCENTRATION OF BAND 6 IN MALE AND FEMALE C57B1/6 MICE PRE- AND POSTPHENYLHYDRAZINE TREATMENT*

Mouse	Sex	Band 6 Pretreatment	Band 6 Postphenylhydrazine	Post-treatment Hematocrit
1	Male	2530	2280	7
2	Male	2630	2190	6
3	Male	2440	2290	17
4	Male	2800	2200	14
5	Male	2500	2140	11
6	Male	2930	1940	15
Mean		2678 ± 194	2170 ± 95	
1	Female	1561	826	18
2	Female	1610	774	10
3	Female	1380	545	9
4	Female	1260	890	15
5	Female	1260	1095	16
6	Female	1225	844	10
7	Female	1248	840	11
8	Female	1250	1199	13
Mean		1349 ± 233	877 ± 186	

* One tenth mg of phenylhydrazine per g of mouse weight divided into four equal daily dosages. All values are corrected to 500 μg plasma protein, and the activity is expressed directly as integrated area under the optical density trace.

Discussion

The high resolution of the vertical flat bed discontinuous electrophoretic technique and the subsequent quantitative recovery of protein by electrophoretic elution of the excised protein zones appears to provide a promising tool for the purification of erythropoietin. An added advantage in carrying out the electrophoretic separation in the optically corrected Tiselius cells is that the protein zones may be located precisely from the schlieren pattern reproduced 1:1 on Polaroid film without any loss or destruction of the protein. When separations are carried out in intact cells in an instrument such as the Spinco model H electrophoresis apparatus separation and behavior of the protein zones may be observed visually with the schlieren optical system during electrophoresis. Also, by employing a buffer tank in which the sample spacer and lower gel are totally immersed in cold buffer, the chance of protein denaturation by ohmic heating is greatly diminished. Buffer temperatures as low as 1° C. have been employed without gel distortion or loss of resolution.

Results with the Step III material suggested that band E separated by this procedure was of questionable purity both by molecular weight and schlieren patterns of the electrophoretic separation, although sedimentation studies showed a single peak. Additionally, since the albumin concentration of different lots of Step III material varied between 30 to 50% indicating a lack of uniformity between preparations, we have for the present abandoned further attempts to purify Step III erythropoietin with this technique.

On initial electrophoresis the location of the erythropoietic activity in the band-6 esterase isozyme suggested that these were one in the same protein. The previous finding that the concentration of the band-6 esterase was directly controlled by testosterone[8] tended to support this view, based on reports in the literature by Fried and Gurney[9,10] demonstrating that erythropoietin production was stimulated by testosterone. The demonstration that this esterase is a cholinesterase by virtue of its eserine sensitivity[11] is in accordance with the observation of Davis[12] that acetylcholinesterase injection into rats caused stimulation of erythropoiesis. On the other hand, there was a decrease in the esterase activity of this band following phenylhydrazine-induced anemia in both sexes. Also, concentration and reelectrophoresis of the initial eluate from this band indicated that some six proteins were present, three of which were esterases. These observations would suggest that the band-6 esterase which is an albumin based on two dimensional starch gel electrophoresis[11] may well not be the erythropoietin per se.

Although it appears that the mouse plasma erythropoietin may not be completely purified with one electrophoretic separation step, the isogenic mouse system appears to be an ideal one in which to attempt to determine the structure, function, and origin of the various components isolated from the initially separated band-6 esterase. These proteins are being purified further with this procedure from phenylhydrazine-treated anemic and polycythemic mice, in order to assess the interrelationships of the proteins in both physiologic conditions and to determine which protein, or proteins, have erythropoietic activity.

Summary

Further purification of Step III sheep erythropoietin was accomplished by separation with a discontinuous vertical flat-bed electrophoresis technique in acrylamide gel followed by electrophoretic elution of the protein zones. A 20% recovery of the initial activity was effected with a specific activity of 2.5 units per mg of the isolated protein zone. Two proteins were evident in this band, which did not separate electrophoretically. An apparent protein complex was isolated from anemic mouse plasma which had both erythropoietin and esterase activity. While 64.5% of the initial anemic plasma activity was recovered in the electrophoretic eluate of this protein band, reelectrophoresis of the concentrated eluate showed that six protein bands were present in the initial isolate, of which three were esterases.

Acknowledgment

The authors wish to express their gratitude to Dr. A. P. Pfuderer for the sedimentation coefficient and molecular weight determinations and for his valuable assistance in interpreting these data.

References

1. Lowy, P. H. & H. Borsook. 1962. Preparation and properties of erythropoietin concentrates from rabbit plasma and human urine. Erythropoiesis. : 33. Grune & Stratton.
2. Goldwasser, E. W., F. White & K. B. Taylor. 1962. On the purification of sheep plasma erythropoietin. Erythropoiesis. : 43. Grune and Stratton.
3. Allen, R. C. & D. J. Moore. 1966. A vertical flat-bed discontinuous electrophoresis system in acrylamide gel. Anal. Biochem. In press.
4. Allen, R. C., R. A. Popp & D. J. Moore. 1965. Separation and relative quantitation of mouse plasma esterases with disc electrophoresis. J. Histochem. Cytochem. **13:** 249–254.
5. Allen, R. C. & G. R. Jamieson. 1966. An automated microdensitometer for the quantitation of pherograms and zymograms in acrylamide gels. Anal. Biochem. In press.
6. Warburg, O. & W. Christian. 1941. Isolieruns und Krystallisation des Garungsferment Enolase. Biochem. Z. **310:** 384–421.
7. DeGowin, R. L., D. Hofstra & C. W. Gurney. 1962. The mouse with hypoxia-induced erythremia, an erythropoietin bioassay animal. J. Lab. Clin. Med. **60:** 846–852.
8. Allen, R. C. & D. J. Moore. 1966. Sex-associated quantitative differences in the plasma esterases of inbred mice. Endocrinology **78:** 655–658.
9. Fried, W. & C. W. Gurney. 1965. Erythropoietic effect of plasma from mice receiving testosterone. Nature **206:** 1160–1161.
10. Fried, W. & C. W. Gurney. 1965. Use of mild plethora to demonstrate an erythropoietic effect from small amounts of androgens. Proc. Soc. Exp. Biol. Med. **120:** 519–521.
11. Allen, R. C. & R. L. Hunter. Unpublished data.
12. Davis, J. E. 1960. Erythropoietic stimulating action of acetylchoninesterase. Proc. Soc. Exp. Biol. Med. **104:** 698–699.

THE COMMERCIAL PRODUCTION OF ERYTHROPOIETIN FROM ANEMIC SHEEP PLASMA*

R. H. Painter, W. R. Bruce and E. Goldwasser

Connaught Medical Research Laboratories and
Department of Medical Biophysics, University of Toronto, Toronto, Canada and
Argonne Cancer Research Hospital, University of Chicago, Chicago, Ill.

White *et al.*[1] developed a process for preparing erythropoietin concentrate from the plasma of sheep which were made anemic with phenylhydrazine. They obtained an average yield of approximately 2,000 units of concentrate per sheep. We have been able to increase this yield to over 10,000 units per sheep by instituting a number of modifications in the procedures for preparing and treating animals and for processing the concentrate. The improvements make it possible to reduce the cost of preparing the concentrate and allow the preparation of quantities in the order of millions of units.

Since it had been shown by White *et al.*[1] that the erythropoietin concentration in blood rises steeply when the hematocrit falls below 15%, it seemed important to us to achieve conditions for reproducibly lowering the hematocrit below this level. To achieve this, we introduced a number of modifications in their method. Animals were rendered anemic by phenylhydrazine (PH) which was injected subcutaneously on alternate days as before. However, the hematocrit of each animal was determined at least every other day and the dose of PH, initially in the range of 16 mg/kg bodyweight, was adjusted as the anemia progressed so as to lower the hematocrit steadily to the desired level. In this way each animal was, in effect, "titrated" to a severe state of anemia. Once the hematocrit fell below 10%, the animal was exsanguinated. Our early results with normal sheep treated in this manner were erratic. Many of the animals died abruptly before becoming anemic, as was observed previously by White *et al.*[1] Since the deaths were frequently associated with gastric and intestinal parasite infections, we turned to animals from a specific pathogen-free (SPF) flock which was free of parasites. With these animals we had no unexpected deaths and all animals had profound anemia when bled out. A further modification in our preparation of anemic sheep was prompted by recent experiments on the production of erythropoietin by rats. Hogson[2] has found that total body radiation, which inhibited the erythropoietic response, facilitated the preparation of highly anemic animals and thus increased the yield of plasma erythropoietin. For our experiments, therefore, sheep were irradiated with 800 rads ^{60}Co γ-rays (midline air dose given bilaterally at a dose rate of 15 rads/min. A further increase in the yield of plasma was achieved by infusing Ringer's-Lactate solution during the bleed-out so as to flush the residual blood from the animal. Each animal was bled out from the carotid artery under local anesthesia and it was a simple matter at this time to infuse 1–2 of Ringer's-Lactate solution into the jugular vein before the animal expired.

The result of the modified procedure was a significant increase in yield of erythropoietin per sheep. The values of hematocrits for two typical SPF sheep treated as described above are shown in FIGURE 1. These animals were bled out at seven and nine days when their hematocrits had reached 8%. Each animal yielded about 10,000 units. TABLE 1 gives the yield of erythropoietin in the plasma of

* This work was partially financed by a grant of the Medical Research Council of Canada (MA–1361).

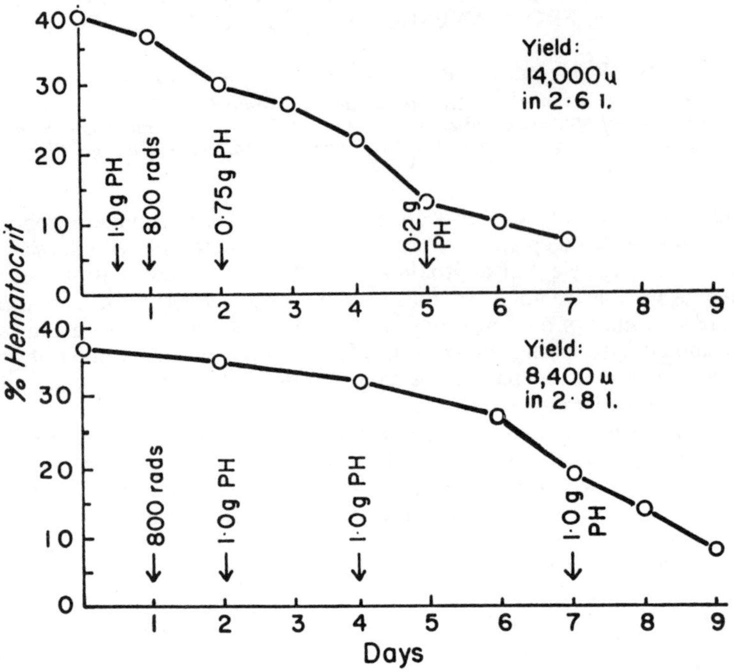

FIGURE 1. Typical hematocrits for two specific pathogen-free sheep treated with radiation and phenylhydrazine (PH) on the days indicated. Animals were bled out and Ringer's-Lactate infused when their hematocrits fell below 10%.

groups of animals prior to and after instituting the perfusion at bleed-out. The data suggest that this procedure increases the yield though the variation among the data make it difficult to assess the magnitude of the increase.

The procedure followed in processing blood to Step I is illustrated by the following method.

Method for Concentration of Erythropoietin from Anemic Sheep Blood

a. Centrifuge to remove cells.
b. Dialyze against distilled water, until specific resistance is greater than 4,000 ohms/cm.
c. Titrate to pH 4.5, with 2 N HCl.
d. Adsorb on a mixture of DEAE cellulose and cellulose phosphate, at pH 4.5.
e. Wash unadsorbed plasma from column with water.
f. Elute activity with 0.4 *M* Na_2HPO_4, 0.5 *M* NaCl.
g. Dialyze eluate to remove salts.
h. Freeze dry Step I material.

Sodium citrate and heparin were used as anticoagulants. The latter prevented clotting during the dialysis step. The activity was adsorbed from the dialyzed and titrated plasma by passing it through a column containing a mixture of equal

TABLE 1

YIELD OF ERYTHROPOIETIN FROM GROUPS OF PHENYLHYDRAZINE TREATED + IRRADIATED SPF SHEEP (AVERAGE WT. 75 KG) SHOWING EFFECT OF INFUSING RINGER'S-LACTATE SOLUTION DURING BLEED-OUT.*

Hematocrit		Yields per Sheep		
Initial Percent	Final Percent	Plasma Volume liters	Plasma Potency u/ml	Total Units
Not Infused**				
35	7.5	1.42	5.6	7,933
(32–39)	(6–9)	(0.86–2.38)	(1.1–24)	(1,100–29,640)
Infused†				
35	7.4	2.76	4.3	11,900
(30–40)	(6–9)	(1.62–4.20)	(1.6–14.6)	(3,600–28,900)

* Ranges of experimental values are shown in parenthesis.

** Average of seven consecutive animals.

† Average of ten consecutive animals.

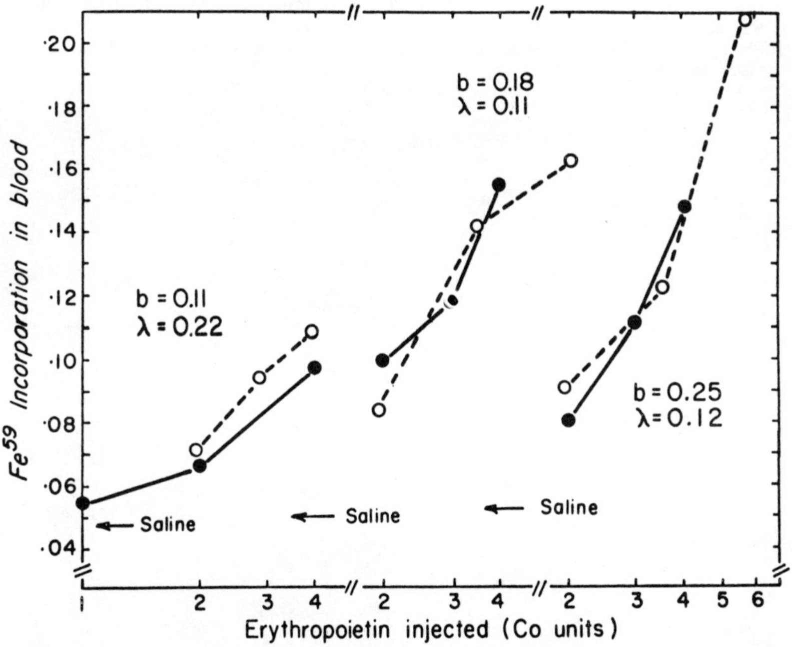

FIGURE 2. The incorporation of radioiron in the blood of starved rats following the injection of erythropoietin standard B (solid symbols) and the Step I material described here, (open symbols). Five rats were used in the determination of each point in the first assay, 10 in each of the other two assays. The procedure used in the assays was that of Freid *et al.*[3], as described in White *et al.*[1]

The slope "b" is the increase in incorporation per tenfold increase in dose. "λ" is the ratio of standard deviation over slope (s/b) used to compare the accuracy per animal of the relative potency by different assays.[4]

parts of DEAE and cellulose phosphate suspended in distilled water and titrated to pH 4.5. The combined resins were used since adsorption on either one allowed a recovery of only 50% of the starting activity. When the resins were combined, the yield was consistently in the region of 85–100%.

The lyophilized Step I product was a brown fluffy powder containing about 75% by weight of protein. It had a specific activity when assayed by the starved rat method against the International Reference Preparation (standard B) of 0.5 units/mg protein (see FIGURE 2). Solubility of the product was in excess of 30 units/ml in water. Some 250,000 units of this material are now on hand and plans are underway for preparing material of higher potency.

Acknowledgments

We thank Dr. P. Mary Cotes, National Institutes for Medical Research, Mill Hill, London, for supplying us with the preparation of standard erythropoietin potency.

References

1. WHITE, W. F., C. W. GURNEY, E. GOLDWASSER & L. O. JACOBSON. 1960. Studies on Erythropoietin. *In* Recent Progress in Hormone Research. **16:** 219.
2. HODGSON, G. Personal communication.
3. FRIED, W., L. F. PLZAK, L. O. JACOBSON & E. GOLDWASSER. 1957. Studies on erythropoiesis. III. Factors controlling erythropoietin production. Proc. Soc. Exper. Biol. Med. **94:** 237.
4. FINNEY, D. J. 1952. *In* Statistical Methods in Biological Assay. : 184. Charles Griffin & Co. London.

PART III. SITES OF ERYTHROPOIETIN PRODUCTION AND APPEARANCE IN TISSUE FLUIDS AND EXTRACTS

EFFECTS OF TESTOSTERONE, COBALT AND HYPOXIA ON ERYTHROPOIETIN PRODUCTION IN THE ISOLATED PERFUSED DOG KIDNEY*

James W. Fisher** and J. W. Langston

University of Tennessee Medical Units, Memphis, Tenn.

Introduction

Hypoxia[1-4] and cobalt[5] have been demonstrated to stimulate the release or production of erythropoietin in the isolated perfused kidney. Elevated plasma levels of erythropoietin have also been reported following renal artery constriction.[6,7] Erythropoietin titers in renal venous blood were also found to be higher than renal arterial blood in dogs following acute hypoxia.[8] On the other hand, other workers were unable to stimulate erythropoietin production in isolated kidneys perfused with blood at moderately reduced oxygen tension.[9]

Testosterone has been shown to stimulate erythropoiesis in polycythemic mice.[10,11] The erythropoietic effects of testosterone were also found to be more marked in the midly plethoric mouse than in polycythemic mice.[12]

The present studies were initiated to reassess the role of oxygen levels in blood on erythropoietin production and to study further the effects of cobalt on erythropoietin formation in isolated perfused kidneys. In order to clarify the mechanism by which testosterone stimulates erythropoiesis, the effects of this hormone on erythropoietin production in the isolated perfused kidney was also studied.

Materials and Methods

Male and female mongrel dogs weighing 15–25 kg were used in the perfusion systems in these studies. However, only female dogs were used in the testosterone studies because female dogs have been shown to be more responsive to the erythropoietic effect of testosterone.[11] All surgical procedures were carried out under pentobarbital (30 mg/kg) anesthesia. Renal blood flow was measured at hourly intervals by allowing the blood from the cannula in the renal vein to drain directly into a graduated cylinder for one minute. Oxygen saturation values were determined hourly on renal arterial and venous blood with the use of a Water's Model X-350 Cuvette Oximeter. Blood pO_2, pCO_2 and pH were measured with an Instrumentation Laboratory meter with a Clark-Severinghaus electrode. The oximeter and the C-S electrode were calibrated initially and checked at periodic intervals by Van Slyke analyses. Microhematocrits were determined using heparinized capillary tubes. The arterial pressure was measured every 30 min with the use of a Grass polygraph and Statham pressure transducer. A Davol heart-lung perfusion pump with single-ended ventricles and two 20-ml actuators was used to circulate the blood through the perfusion systems.

The plasma samples were assayed in polycythemic mice via a modification of the method of DeGowin *et al.*[13] Male Swiss-Webster strain mice were injected s.c. with 1 mg of iron dextran prior to being placed at 0.5 atmosphere for three

* This work was supported by USPHS grant AM–02973.

** USPHS Career Award Program grant GM–5990.

weeks. On the day the mice were removed from the low pressure tank, each mouse was injected intraperitoneally with 1 ml donor mouse blood at hematocrit 70. On the fifth day out of the tank each mouse was injected with 1 ml of plasma three times at 5-hour intervals. Each mouse was injected with 0.5 μc of ^{59}Fe citrate on the seventh posthypoxia day and ^{59}Fe incorporation in RBC was determined three days later. Blood volume of polycythemic mice was estimated to be 8% of body weight and mice with hematocrits of less than 55% on the day of the kill were discarded from the assay. Six to eight mice were used for each dog plasma sample assayed. The plasma samples were dialyzed for 36–48 hr against 0.85% saline and adjusted to pH 7.2 before being injected s.c. in the mice. The plasma samples containing cobalt were dialyzed at 4° C against Dowex-50 resin for 24 hr to remove the cobalt prior to erythropoietin assay. Each plasma sample was analyzed for cobalt by a modification of the technique of Almond[14] and none was found to contain more than 0.1 μm cobalt per ml which is insufficient to stimulate ^{59}Fe incorporation in polycythemic mice. An occasional plasma sample showed more than the usual amount of hemolysis. These samples were passed through a DEAE cellulose column at pH 4.5 and eluted with a phosphate buffer at pH 9.5 according to Step I of the technique of White *et al.*[15] Urine produced by the kidneys was collected throughout the perfusion by allowing the ureteral cannula to drip into a graduated cylinder.

A schematic diagram of perfusion systems nos. 1 and 2 are shown in FIGURE 1.

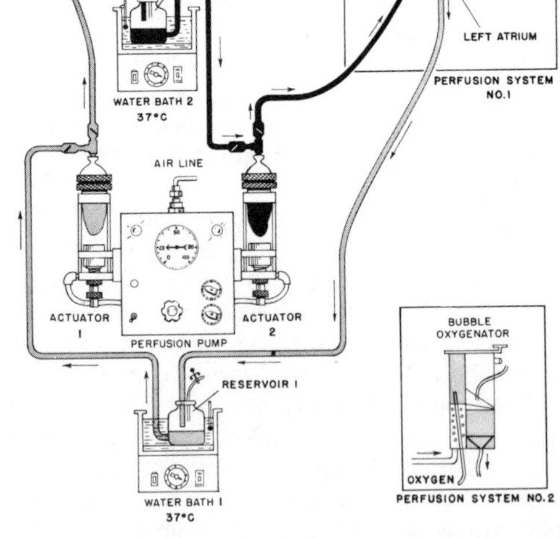

FIGURE 1. Diagram of isolated kidney perfusion systems where the dogs' own lungs were used to oxygenate the blood perfusate (perfusion system no. 1) or when a bubble oxygenator was used in the system (perfusion system no. 2). [A] indicates point where blood pressure was measured and [B] is the point in the system where renal blood flow was measured.

The only essential difference between the two systems is that in perfusion system no. 1 the dogs' own lungs were used to oxygenate the blood, whereas in perfusion system no. 2 an Abbott Pulmo Pak bubble oxygenator with a Saran antifoam column was used to oxygenate the blood. In perfusion system no. 1 where the dog lungs were used the trachea was cannulated and the lungs ventilated 14 times per minute with a tidal volume of 300–400 ml with the use of a Harvard respirator. Normal air was used to ventilate the lungs when the blood was being maintained at a normal oxygen tension while 95% N_2–5% O_2 was used when the blood perfusate was maintained at a low oxygen tension. Approximately 1000 ml of blood was removed via the carotid artery from an anesthetized dog which had been previously heparinized with 3 mg sodium heparin per kg. Five hundred mg streptomycin sulfate, 300,000 units procaine penicillin and 100,000 units sodium penicillin were added to the blood to inhibit bacterial growth during perfusion. Four hundred mg of glucose in saline were added to the perfusion system every hour. The chest was opened through an incision in the third intercostal space. The venous blood was returned to the perfusion system through a cannula tied with a purse string suture in the wall of the left atrium. A glass arterial cannula was placed in the pulmonary artery. The ascending aorta was then clamped with a heavy right angle hemostat. The blood was allowed to circulate through the lungs for 15–20 min before the kidney was connected to the system to remove pressor substances in the perfusate which would interfere with renal blood flow. The left kidney was then removed through a midline abdominal incision and plastic cannulae were placed in the renal artery, renal vein and ureter. The kidney was flushed out with approximately 30 ml warm heparinized blood and then connected to the perfusion system. All kidneys were immersed in Tyrode's solution which was maintained at 37° C in a water bath throughout the perfusion. Plasma samples were removed from the perfusion system initially and after three and four hr of perfusion.

The procedures used in perfusion system no. 2 were the same as those described for system no. 1 except that a bubble oxygenator was used instead of the dogs' lungs and a gas mixture containing 95% O_2–5% CO_2 was bubbled through the blood throughout the perfusion. When the kidney was perfused with hypoxic blood in system no. 2, the bubble oxygenator was excluded from the system. The perfusions were carried out for five hr in system no. 2. However, the perfusion time was only four hr in system no. 1 because after this time the dog lungs failed to adequately oxygenate the blood.

When the effects of testosterone were studied in the isolated perfused kidney where the bubble oxygenator was used to oxygenate the blood (perfusion system no 2), testosterone succinate (.2 mg/ml or 100 mg/500 ml blood) was added directly through the renal arterial perfusion cannula. The initial plasma sample for erythropoietin assay was removed after the testosterone had mixed in the perfusion system for approximately 10 minutes. The effects of testosterone were also studied in perfusion system no. 1, where the dogs' own lungs were used to oxygenate the blood, by pretreating the dogs for seven days with daily i.m. dosages of 25 mg/kg testosterone propionate in cottonseed oil. The kidneys were removed from the dog, flushed with donor dog blood and perfused for four hr with blood at a normal oxygen tension. A plasma sample was removed from the dog after treatment for seven days with testosterone for erythropoietin assay. Following perfusion the dog kidneys were sectioned, stained with hematoxylin and eosin, and examined microscopically. The procedure of analysis of variance was used for the statistical analyses.[16]

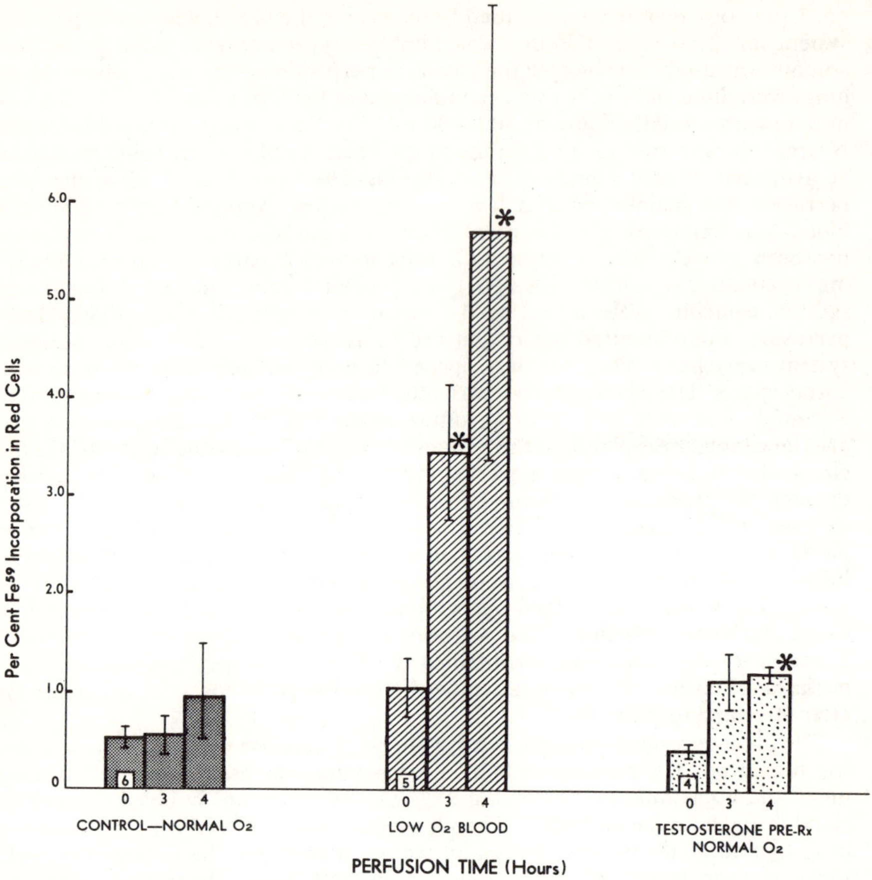

FIGURE 2. Mean ^{59}Fe incorporation in red cell values in polycythemic mice (5–7 mice in each experiment) injected with dog plasma from perfusion system no. 1. Number enclosed at the bottom of each bar indicates number of perfusion experiments in each group and vertical lines at top is the standard error of the mean. * Indicates significantly different at 1% level from 0 time value before perfusion. Mean ^{59}Fe incorporation in polycythemic mice receiving saline as controls (45) was 0.65 ± .07% and 1.0 units Standard B (36) 9.31 ± .91.

Results

TABLE 1 shows the results of 15 separate kidney perfusion studies using a lung-kidney preparation (perfusion system no. 1). High renal blood flows were maintained throughout the 4-hour perfusion. However, there was a progressive decline in renal blood flow during the fourth hour and a gradual increase in pressure, probably due to mild intrarenal vasoconstriction. As seen in FIGURE 2, a slight but not significant rise in erythropoietin titers in the perfusate of kidneys perfused with normal oxygen saturation blood was seen after four hr perfusion. On the other hand, all of the perfusates from kidneys perfused with hypoxic blood showed a significant increase in erythropoietin titers after three and four hr when compared with the O time control values. Erythropoietin titers in the plasma from perfused kidneys which were removed from dogs following seven

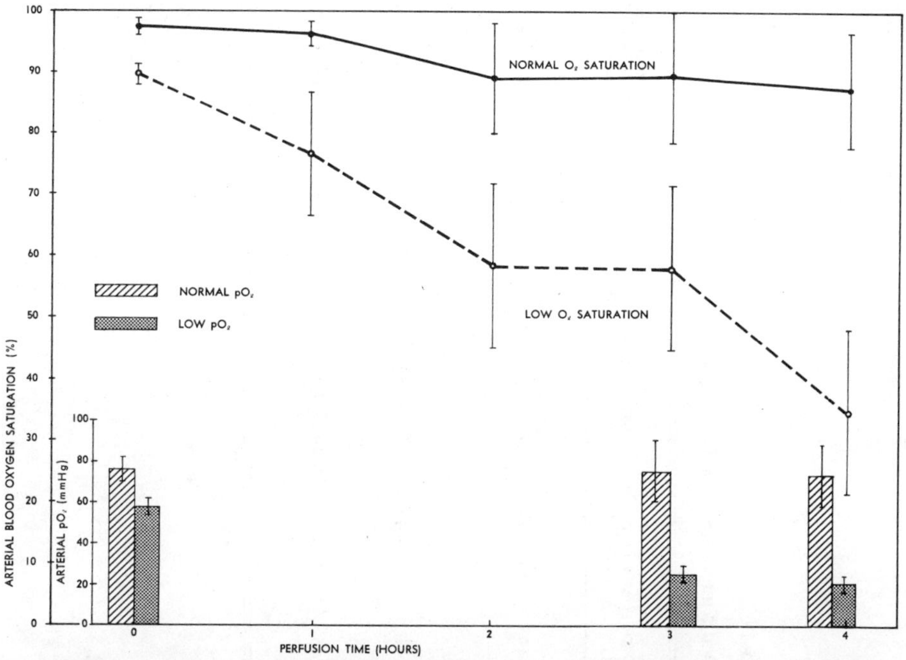

FIGURE 3. Mean hourly arterial blood oxygen saturation and mean oxygen tension values in perfusates from kidneys perfused with blood at normal and low oxygen levels (perfusion system no. 1). Each point in the normal group is the mean of six perfusion experiments while each point in the low saturation and pO_2 groups is the mean value for five experiments. The lines over each pO_2 bar or at each point on the saturation curves represents the standard error of mean.

days treatment with testosterone were significantly elevated after four hr perfusion when compared with the mean O time control value. As seen in TABLE 2, kidneys removed from the testosterone-treated dogs before perfusion were significantly larger and plasma levels of erythropoietin were significantly higher than those of normal controls.

The histological appearance of all perfused kidneys showed varying degrees of glomerular congestion with albuminous fluid and red cells in Bowman's space and the tubular lumen. The glomerular congestion may have been due to some permeability change in the capillary tuft due to ischemia and the gradual increase in pressure during the perfusion. Slight cloudy swelling was occasionally seen in tubular epithelium. However, there was approximately the same degree of kidney congestion in all kidney perfusion experiments with oxygenated, hypoxic or blood perfusates containing cobalt or testosterone. It was not possible to correlate the degree of congestion with the amount of erythropoietin produced.

FIGURE 3 shows the more marked decline in oxygen saturation and pO_2 values in the blood perfusates of the lung-kidney perfusion system where the lungs were ventilated with mixtures of 95% nitrogen–5% oxygen, 95% oxygen–5% CO_2, or normal air to maintain the desired pO_2 and oxygen saturation levels in the blood. The oxygen saturation curve of the blood where testosterone was added

TABLE 1

DATA ON ISOLATED PERFUSED DOG KIDNEYS (SYSTEM NO. 1)

	No. Experiments	Renal Blood Flow (ml/min)	Perfusion Pressure (mm Hg)	Hematocrit (%)	Arterial pCO_2 (mm Hg)	pH	Arterial pO_2 (mm Hg)	Arterial O_2 Saturation (%)	Mean Hourly A-V Difference, O_2 Sat. (%)
Normal O_2 Sat.	6	71 → 47	113 → 172	40 → 45	20 → 38	7.68 → 7.29	75 → 71	96 → 86	16 ± .91
Normal O_2 Sat. + Testosterone Pretreatment	4	68 → 37	136 → 169	39 → 42	20 → 48	7.58 → 7.30	65 → 109	92 → 80	15.9 ± 3.6
Low O_2 Sat.	5	69 → 44	115 → 167	39 → 45	23 → 27	7.49 → 7.27	58 → 17	89 → 30	15 ± 5.1

± = Standard error of mean.
→ = Arrow indicates mean value at start and finish of perfusion.

TABLE 2

EFFECTS OF TESTOSTERONE TREATMENT ON KIDNEY WEIGHT AND PLASMA LEVELS OF ERYTHROPOIETIN IN DOGS USED IN PERFUSION SYSTEM NO. 1

Treatment	No. Dogs	Mean Body Weight (kg)	Kidney Wt. (g/kg)	Per Cent ^{59}Fe Incorporation in RBC of Polycythemic Mice
Control	9	15.5 ± .58	3.08 ± .16	.66 ± .09
Testosterone†	5	11.0 ± .83	4.52 ± .40*	1.39 ± .29*

± = Standard error of mean.
* Indicates significantly different from control at 1% level.
† Each dog injected daily for seven days with 25 mg/kg testosterone propionate in cottonseed oil s.c.

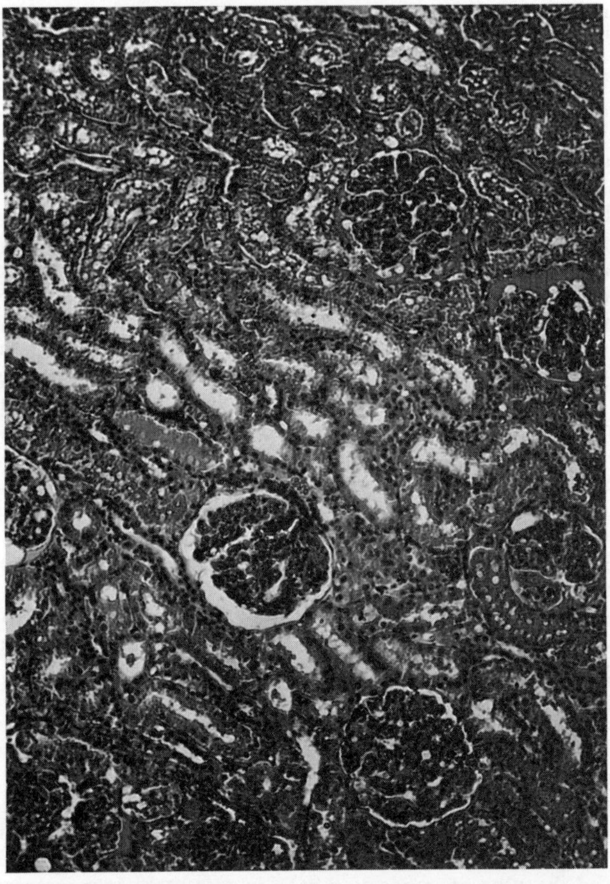

FIGURE 4. Photomicrograph (60×) of dog kidney after five hr perfusion (system no. 2) with blood at normal oxygen saturation. Note fluid in Bowman's space and tubular lumen. This type of glomerular congestion was seen to some extent in all perfused kidneys.

TABLE 3

EFFECTS OF HYPOXEMIA, COBALT AND TESTOSTERONE ON ERYTHROPOIETIN PRODUCTION IN THE ISOLATED PERFUSED DOG KIDNEY USING AN ARTIFICIAL LUNG TO OXYGENATE THE BLOOD PERFUSATE (PERFUSION SYSTEM NO. 2)

Compound Added to Perfusate	No. Experiments	Per Cent ^{59}Fe Incorporation in RBC of Polycythemic Mice		
		0 Hr	3 Hr	5 Hr
		Normal O_2 Saturation		
None	7	1.8 ± .11	1.53 ± .14	1.11 ± .09
Cobalt	5	.64 ± .22	1.0 ± .30	2.92 ± .71*
Testosterone	6	.53 ± .12	——	1.32 ± .92
		Low O_2 Saturation		
None	5	.65 ± .06	1.41 ± .06*	3.84 ± 1.1*
Cobalt	6	1.4 ± .19	5.9 ± 1.0*	4.5 ± .94*

± = Standard error of mean.

* Indicates significantly different at 1% level from 0 time value before perfusion. Mean ^{59}Fe incorporation in RBC of polycythemic mice receiving saline as controls (59) was .89 ± .18% and 1.0 unit Standard B (59) was 13.95 ± 1.0%.

was not significantly different from that of the normal oxygen saturation curve seen in FIGURE 3.

TABLE 3 shows the erythropoietin values in the perfusates of 29 kidneys perfused with blood oxygenated with a bubble oxygenator (system no. 2), with and without cobalt and oxygenated blood containing testosterone. Erythropoietin values are also shown for kidneys perfused in this system with unoxygenated blood alone and unoxygenated blood containing cobalt. Significant increases were seen in erythropoietin values in perfusates after five hr of perfusion with oxygenated blood containing cobalt. When testosterone was added directly to the perfusate at normal oxygen levels a slight but not significant increase in erythropoietin titers was seen. In addition, unoxygenated blood with and without cobalt showed significant increases in erythropoietin titers after three and five hours. The most marked increase in ^{59}Fe incorporation was seen after three hr with plasma from the perfusion system where a combination of hypoxemia and cobalt were used. The perfusates from kidneys perfused with oxygenated blood alone did not demonstrate a rise in erythropoietin levels. As shown in TABLE 4, renal blood flow rates were less than those seen in perfusion system no. 1 where the dogs' own lungs were used to oxygenate the blood.

The results of the histological studies of the kidneys were similar to those from perfusion system no. 1 in that we were unable to correlate a degenerative change in the kidney with erythropoietin production. In fact the histology of three of the kidneys perfused with blood at low oxygen tensions were nearly normal, yet marked elevations of erythropoietin titers in their perfusate were seen. On the other hand, two of the kidneys having 4+ glomerular congestion and two showing 1^+–4^+ congestion, which were perfused for five hr with blood at a normal oxygen saturation, failed to show a rise in erythropoietin titers in their perfusates. FIGURES 4 and 5 are photographs of histological sections from kidneys perfused with blood at normal or low oxygen tension. From 0–40% of the glomeruli in the perfused kidneys showed the type of congestion seen in FIGURE 4. It is interesting to note in a photomicrograph of glomeruli (FIGURE 5) from a kidney perfused for five hr with hypoxic blood that congestion is minimal. Although the renal blood flows

TABLE 4

DATA ON ISOLATED PERFUSED DOG KIDNEYS (SYSTEM NO. 2)

Compound Added to Perfusate	No. Experiments	Renal Blood Flow (ml/min)	Perfusion Pressure (mm Hg)	Arterial O_2 Saturation (%)	Hematocrit (%)	Mean Hourly A-V Difference O_2 Sat. (%)
Normal O_2 Saturation						
None	7	32 → 19	82 → 166	99 → 91	41 → 41	24 ± 3.6
Cobalt	5	29 → 16	74 → 135	98 → 97	41 → 37	26 ± 3.2
Testosterone	6	31 → 14	78 → 173	93 → 84	33 → 35	16 ± 6.6
Low O_2 Saturation						
None	5	23 → 14	98 → 153	89 → 8	36 → 41	—
Cobalt	6	36 → 10	86 → 133	99 → 44	38 → 41	13 ± 2.3

± = Standard error of mean.

→ = Arrow indicates mean value at start and finish of perfusion.

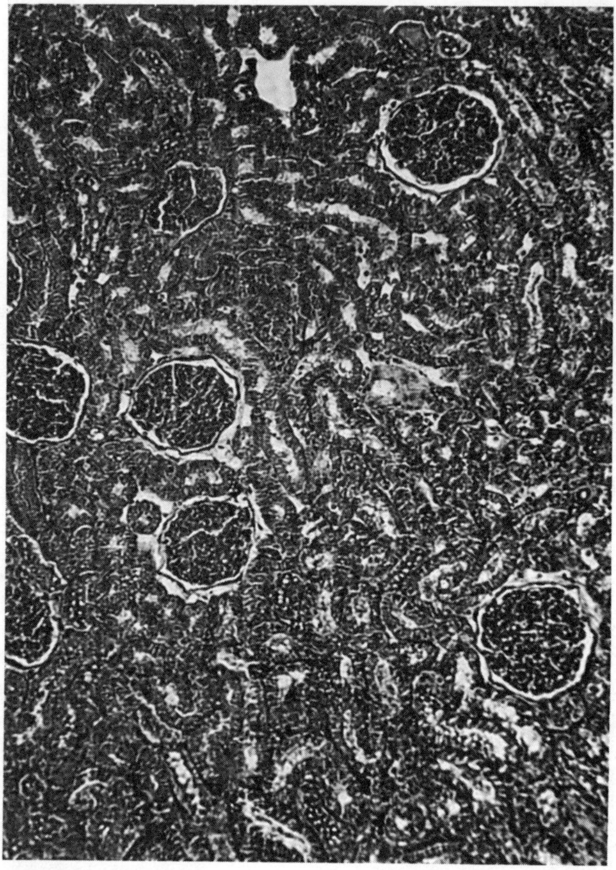

FIGURE 5. Photomicrograph (60×) of dog kidney after five hr perfusion (system no. 2) with blood at low oxygen saturation. Note normal appearance of glomeruli and tubules.

were higher in the experiments where the dogs' own lungs were used (system no. 1), the degree of glomerular congestion appeared to be slightly less when the bubble oxygenator (system no. 2) was used to oxygenate the blood.

FIGURE 6 compares the decline in mean hourly oxygen saturation values in the perfusates from kidneys perfused with unoxygenated blood with and without cobalt. The decrease in oxygen saturation values in the unoxygenated blood containing cobalt was much less rapid and did not reach values as low as those when unoxygenated blood alone was used in the system. This is probably a reflection of the inability of the kidney to extract oxygen from the blood perfusate due to some effect of cobalt on the kidney in this system.

The urine flow ranged between 0.1–0.2 ml/min when the bubble oxygenator was used and was usually bloody and albuminous. When the dogs' own lungs were used to oxygenate the blood the rate of urine production was 0.2–0.3 ml/min and was usually clear. Some kidneys failed to produce urine in both systems.

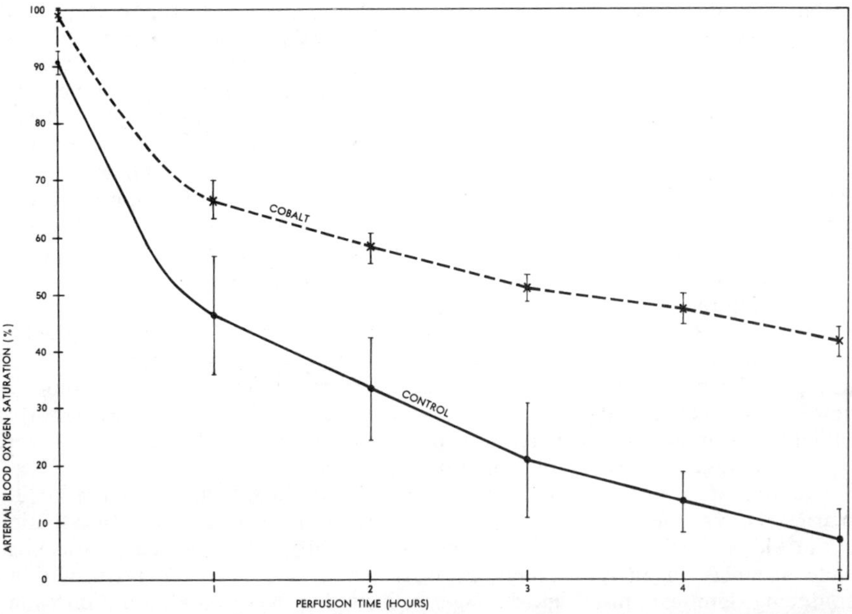

FIGURE 6. Mean hourly blood oxygen saturation values on perfusates of isolated kidneys perfused with hypoxic blood alone or hypoxic blood containing cobalt (perfusion system no. 2). Each point on the cobalt curve represents the mean of six experiments and the control hypoxemic group five experiments. The standard error of the mean is shown for each point.

Discussion

The isolated perfused kidney was found, in the present studies, to produce erythropoietin in response to cobalt or reduction in oxygen tension of the blood perfusate. Cobalt produced a more marked effect when the kidney was perfused with hypoxic blood. Testosterone produced a slight but significant effect on erythropoietin production in the isolated perfused kidneys from dogs following pretreatment with testosterone.

The mechanism by which cobalt stimulates erythropoietin production in the isolated kidney is still unclear. However, our finding that the kidney perfused with hypoxic blood containing cobalt utilizes oxygen at a lesser rate than kidneys perfused with hypoxic blood alone adds further support for a concept of histotoxic hypoxia. Cobalt has been demonstrated to cause a shift in the lactic dehydrogenase-isoenzyme pattern in rabbit kidneys and this was suggested to be due to a local deficiency of oxygen.[17] Our finding that cobalt is more effective in stimulating kidney erythropoietin production on a background of hypoxia may be due to an effect of cobalt in increasing the sensitivity of the kidney to hypoxia. We have found that renal hypoxia as a result of renal artery constriction also enhances the stimulatory effect of cobalt on erythropoietin production.[18]

Our demonstration of a slight effect of testosterone on erythropoietin production in the isolated perfused kidney may support the view that testosterone stimulates erythropoiesis, at least in part, by increasing erythropoietin production and points to the kidney as the site of action. Testosterone's effect on erythropoietin production in the isolated perfused kidney may be more marked if the dogs are treated for a longer period of time or with a different dosage before kidney perfusion. The mechanism of testosterone's effect on kidney erythropoietin production is not known. Testosterone is known to increase plasma levels of an esterase enzyme in female mice.[19] Androgens may elevate the level of this enzyme in the kidney and result in an increased production of erythropoietin. It has been reported previously that testosterone produces an increase in kidney weight.[20] This effect may be related to its mechanism of action on erythropoietin production. Our findings do not preclude the possibility that testosterone, in addition to stimulating erythropoietin production, could potentiate the action of erythropoietin on erythroid cells or else stimulate erythropoiesis directly. Other workers have demonstrated that erythropoietin's effect on iron incorporation in red cells is enhanced by testosterone[11] and that testosterone stimulates erythropoiesis in vitro in bone marrow cultures.[21]

The reasons for the failure of Erslev *et al.*[9] to produce erythropoietin in the isolated perfused kidney in response to hypoxia similar to that of other workers[1-4,8] may have been due to insufficient hypoxia and/or a shorter perfusion time. In view of the fact that oxygen tension or saturation values were only reported initially and at the end of perfusion, the total time in which the kidneys were exposed to very low oxygen tension blood is not known.

The present experiments do not prove or disprove the hypothesis that reduction in arterial oxygen tension is the physiological trigger for erythropoietin production in the kidney. However, they do show that erythropoietin can be produced in some instances in an isolated kidney in response to localized hypoxia without producing significant histologic damage. Admittedly, the oxygen saturation values in our blood perfusates stimulating erythropoietin production were much lower than those reported for normal dog renal venous blood.[22] However, it is possible that under certain conditions, such as anemia, lower oxygen tension of blood may be found in critical areas of the renal vasculature due to shunting of blood through medullary shunts similar to those described by Trueta.[23]

Summary

Isolated dog kidneys were perfused with blood at normal and reduced oxygen tensions and with blood containing testosterone or cobalt. Erythropoietin titers were found to be significantly increased in the blood perfusates from kidneys perfused with blood at lowered oxygen tensions while no change in erythropoietin was seen when kidneys were perfused with blood at a normal oxygen tension. Testosterone produced a slight increase in erythropoietin production in perfused kidneys from dogs pretreated for several days with testosterone before perfusion. Cobalt produced significant increases in erythropoietin levels in the perfusates with normal as well as reduced oxygen tension blood, but its effect was more marked when the kidneys were perfused with hypoxic blood. In studies of the histology of all kidneys perfused, most of the kidneys demonstrated varying degrees of glomerular congestion. No correlation was found between erythropoietin elaboration and renal congestion or other degenerative cellular changes in the kidney. Therefore, it is concluded that increased erythropoietin production in the isolated perfused kidney in response to cobalt, testosterone or hypoxic blood is a direct effect of these stimuli on the kidney rather than a release of erythropoietin from injured and disintegrating cells.

Acknowledgments

The authors gratefully acknowledge the technical assistance of Mrs. Judy Parker and Mr. Carroll Osburn in these studies and are also indebted to Dr. Y. C.

Kim, Pathology Dept., Baptist Memorial Hospital, Memphis, for the histological evaluation of the kidneys.

References

1. Kuratowska, Z., B. Lewartowski & E. Michalski. 1961. Studies on the production of erythropoietin by isolated perfused organs. Blood **18:** 527.
2. Reissmann, K. R. & T. Nomura. 1962. Erythropoietin formation in isolated kidneys and liver. *In* Erythropoiesis. : 71.Grune and Stratton. New York, N. Y.
3. Zangheri, E. O., H. Campana, F. Ponce, J. C. Silva, F. O. Fernandez & F. R. E. Suarez. 1963. Production of erythropoietin by anoxic perfusion of the isolated kidney of a dog. Nature **199:** 572.
4. Pavlovic-Kentera, V., D. P. Hall, C. Brogassa & R. D. Lange. 1965. Unilateral renal hypoxia and production of erythropoietin. J. Lab. Clin. Med. **65:** 577.
5. Fisher, J. W. & B. J. Birdwell. 1961. The production of an erythropoietic factor by the in situ perfused kidney. Acta Haemat. **26:** 224.
6. Takaku, F., K. Hirashima & K. Nakao. 1962. Studies on the mechanism of erythropoietin production. I. Effect of unilateral constriction of the renal artery. J. Lab. Clin. Med. **59:** 815.
7. Fisher, J. W., R. Schofield & D. D. Porteous. 1965. Effects of renal hypoxia on erythropoietin production. Brit. J. Haemat. **11:** 382.
8. Abbrecht, P. H. & R. L. Malvin. 1966. Renal production of erythropoietin in the dog. Am. J. Physiol. **210:** 237.
9. Erslev, A. J., R. W. Solit, R. C. Camishion, S. Amsel, J. Ilda & W. S. Ballinger II. 1965. Erythropoietin in Vitro. III. Perfusion of a lung-kidney preparation. Am. J. Physiol. **208:** 1153.
10. Fried, W., R. L. DeGowin & C. W. Gurney. 1964. Erythropoietic effect of testosterone in the polycythemic mouse. Proc. Soc. Exp. Biol. Med. **117:** 839.
11. Naets, J. P. & M. Wittek. 1966. Mechanism of action of androgens on erythropoiesis. Am. J. Physiol. **210:** 315.
12. Fried, W. & C. W. Gurney. 1965. Use of mild plethora to demonstrate an erythropoietic effect from small amounts of androgens. Proc. Soc. Exp. Biol. Med. **120:** 519.
13. DeGowin, R. L., D. Hofstra & C. W. Gurney. 1962. The mouse with hypoxia-induced erythremia, an erythropoietin bioassay animal. J. Lab. Clin. Med. **60:** 846.
14. Almond, H. 1953. Determination of traces of cobalt in soil. Analyt. Chem. **25:** 166.
15. White, W. F., C. W. Gurney, E. Goldwasser & L. O. Jacobson. 1960. Studies on erythropoietin. Rec. Prog. Hor. Res. **16:** 219.
16. Dixon, W. J. & F. J. Massey, Jr. 1957. *In* Introduction to Statistical Analysis. 2nd Ed. : 139. McGraw-Hill Co., Inc. New York, N. Y.
17. Jensen, K. & E. B. Thorling. 1965. Effect of anemia and cobalt on lactic dehydrogenase isoenzymes in kidney tissues of rabbits and its possible relation to the erythropoietin production. Acta Path. Microbiol. Scandinav. **63:** 385.
18. Fisher, J. W. & B. L. Roh. 1964. Influence of alkylating agents on kidney erythropoietin production. Cancer Res. **24:** 983.
19. Allen, R. C. & D. J. Moore. 1966. Sex-associated quantitative differences in the plasma esterases of inbred mice. Endocrinology **78:** 655.
20. Selye, Hans. 1939. The effect of testosterone on the kidney. J. Urology **42:** 637.
21. Reisner, E. H. 1966. Tissue culture of bone marrow. II. Effect of steroid hormones on hematopoiesis in vitro. Blood **27:** 460.
22. Aukland, K. 1962. Hemoglobin oxygen saturation in the dog kidney. Acta Physiol. Scand. **56:** 315.
23. Trueta, P., A. E. Barclay, K. J. Franklin, P. M. Daniel & M. M. L. Pritchard. 1947. Studies on the renal circulation. Charles C. Thomas, Inc. Springfield, Ill.

EFFECTS OF HYPOTHALAMIC STIMULATION ON ERYTHROPOIESIS AND ON THE PRODUCTION OF ERYTHROPOIESIS-STIMULATING FACTORS IN INTACT AND NEPHRECTOMIZED RABBITS

Sverre Halvorsen

Pediatric Research Institute, Rikshospitalet, and Neurophysiological Laboratory, Anatomical Institute, University of Oslo, Norway

Introduction

The role of the central nervous system (CNS) in the regulation of erythropoiesis is much debated. We have been interested in this problem for several years and our working hypothesis has been that specialized cells in the nervous system may record the variations in oxygen tension and by nervous or humoral routes, stimulate the erythropoiesis-stimulating factor (ESF) producing organ(s). This point of view gained prominence after it was convincingly shown that the kidney is not the sole organ either of recording variations in oxygen tension or of producing ESF.[1] Since previous data[2–4] pointed to the hypothalamus as an active area in this regulation, we have so far been concerned with only this region. The problem has been attacked with conventional neurophysiological methods, i.e., stimulation and ablation experiments.

Electrical stimulation of the hypothalamic area increased the reticulocytes and red cell mass in about one-third of the stimulated rabbits[5] and in about the same number we demonstrated increased amounts of ESF in the plasma.[6] This latter finding has been confirmed by Mirand *et al.*[7] in monkeys. Feldman *et al.*[8] found reticulocytosis and increased radioiron incorporation into newly formed red cells following electrical stimulation of the posterior hypothalamus in rats but did not find any increase of ESF in plasma. They used, however, a much shorter stimulation period than in our experiments, totalling six hr in four days. Large symmetrical lesions in the posterior hypothalamus reduced the reticulocyte response to hypoxia, and this response was not normalized when ACTH, GH, thyroxin and testosterone were given prior to repeated hypoxic tests.[9] In addition, we have compared the effects of hypothalamic stimulation with the effect of pituitary and target organ hormones.[10] Although reticulocytosis was produced with GH and increased red cell mass with a combination of hormones (ACTH, GH, thyroxin and testosterone), we have not found any increase of ESF in plasma after a 14-day period of injections of the tested hormones, as we did with hypothalamic stimulation.

The data referred to do not provide conclusive evidence of a primary influence of the CNS on erythropoiesis because, among others, data on hormone levels and on oxygen tension, saturation and consumption are lacking; however, they strongly suggest that the hypothalamic area is also of primary importance in this respect. The mechanisms of the CNS may be several, the main possibilities being, in our opinion, either an effect through the pituitary gland, through a humoral substance produced in the hypothalamus itself, and/or through the autonomic nervous system on blood flow in the kidneys, or other ESF-producing organs, or in the bone marrow itself. In the present report data on the effect of vasodilators and of nephrectomy on the production of erythropoietic factors and on erythropoiesis following hypothalamic stimulation will be presented.

Materials and Methods

Sixteen male, adult rabbits weighing between 2.5 and 3.5 kg have been used in the studies. Bipolar electrodes were introduced in 13 rabbits during Nembutal narcosis by means of the stereotaxic coordinates described by Sawyer *et al.*[11] The unanesthetized rabbits were stimulated for different periods of time as indicated in the Tables. The stimulation parameters were as previously used.[5] Phenoxybenzamin, 2 mg/kg body weight was given intravenously before hypothalamic stimulation in two rabbits. Blood was withdrawn in heparinized syringes before, during and after the stimulation, the plasma pipetted off and stored at −20° C until used. The erythrocytes were reinjected in order to minimize the blood loss. The plasma was examined for ESF by means of hypoxia- and transfusion-induced polycythemic mice of the NMRI/BOM strain. Bilateral nephrectomy was performed in Nembutal narcosis in eight rabbits. Two days after the nephrectomy they were given peritoneal dialysis in Nembutal narcosis. In the nephrectomized rabbit's bone marrow aspirations were performed before, and two and four days after the operation.

Results

TABLE 1 illustrates two experiments performed in order to repeat our previous studies with the present methods. Rabbit no. 2 was stimulated electrically 4–6 hr daily through 12 days. The reticulocyte levels increased to 3–4 times the initial level, and the reticulocyte curve after termination of the stimulation was very similar to the reticulocyte response following eight hr of hypoxia in intact rabbits.[9] Plasma withdrawn after 9 and 12 days of stimulation increased the ^{59}Fe erythrocyte uptake in the recipient polycythemic mice to 4.2%. Above 2.5% is a significant elevation with our method. After the stimulation was stopped, the uptake was 0.5% indicating that no permanent damage had developed in the rabbit which could secondarily increase erythropoietin production. Rabbit no. 7 was hypertransfused to 18 g hemoglobin before start of the hypothalamic stimulation. In this rabbit there was no significant increase in reticulocytes, but following

TABLE 1

RETICULOCYTE COUNTS AND PLASMA ERYTHROPOIETIC FACTORS AFTER HYPOTHALAMIC STIMULATION

Rabbit No.	Experimental situation	Day of Sampling	Stimulation per Day (Hours)	Reticulocytes percent	^{59}Fe percent Uptake ± SE
2	Hypothalamic stimulation	1	4–6	1.1	1.51 (1)
		3	4–6	1.9	2.10 ± 0.83 (6)
		7	4–6	1.7	1.73 ± 0.13 (3)
		10	4–6	3.2	4.10 ± 2.08 (3)
		13	4–6	3.1	3.78 ± 2.03 (4)
	No stimulation	17		4.2	
		21		1.9	0.98 ± 0.09 (4)
7	Hypertransfused Hypothalamic stimulation	1	4–6	0.3	1.30 ± 0.18 (4)
		4	4–6	0.4	
		6	20	0.5	3.48 ± 1.52 (2)
		9	4–6	0.8	0.50 ± 0.04 (4)
		12	4–6	0.8	1.06 ± 0.06 (5)
			Saline controls		0.92 ± 0.20 (6)
			Rabbit plasma controls		1.09 ± 0.13 (22)

TABLE 2

EFFECT OF HYPOTHALAMIC STIMULATION ON THE RETICULOCYTE COUNTS DURING AND EIGHT DAYS AFTER THE STIMULATION AND ON THE PLASMA LEVEL OF ERYTHROPOIETIC FACTORS BEFORE AND AT THE END OF THE HYPOTHALAMIC STIMULATION*

Rabbit No.	Duration of Stimulation (Days)	Reticulocytes percent Initial	Reticulocytes percent Highest	^{59}Fe percent uptake ± SE Before	^{59}Fe percent uptake ± SE After
1	Sham-stimulated	0.6	1.4	1.36 ± 0.37 (4)	1.26 ± 0.38 (4)
3	3			0.75 ± 0.22 (4)	1.50 ± 0.52 (7)
4	4	0.7	3.9	0.52 (1)	0.93 (1)
6	4	1.2	6.5	0.56 ± 0.04 (4)	0.86 ± 0.04 (4)
7	1	0.7	3.5	1.52 ± 0.38 (4)	1.35 ± 0.37 (4)
	After phenoxyzenzamin 2 mg/kg body weight i.v.				
6	3	1.7	4.8		
7	1	0.7	2.7	1.30 ± 0.18 (4)	5.22 ± 1.98 (4)
			Saline controls	0.92 ± 0.20 (6)	
			Rabbit plasma controls	1.09 ± 0.13 (22)	

* The numbers in the parentheses indicate the number of polycythemic mice tested in each assay.

20 hr continuous stimulation, the ^{59}Fe erythrocyte uptake in the recipient mice was 3.5%.

A 14-day stimulation period is, however, difficult to use in further experimentation and shorter periods have been tested. TABLE 2 illustrates such experiments. In rabbit no. 1 electrodes were implanted in the hypothalamus, the rabbit was kept under the same conditions as during stimulation, but no stimulation was applied. In this sham-stimulated rabbit neither significant reitculocytosis nor increase in erythropoietic factors occurred. In rabbits nos. 4, 6 and 7 a significant reticulocytosis occurred both with and without phenoxybenzamin. Plasma from these rabbits did not significantly increase the ^{59}Fe erythrocyte uptake in the recipient mice, except in one experiment with phenoxybenzamin. The reticulocyte curve after the stimulation again paralleled the curve following hypoxia in intact rabbits (FIGURE 1), indicating that the effect in the erythroid series must be close to the stem cell. An early release of reticulocytes might explain part of the reticulocytosis, but can hardly explain this prolonged curve after termination of the stimulation unless the release of cells through a feedback mechanism affects differentiation and maturation of earlier forms.

Although increased levels of erythropoietic factors were only occasionally achieved following a short stimulation period, this model might prove useful in further studies. TABLE 3 documents the results in nephrectomized rabbits. Three control rabbits were kept alive for 96 hr following bilateral nephrectomy with one peritoneal dialysis after 48 hr. Although the rabbits lost their appetite, they were active throughout this period. The hemoglobin dropped to levels between 9.2 and 12.3 g. The percentage of erythroid cells in the bone marrow was slightly reduced but both two and four days after nephrectomy all stages of erythroid cells were represented, indicating that erythropoiesis was continuing after the loss of an eventual erythropoietic factor from the kidney. The plasma levels of ESF were slightly, although significantly elevated in one rabbit (no. 14) while two others showed borderline responses and no increase 12 hr after being bled 10 ml/kg body weight (No. 16). The reticulocyte counts did not show any characteristic changes.

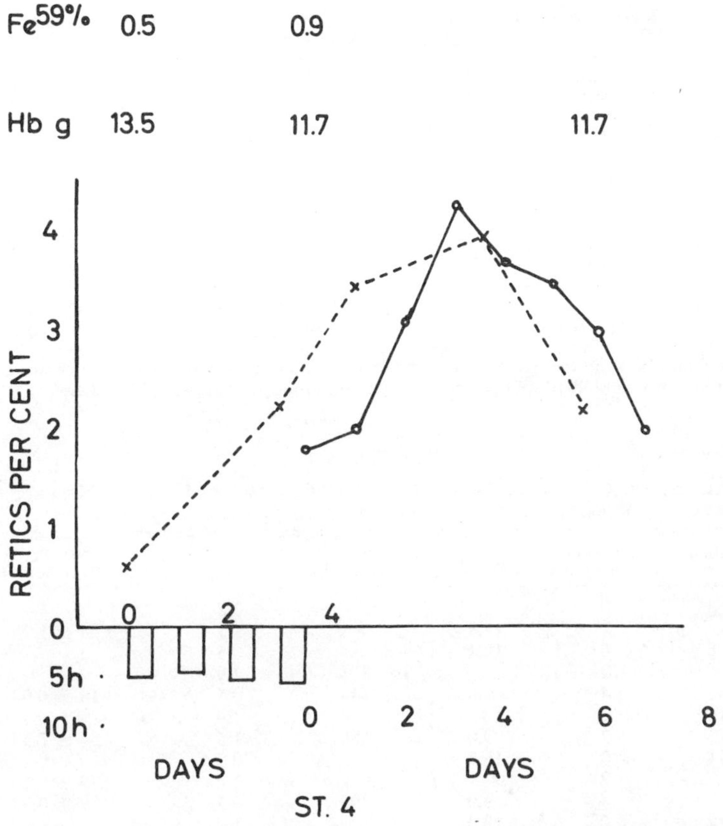

FIGURE 1. The reticulocyte response in rabbit no. 4 to a 4-day period of hypothalamic stimulation (stippled line) compared with the mean reticulocyte response of five intact rabbits to eight hr hypoxia given at day 0 (solid line). The hemoglobin values and the ESF levels before and after the stimulation are also indicated.

TABLE 4 shows the results of hypothalmic stimulation in four nephrectomized rabbits and in one rabbit with implanted electrodes, nephrectomized and sham-stimulated. The reticulocytes did not change significantly in these rabbits. The hemoglobin dropped to between 9 and 10 g and the serum urea rose to between 260 and 480 mg/100 ml. The bone marrows showed definite erythropoiesis both two and four days postnephrectomy; details will be presented separately together with the localization of the electrodes in the hypothalamus. The plasma levels of ESF were increased in two rabbits and not increased in two others. In the sham-stimulated rabbit there was also an increase in plasma ESF. This rabbit had respiratory difficulties and died two days after nephrectomy and the sample of blood was taken shortly after death.

Summary and Conclusions

The present study in intact rabbits confirms the previous findings of reticulocytosis and elevated plasma levels of erythropoietic factors following hypothalmic

TABLE 3

RETICULOCYTE COUNTS AND PLASMA ERYTHROPOIETIC FACTOR LEVELS FOLLOWING NEPHRECTOMY*

Rabbit No.	Day after Nephrectomy	Hb, g	Ur + mg/100 ml	Reticulocytes Percent	^{59}Fe Percent Uptake ± SE
14	0	15.7		0.5	
	4	12.3	324	0.5	2.86 ± 0.72 (11)
15	0	14.0		1.8	0.79 ± 0.36 (2)
	4	10.0	880	1.3	1.95 ± 0.22 (2)
16	0	14.8		0.7	
	4 Bled	11.7	376	1.0	1.98 ± 0.69 (5)
	4.5	9.2			1.79 ± 0.63 (9)
			Saline controls		0.92 ± 0.20 (6)
			Rabbit plasma controls		1.06 ± 0.13 (22)

* The numbers in the parentheses indicate number of polycythemic mice in each assay. Rabbit no. 16 was bled 10 ml/kg body weight and blood withdrawn 12 hr later.

TABLE 4

RETICULOCYTE COUNTS AND PLASMA ERYTHROPOIETIC FACTOR LEVELS IN NEPHRECTOMIZED RABBITS FOLLOWING 4–6 HR DAILY HYPOTHALAMIC STIMULATION

Rabbit No.	Day after Nephrectomy	Hb, g	Ur + mg/100 ml	Reticulocytes Percent	^{59}Fe Percent Uptake ± SE
8*	0			0.2	
	2	14.8		1.5	9.84 ± 1.98 (2)
6	0	12.1		0.5	
	2		308	1.9	
	4	9.0	444	0.5	3.10 ± 0.94 (6)
10	0	14.5		1.9	
	2	9.0	480	1.5	7.54 ± 2.37 (2)
11	0	15.1		0.5	
	2			1.2	0.79 ± 0.18 (2)
	4	9.0	392	0.5	1.39 ± 0.31 (4)
12	0	13.4		1.4	
	2	13.4	260		1.39 ± 0.65 (2)
			Saline controls		0.92 ± 0.20 (6)
			Rabbit plasma controls		1.06 ± 0.13 (22)

* Rabbit 8 was sham-stimulated only. The numbers in parentheses indicate number of polycythemic mice in each assay.

stimulation and further supports the hypothesis that the CNS has an important role in the regulation of erythropoiesis. The reticulocytosis was observed both after short and long stimulation periods while the increased levels of ESF were found either after several days of stimulation or after a single long stimulation period (20 hr). The reticulocytosis and the increased levels of ESF were not always correlated. This may be due to utilization of ESF but may also indicate that different mechanisms are operating. Feldman *et al.*[8] found reticulocytosis, but no elevation, of ESF in plasma. The difference in this respect between their results and ours may be due to species variations but may also be due to the much shorter stimulation period used in their experiments. Phenoxybenzamin did not reduce the effect of hypothalamic stimulation in our work.

In the nephrectomized rabbits the hemoglobin dropped while the reticulocytes remained unchanged. All stages of erythroid cells were represented in the bone marrows of both stimulated and nonstimulated rabbits two and four days post-nephrectomy. The data thus indicate that in the rabbit the bone marrow functions after nephrectomy as previously demonstrated by Erslev.[12] With nonstimulated, nephrectomized rabbits there was a slight, but significant, increase of ESF in plasma in one rabbit while the other two showed borderline responses. The rabbits were slightly anemic and it is possible that this anemia is the stimulus for production of erythropoietic factors. Another possibility is that a compensatory increase in nonrenal erythropoietic factors occurs at this stage following nephrectomy. Electrical stimulation of the hypothalamus in the nephrectomized rabbits also increased the plasma leavels of ESF. The increase was similar to the increase in the control rabbits and the data are insufficient to indicate any difference between the groups. The question of whether the hypothalmic stimulation acts through the kidneys cannot therefore be answered adequately on the basis of these data. Since the rabbit has only moderately reduced erythropoiesis in the bone marrow after nephrectomy, and a possible compensatory increase in nonrenal erythropoietic factors, it is probably not the best experimental animal to test the effect of hypothalmic stimulation following nephrectomy. However, the study does provide further evidence that ESF may be produced in the absence of the kidneys.

References

1. Nathan, D. G., E. Schupak, F. Stohlman, Jr. & F. Merrill. 1964. Erythropoiesis in anephric man. J. Clin. Invest. **43**: 2158.
2. Seip, M. 1953. Reticulocyte studies. Grundt Tanum. Oslo, Norway.
3. Komyia, E. 1956. Die zentralnervöse Regulation des Blutbildes. Georg Thieme. Stuttgart, Germany.
4. Baciu, I. 1964. Système nerveux et mécanismes humoraux dans la régulation de l'érythropoïèse. Rev. Rhum. **1**: 149.
5. Seip, M., S. Halvorsen, P. Andersen & B. R. Kaada. 1961. Effects of hypothalamic stimulation on erythropoiesis in rabbits. Scand. J. Clin. Lab. Invest. **13**: 553.
6. Halvorsen, S. 1961. Plasma erythropoietin levels following hypothalamic stimulation in the rabbit. Scand. J. Clin. Lab. Invest. **13**: 564.
7. Mirand, E. A., J. T. Grace, G. S. Johnston & G. P. Murphy. 1964. Effects of hypothalamic stimulation on the erythropoietic response in the *Rhesus* monkey. Nature **204**: 1163.
8. Feldman, S., E. A. Rachmilewitz & G. Izak. 1966. The effect of central nervous system stimulation on erythropoiesis in rats with chronically implanted electrodes. J. Lab. Clin. Med. **67**: 713.
9. Halvorsen, S. 1964. Effects of hypothalamic lesions on the erythropoietic response to hypoxia in rabbits. Acta Physiol. Scand. **61**: 1.
10. Halvorsen, S. 1966. The central nervous system in regulation of erythropoiesis. Acta Haemat. (Basel) **35**: 65.
11. Sawyer, C. H., J. W. Everett & J. D. Green. 1954. The rabbit diencephalon in stereotaxic coordinates. J. Comp. Neurol. **101**: 801.
12. Erslev, A. J. 1958. Erythropoietic function in uremic rabbits. Arch. Int. Med. **101**: 407.

EXTRA-RENAL AND RENAL CONTROL OF ERYTHROPOIETIN PRODUCTION*

E. A. Mirand

Roswell Park Memorial Institute, New York State Department of Health, and State University of New York at Buffalo, Buffalo, N. Y.

It is now accepted that erythropoiesis is under humoral control and that hypoxia, the fundamental stimulus for erythropoiesis, results in the production of a circulating factor called erythropoietin.[1–4] The kidney is believed to be the major site of production of erythropoietin.[1–4] However, erythropoietin can be produced in the absence of the kidney, as shown by Mirand *et al.*[2,3] and Erslev,[5] and which was later confirmed by others.[6,7] Moreover, Nathan *et al.*[8] have shown that erythropoiesis continues in anephric man. The location of the extrarenal sites of erythropoietin production has not yet been ascertained, although the pituitary,[9] liver,[10] spleen,[11] and other organs have been suggested. How and where erythropoietin is released from the kidney and other sites of production is not specifically known. It is well established, however, that endocrine glands are under the influence of the central nervous system and that certain functions of the nervous system are in turn affected by endocrine substances. For instance, the hypothalamus is the focal point at which neural stimuli converge to influence adenohypophyseal secretions. Although no consensus has been reached as to the specificity or localization of the hypothalamic areas involved in ACTH, TSH, LH, FSH and growth hormone production, most workers in the field of pituitary physiology agree with the concept proposed by Harris[12] that the diencephalon exerts its effect on anterior pituitary hormones through secretion of some neurohumoral substance(s) transmitted to the hypophyseal cells by means of the hypophyseal portal circulation.

The participation of the central nervous system in the regulation of erythropoiesis has been reported by many investigators.[13–18] Both electrical stimulation of and injury to the hypothalamic complex have been reported to induce increases in the numbers of circulating erythrocytes and reticulocytes, and in hemoglobin levels.[13–18] The more recent investigations of Halvorsen[19–22] and Seip[23] indicate that the hypothalamus may participate in the regulation of erythropoiesis in rabbits. They noted that electrical stimulation of the hypothalamus increased the reticulocyte level and red cell mass in some of their rabbits. Plasma from such rabbits induced an increase in erythrocyte uptake of ^{59}Fe and in the number of circulating reticulocytes when injected into starved or polycythemic mice.[22] Piliero[24,25] investigated the erythropoietic response to long-term hypoxia in rats with hypothalamic lesions and found no differences between the operated and sham-operated animals.

It is the purpose of this communication to present our findings on (1) the effect of electrical stimulation of the hypothalamus on erythropoietin production in rhesus monkeys and in rats; (2) the ability of hypothalamic-lesioned monkeys and rats to produce erythropoietin (EPF) by bleeding or under hypoxia; and (3) erythropoietin activity in patients with renal abnormalities.

* This investigation was supported in part by research grants (AI–04506, CA–02728, CA–07745 and 1 MO1–FR00262) from the National Institutes of Health, Public Health Service, and the John A. Hartford Foundation, Inc.

The Effect of Electrical Stimulation on the Hypothalamus

Monkeys. Rhesus monkeys in normal health and nutrition were used in these studies. The monkeys were nonuremic and nonanemic. The monkeys were treated in the following manner: Group I–electrical stimulation was applied to intact monkeys in the area of (1) the supraoptic nucleus, (2) the preoptic nucleus, (3) the posterior median eminence, (4) the mammillary nucleus, and (5) the anterior commissure; Group II–hypophysectomized male monkeys received electrical stimulation in the area of (1) the supraoptic nucleus and (2) the posterior median eminence; Group III–gonadectomized male monkeys received electrical stimulation in the area of (1) the supraoptic nucleus and (2) the posterior median eminence.

The stimulating electrodes were nickel chromium wire electrodes stereotaxically inserted into the brains of rhesus monkeys under general anesthesia (pentobarbital sodium). The electrodes were fixed utilizing the stereotaxic localization coordinates of Synder and Lee[26] and a correction factor for the skull cap based on animal body-weight charts was used. These electrodes were fully insulated except at the tip and were 0.09 mm in diameter. Forty-eight hours following electrode insertion, stimulation was applied with a BRS (Behavior Research Systems) constant current stimulator. The following currents were individually used on each electrode: a current varying from 0.6 to 0.7 ma was administered for a 300 m sec duration every 30 sec for ½ to 8-hour periods on four consecutive days unless otherwise stated.

Blood was collected before and during the period of stimulation; care was taken, however, to prevent monkeys from becoming anemic. In some instances, following completion of stimulation of the brain, a lesion was burned in each area to assist in the later anatomical localization of the position of the electrode. The brain was fixed in buffered formalin solution, and serial sections and multiple staining procedures were used to locate the lesion.

Five-week-old Ha/ICR Swiss male mice, 30–35 g in weight, were used to assay plasma for EPF.[27] Each assay animal was injected i.p. with a total of 2.5 cc of isologous washed RBC's to induce polycythemia. The hematocrits had to be in the 75–85% range before the animals could be used for erythropoietin assay. This degree of hypertransfusion assures the cessation of erythropoiesis. Polycythemic mice were injected s.c. with 0.5 cc of rhesus plasma on three consecutive days.

Table 1

Plasma Erythropoietin Levels in Rhesus Monkeys Subjected to Hypothalamic Stimulation in the Area of Supraoptic Nucleus

Animal	Duration of Stimulation (Hours)	Percent 24 hr Blood ^{59}Fe Uptake in Polycythemic Mice		
		Prestimulatory Plasma	Stimulatory Plasma	Sham Control
		S.D.*	S.D.	S.D.
(A) *Experimental*				
(1) Male	1	0.46 ± 0.09	1.59 ± 0.30	
(2) Male	2	0.38 ± 0.03	5.08 ± 0.66	
(3) Male	4	0.53 ± 0.07	3.29 ± 0.50	
(4) Male	8	0.65 ± 0.02	3.86 ± 0.90	
(B) *Sham Control* (8 hr)				
(1) Male	—			0.55 ± 0.06

* S.D. = Standard Deviation.

TABLE 2

PLASMA ERYTHROPOIETIN LEVELS IN RHESUS MONKEYS SUBJECTED TO HYPOTHALAMIC STIMULATION IN THE AREA OF PREOPTIC NUCLEUS

Animal	Duration of Stimulation (Hours)	Percent 24 hr Blood ^{59}Fe Uptake in Polycythemic Mice		
		Prestimulatory Plasma	Stimulatory Plasma	Sham Control
		S.D.*	S.D.	S.D.
(A) *Experimental*				
(1) Female	½	0.39 ± 0.11	0.90 ± 0.10	
(2) Female	1	0.52 ± 0.11	1.14 ± 0.16	
(3) Male	1½	0.38 ± 0.13	2.05 ± 0.48	
(4) Male	8	0.43 ± 0.15	2.66 ± 0.41	
(B) *Sham Control* (8 hr)				
(1) Female				0.38 ± 0.07
(2) Male				0.54 ± 0.14

* S.D. = Standard Deviation.

On the fourth day, 0.5 μc of ^{59}Fe in 0.2 ml of saline were injected i.v. and, on the fifth day, 24-hour ^{59}Fe uptakes by the blood were determined.

The results in TABLE 1 show that stimulation of the supraoptic nucleus in four monkeys, one to eight hr on four consecutive days, induced the release of high levels of plasma erythropoietin. The levels of ^{59}Fe uptake by the blood were 3–13 times greater than the prestimulatory levels in these animals and levels in sham control animals.

Significant levels of plasma erythropoietin were obtained following stimulation in the area of the preoptic nucleus for one-half to eight hr on four consecutive days (TABLE 2). The stimulation of the posterior median eminence for one to three hr on four consecutive days produced the highest levels of plasma EPF (TABLE 3). Stimulation of other areas of the hypothalamus, i.e., the mammillary nucleus and the anterior commissure for four to eight hr on four consecutive days did not produce significant levels of plasma EPF (TABLE 4). TABLE 4 also shows that although stimulation of some areas produced high levels of plasma EPF in some monkeys, in many more instances there was no increase in plasma EPF levels. The reason for this is unknown. Perhaps the amount of stimulation of the hypothalamus was too little or too great to release erythropoietin in the plasma. The functional state of the animal may determine the amount of stimulation required. Also, there is variation in the localization of the nuclei and tracts in the hypothalamus from one animal to another. Therefore, we may not have stimulated similar areas in all animals.

Since it is known that specific areas of the hypothalamus regulate pituitary function,[28,29] it was deemed advisable to determine if EPF is released via a hypothalamic-pituitary-kidney pathway. Eight monkeys were hypophysectomized and two areas, the supraoptic nucleus and posterior median eminence, were stimulated. Only one hypophysectomized monkey, stimulated in the posterior median eminence, gave us a high level of plasma EPF (4.85 ± 0.58% ^{59}Fe uptake vs. sham control 0.54 ± 0.04%) (TABLE 5). From this finding it appears that the hypothalamus can directly affect the target organ producing erythropoietin.

Testosterone[30] has been shown to influence the production of EPF. For this reason, eight male monkeys were gonadectomized and the areas of the supraoptic

TABLE 3

PLASMA ERYTHROPOIETIN LEVELS IN RHESUS MONKEYS SUBJECTED TO HYPOTHALAMIC STIMULATION IN THE AREA OF POSTERIOR MEDIAN EMINENCE

Animal	Duration of Stimulation (Hours)	Percent 24 hr Blood ^{59}Fe Uptake in Polycythemic Mice		
		Prestimulatory Plasma	Stimulatory Plasma	Sham Control
		S.D.*	S.D.	S.D.
(A) *Experimental*				
(1) Male	1	0.40 ± 0.09	5.44 ± 0.98	
(2) Female	2	0.62 ± 0.12	6.87 ± 1.34	
(3) Male	3	0.43 ± 0.07	9.40 ± 2.19	
(B) *Sham Control* (3 hr)				
(1) Male				0.60 ± 0.07
(2) Female				0.51 ± 0.05

* S.D. = Standard Deviation.

TABLE 4

PLASMA ERYTHROPOIETIN (EPF) LEVELS IN RHESUS MONKEYS SUBJECTED TO STIMULATION IN VARIOUS AREAS OF HYPOTHALAMUS

Duration of Stimulation (Hours)	Area Stimulated	Number of Animals	Number Positive for EPF	Number Negative for EPF
½ – 8	Preoptic nucleus	14	4	10
½ – 8	Supraoptic nucleus	15	4	11
1 – 3	Posterior median eminence	7	3	4
4	Mammillary nucleus	1	—	1
8	Anterior commissure	1	—	1
		38	11	27

TABLE 5

PLASMA ERYTHROPOIETIN (EPF) LEVELS IN HYPOPHYSECTOMIZED MALE RHESUS MONKEYS SUBJECTED TO STIMULATION IN VARIOUS AREAS OF THE HYPOTHALAMUS

Duration of Stimulation (Hours)	Area Stimulated	Number of Animals	Number Positive for EPF	Number Negative for EPF
2	Supraoptic nucleus	1	—	1
4		2	—	2
8		1	—	1
2	Posterior median eminence	1	—	1
4		1	—	1
8		2	1*	1

* 4.85% blood ^{59}FE uptake. (S.D. ± 0.58).

TABLE 6

PLASMA ERYTHROPOIETIN (EPF) LEVELS IN GONADECTOMIZED MALE RHESUS MONKEYS SUBJECTED TO HYPOTHALAMIC STIMULATION

Duration of Stimulation (Hours)*	Area Stimulated	Number of Animals	Number Positive for EPF	Number Negative for EPF
4	Supraoptic nucleus	2	—	2
8		2	—	2
4	Posterior median eminence	2	—	2
8		2	—	2

* Stimulation administered only once for 4 or 8 hours.

nucleus and posterior median eminence were stimulated. No significant increase in EPF levels was detected. It must be pointed out, however, that stimulation was carried out for four to eight hr on only one day, instead of on four successive days (TABLE 6).

Plasma which was collected from non-anemic monkeys with hypothalamic lesions in the areas of the posterior median eminence and the supraoptic nucleus failed to produce an increase in 24 hour ^{59}Fe uptake by the blood when assayed in polycythemic mice. Values were comparable with control values. Two monkeys with lesions in the posterior median eminence and with hematocrit values of 28% and 30% did not have significant levels of plasma EPF.

Rats. Weanling male rats weighing between 66 and 83 g were treated as follows: Electrolytic lesions were made in the hypothalamus in (1) the supraoptic nucleus, (2) the ventromedial nucleus, (3) the dorsomedial nucleus and (4) the mammillary nucleus. Sham-operated rats served as controls (TABLE 7).

Adult rats of the same strain and sex, but weighing between 268 and 337 g, were grouped and treated similarly (TABLE 8).

The hypothalamic lesions were placed with a Horsley-Clarke Stereotaxic instrument (Baltimore Instrument Co.) using a Spar varnish-coated stainless steel electrode of 0.25 mm diameter, from the bared tip of which an anodal current of 1.5 ma was allowed to flow for 10 seconds. The coordinates used for placing the electrodes were those mapped by Bernardis and Skelton.[31] The sham-operated animals were similarly treated except for electrical stimulation.

The rats were accommodated in single cages in a room kept at 74° F and given tap water and lab chow ad libitum. Two weeks following the hypothalamic opera-

TABLE 7

EFFECTS OF LOW OXYGEN ATMOSPHERE (10%) UPON PLASMA ERYTHROPOIETIN LEVELS IN HYPOTHALAMIC-LESIONED AND SHAM-OPERATED YOUNG RATS

Pooled Plasmas from Rats with Lesions at the Site of:		Percent 24 hr Blood ^{59}Fe Uptake in Polycythemic Mice
		S.D.**
(A)	(1) Supraoptic nucleus*	4.03 ± 1.5
	(2) Ventromedial nucleus	3.05 ± 1.5
	(3) Dorsomedial nucleus	0.77 ± —
	(4) Mammillary nucleus	0.50 ± 0.20
(B)	Sham controls	1.45 ± 0.72

* Approximately in the vicinity.
** S.D. = Standard Deviation.

tion, they were subjected to low oxygen atmosphere (10%) for 36 hr, after which they were anesthetized with ether, exsanguinated and their plasma collected for assay in polycythemic mice. The brains were removed, trimmed, weighed, and placed in 10% formalin; after several weeks, they were prepared for localization of hypothalamic lesions as described in the atlas of Groot.[32] Only rats with perfectly situated lesions were included in the tabulation of results; rats with asymmetrical lesions were grouped separately.

TABLE 7 shows the results of hypothalamic-lesioned and sham-operated young rats exposed to low oxygen atmosphere (10%). Rats with lesions in the dorsomedial and mammillary nuclei did not produce detectable EPF under hypoxia, whereas rats with lesions in the supraoptic and ventromedial nuclei did.

Adult rats with lesions in the mammillary nucleus, like young rats, did not produce EPF under hypoxia (TABLE 8). Unlike the young rats, however, adult rats with lesions in the supraoptic or ventromedial nuclei showed some decrease in ability to produce erythropoietin in low oxygen atmosphere (TABLE 8).

Stimulation of the hypothalamus in the area of the ventromedial nucleus in adult rats has failed to produce detectable levels of plasma EPF to date (TABLE 9). Further studies on the effects of stimulation of other areas of the hypothalamus are in progress and await confirmation of localization of the lesions and plasma assays.

Studies on the role of the central nervous system in the regulation of erythropoiesis are admittedly difficult to interpret because stimulation of the hypothalamus, or lesions made in the hypothalamus, can induce reactions in experimental animals which may have a secondary effect on erythropoiesis. This is particularly serious when changes in the hemoglobin, RBC or hematocrit levels are used as parameters since it is known that pronounced plasma volume alterations do occur when one interferes with the hypothalamic-pituitary axis. Realizing this state of affairs, Halvorsen's studies in rabbits[19–21] and ours in monkeys,[33] as well as those in this report, reveal increases in plasma EPF levels following stimulation of the hypothalamus. Seip *et al.*[23] also noted an increase in reticulocytes and red cell mass in 8 out of 28 rabbits following stimulation of the hypothalamus. Lesions in the hypothalamus have impaired the ability of animals to produce erythropoietin under hypoxia. This has been borne out by our studies and those by Baciu *et al.*[34] in the rat, as well as by studies by Halvorsen[21]

TABLE 8

EFFECTS OF LOW OXYGEN ATMOSPHERE (10%) UPON PLASMA ERYTHROPOIETIN LEVELS IN HYPOTHALAMIC-LESIONED AND SHAM-OPERATED ADULT RATS

Pooled Plasmas from Rats with Lesions at the Site of:		Percent 24 hr Blood ^{59}Fe Uptake in Polycythemic Mice
		S.D.**
(A)	(1) Supraoptic nucleus	1.18 ± 0.23
	(2) Supraoptic nucleus*	0.50 ± 0.13
	(3) Ventromedial nucleus	1.80 ± 0.39
	(4) Ventromedial nucleus*	1.01 ± 0.04
	(5) Mammillary nucleus	0.64 ± 0.12
	(6) Mammillary nucleus*	0.18 ± 0.09
(B)	Sham controls	4.14 ± 0.55
(C)	Nonsham controls	3.98 ± 0.24

* Approximately in the vicinity.
** S.D. = Standard Deviation.

TABLE 9

PLASMA ERYTHROPOIETIN LEVELS IN ADULT RATS SUBJECTED TO HYPOTHALAMIC STIMULATION IN THE AREA OF THE VENTROMEDIAL NUCLEUS

Animals	Duration of Stimulation (Minutes)	Percent 24 hr Blood ^{59}Fe Uptake in Polycythemic Mice
		S.D.*
(A) Experimental	5	0.59 ± —
	15	0.45 ± 0.11
	30	0.47 ± 0.13
	60	0.64 ± 0.48
(B) Sham controls	15	0.84 ± 0.34
	30 and 60	0.67 ± 0.12

* S.D. = Standard Deviation.

and Hollan[16] and Linke[35] in the rabbit. In Halvorsen's studies with rabbits, lesions in the middle and ventral hypothalamus reduced the reticulocyte response to hypoxia but the usual hypoxic response was obtained when ACTH was given prior to repeated exposure to hypoxia. Also, he found that lesions in the posterior hypothalamus reduced the response to hypoxia, and the usual hypoxic response was not obtained when pituitary hormones were given prior to repeated exposure to hypoxia. By contrast, lesions to the anterior hypothalamus did not reduce the reticulocyte response to hypoxia. Baciu *et al.*[34] found reduced erythropoietic response to hypoxia in rats with lesions in the anterior hypothalamus. Their results are in contrast with Halvorsen's. However, one must keep in mind the size of the lesion[22] and species[36] and age differences,[37] in relating any specific area to the hypothalamic control of hormones. Piliero *et al.*[24,25] studied the influence of long-term hypoxia upon erythropoiesis in hypothalamic-lesioned rats, and found that there was no derangement in the response to hypoxia. The lesions in their series appeared to be small and this might account for their negative results. From our studies and those mentioned above, both the ablation and the stimulation experiments indicate that the hypothalamus plays a prominent role in the regulation of erythropoiesis.

The question remains as to how the hypothalamus exerts its influence on erythropoiesis. There are three possible pathways by which the hypothalamic area may exert its control on erythropoiesis: (1) through specific nervous or humoral stimuli affecting erythropoietin-producing target organ(s) directly or indirectly; (2) through the hypothalamus, causing release of pituitary secretions which have been reported to have either a primary or a secondary influence on erythropoiesis (thyroxin,[38] androgens,[27,30,39–41] growth hormone,[42–44] and prolactin[45] have been found to stimulate erythropoiesis and/or erythropoietin production, or to interact with erythropoietin in an additive manner[30,46]); and (3) through the autonomic nervous system. Hypothalamic stimulation or lesions interfere with the function of the autonomic nervous system; both may influence the cardio-pulmonary function and induce hypoxemia and, also, both may affect renal circulation and therefore, affect erythropoietin production. Trueta[47] caused a severe and transient renal vasoconstriction by electrical stimulation of the splanchnic nerves and Gomori *et al.*[48] showed that both cerebral and local regulatory mechanisms operate in the control of renal circulation. If Gomori's findings are confirmed, both renal and cerebral hypoxia may cause changes in renal circulation, which may account for the difference in erythropoietin production.

Takaku *et al.*[49] reported that bilateral resection of the splanchnic nerves in rats markedly inhibited the reticulocytosis and elevation of plasma EPF levels following hemorrhage. Also, bilateral splanchnic nerve resection reduces renal blood flow. The findings of Mirand *et al.*[50] and Murphy *et al.*[51] on the alterations in erythropoietin activity in monkeys bearing ischemic and infarcted autotransplanted and homotransplanted kidneys appear to minimize Takaku's idea that the splanchnic nerves influence erythropoietin production through a regulatory influence on renal blood flow. Neither do the studies of Baciu *et al.*[52] on transplanted kidneys in the dog provide support for Takaku's concept. However, one cannot rule out conclusively the role of the splanchnic nerves, for any impairment of the nervous system might call upon other mechanisms to release erythropoietin from the site(s) of production.

The mechanism by which the hypothalamus exerts its influence on erythropoietin production and erythropoiesis is not understood by us at present. However, merely as a working hypothesis, we feel, as does Halvorsen,[22] that there may be a specific group of cells located in various areas of the hypothalamus capable of monitoring variations in oxygen tension; stimulation of the kidney and other target organ(s) by nervous and/or humoral routes then results in erythropoietin production. Since we are inclined to favor a humoral route, the hypothalamus may directly affect erythropoietin-producing organ(s) by putting out a hypothalamic erythropoietin-releasing factor, ERF. This ERF factor would then directly signal erythropoietin-producing cells in target organ(s) to manufacture EPF. We feel that the effect of ERF from the hypothalamus might be direct since stimulation of the posterior median eminence in a hypophysectomized monkey resulted in the release of a high level of plasma EPF.

Hypothalamic-releasing factors have been reported for ACTH,[53,54] TSH,[55] LH,[54] FSH[56] and growth hormone.[57] FSH-releasing factor, reported by Igarashi and McCann,[58] appears to be present in the rat stalk median eminence complex, and to be a small peptide[29,59] which differs from vasopressin and corticotrophin-releasing factor.[59]

Reissmann and Nomura,[60] as well as others, have shown erythropoietin formation in isolated kidneys and liver. This might be regarded as evidence against the central nervous system playing a role in the regulation of erythropoietin production; however, this does not necessarily mean that under physiological conditions the kidney and other erythropoietin target organs are not under the control of the hypothalamus by an erythropoietin-releasing factor.

Although the exact mechanism(s) by which the hypothalamus controls erythropoietin production and erythropoiesis has not been substantiated by facts, one cannot ignore the findings reported herein on the role of the central nervous system in regulating erythropoiesis.[13–22,33,64] As stated too by Halvorsen,[22] future studies are needed, using differential ablation of various areas of kidney and using hypophysectomized and/or nephrectomized animals, with simultaneous recordings of arterial oxygen saturation, oxygen tension, and blood flow in the target organs to determine the mechanism(s) by which the hypothalamus exerts its influence on erythropoiesis. In addition, hypothalamic extracts should be studied in vitro and in vivo to determine the existence of hypothalamic erythropoietin-releasing factor, as proposed in this communication.

Erythropoietin-Like Activity in Patients with Renal Abnormalities

Patients with secondary polycythemia as the result of renal abnormalities have been shown in some instances to possess high levels of EPF in their plasma. Patients with hydronephrosis and multiple renal cysts, carcinoma of the kidney, and also lung cancer, show high levels of plasma EPF (TABLE 10). Plasma EPF levels are decreased following removal of carcinoma of the kidney. Patients with cystic kidneys may have high levels of EPF in the plasma, urine, and cystic fluid or may have an enormous amount of EPF in the cystic fluid without having a high level of EPF in the plasma (23.25% ^{59}Fe uptake in the cystic fluid, 0.49% in the plasma) (TABLE 11).

Young children with Wilms' tumors have been shown to have high levels of erythropoietin activity in the plasma but not in the urine, and EPF levels are decreased following removal of the tumor (TABLE 12).

Since we have seen that patients with carcinoma of the kidney sometimes have high levels of plasma EPF, similar studies were carried out in rats with experimentally-induced renal carcinoma. Rats given single injections of a small amount of dimethylnitrosamine develop renal adenocarcinoma. These tumor-bearing rats, which are not anemic, show significant elevation of plasma EPF (TABLE 13). This

TABLE 10

PLASMA ERYTHROPOIETIN IN PATIENTS WITH RENAL ABNORMALITIES

Sex	Age	Diagnosis	Hematocrit	Percent 24 hr Blood ^{59}Fe Uptake in Polycythemic Mice: Healthy Control	Patient studied: Preoperative	Patient studied: Postoperative
1. Female	58	Hydronephrosis and multiple cysts	58	0.35	1.56	—
2. Male	61	Bilateral hydronephrosis and lung cancer	61	0.41	3.14	—
3. Male	52	Carcinoma of kidney	66	0.52	7.41	0.68 (7) *
4. Male	58	Hydronephrosis and multiple cysts	78	0.29	3.09	—
5. Male	62	Carcinoma of kidney and metastasis to lung	70	0.42	1.84	0.35 (21) *

* Number in ( ) means Postoperative day.

TABLE 11

ERYTHROPOIETIN ACTIVITY IN PATIENTS WITH CYSTIC KIDNEYS

Sex	Age	Hematocrit	Percent 24 hr Blood ^{59}Fe Uptake in Polycythemic Mice: Plasma	Urine	Cystic Fluid
1. Female	57				
Preoperative		66	1.88*	1.27	—
At operation		62	—	—	3.18
Postoperative (12 days)		41	0.43*	0.47	—
2. Male	62				
Preoperative		43	0.38	—	—
At operation		41	—	—	3.29
Postoperative (3 days)		39	0.35	—	—
Postoperative (8 days)		38	0.23	—	—
3. Male					
Preoperative			0.49	—	—
At operation			—	—	23.25

* Deproteinized.

TABLE 12

PLASMA ERYTHROPOIETIN IN PATIENTS WITH WILMS' TUMORS

Sex	Age	Hematocrit	Percent 24 hr Blood ^{59}Fe Uptake in Polycythemic Mice		
			Healthy Control	Patient Studied	
				Preoperative	Postoperative
1. Female	3	40	0.25	1.79	0.49 (3) *
2. Male	3	39	0.33	4.97	0.38 (5) *
3. Male	5	35	0.28	0.64	—
4. Female	5	36	0.34	1.39	0.37 (10) *

* Number in ( ) means Postoperative day. Note: No erythropoietin activity found in urine.

TABLE 13

PLASMA ERYTHROPOIETIN IN NONANEMIC RATS WITH DIMETHYLNITROSAMINE (DMN)-INDUCED RENAL ADENOCARCINOMAS

Pooled Plasmas	Percent 24 hr Blood ^{59}Fe Uptake in Polycythemic Mice
	S.D.*
(A) DMN-induced renal tumor rats at 14, 15, 16, 17 months	1.33 ± 0.19
(B) Control rats at 14, 15, 16, 17 months	0.31 ± 0.06

* S.D. = Standard Deviation.

TABLE 14

PLASMA ERYTHROPOIETIN IN PATIENTS WITH POLYCYTHEMIA VERA

Sex	Age	Hematocrit	Percent 24 hr Blood ^{59}Fe Uptake in Polycythemic Mice	
			Healthy Control	Patient Studied
1. Male	58	72	0.34	0.39 0.38*
2. Male	73	69	0.38	0.48
3. Male	66	73	0.35	0.41 0.38*
4. Male	49	78	0.29	0.35 0.41*
5. Male	59	71	0.37	0.34 0.28*

* Deproteinized.

experimental model could be useful for studying in greater detail some of the hemodynamic factors which regulate EPF production, and in explaining the role of the kidney, particularly in abnormal states, in this process.

These clinical findings support the existence of a relationship between the kidneys and the elaboration of erythropoietin-like substance. Similar findings have been reported by Lange and Gallagher,[6] Gurney,[61] Rosse *et al.*,[62] and many others. Of interest is the elevation of erythropoietin levels in association with Wilms' tumor and the decrease in erythropoietin levels that occurs following the removal of the primary tumor. This was also reported recently by Thurman *et al.*[63]

Polycythemia Vera

We have never been able to detect increased levels of EPF in the plasma and urine from patients with polycythemia vera. Most patients with secondary polycythemia do have high levels of EPF in the plasma and even in the urine. We have studied a number of patients during the past several years, and the data included in TABLE 14 are representative of our findings. Perhaps, through serial phlebotomies and a lowering of the hematocrit to normal or anemic levels, one can detect erythropoietin. Studies are in progress to determine this.

Summary

1. Both electrical stimulation of and injury to the hypothalamic complex affects the regulation of erythropoietin production in monkeys and in rats. How the hypothalamic complex exerts its influence on erythropoietin production is unknown; however, it is postulated that this might be done through specific nervous and/or humoral stimuli affecting erythropoietin-producing organs.

2. Erythropoietin-like activity in patients with renal abnormalities is presented. These findings further support the concept that the kidney is implicated in erythropoietin production.

Acknowledgments

We extend thanks to Drs. Gerald Murphy, Gerald Johnston, L. Bernardis, G. Owens and P. Trudel, and to Edmund Dywinski, Andres Bulba, Joyce Jividen, Ruth Deckert, Basilius Sywenkyj, A. G. Mirand, C. O'Leary, and W. Trudel for services rendered.

References

1. Jacobson, L., E. Goldwasser, W. Fried & L. Plzak. 1957. Role of the kidney in erythropoiesis. Nature **179:** 633–634.
2. Mirand, E. A. & T. C. Prentice. 1957. Presence of plasma erythropoietin in hypoxic rats with or without kidneys and/or spleen. Proc. Soc. Exp. Med. **96:** 49–51.
3. Mirand, E. A., T. C. Prentice & W. R. Slaunwhite. 1959. Current studies on the role of erythropoietin in erythropoiesis. Ann. N. Y. Acad. Sci. **77:** 677–702.
4. Gordon, A. S. 1959. Hemopoietine. Physiol. Rev. **39:** 1–40.
5. Erslev, A. 1960. Erythropoietic function in uremic rats. II. Effect of nephrectomy on red cell production and iron metabolism. Acta Haemat. **23:** 226–235.
6. Jacobson, L. O. 1962. Sites of formation of erythropoietin. *In* Erythropoiesis. L. O. Jacobson & M. Doyle, Eds. : 69–70. Grune & Stratton. New York, N. Y.
7. Lange, R. D. & N. I. Gallagher. 1962. Clinical and experimental observations on the relationship of the kidney to erythropoietin production. *In* Erythropoiesis. L. O. Jacobson & M. Doyle, Eds. : 361–373. Grune & Stratton. New York, N. Y.
8. Nathan, D. G., E. Scheipak, F. Stohlman, Jr. & F. Merrill. 1964. Erythropoiesis in anephric man. J. Clin. Invest. **43:** 2158–2164.
9. Van Dyke, D. 1959. The pituitary erythropoietic factor. Ann. N. Y. Acad. Sci. **77:** 543–550.
10. Burke, W. T. & B. S. Morse. 1962. Studies on the production and metabolism of erythropoietin in rat liver and kidney. *In* Erythropoiesis. L. O. Jacobson & M. Doyle, Eds. : 111–119. Grune & Stratton. New York, N. Y.
11. de Franciscis, P., G. de Bella & S. Cifaldi. 1965. Spleen as a production site for erythropoietin. Science **150:** 1831–1833.
12. Harris, G. W. 1948. Neural control of pituitary gland. Physiol. Rev. **28:** 139–179.
13. Beer, A. G. 1942. Über die nervös-humorale Regulation des Blutes. Folia haemat., Lpz. **66:** 222–298.
14. Seip, M. 1953. Reticulocyte Studies. Grundt Tanum. Oslo, Norway.
15. Komyia, E. 1956. Die zentralnervöse Regulation des Blutesbildes. Georg Thieme. Stuttgart, Germany.
16. Hollan, S. R. 1963. Über die neurale Regulation der Blutzellen. Folia haemat., Lpz. **80:** 138–152.
17. Remmele, W. 1963. Die humorale Steuerung der Erythropoiese. Springer. Berlin, Germany.

18. Baciu, L. 1964. Système nerveux et mécanismes humoraux dans la régulation de l'érythropoïèse. Rev. Rhum. **1**: 149–160.
19. Halvorsen, S. 1961. Plasma erythropoietin levels following hypothalamic stimulation in the rabbit. Scand. J. Clin. Lab. Invest. **13**: 564–575.
20. Halvorsen, S. 1963. Effects of ACTH on erythropoiesis in the rabbit. Acta Physiol. Scand. **58**: 30–39.
21. Halvorsen, S. 1964. Effects of hypothalamic lesions in the erythropoietic response to hypoxia in rabbits. Acta Physiol. Scand. **61**: 1–19.
22. Halvorsen, S. 1966. The central nervous system in regulation of erythropoiesis. Acta Haemat. **35**: 65–79.
23. Seip, M., S. Halvorsen, P. Anderson & B. R. Kaada. 1961. Effects of hypothalamic stimulation on erythropoiesis in rabbits. Scand. J. Clin. Lab. Invest. **13**: 553–563.
24. Piliero, S. J., P. T. Medici & A. Orr. 1962. Influence of hypoxic stimuli upon erythropoiesis in hypothalamic lesioned animals. Acta Haemat. **28**: 101–112.
25. Piliero, S. J., P. T. Medici & A. Orr. 1962. Influence of hypoxic stimuli upon erythropoiesis in hypothalamic-lesioned animals. *In* Erythropoiesis. L. O. Jacobson & M. Doyle, Eds. : 258–262. Grune & Stratton. New York, N. Y.
26. Snyder, R. S. & J. C. Lee. 1961. Stereotaxic Atlas of the Monkey Brain. University of Chicago Press. Chicago, Ill.
27. Mirand, E. A. 1965. Studies on erythropoietin in tamarins. Invest. Urol. **2**: 579–588.
28. Harris, C. W. 1964. The development of ideas regarding hypothalamic-releasing factors. Metabolism **13**: 1171–1175.
29. Guillemin, R. 1964. Hypothalamic polypeptides releasing pituitary hormones. Metabolism **13**: 1206–1210.
30. Mirand, E. A., A. S. Gordon & J. Wenig. 1965. Mechanism of testosterone action in erythropoiesis. Nature **206**: 270–272.
31. Bernardis, L. L. & F. R. Skelton. 1965. Stereotaxic localization of supraoptic, ventromedial and mammillary nuclei in the hypothalamus of weanling to mature rats. Amer. J. Anat. **116**: 69–74.
32. de Groot, J. 1959. The rat forebrain in stereotaxic coordinates. Verhandel. Kinil. Ed. Akad. Wetench., Afd. Natuurk LII, No. **4**: 1–40.
33. Mirand, E. A., J. T. Grace, G. S. Johnston & G. P. Murphy. 1964. Effects of hypothalamic stimulation on the erythropoietic response in the rhesus monkey. Nature **204**: 1163–1165.
34. Baciu, I., V. Soltuz, N. Stoica & N. Radigan. 1964. Localisation dans l'hypothalamus des centres régulateurs de l'érythropoïèse. Proc. Xth Congr. int. Soc. Haemat., Stockholm. M 28.
35. Linke, P. G. 1958. Zentralnervöse Regulierung der Retikulocytenzahl im peripherem Blut. Folia haemat., Lpz. **76**: 282–290.
36. Kragt, C. & J. Meites. 1965. Stimulation of pigeon prolactin release by pigeon hypothalamic extract in vitro. Endocrinol. **76**: 1169–1176.
37. Pecile, A., E. Güller, G. Falconi & L. Martini. 1965. Growth hormone-releasing activity of hypothalamic extracts at different ages. Endocrinol. **77**: 241–246.
38. Meineke, H. A. & R. C. Crafts. 1964. Evidence for a noncalorigenic effect of thyroxin on erythropoiesis as judged by radioiron utilization. Proc. Soc. Exp. Med. **117**: 520–524.
39. Mirand, E. A. & A. S. Gordon. 1966. Mechanism of estrogen action in erythropoiesis. Endocrinol. **78**: 325–332.
40. Fried, W. R., R. de Gowin & C. W. Gurney. 1964. Erythropoietic effect of testosterone in the polycythemic mouse. Proc. Soc. Exp. Med. **117**: 839–842.
41. Naets, J. P. & M. Wittek. 1966. Mechanism of action of androgens on erythropoiesis. Amer. J. Physiol. **210**: 315–320.
42. Halvorsen, S. In press. Effects of growth hormone on erythropoiesis in the intact rabbit and polycythemic mouse. Acta Physiol. Scand.
43. Fisher, J. W., B. L. Roh, C. Couch & W. D. Nightingale. 1964. Influence of cobalt, sheep erythropoietin and several hormones on erythropoiesis in bone marrows of isolated perfused hind limbs of dogs. Blood **23**: 87–98.
44. Crafts, R. C. & H. A. Meineke. 1959. The anemia of hypophysectomized animals. Ann. N. Y. Acad. Sci. **77**: 501–517.
45. Jepson, J. H. & L. Lowenstein. 1964. Effect of prolactin on erythropoiesis in the mouse. Blood **24**: 726–738.
46. Evans, E. S., D. C. Van Dyke & L. L. Rosenberg. 1964. Interaction of the ESF with calorigenic hormones. Endocrinol. **75**: 758–764.
47. Trueta, J. 1947. Studies of the Renal Circulation. C. C. Thomas. Springfield, Ill.

48. GOMORI, P., A. G. KOVÁCH, T. M. TÁKACS, M. FOLDI, G. SZABO, Z. NAGY & W. WILTNER. 1960. The control of renal circulation in hypoxia. Acta Med. hung. **16:** 43–60.
49. TAKAKU, F., K. HIROSHIMA & S. OKINAKA. 1962. Studies on the mechanism of erythropoietin production. II. Effect of bilateral section of the splanchnic nerve. J. Lab. Clin. Med. **59:** 821–825.
50. MIRAND, E. A., G. S. JOHNSTON, H.-J. HUSER & G. MURPHY. 1965. Renal transplantation in the rhesus monkey. V. Alteration in erythropoietin activity. Invest. Urol. **2:** 574–577.
51. MURPHY, G. P., E. C. MELBY, E. A. MIRAND, H.-J. HUSER & C. S. WELDON. 1965. Renal transplantation in the rhesus monkey. VI. Observations in homotransplanted animals. Invest. Urol. **3:** 245–267.
52. BACIU, I., C. OPRISIU, M. DOROFTIEU, E. ROSENFELD, M. RUSU & C. CHEREBETEIU. 1963. Le rein et la production de l'érythropoïétine. J. Physiol. Paris. **55:** 557–567.
53. VERNIKOS-DANELLIS, J. 1964. Estimation of corticotrophin-releasing activity of rat hypothalamus and neurohypophysis before and after stress. Endocrinol. **75:** 514–520.
54. MCCANN, S. M., A. V. SCHALLY, R. NALLAR & C. Y. BOWERS. 1964. Evidence for separate corticotrophin and luteinizing hormone-releasing factors in hypothalamic extracts. Proc. Soc. Exp. Med. **117:** 435–437.
55. DUCOMMUN, P., E. SAKÍZ & R. GUILLEMIN. 1965. Increase of plasma TSH concentration following injection of purified hypothalamic TRF. Endocrinol. **77:** 792–796.
56. KUROSHIMA, A., Y. ISHIDA, C. BOWERS & H. SCHALLY. 1965. Stimulation of release of follicle-stimulating hormone by hypothalamic extracts in vitro and in vivo. Endocrinol. **76:** 614–619.
57. SCHALLY, H. V., S. L. STEELMAN & C. Y. BOWERS. 1965. Effect of hypothalamic extracts on release of growth hormone in vitro. Proc. Soc. Exp. Med. **119:** 208–212.
58. IGARASHI, M. & S. M. MCCANN. 1964. A new sensitive bioassay for follicle-stimulating hormone (FSH). Endocrinol. **74:** 440–445.
59. IGARASHI, M., R. NALLAR, V. D. RAMIREZ & S. M. MCCANN. 1964. Purification of hypothalamic gonadotrophin-releasing factors by gel filtration sephadex. Fed. Proc. **23:** 151.
60. REISSMANN, K. R. & T. NOMURA. 1962. Erythropoietin formation in isolated kidneys and liver. *In* Erythropoiesis. L. O. Jacobson & M. Doyle, Eds. : 71–77. Grune & Stratton. New York, N. Y.
61. GURNEY, C. W. 1962. Relationship of erythropoietin production to renal abnormalities. *In* Erythropoiesis. L. O. Jacobson & M. Doyle, Eds. : 359–360. Grune & Stratton. New York, N. Y.
62. ROSSE, W. F., T. A. WALDMANN & P. COHEN. 1963. Renal cysts, erythropoietin and polycythemia. Amer. J. Med. **34:** 76–81.
63. THURMAN, W. G., H. GRABSTOLD & P. H. LIEBERMAN. 1966. Elevation of erythropoietin levels in association with Wilms' tumor. Arch. Intern. Med. **117:** 280–283.
64. FELDMAN, S., A. RACHMILEWITZ & G. IZAK. 1966. The effect of central nervous system stimulation on erythropoiesis in rats with chronically implanted electrodes. J. Lab. & Clin. Med. **67:** 713–725.

ERYTHROCYTOSIS, JUXTAGLOMERULAR APPARATUS (JGA), AND ERYTHROPOIETIN IN THE COURSE OF EXPERIMENTAL UNILATERAL HYDRONEPHROSIS IN RABBITS*

W. J. Mitus, Keisuke Toyama and Mark J. Brauer

Blood Research Laboratory, New England Medical Center Hospitals, and Tufts University School of Medicine, Boston, Mass.

Experimentally induced unilateral hydronephrosis leads to erythrocytosis in approximately 60 percent of rabbits. Erythrocytosis usually appears between the 35th and 67th postoperative day, lasts a variable period of time and eventually subsides.[1] Our recent experiments have shown that the development of erythrocytosis is closely related to the degree of hydronephrotic pressure.[2] Animals with hydronephrotic pressure of up to 330 mm of H_2O develop erythrocytosia while animals with pressures of over 340 mm H_2O do not. Periodic removals of urine from the hydronephrotic kidney with resulting decrease of pressure was associated with the development of erythrocytosis in a high percentage of animals. It would appear that periodic release of pressure protected renal parenchyma from pressure atrophy. While nonerythrocytotic animals had invariably marked atrophy of renal tissue, erythrocytotic animals showed only moderate narrowing of renal parenchyma.

Studies of Osnes,[3] Hirashima and Takaku,[4] Oliver and Brody,[5] Demopoulas *et al.*,[6] as well as our own,[7] suggested the association of juxtaglomerular apparatus (JGA) with the regulation of erythropoiesis, but Goldfarb and Tobian[8,9] did not find any correlation between the two. The purpose of our present study was to correlate serially the development of erythrocytosis with changes in the granularity of the juxtaglomerular apparatus and with the plasma erythropoietin levels in the rabbits with unilateral hydronephrosis.

Materials and Methods

The left ureter was ligated using a previously described method[1] in 68 male adult New Zealand rabbits. Hematologic studies, including hemoglobin (Hb), micro-hematocrit and reticulocyte count, were done at weekly intervals. Blood volume studies using the ^{51}Cr method were performed in all animals at the beginning of the experiment and again just prior to sacrificing. Rabbits were sacrificed in groups of four to ten animals at 5- or 10-day intervals following operation, the kidneys were removed, weighed and measured and stained with hematoxlin and eosin, PAS and Bowie's stain for granules of the juxtaglomerular apparatus.[10] The index of granularity was estimated by the method of Hartroft and Hartroft.[11] Plasma was separated from the cells by centrifugation and frozen for subsequent erythropoietin studies. Erythropoietin bioassay was performed in 15 plasmas from rabbits at various stages according to the method of De Gowin *et al.*[12] 0.5 ml of plasma was injected subcutaneously into assay animals. Post-mortem renal angiography using barium sulfate (micropaque) at the pressure of 120 cm H_2O was done in seven animals. Blood pressure was measured in the central artery of the ear in eight normal and nine hydronephrotic rabbits. Blood urea nitrogen (BUN), Na, K and Cl were measured in 11 normal and 12 hydronephrotic animals.

Results

FIGURE 1 shows mean hemoglobin levels and mean JGA indices in the course of unilateral hydronephrosis in 68 rabbits. There is a distinct rise of hemoglobin

* Aided by grant no. CA 04168 from the National Cancer Institute.

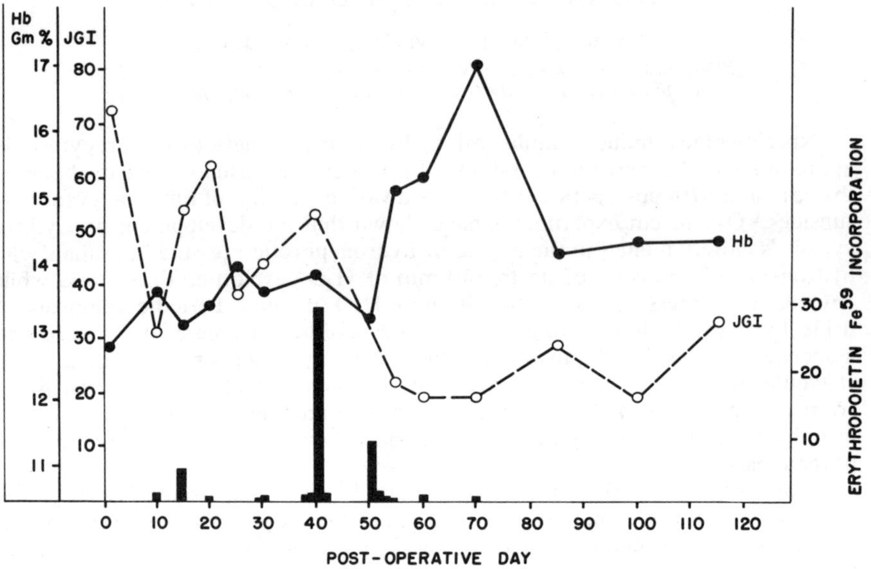

FIGURE 1. Means of hemoglobin, JGA index of granularity and individual plasma erythropoietin levels in the course of unilateral hydronephrosis in rabbits.

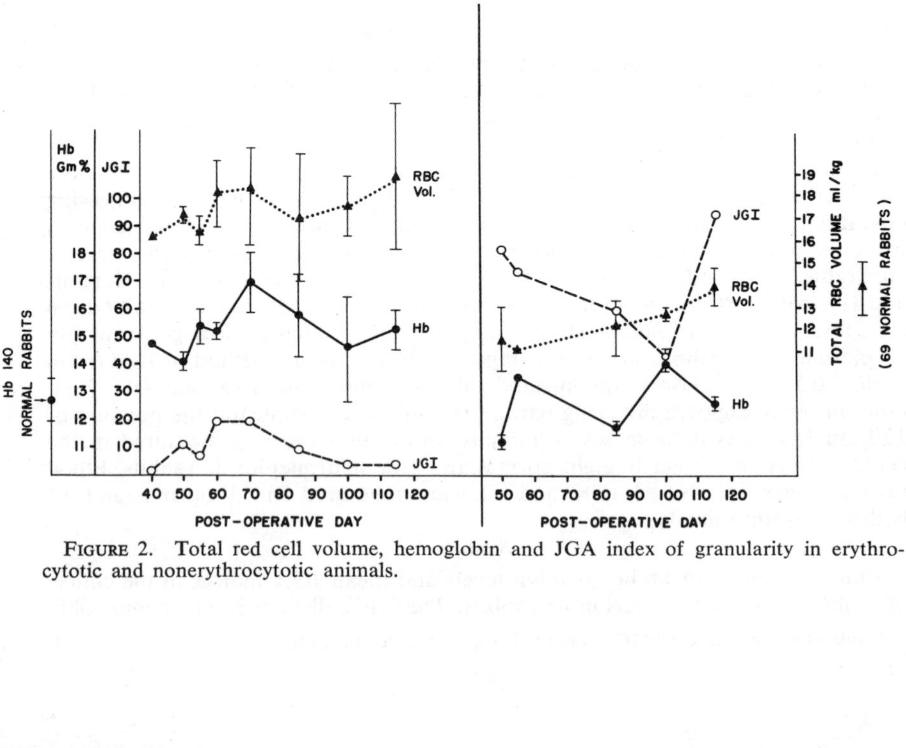

FIGURE 2. Total red cell volume, hemoglobin and JGA index of granularity in erythrocytotic and nonerythrocytotic animals.

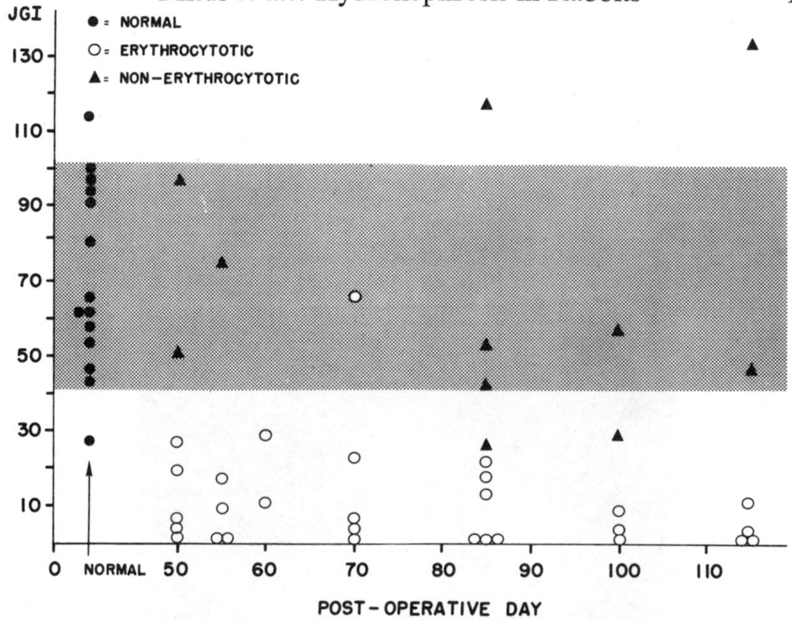

FIGURE 3. Individual indeces of JGA granularity in erythrocytotic and nonerythrocytotic rabbits.

mean between the 50th and 60th postoperative day reaching a peak of 17 g% at the 70th day. Normal hemoglobin values in 140 rabbits is 12.8 ± SD 0.7. The JGA index of granularity shows an inverse relationship with the hemoglobin levels. At the time when the hemoglobin level becomes elevated, the JGA index falls to below normal levels, but subsequently, as the hemoglobin returns to normal, it rises again.

FIGURE 2 shows hemoglobin, total red cell volume and JGA indices in animals which developed erythrocytosis and in those which did not. In the erythrocytotic animals the indices of granularity of JGA are low, while in nonerythrocytotic animals they are within normal range.

FIGURE 3 demonstrates individual JGA indices. All except one of the erythrocytotic animals have low JGA indices while all except two nonerythrocytotic animals have normal or high indices. These two animals have levels which are just below normal range. The mean for 29 erythrocytotic animals is 10.3 with a range of 0–66. The mean for 11 nonerythrocytotic animals is 68.2 with a range of 25–144.

Plasma erythropoietin levels in 15 rabbits are shown in FIGURE 1. There is a distinct elevation of 29% and 8.8% of ^{59}Fe incorporation into RBC in two of the animals between the 40th and 50th postoperative day and a smaller elevation of 4.9% at the 15th postoperative day. A normal value of 15 animals in the present study is 0.76 + st. dev. 0.3. Renal angiography (FIGURES 4A & B) shows a distinct decrease of vascularity of the hydronephrotic kidney which is most pronounced in the cortex.

Arterial blood pressure in normal and hydronephrotic animals is shown in TABLE 1. There is no significant difference between these two groups. BUN, creatinine, and electrolytes are shown in TABLE 2. There is a slight increase of BUN and creatinine in hydronephrotic animals but Na, K and Cl are within normal range.

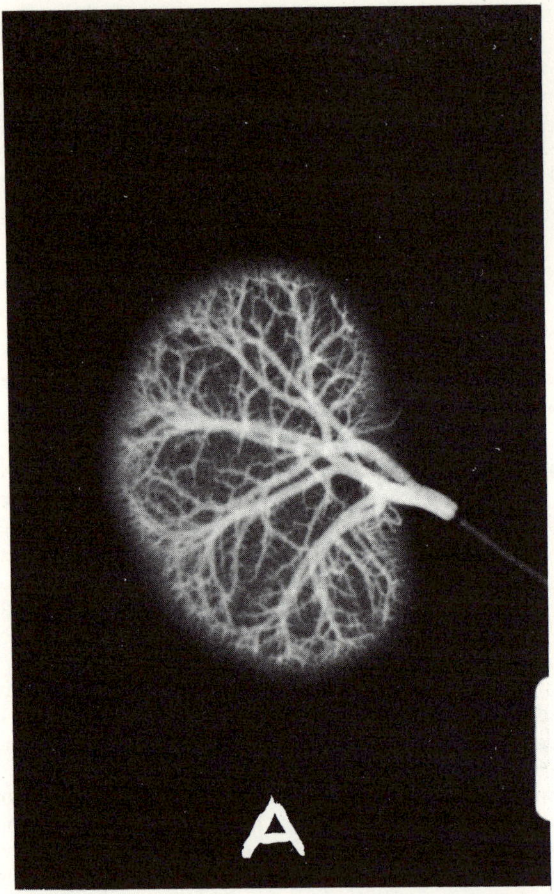

FIGURE 4A. Angiography of normal rabbit kidney.

TABLE 1

ARTERIAL BLOOD PRESSURE IN NORMAL AND HYDRONEPHROTIC RABBITS

	Normal (Eight animals)	Hydronephrosis	
		Erythrocytosis (Five animals)	No Erythrocytosis (Four animals)
	119.7 mm H_2O	117.5 mm H_2O	117.5 mm H_2O
Range	(105.5–128.5)	(105.0–128.5)	(108.5–129.0)

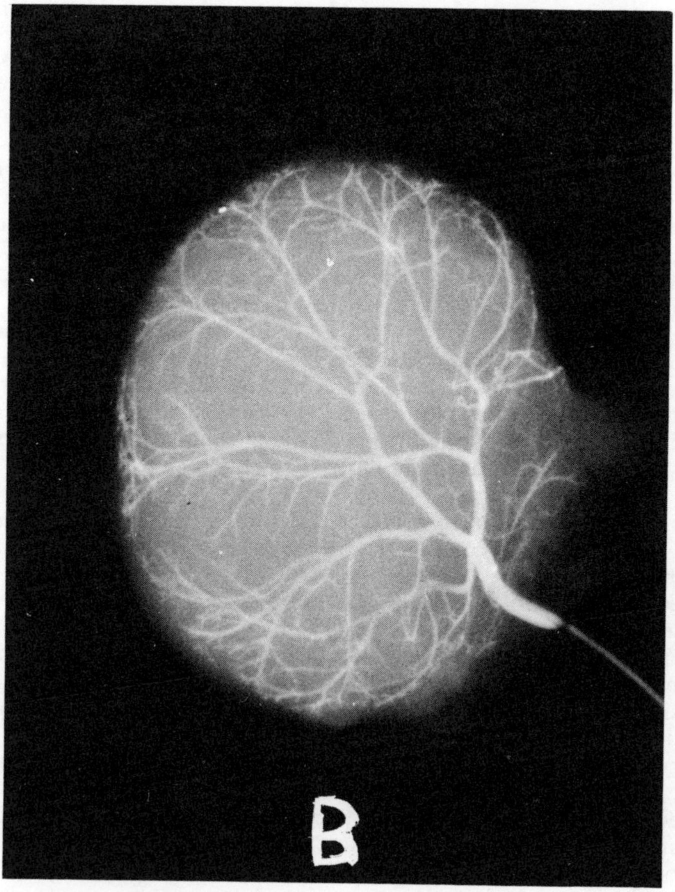

FIGURE 4B. Hydronephrotic rabbit kidney.

TABLE 2

SODIUM, POTASSIUM, CHLORIDE, BLOOD UREA NITROGEN (BUN) AND CREATININE LEVELS IN PLASMA OF NORMAL AND HYDRONEPHROTIC RABBITS

	Normal Eleven Animals	Erythrocytosis Five Animals	Nonerythrocytosis Seven Animals
Na, mEq/l	144 ± 5	141 ± 3	145 ± 2
K, mEq/l	4.7 ± 0.5	4.7 ± 0.9	4.5 ± 0.9
Cl, mEq/l	101 ± 4	101 ± 3	102 ± 2
BUN, mg %	19 ± 4	22 ± 3	25 ± 5
Creatinine, mg %	1.1 ± 0.2 (Four animals)	1.5 ± 0.1	1.4 ± 0.3

Discussion

Changes which occur in the course of unilateral hydronephrosis can be conveniently discussed in three periods, the preerythrocytotic, erythrocytotic and posterythrocytotic. Following the ligation of ureter approximately 40–50 days elapse before a mean of hemoglobin and of total red cell volume shows an elevation. During this preerythrocytotic period distinct elevation of plasma erythropoietin levels was found in some of the animals. Elevations were most marked just prior to the development of erythrocytosis. In view of previous studies which showed relationship between the increased erythropoietic activity and increased granularity of the JGA[4–6] one would expect an increase of granularity of the JGA during the preerythrocytotic phase. However, in our study, no such increase was detected. It is possible that a rather wide range of normality for JGA indices did not permit more subtle elevations to be noted.

In the erythrocytotic phase, erythropoietin levels were within normal range, but the JGA index of granularity showed a distinct decrease. The state of erythrocytosis is known to decrease erythropoietic activity. In our erythrocytotic animals this was associated with a low JGA index of granularity, indicating that the two findings are related. On the other hand the animals which did not develop erythrocytosis and in whom erythropoietic activity was proceeding at a normal pace had normal JGA indices.

In the posterythrocytotic phase when Hb and total red cell volume levels returned to normal, the JGA index also became normal, again suggesting close relationship.

Changes in the granularity of the JGA were previously reported in association with changes in the blood pressure[13] and in changes in the electrolites and most notably in sodium levels.[11,14] In our animals gross changes in the blood pressure or sodium levels could be excluded. Thus, the changes observed in the granularity of the JGA were most likely related to the variations in the hematologic status of the animals.

Changes which occur in the hydronephrotic kidney and most notably, vascular changes, lead to ischemia and hypoxia of renal tissue. Hypoxia causes stimulation of the secretion of the erythropoietic principle and results in increased erythropoiesis and erythrocytosis. Variations of granularity of the JGA which occur in the course of hydronephrosis suggest strongly that this organ plays a role in this mechanism of erythrocytosis.

References

1. Mitus, W. J., P. Galbraith, M. Gollerkeri & K. Toyama. 1964. Experimental renal erythrocytosis. I. Effects of pressure and vascular interference. Blood **24:** 343–355.
2. Toyama, K. & W. J. Mitus. 1966. Experimental renal erythrocytosis. III. Relationship between pressure and production of erythrocytosis. J. Lab. Clin. Med. **68:** 740.
3. Osnes, S. 1958. An erythropoietic factor produced in the kidney. Brit. Med. J. **2:** 1387.
4. Hirashima, K. & F. Takaku. 1962. Experimental studies on erythropoietin. II. The relationship between juxtaglomerular cells and erythropoietin. Blood **20:** 1–8.
5. Oliver, W. J. & G. L. Brody. 1965. Effect of prolonged hypoxia upon granularity of renal juxtaglomerular cells. Circulation Res. **16:** 83–88.
6. Demopoulos, H. B., B. Highman, P. D. Altland, M. A. Gerving & G. Kaley. 1965. Effects of high altitude on granular juxtaglomerular cells and their possible role in erythropoietin production. Amer. J. Path. **46:** 497–509.
7. Mitus, W. J. & K. Toyama. 1965. Experimental renal erythrocytosis. Role of the juxtaglomerular apparatus. Arch. Pathol. **78:** 658–664.
8. Goldfarb, B. & L. Tobian. 1962. The interrelationship of hypoxia, erythropoietin, and the renal juxtaglomerular cell. Proc. Soc. Exper. Biol. Med. **111:** 510–511.

9. GOLDFARB, B. & L. TOBIAN. 1963. Effect of high oxygen concentrations on erythropoietin and the renal juxtaglomerular cell. Proc. Soc. Exper. Biol. Med. **113**: 35–36.
10. PITCOCK, J. A. & P. M. HARTROFT. 1958. The juxtaglomerular cells in man and their relationship to the level of plasma sodium and to the zona glomerulosa of the adrenal cortex. Amer. J. Path. **34**: 863–873.
11. HARTROFT, P. M. & W. S. HARTROFT. 1953. Studies on renal juxtaglomerular cells. I. Variations produced by sodium chloride and desoxycorterone acetate. J. Exper. Med. **97**: 415–427.
12. DE GOWIN, R. L., D. HOFSTRA & C. W. GURNEY. 1962. The months with hypoxia-induced erythremia, an erythropoietin bioassay animal. J. Lab. Clin Med. **60**: 846-852.
13. TOBIAN, L., J. LANECK & A. TOMBOULIAN. 1959. Correlation between granulation of juxtaglomerular cells and extractable renin in rats with experimental hypertension. Proc. Soc. Exper. Biol. Med. **100**: 94–96.
14. HARTROFT, P. M. 1952. Effect of a depressor and a pressor substance on renal juxtaglomerular cells and blood pressure in rats fed varying amounts of sodium chloride. Anat. Rec. **115**: 319 (Abtract).

THE RENAL ERYTHROPOIETIC FACTOR. I. STUDIES ON ITS PURIFICATION AND PROPERTIES*

Joseph F. Contrera and Albert S. Gordon

Department of Biology, Graduate School of Arts and Science, New York University, New York, N. Y.

The extraction of erythropoietin (erythropoiesis-stimulating factor or ESF) from the kidneys of hypoxic and anemic rats with hypotonic phosphate buffer at pH 6.8 has recently been reported.[1] Such extracts possessed more erythropoietic activity than could be accounted for by that determined to be present in residual trapped plasma. We have recently developed a two-step extraction procedure in which most residual plasma is separated from particulate-bound erythropoietic material.[2,3] This method resulted in a hypotonic extract with a specific activity roughly twice that obtained with the one-step method. Incubation of the two-step hypotonic extract with an equal volume of normal rat serum was attended by a two-to-three-fold increase in erythropoietic activity.

Subcellular fractionation by differential centrifugation of kidneys of hypoxic rats revealed that the extract of the light mitochondrial fraction contained material which had little or no activity when injected intraperitoneally into assay mice. Upon incubating this light mitochondrial extract (LME) with an equal volume of normal rat serum for 30 min, significant erythropoiesis-stimulating activity appeared in the incubation mixture.[2,3] It was postulated that a renal erythropoietic factor (REF) was present in extracts obtained from a particulate fraction of the kidney which has the ability to produce the ESF or become erythropoietically active in the presence of normal serum.

Kuratowska *et al.*[4] have reported a factor from saline-perfused, isolated anoxic kidneys which engendered erythropoietic activity when added to normal serum. In a more recent report,[5] the factor was stated to be present in the nuclear fraction of the kidney. The methods used by Kuratowska[5] differed considerably from those used in the present study. In the centrifugation scheme that she employed, the light mitochondrial fraction was not collected, and it would be expected that the lysosomes present in this fraction would be present as contaminants in both the mitochondrial and microsomal fractions.[6] Incubation of these latter fractions for relatively long periods (two hr) would result in the release of lysosomal contents and the degradation of the active material contained within the fractions. The present report indicates that the REF is inactivated by proteolytic enzymes present in the lysosomes during extended periods of incubation. The method employed by Kuratowska would therefore not detect REF present in fractions containing lysosomal contamination.

Another difference is that Kuratowska employed intact particles, whereas we incubated extracts of the subcellular particles. Extracts of the nuclear fraction of kidneys of hypoxic rats showed no ESF or REF activity in our hands.

The present study is concerned with the purification of the REF present in the light mitochondrial extract (LME) and its interaction with normal rat serum.

Assay Procedures

Erythropoietic activity of all preparations was determined in hypoxia-induced polycythemic mice[8,9] and potency was expressed in terms of Units (U) of Ery-

* Supported by grant 5–R01–HE03357–09 from the National Heart Institute of the National Institutes of Health, U.S.P.H.S.

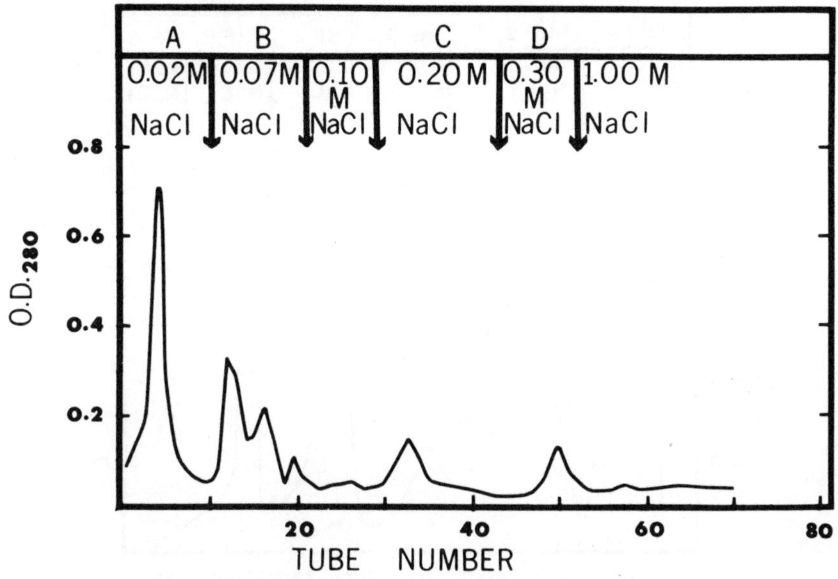

FIGURE 1. Effluent diagram of light mitochondrial extract chromatographed on DEAE ion exchange cellulose at pH 6.8. Each tube represents 10 ml of effluent.

thropoietin Standard A. The assay mice were made polycythemic by exposure to 0.4 atm of air, 16 hr a day for approximately 200 hr. Five mice were used at each dose level for all materials tested. Assay mice received their entire dose of sample (up to 2.0 ml) i.p. on the third posthypoxia day. On the fifth day the mice were injected i.v. with an amount of ^{59}Fe registering approximately 150,000 cpm. The calculation of ESF concentration was done according to the methods outlined by Bliss.[7] This assay procedure, recently further developed in our laboratory, now permits detection of quantities of ESF as low as 0.02 U (unpublished observations). Assay values provided in the Tables represent data extrapolated down to U per ml of extract or incubation mixture.

Incubation Technique

In experiments involving the addition of normal rat serum to two-step extracts of kidney, one volume of serum was added to one volume of extract. Unless otherwise indicated, all incubations were conducted at 37° C in buffered saline at pH 6.8. All reaction flasks were left open to the atmosphere. In some experiments, reactions were stopped by plunging the reaction vessels into an acetone-dry ice mixture.

Chromatographic Purification of Light Mitochondrial Extract

The LME was obtained from the kidneys of adult male Long-Evans rats rendered hypoxic by continuous exposure to 0.4 atm for 16 hr. Their kidneys were fractionated by a centrifugation scheme which was essentially that of La Bella *et al.*[10] and employed by us in fractionation of the kidney.[2,3]

Ten ml of LME having a protein concentration of 5 mg/ml were diluted to 20 ml with distilled water, and chromatographed on a 2 × 20 DEAE column. The column was eluted with NaCl solutions of increasing molarity (0.02–1.00 *M*) buffered at pH 6.8 with 0.005 *M* phosphate buffer (FIGURE 1).

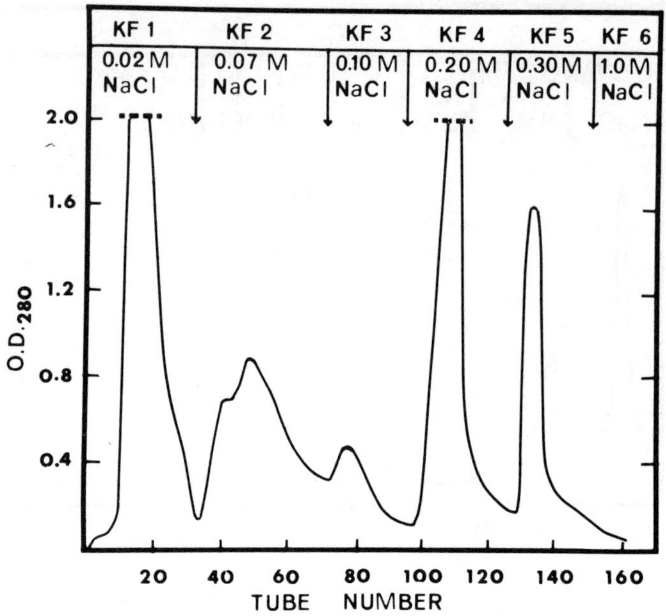

FIGURE 2. Effluent diagram of two-step extract of hypoxic rat kidneys chromatographed on DEAE ion exchange cellulose at pH 6.8. Each tube represents 10 ml of effluent.

TABLE 1

DEAE FRACTIONATION OF LIGHT MITOCHONDRIAL EXTRACT FROM KIDNEYS OF HYPOXIC RATS

Fraction	Volume of Fraction Incubated* with NRS** (ml)	Units ESF† Produced/ml Fraction	Protein Conc. of Fraction (mg/ml)	Units ESF Produced/mg Protein of Fraction
A	1.0	N.D.	0.4	—
B	1.0	0.06	0.4	0.15
C	2.0	N.D.	0.2	—
D	1.0	0.05	0.1	0.50††
Light mitochondrial extract (starting material)	1.0	0.08	5.0	0.02

* All were incubated with 1.0 ml of normal rat serum for 30 min at 37° C and pH 7.0.
** Normal Rat Serum.
† Erythropoietin.
†† Fraction D represents a 25-fold purification over the starting material.

The LME was resolved into four distinct components labeled LME-A to D. There was some similarity between the LME effluent diagram shown in FIGURE 1 and the two-step kidney extract effluent diagram (FIGURE 2).

Incubation Studies

The chromatographic fractionation of the two-step hypotonic extract of the kidney revealed the presence of two erythropoietically significant elution areas. The material eluted with 0.10 *M* NaCl stimulated erythropoiesis, but possessed no REF activity. The mobility and stability of this fraction were similar to those of ESF obtained from the plasma of hypoxic rats. It was postulated that the

TABLE 2

INCUBATION STUDIES WITH PURIFIED LME* FRACTION D

Volume Fraction D / Volume NRS**	Total Volume of Incubation Mixture (ml)	Incubation Time (min)	Total ESF† Produced (Units)	Units ESF Produced/ml Fraction D	Units ESF Produced/mg Fraction D
0.10	40.0	0	N.D.‡	—	—
0.10	40.0	10	0.80	0.40	4.00
0.10	40.0	30	0.40	0.20	2.00
0.10	40.0	90	N.D.	—	—
0.01	10.0	60	0.10	2.00	20.00
0.10	10.0	60	N.D.	—	—
0.50	10.0	60	N.D.	—	—

* Light Mitochondrial Extract of hypoxic rat kidneys.
** Normal Rat Serum.
† Erythropoietin.
‡ Nondetectable erythropoietic activity.

material eluted with 0.10 *M* NaCl (KF-3) was composed of ESF derived partly from contaminating residual plasma, and partly from ESF produced or activated by the interaction of residual plasma with some REF released during the homogenization of the kidney. REF activity was found in the 0.20 *M* NaCl fraction (KF-4).[3]

All LME fractions were found to be inactive when 1 or 2 ml of each were injected i.p. into assay mice. When each fraction was incubated with normal rat serum for 30 min at pH 7.0, fraction D was found to contain the REF in the highest specific activity (TABLE 1). This fraction was capable of generating approximately 0.50 U of ESF per mg of fraction D protein, when incubated in a 1 to 1 ratio (volume/volume) with normal rat serum for 30 minutes. Similarly treated crude LME produced 0.O2 U ESF per mg of crude LME protein. The fractionation procedure therefore resulted in a 25-fold purification of the LME. It is of interest to note the absence of any erythropoietic material in the 0.10 *M* NaCl elution region which would correspond to the area of residual ESF.

The data presented in TABLE 2 indicate that minute quantities of fraction D were sufficient to produce significant amounts of ESF upon interacting with normal rat serum. When 0.10 ml of fraction D was incubated per ml of normal serum, about 0.40 U of ESF were engendered per ml of fraction D. This is equivalent to 4.00 U of ESF generated/mg fraction D protein. When fraction D was incubated with 100 times its volume of serum (0.01 ml fraction D per ml of normal serum), it was calculated that 2.00 U of ESF could be produced per ml of fraction D. This is equivalent to 20.00 U of ESF generated per mg protein of fraction D. Incubation of as little as 0.005 mg of fraction D with 5.00 ml of serum resulted in the production of 0.1 U of ESF.

A study of the time course of the interaction of 2 ml LME fraction D with 20 ml of serum indicated that maximum ESF production occurred at 10 min of incubation. Within 30 min the incubation mixture had lost half of its former activity. Longer periods of incubation resulted in a reduction of the ESF activity to nondetectable levels. In this respect the time course of the interaction of the REF present in fraction D with serum was similar to that followed by crude LME. The partial purification of the LME did not eliminate the inactivation of ESF that occurred during incubation with normal serum.

Protease activity has been detected in the LME, and is believed at least partly responsible for the inactivation of ESF. Straus[11,12] has reported that droplets from normal rat kidneys had a large range in size, the smallest of which sedimented at

TABLE 3

INCUBATION STUDIES OF LIGHT MITOCHONDRIAL EXTRACT (LME) OF KIDNEY WITH NORMAL RAT SERUM

NRS* (ml)	Hypoxic LME (ml)	Time of Incubation (min)	Units ESF** Produced/ml LME
1.0	1.0	5	1.10
1.0	1.0	10	0.09
1.0	1.0	15	0.10
1.0	1.0	30	0.11
0.0	0.1	30	N.D.†
0.1	0.1	120	N.D.
0.1	0.1	240	N.D.
2.0	1.0	30	0.20
2.0	0.1	30	1.27
2.0	0.1	120	0.50
2.0	0.1	240	0.50
15.0	0.1	30	6.00
0.1	2.0	30	0.03
0.1	2.0	120	0.03
0.1	2.0	240	0.03
2.0	—	30	N.D.
—	2.0	30	N.D.

* Normal Rat Serum
** Erythropoietin
† Nondetectable erythropoietic activity

15,000 × g at 30 minutes. Such particles contained hydrolytic enzymes similar to those found in the lysosomes. The method of preparation of the LME in the present study would include such lysosome-like particles.

Due to the inactivation of ESF which is most apparent during prolonged incubations, the largest yield of ESF is produced when serum is incubated with excess LME for short durations. In this connection, the crude LME (TABLE 3) should be incubated in at least a 1 to 1 ratio (volume/volume) with normal serum for not more than 30 minutes. By incubating the serum with excess LME, the ESF generating or activating process proceeds more rapidly than the inactivating reaction.

The data also indicate (TABLE 3) that the total quantity of ESF produced is dependent on the volume of serum present if time and LME concentration are kept constant.

The evidence suggests that the REF may be an enzyme, present in some subcellular granule of the kidney, which acts on a serum protein substrate to produce the ESF. Another possibility is that the REF represents the active center or core of the ESF molecule, which must complex with a serum carrier to become physiologically active.

Summary

Ion-exchange chromatography of the light mitochondrial extract (LME) of the kidneys of hypoxic rats resulted in a 25-fold purification of the renal erythropoietic factor (REF) contained within this extract. The LME possessed no component which corresponded to residual ESF in either mobility on the column or in erythropoietic behavior. The REF was therefore present in the LME in the absence of ESF.

The incubation of purified REF in quantities as low as 0.005 mg with normal rat serum was found to produce significant erythropoietic activity.

An ESF inactivation process occurred during the incubation of either crude or purified LME with serum. This inactivation was most apparent in incubations lasting more than 30 minutes.

The total quantity of ESF produced in an incubation mixture was dependent on the amount of serum available, when the quantity of LME and the period of incubation were kept constant.

The REF may be either an enzyme acting on a serum substrate to produce ESF, or an ESF precursor which is required to complex with a serum carrier in order to acquire erythropoiesis stimulating activity.

Acknowledgment

We thank the National Heart Institute for supplies of Step IV sheep erythropoietin.

References

1. CONTRERA, J. F., J. F. CAMISCOLI, A. H. WEINTRAUB & A. S. GORDON. 1965. Extraction of erythropoietin from kidneys of hypoxic and phenylhydrazine-treated rats. Blood **25:** 809–816.
2. CONTRERA, J. F. & A. S. GORDON. 1966. Erythropoietin: Production by a particulate fraction of rat kidney. Science **152:** 653–654.
3. CONTRERA, J. F., A. S. GORDON & A. H. WEINTRAUB. 1966. Extraction of an erythropoietin-producing factor from a particulate fraction of rat kidney. Blood **28:** 330–343.
4. KURATOWSKA, Z., B. LEWARTOWSKI & B. LIPINSKI. 1964. Chemical and biological properties of an erythropoietin-generating substance obtained from perfusates of isolated anoxic kidneys. J. Lab. Clin. Med. **64:** 226–237.
5. KURATOWSKA, Z. 1965. On the subcellular localization of the erythropoietic renal factor. Bull. Acad. Polon. Sci. **8:** 385–390.
6. DE DUVE, C. 1964. Principles of tissue fractionation. J. Theoret. Biol. **6:** 33–59.
7. BLISS, C. I. 1952. The Statistics of Bioassay. Academic Press. New York, N. Y.
8. GORDON, A. S. & A. H. WEINTRAUB. 1962. Assay of the erythropoietic stimulating factor (ESF). *In* Erythropoiesis. L. O. Jacobson and M. Doyle, Eds. : 1–16. Grune & Stratton, New York, N. Y.
9. WEINTRAUB, A. H., A. S. GORDON & J. F. CAMISCOLI. 1963. Use of the hypoxia-induced polycythemic mouse in the assay and standardization of erythropoietin. J. Lab. Clin. Med. **62:** 743–752.
10. LA BELLA, F. S., R. J. REIFFENSTEIN & G. BEAULIEU. 1963. Subcellular fractionation of bovine posterior pituitary glands by centrifugation. Arch. Biochem. Biophys. **100:** 399–408.
11. STRAUS, W. 1954. Isolation and biochemical properties of droplets from the cells of rat kidney. J. Biol. Chem. **207:** 745–755.
12. STRAUS, W. 1956. Concentration of acid phosphatase, ribonuclease, desoxyribonuclease, glucuronidase, and cathepsin in "droplets" isolated from the kidney cells of normal rats. J. Biophys. Biochem. Cytol. **2:** 513–521.

STUDIES ON THE SITE OF PRODUCTION OF ERYTHROPOIETIN*

Robert Katz, George W. Cooper, Albert S. Gordon and Esmail D. Zanjani

Departments of Biology, Graduate School of Arts and Science, New York University, and The City College of The City University of New York, New York, N. Y.

Introduction

The importance of the kidney in the production of erythropoietin (erythropoiesis-stimulating factor or ESF) has been clearly established through evidence obtained from at least three independent avenues of investigation: (1) Studies with anephric animals in which the renal dependency of the circulating ESF has been demonstrated;[1,2] (2) in vitro perfusion experiments with isolated anoxic kidneys in which erythropoietic activity was detected in the perfusates;[3,4] and (3) the extraction of erythropoietically active fractions from renal tissues of hypoxic animals.[5,6]

These data, however, do not clarify whether the kidney is the site of synthesis or site of activation of the ESF. The implication that the active erythropoietic principle may, in fact, be the product of two essential components of intra- and extra-renal origin stems from the work of Kuratowska *et al.*[7] and Contrera and Gordon.[8] Both groups of investigators have given evidence for a renal factor whose erythropoietic activity is expressed only when previously incubated with serum or a serum fraction.

An exploration of this fundamental problem has been undertaken employing radioisotopic tracer techniques. Attempts were made to correlate the rates of protein synthesis in the livers and kidneys of hypoxic rats with the appearance of the ESF in the circulation. The isotopes of three compounds, d-glucosamine-^{14}C, l-leucine-^{3}H and l-isoleucine-^{14}C, previously identified as major components of Step IV sheep plasma erythropoietin,[9] were employed. Extirpation studies were also conducted in a separate series of experiments to evaluate the role of the liver in the production of the ESF.

Materials and Methods

Male Long-Evans rats, weighing 240–260 g, were used as the experimental animals. Hypoxia was produced by subjecting animals to reduced barometric pressures of 0.42 atmospheres. In all radioisotopic experiments the isotope/s were administered i.v. exactly one hour prior to exsanguination. This necessitated removing the animals from the decompression chamber for a brief interval of time (10–15 min) in order to inject the isotope/s; the animals were then immediately returned to the decompression chamber and retained there until sacrifice time. Glucosamine-^{14}C (4 μc) and leucine-^{3}H (10 μc) were administered simultaneously to animals which had been exposed to 16 hr of hypoxia. Isoleucine-^{14}C (13.2 μc) was given alone to animals subjected to varying intervals of hypoxia covering a total period of 18½ hours. Isotopic incorporation was measured in the proteins extracted from liver and kidney cellular fractions,[10] as well as from plasma, using a modified Schoeniger combustion technique.[11,12] Total protein determinations were made with the biuret method.[13] Plasma titers of the ESF were estimated by employing the plethoric mouse assay described by Gordon and Weintraub.[14] Control samples were obtained from animals given

* Supported by Grant 5–R01–HE03357–09 from the National Heart Institute of the National Institutes of Health, U.S.P.H.S.

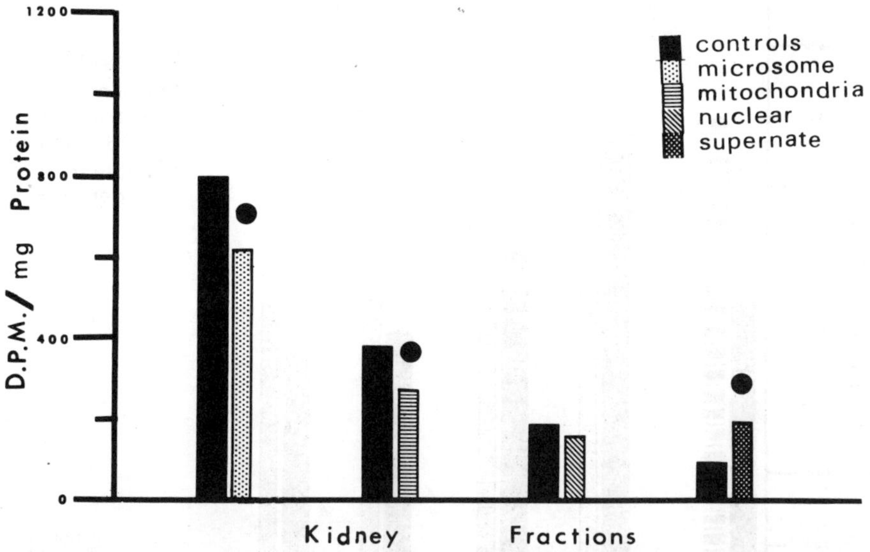

FIGURE 1. D-glucosamine-^{14}C incorporation into proteins of kidney subcellular fractions following exposure to 16 hr hypoxia. Four μc isotope injected one hour prior to exsanguination. Values represent means of four animals. Black dot indicates $P < .05$ compared to corresponding control sample. Control samples from animals maintained at atmospheric pressures.

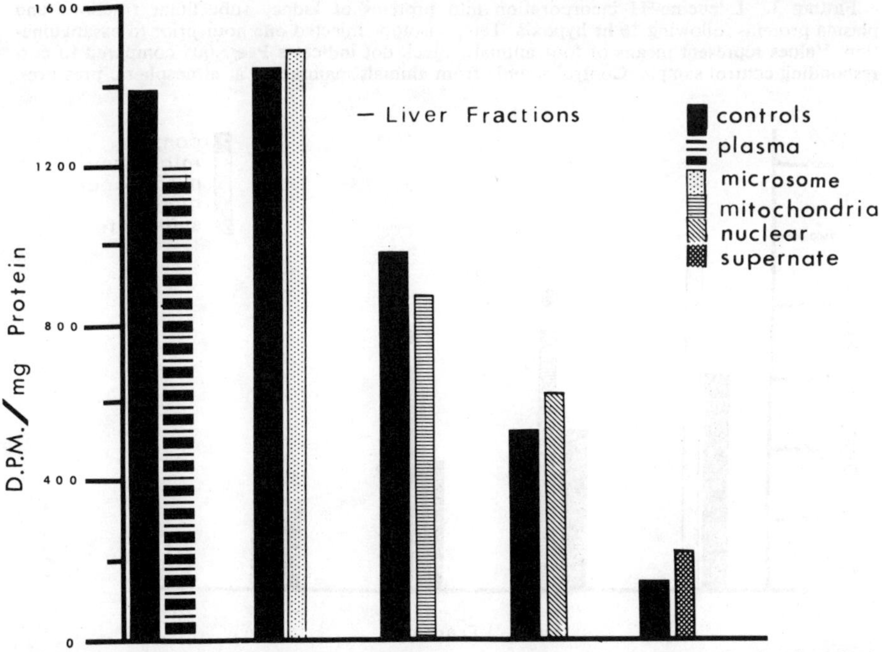

FIGURE 2. D-glucosamine-^{14}C incorporation into proteins of liver subcellular fractions and plasma proteins following 16 hr hypoxia. Four μc isotope injected one hour prior to exsanguination. Values represent means of four animals. Control samples from animals maintained at atmospheric pressures.

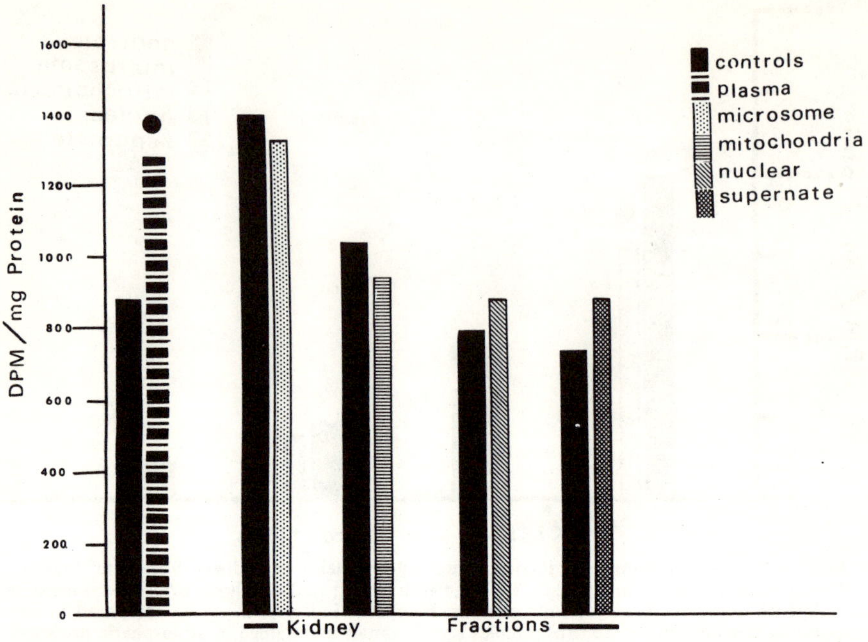

FIGURE 3. L-leucine-^{3}H incorporation into proteins of kidney subcellular fractions and plasma proteins following 16 hr hypoxia. Ten μc isotope injected one hour prior to exsanguination. Values represent means of four animals. Black dot indicates $P < .005$ compared to corresponding control sample. Control sample from animals maintained at atmospheric pressures.

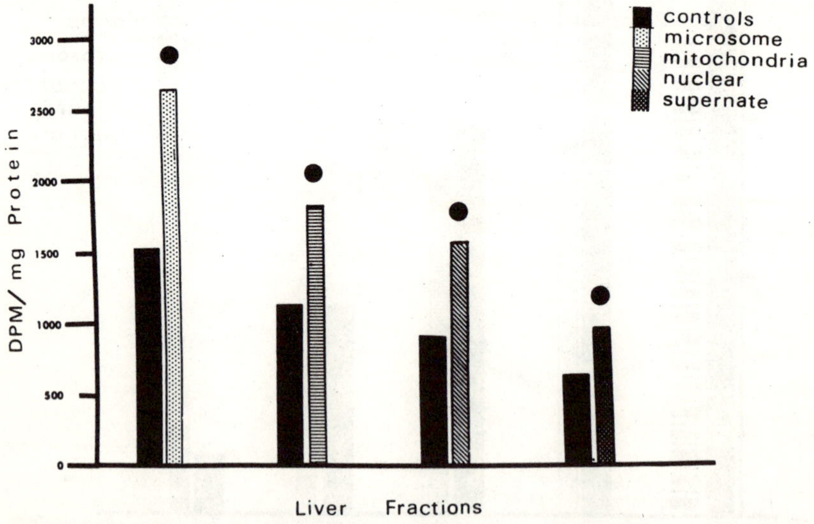

FIGURE 4. L-leucine-^{3}H incorporation into proteins of liver subcellular fractions following 16 hr hypoxia. Ten μc isotope injected one hour prior to exsanguination. Values represent means of four animals. Black dot indicates minimum P value of $P < .01$ compared to corresponding control sample. Control samples from animals maintained at atmospheric pressures.

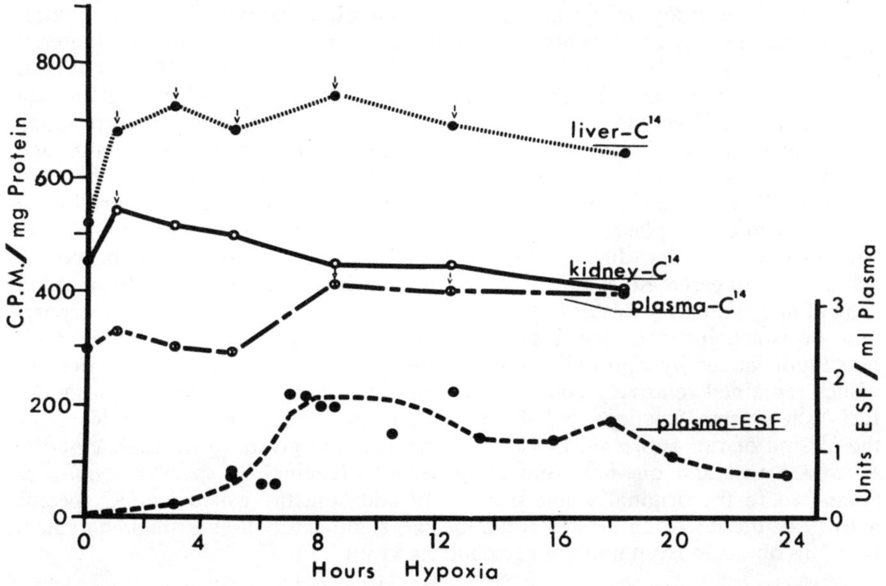

FIGURE 5. L-isoleucine-^{14}C incorporation into proteins of liver and kidney particulate fraction (material deposited between 960–110,000 × g) and plasma proteins following varying intervals of hypoxia. Isotope (13.2 μc.) injected one hour prior to exsanguination. Each point represents mean of five animals. Arrows indicate minimum P values of $P < .02$ relative to corresponding control at zero hours of hypoxia.

identical isotopic schedules but maintained at atmospheric pressures. ESF-rich plasma fractions were prepared from alcoholic extracts of plasma according to the method of Lowy and Borsook.[15]

The ability to produce the ESF was compared in three different groups of animals exposed to eight hr of continuous hypoxia: Group 1 eviscerated rats[16] in which only the kidneys, adrenals and urinary bladder were left intact in the abdominal cavity; Group 2: intact animals (nonoperated controls); Group 3: surgical controls in which only the spleen, pancreas and stomach were extirpated. Salivary glands were removed from animals in group 1 and group 3 to prevent lung congestion. All groups received a single injection of 10 ml of 5 percent glucose (4 ml i.m.; 6 ml s.c.). In separate experiments the erythropoietic activity of plasma from partially hepatectomized (approximately 85 percent of liver removed) and sham-operated animals was compared after five hr of continuous hypoxia.

Results

Following 16 hr of hypoxia, the plasma of the rats contained 0.70 units ESF/ml plasma. Nevertheless, the incorporation of glucosamine was slightly, but significantly, increased in only the supernate fractions (materials not deposited at 110,000 × g) of kidneys from hypoxic animals (FIGURE 1). No significant changes were noted in glucosamine uptake into either plasma proteins or any liver subcellular fractions during hypoxia (FIGURE 2). While the patterns of leucine incorporation into the kidney subcellular fractions were not significantly altered following hypoxia, the uptake of this amino acid into the plasma proteins and all liver subcellular fractions was significantly increased (FIGURES 3 &4).

In the kinetic study, where animals were exposed to hypoxia for varying intervals of time, isoleucine incorporation into liver particulate fractions (all material deposited between 960–110,000 × g) rose significantly during the first hour of hypoxia and the high incorporation rate was then sustained during the rest of the period of hypoxic stimulation (FIGURE 5). However, renal incorporation of isoleucine increased significantly only during the first hour of hypoxia, although somewhat elevated incorporation rates were observed until the fifth hour of hypoxia. Of particular interest were the findings that both the incorporation of isoleucine into the plasma proteins and the plasma titers of the ESF closely paralleled each other during hypoxic stimulation and also both appeared to reflect the increased isoleucine incorporation which occurred in the liver. After a lag of approximately five hr both the levels of the plasma ESF and the incorporation of isoleucine into the plasma proteins climbed sharply, reaching their maximum values by approximately the eighth hour of hypoxia; thereafter the values remained relatively constant for the next 10 hr of hypoxia (FIGURE 5). ESF-rich plasma fractions (65–81 percent EtOH precipitates) extracted from the plasma of rats subjected to 12 hr of hypoxia and given 10 μc isoleucine-^{14}C showed a two and one-half fold increase in isoleucine-^{14}C specific activity as compared to the original whole plasma. In addition, the isoleucine-^{14}C specific activity of the ESF-rich plasma fractions was significantly higher than equivalent fractions obtained from nonhypoxic controls (TABLE 1).

TABLE 1

RADIOACTIVITY OF ETHANOL PLASMA FRACTIONS PREPARED FROM RATS GIVEN 10 μC L-ISOLEUCINE-^{14}C

Plasma Sample	Hours Hypoxia	CPM-^{14}C/mg Protein Means ± S.E.m.*	P Values as Compared to Controls**
Whole plasma	0	241.2 ± 17.2	
Whole plasma	12	315.7 ± 11.5	$P < .01$
0–55 percent EtOH ppt.	0	257.2 ± 15.9	
0–55 percent EtOH ppt.	12	353.5 ± 23.1	$P < .01$
55–65 percent EtOH ppt.	0	250.8 ± 20.2	
55–65 percent EtOH ppt.	12	354.6 ± 8.79	$P < .005$
65–81 percent EtOH ppt.†	0	646.9 ± 57.2	
65–81 percent EtOH ppt.†	12	857.4 ± 35.8	$P < .02$

* Means of five animals
** Compared to zero hours of hypoxia
† ESF-rich plasma fractions

TABLE 2

PLASMA LEVELS OF THE ESF IN SURGICALLY TREATED RATS EXPOSED TO HYPOXIA

Donor Rats	No. Rats	Hours Hypoxia	Units ESF/ml Plasma ± S.E.m
Nonoperated Controls	15	8	0.77 ± 0.05
Eviscerated	16	8	0.36 ± 0.07*
Surgical Controls	12	8	2.53 ± 0.36
Sham-operated controls	3	5	0.54 ± 0.14
Partially hepatectomized	3	5	0.20 ± 0.03**

* $P < .001$ vs Surgical Controls
$P < .005$ vs Nonoperated Controls
** $P < .05$ vs Sham-Operated Controls

In the extirpation studies, eviscerated animals showed markedly reduced plasma levels of the ESF as compared to either those of nonoperated or surgical controls following eight hr of hypoxia. Also, the erythropoietic activity of plasma from partially hepatectomized animals was significantly lower than that of sham-operated controls following five hr of hypoxia (TABLE 2).

Discussion

The synthesis of the polysaccharide and polypeptide moieties of the ESF in rats during exposure to hypoxia was related to the incorporation of d-glucosamine-^{14}C, l-leucine-^{3}H and l-isoleucine-^{14}C into kidney, liver and plasma proteins. In view of the established role of the kidney in the production of the ESF,[1–5] it was anticipated that the appearance of the ESF in the circulation during hypoxia would be associated with an increased rate of glycoprotein synthesis, particularly in the kidney. Contrary to expectations, however, the uptake of glucosamine into kidney, liver and plasma proteins gave no indication of an increased rate of glycoprotein synthesis during hypoxia although the plasma titers of the ESF were elevated. Even more surprising were the results obtained in the leucine and isoleucine incorporation experiments. These studies indicated that general protein synthesis was enhanced during hypoxia, however the liver, rather than the kidney, was most actively engaged in protein synthesis. Indeed, a qualitative relationship could be demonstrated in the isoleucine kinetic studies between the rate of liver protein synthesis, the incorporation of isoleucine into plasma proteins and the plasma titers of the ESF. On the other hand, the brief period of increased isoleucine incorporation into kidney proteins during only the first to, at most, the fifth hour of hypoxia did not correspond to either the incorporation of isoleucine into the plasma proteins or the appearance of the plasma ESF. The increased isoleucine uptake into the ESF-rich plasma fractions following 12 hr of hypoxia could hardly be due to kidney protein synthesis.

To reconcile these data with the known role of the kidney in the production of the ESF, consideration was given to the proposal of Gordon[17] which suggests a cooperative kidney-liver axis being required for the ESF production. Accordingly, it was postulated that during the initial phases of hypoxia the kidney is stimulated to elaborate an activator or enzyme which converts a plasma substrate of liver origin into the active ESF. Assuming the renal factor acts enzymatically, the relatively small amounts of enzyme required to activate large quantities of substrate could reflect the brief period of increased protein synthesis which occurred in the kidney during the initial phases of hypoxia. The large quantities of substrate needed to maintain the observed high levels of the plasma ESF could be furnished by the liver and would correspond to the sustained rate of protein synthesis noted in this organ during hypoxia.

The inability to demonstrate an augmented rate of glucosamine incorporation during hypoxia might be explained in terms of a specific polypeptide substrate being produced by the liver in response to hypoxia which is subsequently complexed with a nonspecific glycoprotein. It is also conceivable that hypoxia merely induces a selective shift in the type of polypeptide moiety to be incorporated into a glycoprotein without causing any increase in total glycoprotein synthesis.

The basic concept requiring both a renal factor and a plasma substrate is in accord with the findings of Kuratowska *et al.*[7] and Contrera and Gordon[8] who have reported isolating renal factors which generate erythropoietic activity only when previously incubated with serum or a serum component. The tenet of a kidney-liver axis for the production of the ESF also predicts that the capacity to produce the ESF is contingent on the presence of the liver. The findings of significantly reduced titers of the plasma ESF in eviscerated and partially hepatectomized animals, therefore, lends strong support to this hypothesis. The low but significant levels of the ESF found in the eviscerated and partially hepatectomized animals probably represents the conversion of residual quantities of the plasma substrate into ESF by the renal factor which would still be produced during hypoxia. This suggestion is not inconsistent with the reactions between the isolated renal factors and serum previously reported.[7,8]

The possibility that the lowered erythropoietic activity of plasma from eviscerated animals might have been the result of some inherent toxic factor elaborated by these animals was precluded by the fact that the activity of known quantities of exogenous ESF was not diminished when assayed after previous incubation with plasma from eviscerated rats. These animals were maintained at atmospheric pressures for 10 hr after evisceration. The high levels of the ESF found in the plasma of the hypoxic surgical controls probably resulted from a superimposed hypoxic stimulus as a result of small blood losses occurring during the operative procedure. Supporting this premise were the findings that plasma from surgical controls maintained at atmospheric pressures for eight hr contained from 0.3 to 0.5 units ESF/ml plasma.

Summary

Radioisotope studies employing d-glucosamine-^{14}C, 1-leucine-^{3}H and 1-isoleucine-^{14}C were conducted to monitor the rates of protein synthesis in the liver and kidneys of rats exposed to varying periods of reduced barometric pressure (0.42 atm). The uptake of glucosamine-^{14}C into either liver or kidney glycoproteins was not found to be influenced by hypoxia. The incorporation of isoleucine-^{14}C into the kidney proteins was significantly increased only during the first few hours of hypoxia. However, the incorporation of leucine-^{3}H and isoleucine-^{14}C into liver and plasma proteins was consistently elevated during hypoxia, and this correlated with increased titers of ESF in the plasma.

Extirpation studies demonstrated that the capacity to produce ESF was markedly reduced in hypoxic animals with functionless livers, and was significantly reduced in partially hepatectomized animals exposed to hypoxia.

These results are most readily interpreted within the general framework of a renal activator-liver substrate axis being involved in the production of the active ESF.

Acknowledgment

We thank the National Heart Institute for supplies of Step IV sheep erythropoietin.

References

1. Jacobson, L. O., E. Goldwasser, W. Fried & L. Plzak. 1957. Role of kidney in erythropoiesis. Nature **179:** 633–634.
2. Jacobson, L. O., E. Goldwasser, C. W. Gurney, W. Fried & L. Plzak. 1959. Studies on erythropoietin: The hormone regulating red cell production. Ann. N. Y. Acad. Sci. **77:** 551–573.
3. Kuratowska, Z., B. Lewartowski & E. Michalak. 1961. Studies on the production of erythropoietin by isolated perfused organs. Blood **18:** 527–534.
4. Fisher, J. W. & B. J. Birdwell. 1961. Erythropoietin production by the in situ perfused kidney. Fed. Proc. **20:** 81.
5. Contrera, J. F., J. F. Camiscoli, A. H. Weintraub & A. S. Gordon. 1965. Extraction of erythropoietin from kidneys of hypoxic and phenylhydrazine-treated rats. Blood **25:** 809–816.

6. LAGRUE, G., P. BOIVIN & A. BRANELLEC. 1960. Activité érythropoïétique d'un extrait rénal. Rev. Franc. Études Clin. Biol. **5**: 816–821.
7. KURATOWSKA, Z., B. LEWARTOWSKI & B. LIPINSKI. 1964. Chemical and biological properties of an erythropoietin-generating substance obtained from perfusate of isolated anoxic kidney. J. Lab. Clin. Med. **64**: 226–237.
8. CONTRERA, J. F. & A. S. GORDON. 1966. Erythropoietin: Production by a particulate fraction of rat kidney. Science **152**: 653–654.
9. WHITE, W. F., C. W. GURNEY, E. GOLDWASSER & L. O. JACOBSON. 1960. Studies on erythropoietin. Recent Progr. Hormone Res. **16**: 219–262.
10. ROBINSON, G. B., J. MOLNAR & R. J. WINZLER. 1963. Biosynthesis of glycoproteins. J. Biol. Chem. **239**: 109–136.
11. NATHAN, D. G., T. G. GABUZDA & F. H. GARDNER. 1963. Liquid scintillation counting of ^{14}C-labeled hemoglobin and hemin by a modified Schoeniger technique. J. Lab. Clin. Med. **62**: 511–516.
12. BUSH, E. T. 1964. Liquid scintillation counting of doubly-labeled samples. Anal. Chem. **36**: 1082–1089.
13. GORNALL, A. G., C. J. BARDAWILL & M. M. DAVID. 1949. Determination of serum proteins by means of the buiret reaction. J. Biol. Chem. **177**: 761–766.
14. GORDON, A. S. & A. H. WEINTRAUB. 1962. Assay of the erythropoietic stimulating factor (ESF). *In* Erythropoiesis. L. O. Jacobson and M. Doyle, Eds. : 1–15. Grune and Stratton. New York, N. Y.
15. LOWY, P. H. & H. BORSOOK. 1962. Preparation and properties of erythropoietin concentrates from rabbit plasma and human urine. *In* Erythropoiesis. L. O. Jacobson and M. Doyle, Eds. : 33–42. Grune and Stratton. New York, N. Y.
16. RUSSEL, J. A. 1942. The anterior pituitary in carbohydrate metabolism of the eviscerated rat. Amer. J. Physiol. **136**: 95–104.
17. GORDON, A. S. 1959. Hemopoietine. Physiol. Rev. **39**: 1–50.

THE RENAL MECHANISM OF THE FORMATION AND INACTIVATION OF ERYTHROPOIETIN

Z. Kuratowska

Department of Radiobiology and Health Protection, Institute of Nuclear Research, Warsaw, Poland

The important role of the kidney in the production of erythropoietin has been firmly established during the last few years.[1–5] We have previously reported that: 1) The isolated kidneys release erythropoietin under hypoxic conditions;[3,6] 2) The erythropoietic factor released by kidneys requires the α-globulin from blood plasma for its activity;[7] 3) The renal factor is thermolabile before the interaction with α-globulin and is stabilized by α-globulin.

Studies on the Localization of Erythropoietin in Subcellular Fractions

As a further step in our investigations on the renal erythropoietic factor, experiments were carried out on the presence of erythropoietin in kidney tissue. Since only a few successful experiments concerning the presence of erythropoietin in whole kidney tissue have been published thus far,[8–11] we attempted to find the erythropoietic factor in whole kidney homogenate as well as in the renal subcellular fractions: nuclei, mitochondria, microsomal and soluble fractions. Rabbit kidneys used in these experiments were: 1) normal control rabbit kidneys; 2) kidneys from animals which were injected intravenously with 50 μM of $CoCl_2$ in two divided doses on two days before removing the organs ("stimulated" kidneys); and 3) kidneys removed 20 hr after bleeding the animals an amount of blood equivalent to one-fourth of the animals' own blood volume (so-called "anemic" kidneys).

In addition to the kidneys we tested also the erythropoietic activity of livers and spleens in the same groups of experimental animals.

The methods for the separation of subcellular fractions and assay of the erythropoietic activity have already been described in detail.[12]

The results of the experiments are presented in FIGURE 1. As can be seen marked erythropoietic activity was found in the nuclear fraction of stimulated kidneys after incubation for 2 hr at 37°C with α-globulin from plasma. Significant activity was also found in the nuclear fraction of normal kidney incubated with α-globulin. Since the results on the anemic and stimulated kidneys were very similar, only the stimulated group is included in the Figure. Traces of activity were found in mitochondria of stimulated and anemic kidneys. The whole renal homogenate and soluble fractions were completely inactive in all experiments.

On the other hand it was possible to find low erythropoietic activity in the whole homogenate, nuclear and mitochondrial fractions of the liver (TABLE 1). The activity was not related to incubation with α-globulins and was present in stimulated, anemic and normal livers.

The comparison between the erythropoietic activity, expressed in cobalt units, of some kidney and liver fractions is presented in TABLE 2. The nuclear fraction from the kidney possessed markedly higher erythropoietic activity than that of the liver.

In attempting the cellular localization of the renal erythropoietic factor in the kidney, the nuclear fractions from the cortical and medullary parts of the stimulated kidneys were assayed for erythropoietic activity. TABLE 3 shows that the renal factor is mainly concentrated in the renal medulla.

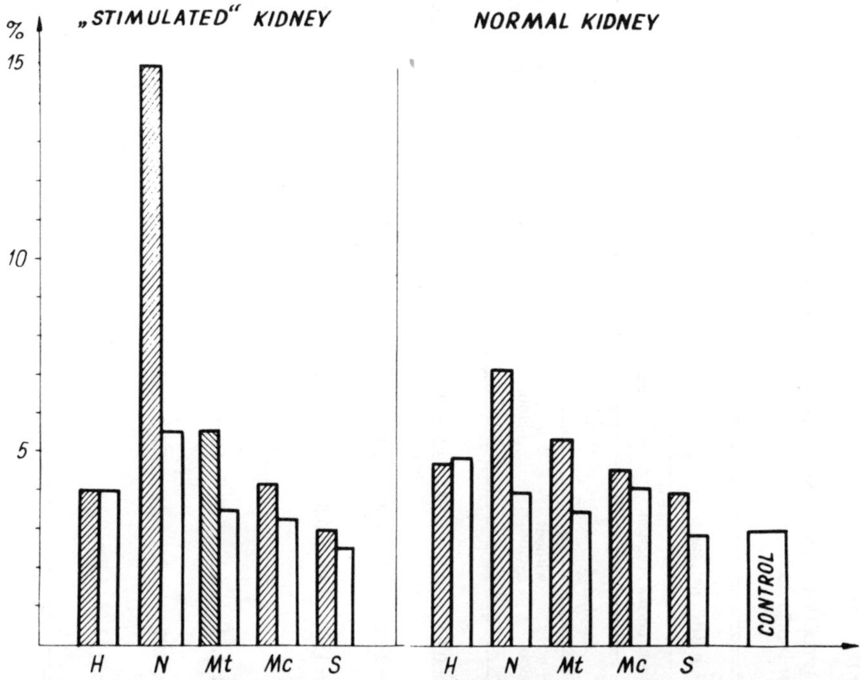

FIGURE 1. The incorporation of ^{59}Fe into RBC of fasted rats (percent of injected dose) after two injections of kidney homogenate (H) and subcellular fractions (N, Mt, Mc and S) incubated with α-globulin (lined bars) and with 0.9% natrium chloride (plain bars).

From these data it may be concluded that the renal erythropoietic factor is spun down with the nuclear fraction of the kidneys stimulated to produce erythropoietin by injection of cobalt or by bleeding. The nuclear factor has the same properties as that described for the perfusate fluid from isolated kidney.[7] The erythropoietic activity found in the liver has different properties and will be discussed later in this report.

Studies on the Presence of an Erythropoietin Inhibitor in a Kidney Cytoplasmic Fraction

The lack of erythropoietic activity in the whole homogenate of the kidney observed in our experiments suggested that a factor may be present in the homogenate which destroyed the activity. The following experiment was performed to throw some light on this problem: 1) The active nuclear fraction (incubated with α-globulins, with standard activity of 4 units from the stimulated kidney was incubated for three hr at 37° C in the presence of the soluble fraction from stimulated or normal kidney, respectively; 2) sheep plasma erythropoietin (Step IV) was incubated for three hr at 37° C with the soluble fraction from normal and stimulated kidneys; and 3) the erythropoietically active samples (nuclear or Step IV) were incubated also under the same conditions without the fraction in the sucrose or buffer as a control, depending on the medium in which the soluble fraction was separated.

The results of the experiments are illustrated in FIGURE 2. The erythropoietic activity of nuclear fraction was completely inhibited after incubation with the

TABLE 1

^{59}Fe INCORPORATION INTO RBC OF STARVED RATS AFTER INJECTIONS OF SUBCELLULAR FRACTIONS FROM THE SPLEEN AND LIVER

	^{59}Fe Incorporation into RBC, percent									
	Homogenate		Nuclear Fraction		Mitochondrial Fraction		Microsomal Fraction		Soluble Fraction	
	Incubated									
	with α-glob.	without α-glob.	with α-glob.	without α-glob.	with α-glob.	without α-glob.	with α-glob.	without α-glob.	with α-glob.	without α-glob.
Normal spleen	3.5 ± 0.52*	3.1 ± 0.78	3.2 ± 1.08	4.2 ± 0.83	4.9 ± 0.98	4.5 ± 0.77	3.5 ± 0.96	3.8 ± 0.88	4.0 ± 0.96	4.1 ± 0.6
$CoCl_2$ spleen	3.8 ± 0.63	3.0 ± 0.45	3.0 ± 0.99	3.2 ± 1.21	4.0 ± 1.31	4.1 ± 0.83	2.8 ± 1.86	3.0 ± 1.02	3.0 ± 0.87	4.0 ± 0.4
Anemic spleen	3.2 ± 0.96	3.2 ± 0.96	4.0 ± 0.83	3.8 ± 1.03	3.5 ± 1.03	4.0 ± 0.89	3.8 ± 1.01	3.5 ± 1.23	4.2 ± 0.72	3.9 ± 0.7
Normal liver	6.5 ± 1.02	6.8 ± 1.28	5.9 ± 0.95	6.2 ± 1.10	6.1 ± 1.03	6.1 ± 0.38	4.0 ± 1.01	4.1 ± 0.96	4.3 ± 1.08	3.2 ± 0.9
$CoCl_2$-liver	6.0 ± 0.98	6.2 ± 1.07	6.1 ± 0.87	6.0 ± 0.90	5.9 ± 0.97	5.8 ± 0.41	4.7 ± 0.48	4.2 ± 1.32	4.0 ± 0.89	3.7 ± 1.0
Anemic liver	6.2 ± 1.03	6.4 ± 0.99	6.0 ± 1.03	5.8 ± 0.88	5.8 ± 0.72	5.8 ± 0.30	4.3 ± 0.72	3.8 ± 0.88	3.9 ± 0.69	3.9 ± 0.6

* Standard deviation of the mean.

TABLE 2

THE COMPARISON OF ERYTHROPOIETIC ACTIVITY OF SOME KIDNEY FRACTIONS WITH THE SAME FRACTIONS OF LIVER

	Nuclear Fraction	Mitochondria	Homogenate
	cobalt units per mg of protein		
Stimulated kidney	0.5–1.0	0.05	0.0
Anemic kidney	0.4	0.03	0.0
Normal kidney	0.3	0.0	0.0
Stimulated liver	0.08	0.07	0.08
Anemic liver	0.0	0.05	—
Normal	0.08	0.17	0.09

soluble fraction from normal kidneys and was decreased from 4.2 units to 1.5 units after incubation with soluble fraction from stimulated kidneys. The activity of sheep erythropoietin was also almost completely inhibited by the soluble fraction of normal kidney and was decreased to 50% of its initial value by the cytoplasmic fraction of stimulated kidney. These experiments have demonstrated the presence of a potent inhibitor of erythropoietin in the cytoplasmic fraction of normal kidney.

Some of the properties of the inhibitor which we have found are:

1) Thermolability: The inhibitory activity of the soluble fraction is destroyed after seven min heating in a boiling water bath. Approximately 30% of the activity was destroyed during 24 hr of incubation at 37° C. The activity of the erythropoietin inhibitor did not change after storage for six months at 20° C.

2) Influence of proteolytic inhibitors: It was not possible to demonstrate an influence of either soy bean inhibitor or salivary gland trypsin inhibitor ("Trasylol"-Bayer) on the erythropoietic inhibitory activity of the soluble kidney fraction.

3) Neuraminidase-like activity of the soluble kidney fraction: We have found that the soluble fraction of the kidney possesses the ability to split off N-acetylneuraminic acid from glycoproteins and further to cleave N-acetylneuraminic acid to mannosamine and pyruvic acid (aldolase activity). During the purification of neuraminidase from the soluble fraction, according to the technique of Cassidy and Coll.,[13] the fraction which was obtained possessed 150 times higher neuraminidase activity than that of the starting material. However, the inhibitory activity of this sample was approximately one-third of that in the whole soluble fraction. At the present time we have succeeded in the isolation of highly purified neuraminidase from rabbit kidney.[14] However, the problem as to whether the renal inhibitor of erythropoietin is specific or is dependent on neuraminidase activity still remains unsolved.

General Conclusions

Based on results of our previous papers as well as the results presented here, we

TABLE 3

ERYTHROPOIETIC ACTIVITY OF NUCLEAR FRACTION OF RENAL CORTEX AND MEDULLA STIMULATED KIDNEY

	Incorporation of ^{59}Fe Percent	Units per mg of Dry Weight
Cortex	6.9	0.09
Medulla	14.1	0.85
Control	3.5	0.0

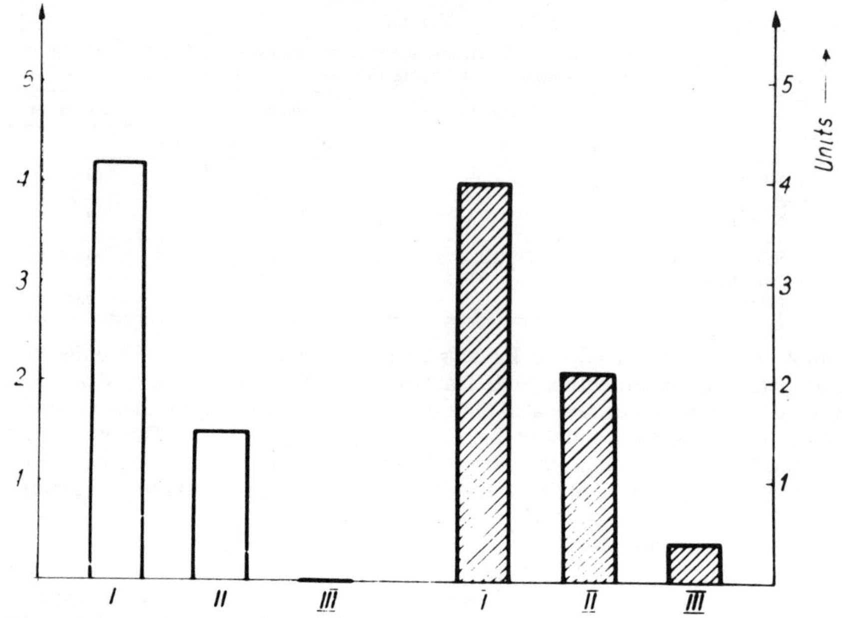

FIGURE 2. Effect of soluble fraction upon erythropoietic activity of renal nuclear fraction (plain bars) and sheep plasma erythropoietin (lined bars). I. Control active sample. II. Active sample incubated with soluble fraction from stimulated kidney. III. Active sample incubated with soluble fraction from normal kidney.

propose the following hypothesis (FIGURE 3): The kidney releases a labile component ("renal erythropoietic factor") which is synthesized in the nuclei or in the other heavy structures or granules adsorbed onto the nuclei which are spun down together. The labile "unbound" component forms an active complex with α-globulin from blood plasma.[7,15,16] This active, relatively stable complex is postu-

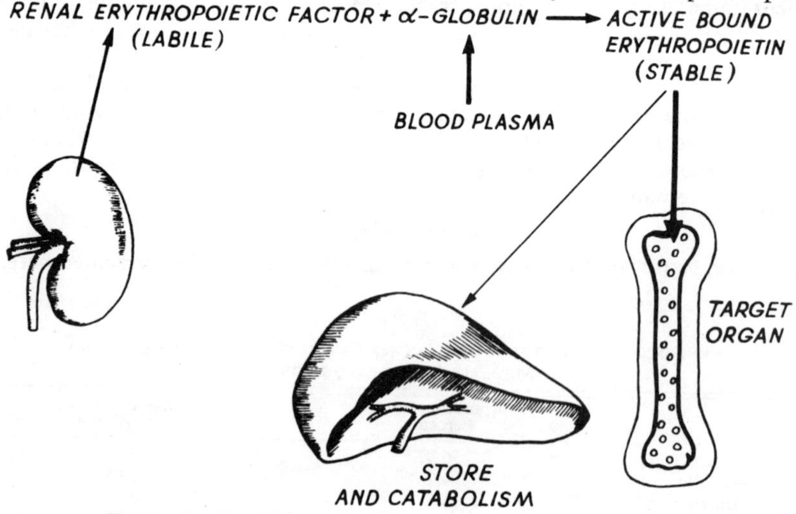

FIGURE 3. Formation of erythropoietin (explanation in text).

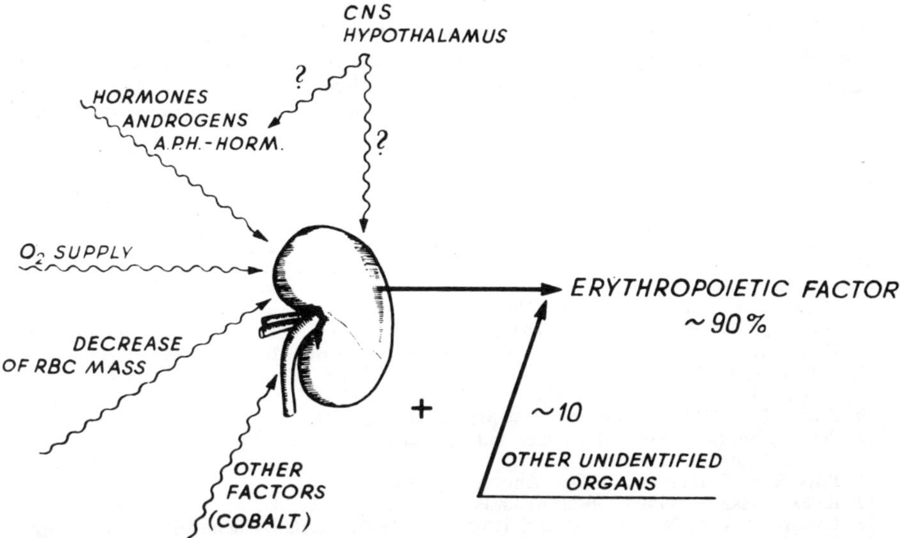

FIGURE 4. Regulation of the production of erythropoietin by the kidney (explanation in text).

lated to be the erythropoietin which is circulating in the blood stream and acts upon the blood-forming organs. The low erythropoietic activity which has been found in liver tissue possesses different properties. It is very similar to plasma "bound" erythropoietin. The liver probably plays a role as a site of storage and catabolism of erythropoietin. The presence of the erythropoietic renal factor in the nuclear fraction of normal kidney is further support for the controversial role of erythropoietin as a physiological substance controlling erythropoiesis in a normal steady state. During an "alarm situation" such as blood loss or hypoxia or after treatment with stimulating agents such as cobalt the level of renal factor increases rapidly. The increased amount of erythropoietic factor in these conditions may depend either on the higher rate of synthesis or on a decrease in the inhibitor. In the experiments presented above the activity of the erythropoietin inhibitor was found to be much higher in normal than in stimulated or anemic kidneys. This suggests that during a state when there is a greater demand for erythropoietin in the organism, both mechanisms may produce a decrease in the inhibitor titer. This may result in an increased rate of erythropoietin synthesis which acts as an efficient control of the erythropoietic system.

The renal mechanism of production and inactivation of erythropoietin seems to be the most important but not the only component controlling and releasing erythropoietin. It has been demonstrated by Lucarelli and Stohlman[17] that tissues other than the kidney in the embryo are responsible for erythropoietin production. A few years ago Jacobson stated that approximately 10% of the erythropoietin is of extrarenal origin. It seems quite possible that in adults other tissues are potentially ready to produce erythropoietin in special conditions. More undifferentiated tissue could play this role, such as that observed in the embryonic period of life or in some types of neoplasms. But certainly in the adult the renal tissue, which is extremely sensitive to hypoxia, must contain a specific receptor cell system, either medullary or glomerular,[18] which responds directly to a hypoxic stimulus by releasing the renal erythropoietic factor. Other stimuli such as a decrease in RBC mass or cobalt may also act directly at the level of kidney tissue. An indirect control mechanism also seems to exist and operate through the influences of hormones and the central nervous system,[19] as shown in FIGURE 4. According to this model the oxygen-kidney system and the renal activator and inhibitor mechanisms are important links in a more complex chain of events.

References

1. ABBERT, P. H. & R. L. MALVIN. 1966. Amer. J. Physiol. **210:** 237.
2. FISHER, J. W. & B. J. BIRDWELL. 1961. Acta Haemat. **26:** 224.
3. KURATOWSKA, Z., B. LEWARTOWSKI & E. MICHALAK. 1960. Bull. Acad. Pol. Sc. (C1.II) **8:** 77.
4. NAETS, J. P. 1960. Blood **16:** 1770.
5. WARTER, J., J. M. MANTZ & B. HAMMANN. 1962. Compt. Rend. Soc. Biol. **156:** 897.
6. KURATOWSKA, Z., B. LEWARTOWSKI & E. MICHALAK. 1961. Blood **18:** 527.
7. KURATOWSKA, Z., B. LEWARTOWSKI & B. LIPINSKI. 1964. J. Lab. Clin. Invest. **64:** 226.
8. HANSEN, P. 1963. Scand. J. Clin. Lab. Invest. **15:** 622.
9. NAETS, J. P. 1960. Proc. Soc. Exp. Med. Biol. **103:** 129.
10. Pennington, D. 1963. Hormones and The Kidney. *In* Mem. Soc. Endocrinology. Acad. Press. London. **13:** 201.
11. PIHA, R. S., E. HYRSKE. 1961. Ann. Acad. Fenn. S.A. 76.
12. KURATOWSKA, Z. 1965. Bull. Acad. Pol. Soc. (Cl.II) **13:** 385.
13. CASSIDY, J. T., G. W. JOURDIAN & S. ROSEMAN. 1965. J. Biol. Chem. **240:** 3501.
14. KURATOWSKA, Z. & T. KUBICKA. Acta Biochem. Pol. In press.
15. GOLDWASSER, E. 1964. X Congress Int. Soc. Haemat. Stockholm.
16. GOLDWASSER, E., W. F. WHITE & K. B. TAYLOR. 1962. *In* Erythropoiesis. L. O. Jacobson & M. Doyle, eds. : 43. Grune & Stratton. New York-London.
17. LUCARELLI, G., D. HOWARD & F. STOHLMAN. 1964. J. Clin. Invest. **43:** 2195.
18. FISHER, J. W., C. TAYLOR & D. D. PORTEOUS. Nature **205:** 611.
19. HALVORSEN, S. 1966. Acta Haemat. **35:** 65.

RENAL TRANSPLANTATION AND EXTRACTS AND ERYTHROPOIESIS

E. E. Muirhead, B. E. Leach and J. W. Fisher
University of Tennessee Medical Units, Memphis, Tenn.

and

Mary Kosinski
Department of Pathology, School of Medicine, Wayne State University, Detroit, Mich.

The kidney as a major source of erythropoietin was first proposed by Jacobson *et al.*[1] in experiments on the rat. Naets[2] confirmed this proposal for the dog. This view has been supported by other investigators.[3–7] While a major role of the kidney in erythropoiesis appears established, the site of erythropoietin production within the kidney remains unsettled. Osteen,[8] Hirashima and Takaku,[9] as well as others, suggested the juxtaglomerular apparatus as the site of erythropoietin production, thus placing this function within the cortex. Fisher *et al.*[10] using the fluorescent antibody technique, also supported a cortical origin for the hormone by detecting fluorescence in the area of the glomerulus. Pennington,[11] on the other hand, derived erythropoietin activity from both cortex and medulla of the hog kidney through the application of extraction procedures. In a preliminary presentation, using a transplantation procedure, Muirhead *et al.*[12] suggested that both renocortical and renomedullary tissue appeared to support erythropoiesis. Since the latter findings could not be confirmed, a different scheme was developed for the transplantation approach. It is the purpose of this presentation to relate the results of the modified transplantation approach as well as to present preliminary results on the separation of erythropoietin from various regions of the kidney.

Materials and Methods

Healthy-appearing male and female mongrel dogs were used in all experiments. The ureterovenous anastomoses and the nephrectomy experiments were performed under pentobarbital anesthesia. The second nephrectomies and bilateral nephrectomy were performed under ether. The animals were not dialyzed during the experiment. In order to prolong life, solid foods and water were excluded from the diet. The animals received daily intravenous injections of 16 ml/kg of physiologic saline and 16 ml/kg of 5% dextrose. In essence, this was the graded fluid increment approach used by Ivy long ago.

^{59}Fe incorporation in red cells[13] was determined by injecting 8 μc of ^{59}Fe citrate intravenously and appropriate standard was prepared. Blood samples were obtained at 30, 60, 120 and 180 minutes for the determination of the rate of disappearance of ^{59}Fe from the plasma (T ½ ^{59}Fe). Additional samples were obtained on the second, third and fourth days. Sequestrene was used as the anticoagulant in these studies. Hematocrits were determined by the method of Wintrobe[14] and corrected with a factor of 0.96. Whole blood and plasma were counted for radioactivity. The plasma volume was determined by extrapolating plasma counts back to zero and using the expression $\text{total net counts injected}/\text{zero time cpm ml of plasma}$. The plasma volume was converted to the blood volume $\left(\text{plasma volume}/(\text{1-corrected hematocrit})\right)$. The difference between the whole blood and plasma counts was considered as the corrected red cell cpm. This maneuver was necessary since the nephrectomized animal retains considerable radioactivity in the circulating plasma. The percent ^{59}Fe incorporation into red cells was determined by $\frac{\text{red blood cell cpm} \times \text{blood volume}}{\text{total count injected}} \times 100$. The blood volume for the first two days of the study was estimated using ^{59}Fe plasma dilution, while on the third day the blood volume was repeated using the Risa ^{131}I method. The latter was considered necessary since the nephrectomized dog is in a hemolytic state[15] which may alter the determination. The two isotopes were measured by a discriminating counter.

In contrast to our previous findings,[12] when the radioiron was injected into four animals 5 to 13 min after nephrectomy, the percent ^{59}Fe incorporation (TABLE 1) at three to four days was between 13 and 98% (mean $\pm$ SE = 54.8 $\pm$ 11). When the injection was made 48 hr after the nephrectomies (four animals), the incorporation was between 9 and 38% (17.5 $\pm$ 6). The scheme was modified and conformed closer to that of Naets.[2] The nephrectomies were performed, 60 to 90 hr later the radioiron was injected, and the rate of ^{59}Fe disappearance from plasma was measured. The incorporation of ^{59}Fe into circulating red cells was determined within an additional three days. Thus, the study covered a period of 132 to 162 hr following nephrectomy. In the sham-operated group, the radioiron was injected 60 to 90 hr after the renal manipulations. For the groups having the ureter anastomosed to the inferior vena cava and the group having renal tissue

TABLE 1

CLEARANCE OF ^{59}FE FROM PLASMA AND SERUM IRON*

Group	Plasma T½ Minutes**	^{59}Fe n	RBC % ^{59}Fe Incorporation** (132–162 hr)	Serum Fe Percent μg**	n
Normal – sham	74 ± 5	8	57 ± 8	130 ± 7 100 ± 2	4
Ureterovenous	100 ± 18	8	51 ± 4	106 ± 7 140 ± 7	7
Bilateral nephrectomy	281 ± 23	21	7.5 ± 1.2	141 ± 16 158 ± 17	8
Whole kidney-cortex transplantation	292 ± 20	8	3.0 ± 1.8	155 ± 9 171 ± 11	3
Medulla transplantation	283 ± 19	16	8.5 ± 2.2	141 ± 9 148 ± 9	15

* The time required for clearance of ^{59}Fe from the circulating plasma, the percent incorporation of ^{59}Fe into circulating erythrocytes and the serum iron concentration are tabulated for the five groups. The mean $\pm$ the standard error of the mean $\left(\frac{SD}{\sqrt{N}}\right)$ are recorded. The upper serum iron value was determined 60–90 hr after the renal manipulation, at the time of the ^{59}Fe injection, while the lower value was determined three days later, at the time the ^{59}Fe incorporation into the erythrocytes (shown in the third column) was determined.

** Mean $\pm$ Standard error of mean $\left(\frac{SD}{\sqrt{N}}\right)$

transplanted to peritoneum or lungs, the radioiron was injected 60 to 90 hr after the unmanipulated kidney was removed.

Renal Autotransplantation in the Dog. One kidney was removed under pentobarbital anesthesia. The kidney was then divided into small fragments, washed in saline and reinjected within 15–20 min, along with an antibiotic mixture, either i.p. or i.v. into the lungs. The transplantation procedure was similar to that described previously.[16] Whole kidney and cortical fragments (eight experiments) were injected i.p. Renal medulla was injected i.v. in 15 experiments and i.p. on six occasions. The remaining kidney was removed 14 days later and the experiment begun.

Ureterovenous Anastomosis. The left ureter was connected to the lower abdominal vena cava by means of a U-shaped polyethylene tube as previously described.[17] In this preparation, urine flows readily and there is no hydronephrosis. The caval urine flow was checked under anesthesia and determined to be satisfactory before sacrifice.

The following additional methods were used: hemoglobin by the cyanmethemoglobin technic, the whole blood urea by Annino's method,[18] serum sodium and potassium by flame photometry and the serum iron by Caraway's method.[19]

Kidney extraction procedure in anemic dogs: Each donor dog had a hematocrit of between 40–45% at the beginning of the experiment and was made anemic by a combination of phenylhydrazine injections and bleeding. Phenylhydrazine hydrochloride was injected i.v. at a dose level of 40 mg/kg and was followed by the withdrawal of 200 ml of blood every other day and replacing the blood volume with Dextran. This procedure was continued until the animal's hematocrit decreased below 20%. Two animals were made anemic by bleeding alone every other day until their hematocrits were reduced to 8 and 10% respectively. All animals were sacrificed by exsanguination and the blood collected. The blood was allowed to clot in a cold room at 4° C. The serum was separated by centrifugation and frozen until assayed for erythropoietic activity.

The kidneys were removed from the animals immediately after sacrifice, and each kidney was flushed with 200 ml of saline to remove most of the blood. In two instances, the hemoglobin was determined by the benzidine method[20] using the last 25 ml of the saline wash, and the concentration was 6 μg of hemoglobin per ml of saline.

Each kidney was sectioned transversely in approximately 0.25-inch slices, and the medulla precisely separated from the cortex. The dissected medulla and cortex were frozen separately and stored in a deep freeze until processed.

Preparation of Extracts. The extraction procedure was similar to that of Gordon *et al.*[21] For each gram of frozen tissue, 3 ml of cold 0.02 *M* phosphate buffer, pH 6.8, was added and homogenized for two minutes in a Waring blendor. This homogenate was centrifuged at 37,000 g for 30 min at 4° C in a Beckman model L centrifuge. The supernatant was collected and stored frozen until assayed for erythropoietic activity. The renomedullary extract did not contain a detectable amount of renin activity when assayed in the 24-hour nephrectomized rat.

Erythropoietin Assay. The erythropoietic activity of each preparation was assayed by determining ^{59}Fe incorporation into red blood cells of polycythemic mice.[22] The mice were made polycythemic by being kept at 0.5 atmospheric pressure for three weeks. Each mouse received 1.0 ml hematocrit 70 blood i.p. on the day they were removed from the low pressure tank. Three ml of each extract were given in three divided doses at 5-hour intervals on the fifth day out of tank. Six to eight mice were used in each group. 0.5 μc ^{59}Fe citrate was given 48 hr later, and the animals were completely exsanguinated 72 hr beyond this time. ^{59}Fe incorporation in red cells was determined for each animal. Mice with hematocrit values less than 55% were discarded from the assay.

RESULTS

Percent Incorporation ^{59}Fe into Erythrocytes (Figure 1 & Table 1)

Normal and Sham-Operated Group (n=8). There were four sham-operated and four normal animals in this group. Together, the percent ^{59}Fe incorporation at the three-day interval (three days after the 60–90 hr wait for the sham group) amounted to 57% ± 8 (mean ± SE). The average incorporation for the normal group was 51% and for the sham group 64%; these two groups did not differ (p¬0.5).

Ureterovenous anastomosis group (n = 10): When the ureter was connected to the vena cava, the incorporation at three days was 51% ± 4. These results did not differ from the normal-sham group (p¬0.6). Since this group did not have a urinary external excretory outlet and was not dialyzed, the degree of acute uremia was the same as in the nephrectomized group.

Bilateral Nephrectomy Group (n=25). The incorporation for this group at the three-day period was 7.5 ± 1.2. Of the 25 examples, ten yielded zero incor-

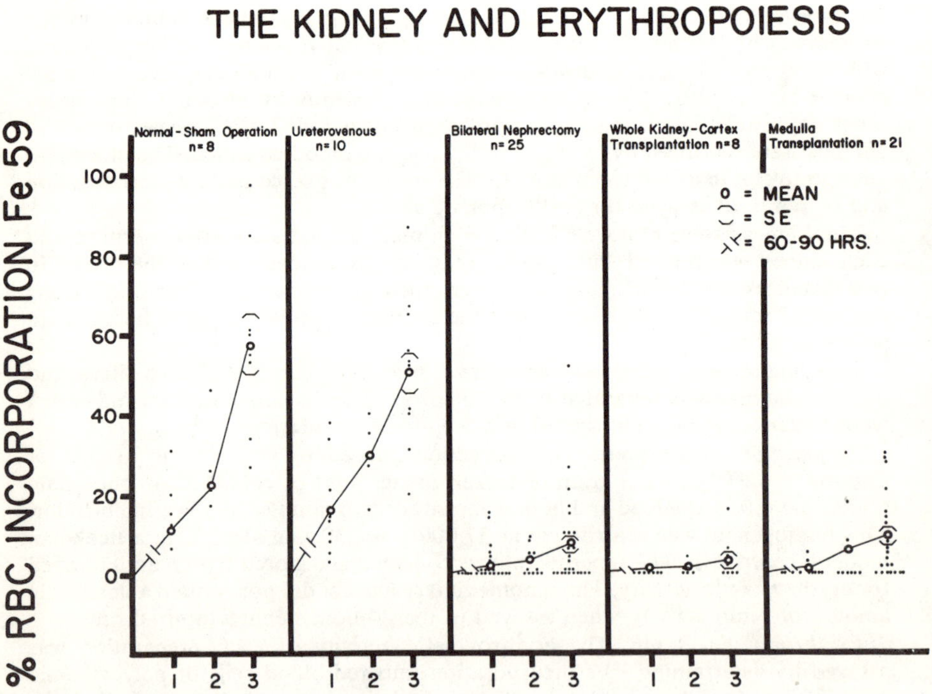

FIGURE 1. The vertical axis depicts the percent incorporation of ^{59}Fe into circulating erythrocytes and the horizontal axis the time in days. The mean value for each of the three days is shown; on the third day the standard error of the mean is added. The 60–90-hour gap represents the waiting period prior to the ^{59}Fe injection. It is to be noted that the animals were not dialyzed.

poration. This meant that the plasma counts usually exceeded the whole blood counts. These results do not necessarily indicate no ^{59}Fe incorporation, partly because of the renoprival hemolytic state. The red cell life-span was not measured in these experiments but it is known that in a high proportion of nephrectomized dogs, there is a high rate of destruction of red cells[15] (Cr 51 T ½ about five days). Had these 10 animals been the ones with a high rate of red cell destruction (a likely possibility), then some degree of ^{59}Fe incorporation would have been masked. Three of the 25 dogs incorporated more than 20% of the injected iron into the red cells, one incorporated 52%. We have no explanation for these rare observations. In general, our results are similar to those reported by Naets for the dog.[2] Naets' animals were dialyzed, ours were not.

The differences between the nephrectomized (renoprival) and the normal-sham and ureterovenous groups were highly significant ($p < .001$).

Renal Transplantation Groups. On six occasions cortical tissue and on two occasions whole kidney tissue was transplanted to the peritoneum. The average ^{59}Fe incorporation was 3% ± 1.8. Four of this group showed zero incorporation at three days. There were 21 experiments in which renal medulla was transplanted. The incorporation at the three-day mark averaged 8.5% ± 2.2. Three animals had incorporation between 20 and 25%. Seven animals of the latter group showed zero incorporation. Possibly the same reasoning for the zero values applies here as for the renoprival group. Although renoprival hemolysis appears significantly improved by the transplantation of renal tissue, it is not entirely prevented.[15] The difference between the renoprival and transplantation groups and between the two transplantation groups was not significant ($p \sim 0.4$ and 0.7, respectively).

Serum Iron Concentration. The serum iron concentration of the sham-operated group decreased between the renal manipulation and the third day (average 130 to 100 $\mu g\%$, see TABLE 1). The serum iron of the ureterovenous group increased during the three-day interval of ^{59}Fe incorporation (106–140 $\mu g\%$). The other groups (renoprival, renoprival plus renal transplantation) had elevated serum iron to a comparable degree throughout the period of ^{59}Fe measurement. Although siderois may have influenced the results to a certain extent, the differences in ^{59}Fe incorporation between the nephrectomized-transplanted groups and the ureterovenous group (both having hyperferremia) were so outstanding as to minimize the significance of this factor. The lack of difference between the normal-sham and ureterovenous groups adds credence to this interpretation.

Disappearance Rate of ^{59}Fe from Plasma. The disappearance of radioiron from the circulating plasma (T ½ in minutes), as shown in TABLE 1, averaged 74 and 100 for the normal-sham operated and ureterovenous groups and 281, 292 and 283 for the bilateral nephrectomy and transplantation groups. Thus, the results of this parameter paralleled those of the ^{59}Fe incorporation into red cells.

Magnitude of Uremia. TABLE 2 gives results of the concentration of hemoglobin in the peripheral blood and the concentration of whole blood urea and serum sodium and potassium. These values were chosen as guides of the magnitude of uremia.

The sham group displayed no major changes (there was a slight lowering of hemoglobin concentration). In general, the other groups displayed little change in hemoglobin and serum sodium concentration, prominent azotemia and hyperkalemia. It is to be noted that during the time of measurement of the ^{59}Fe incorporation, azotemia and hyperkalemia were present and mounting in all test groups, as expected since dialysis was not instituted. Of interest is the comparable level of uremia in the ureterovenous group which incorporated ^{59}Fe and the bilateral

TABLE 2

THE EFFECT OF RENAL MANIPULATION ON THE HEMOGLOBIN, UREA, SODIUM AND POTASSIUM CONCENTRATIONS*

Group	No.	Hemoglobin Concentration g/%	Hematocrit Percent	Blood Urea mg Percent	Serum Na mEq/1	Serum K mEq/1
Sham	4	15 ± 1.4	47.0 ± 2.3	21 ± 2	157 ± 9.7	5.3 ± 0.2
		13.4 ± 1.6	36.0 ± 7.1	19 ± 1.4	153 ± 9.1	5.0 ± 0.8
Ureterovenous	10	12.9 ± 0.55	45.4 ± 2.3	141 ± 14	153 ± 1.2	6.5 ± 0.33
		11.7 ± 0.52	41.3 ± 2.3	234 ± 26	153 ± 2.3	7.7 ± 0.4
Bilateral nephrectomy	23	12.9 ± 0.42	42.5 ± 1.8	148 ± 7	150 ± 1.4	6.7 ± 0.17
		13.1 ± 0.44	44.0 ± 1.8	209 ± 23	153 ± 2.9	7.7 ± 0.28
Whole kidney–cortex transplantation	6	13.8 ± 0.3	43.0 ± 2.0	147 ± 7	151 ± 2.4	6.4 ± 0.36
		13.9 ± 2	45.0 ± 2.4	239 ± 19	151 ± 2.0	8.1 ± 0.35
Medulla transplantation	20	12.0 ± 0.34	40.7 ± 1.7	148 ± 10	151 ± 6	6.7 ± 0.24
		12.4 ± 0.42	38.2 ± 1.2	223 ± 15	153 ± 2.4	8.0 ± 0.34

* The blood findings used in appraising the degree of uremia are shown. The values include the mean and standard error of the mean. The upper value represents results at the time of the ^{59}Fe injection, while the lower value consists of results three days later.

TABLE 3

ERYTHROPOIETIC ACTIVITY OF SERUM, RENOCORTICAL AND MEDULLARY EXTRACTS FROM ANEMIC DOGS*

Exp. No.	Hematocrit Percent	Serum	n	Renocortical Extract	n	Renomedullary Extract	n
1	8	15.0 ± 5**	6	5.3 ± 1.3**	6	2.3 ± 1.0**	5
2	10	9.3 ± 2.7	5	4.7 ± 2.8	6	1.1 ± 0.43	5
3	14	7.6 ± 0.9	5	2.2 ± 0.89	3	0.26 ± 0.05	5
4	24	10.3 ± 3.9	7	0.54 ± 0.2	3	0.5 ± 0.05	2

* Results of the assays for erythropoietin-like activity in erythremic mice of serum and extracts of renal cortex and medulla of anemic dogs are depicted. The mean and standard error are given. Three ml of serum and 3 ml of extracts or the equivalent of 1 g of wet tissue were injected per mouse. The saline controls, derived at the same time as the above data, gave 0.68 ± 0.09 percent ^{59}Fe incorporation (n = 31). One unit of Standard B was determined in our mice to yield 7.65 ± 1.09 percent incorporation (n = 24). The difference between the renocortical and renomedullary results was significant ($p < .05 > .025$).

** Mean ± standard error of mean $\left(\frac{SD}{\sqrt{N}}\right)$ of ^{59}Fe incorporation into erythrocytes.

nephrectomy and transplantation groups which incorporated ^{59}Fe very poorly.

Renocortical and Renomedullary Erythropoietic Activity. TABLE 3 relates the results. The serum erythropoietic activity was elevated as expected (7.6–15% ^{59}Fe incorporation, one unit standard B 7.65%). In each experiment erythropoietic activity was derived from both cortical and medullary tissue. Converted to standard B units, the overall cortical activity averaged 0.37 units per gram wet weight of tissue and the medullary activity 0.13 units. The difference between cortical and medullary activity was significant ($p<.05>.025$).

SUMMARY AND COMMENTS

Radioiron incorporation into circulating erythrocytes was significantly lower following bilateral nephrectomy (renoprival state) than in normal and sham-operated dogs as well as in animals having the ureter anastomosed to the inferior vena cava. The results were similar to those reported by Naets using dialyzed animals. In the present experiments, dialysis was not instituted; thus the degree of uremia was comparable in the renoprival and ureterovenous groups. Acute uremia, then, did not seem to alter the iron incorporation. Transplantation of fragments of cortex and medulla did not alter the depressed level of iron incorporation of the renoprival state. Contrary to earlier data, this type of renal transplantation is not satisfactory for evaluating the support of erythropoiesis by the kidney. These results differ from those of R. Ardaillou *et al.*[23] utilizing the rat. This could represent a species difference.

The erythropoietic activity derived by the extraction of renal tissue of dogs having severe phenylhydrazine-induced anemia was significantly higher in the renal cortex than in the renal medulla. The slight medullary activity could be the result of urinary erythropoietin in tubular fluid as well as that adsorbed to renal tissue and may not represent in situ formation.

The finding of erythropoietic activity in homogenates of renal tissue derived in hypotonic buffer solution confirms, for the dog, the observations of Gordon *et al.*[7,21] for the rat.

In general, the data appear to support the view that erythropoietin is principally of renocortical origin.

References

1. Jacobson, L. O., E. Goldwasser, W. Fried & L. Plzak. 1957. Role of the kidney in erythropoiesis. Nature **179:** 633.
2. Naets, J. P. 1960. The role of the kidney in erythropoiesis. J. Clin. Invest. **39:** 102.
3. Fisher, J. W. & B. J. Birdwell. 1961. The production of an erythropoietic factor by the in situ perfused kidney. Acta Hematol. **26:** 224.
4. Eisler, A. J. 1961. Kidney-bone marrow interaction. Trans. N. Y. Acad. Sci. **24:** 131.
5. Kuratowska, Z., B. Lewartowski & E. Michalak. 1961. Studies on the production of erythropoietin by isolated perfused organs. Blood **18:** 527.
6. Reissman, K. R. 1963. Erythropoietin formation in the kidney. *In* Hormones and the Kidney. P. C. Williams, ed. : 195–200. Academic Press. London-New York.
7. Gordon, A. S. & J. F. Contrera. 1966. Erythropoietin: production by a particulate fraction of rat kidney. Science **152:** 653.
8. Osnes, S. 1958. An erythropoietic factor produced in the kidney. Brit. Med. J. **2:** 1387.
9. Hirashima, K. & F. Takaku. 1962. Experimental studies on erythropoietin. II. Relationship between juxtaglomerular cells and erythropoietin. Blood **20:** 1.
10. Fisher, J. W., G. W. Taylor & D. D. Porteous. 1965. Localization of erythropoietin in glomeruli of sheep kidney by the use of a fluorescent antibody technique. Nature **205:** 611.
11. Pennington, D. G. 1963. Erythropoietin in tissues: features of the renal erythropoietin-producing system. *In* Hormones of the Kidney. P. C. Williams, ed. : 201–219. Academic Press. London-New York.
12. Muirhead, E. E., M. Kosinski, F. Jones & E. Reno. 1962. Erythropoietin and the state of renal tissue. Blood **20:** 782 (abstr.).
13. Huff, R. L., T. G. Hennessy, R. E. Austin, J. E. Garcia, B. M. Roberts & J. H. Lawrence. 1950. Plasma and red cell iron turnover in normal subjects and patients having various hematopoietic disorders. J. Clin. Invest. **29:** 1041.
14. Wintrobe, M. M. 1929. A simple and accurate hematocrit. J. Lab. Clin. Med. **15:** 287.
15. Muirhead, E. E. & F. Jones. 1963. Renoprival hemolysis and its prevention by renal tissue. Blood **22:** 272.
16. Muirhead, E. E., J. A. Stirman & F. Jones. 1960. Renal autoexplantation and protection against renoprival hypertensive cardiovascular disease and hemolysis. J. Clin. Invest. **39:** 266.
17. Muirhead, E. E., F. Jones & J. A. Stirman. 1960. Hypertensive cardiovascular disease of dogy, relation of sodium and dietary protein to ureterocaval anastomosis and ureteral ligation. A.M.A. Arch. Path. **70:** 108.
18. Annino, J. S. 1964. Clinical Chemistry, Principles and Procedures. 3rd ed. : 157. Little, Brown & Co. Boston, Mass.
19. Caraway, W. T. 1963. Macro and micro methods for the determination of serum iron and iron-binding capacity. Clin. Chem. **9:** 188.
20. Miale, J. B. 1958. Laboratory Medicine-Hematology. : 661. C. V. Mosby Co. St. Louis, Mo.
21. Gordon, A. S., J. F. Contrera, J. F. Camiscoli & A. H. Weintraub. 1964. Extraction of erythropoietin from kidneys of phenylhydrazine-treated and hypoxic rats. Blood **24:** 845.
22. Gurney, C. W. & C. Pan. 1958. Studies on erythropoiesis. IX. Mechanism of decreased erythropoiesis in experimental polycythemia. Proc. Soc. Exper. Biol. Med. **98:** 789.
23. Ardaillou, R., Y. Najean, J. Altman & G. Richet. 1960. Etude de l'érythropoïèse chez les rats néphrectomisés et porteurs d'une autogreffe rénale. Rev. Franc. Etudes Clin. Biol. V: 189.

ERYTHROPOIESIS IN RENAL INSUFFICIENCY AND IN ANEPHRIC MAN*

J. P. Naets, M. Wittek, C. Toussaint,
and
J. Van Geertruyden

Laboratoire de Médecine Expérimentale et Laboratoire de Biologie Clinique, Université Libre de Bruxelles et Fondation Médicale Reine Elisabeth, Bruxelles, Belgique

While the role of the kidney in erythropoiesis has been experimentally demonstrated,[1,2] we have only indirect arguments concerning the eventual production of erythropoietin by this organ in man.

The fact that acute anuria is followed by a sudden and marked depletion of the erythroid marrow,[3,4] as opposed to the moderate normoblastic depression observed in chronic renal disease, has led us to think that uremic intoxication is not the main cause of the erythropoietic depression in renal insufficiency, but that the kidney has a predominent role in erythropoiesis independent of its excretory function.[2] Erythropoietin plasma level is not measurable in patients with chronic renal disorders regardless of the severity of anemia, while increased values are generally found in patients with similar anemia but normal renal function.[5,6] On the other hand, polycythemia has been reported in some renal diseases (renal tumors, cysts or hydronephrosis). In certain cases erythropoietin has been detected in plasma and in tumor extracts or cystic fluid.[7,10] These facts corroborate the hypothesis that in man, the kidney is concerned with the elaboration of erythropoietin, if not with the exclusive source of the hormone.

In this study we have presented determinations of erythropoietin plasma levels in patients with chronic uremia or acute anuria, treated or not by extrarenal epuration, nephrectomy or transplantation, and compared the modifications of normoblast percentage observed in the bone marrow after nephrectomy or acute anuria.

Determination of Erythropoietin Plasma Level

Determinations of the erythropoietin plasma level have been performed on hypoxic or transfused polycythemic mice following the methods described by Degowin *et al.*[11,12] The day the plasma was collected, the hematocrit was below 26%, except in some cases indicated in TABLE 1.

In Nondialyzed Patients with Chronic Uremia

The erythropoietin plasma level was measured in 44 patients with chronic renal failure and in 66 nonuremic but similarly anemic patients. In the uremic group, a slight elevation of erythropoietin plasma titer ($\triangle$uptake 1.79–6.89%, M:4.15%) was observed in eight patients (18%). In the nonuremic group, 13 patients (21%) had a moderate ($\triangle$uptake 1.11–3.75%, M:1.9%) and 40 patients (63%) a marked increase ($\triangle$uptake 4.32–50.68%, M:17.0%) in erythropoietin plasma titer.

In Acute Anuria

In 10 anemic patients with acute anuria of various origin that have been investigated, no erythropoietic activity was detectable.

* This work was performed under Contract Euratom U.L.B. – Pise no. 063–4–BIAC.

TABLE 1

ERYTHROPOIETIN PLASMA LEVEL IN HEMODIALYZED, NEPHRECTOMIZED OR TRANSPLANTED PATIENTS

Name	Sex	Diagnosis	After First Hemodialysis				After Bilateral Nephrectomy				After Transplantation				
			Days	Hematocrit %	Urea mg %	Δ ^{59}Fe Uptake %	Days	Hematocrit %	Urea mg %	Δ ^{59}Fe uptake %	Days	Hematocrit %	Urea mg %	Creat. Clear. ml/min	Δ ^{59}Fe Uptake %
Boe	F	Polycyst. dis.	4	25	240	0									
Re	F	Nephrosclerosis	63	30	150	0.02									
Ki	F	Nephrosclerosis	38	27	210	0									
			104	18	113	0.29									
Ke	F	Chron. glom.	41	25	204	0.44									
			107	17	112	0.27									
De	F	Chron. pyelon.	79	32	92	0.34									
			289	26	112	0.39									
V.d.Z.	M	Chron. glom.	60	22	125	0.16									
Boo	M	Chron. glom.	24	22	216	0.69									
Vae	M	Chron. glom.	146	23	135	0.16									
Ya	M	Nephrosclerosis	30	22	153	0									
Im	M	Chron. glom.	205	32	95	0									
Fe	M	Chron. pyelon.	6	21	138	0*	10	22	117	0					
							46	24	80	0.43					
Bog	F	Nephrosclerosis					34	23	63	0					
							72	18	165	0					
Fa	M	Chron. pyelon.	36	24	171	0.02	14	24	170	0	19	20	231	14	0.02
							21	37	165	0	39	22	99	38	0.06
Cap	M	Chron. pyelon.	14	19	100	0	60	27	148	0.23	7	24	255	1	0
							88	25	159	0	19	29	78	40	0
											57	22	30	80	0.76
Car	M	Chron. glom.	145	21	159	0					17	30	82	50	0.18
Mu	M	Chron. glom.	82	22	138	0*					17	32	35	94	0
Sm	M	Chron. glom.									66	25	150	35	0
Du	F	Chron. pyelon.	3	27	147	0.36					21	22	80	55	0
Dr	M	Chron. glom.									18	28	54	70	1.59

* 2 ml of plasma injected instead of 1 ml.

In Uremic Patients Treated by Hemodialysis, Bilateral Nephrectomy or Homotransplantation (TABLE 1)

In 16 uremic patients and in four patients bilaterally nephrectomized for 10 to 88 days (eight determinations) and maintained alive with intermittent hemodialysis, the erythropoietin plasma level was not measurable in spite of severe anemia. After homotransplantation (7–66 days), erythropoietin was measurable in only one of the seven investigated patients. In one patient (Ca), in spite of an evident erythropoietic response (reticulocytes: 74%, marrow normblasts: 43%) following an acute hemolytic crisis that resulted in a sudden drop of the hematocrit from 37 to 21%, no erythropoietin was detectable in the plasma. Urea levels of the assayed plasma samples were generally high since blood was collected for practical reasons immediately before hemodialysis.

Measurement of Normoblast Percentage in the Bone Marrow of Patients with Acute Anuria or Bilateral Nephrectomy

In eight patients, bilateral nephrectomy was performed before renal transplatation in order to palliate malignant hypertension. Blood urea levels varied from 200–250 mg percent before, to 30–70 mg percent after hemodialysis. Repeated counts of normoblasts from 5–100 days following nephrectomy showed a sudden depletion of the erythroid marrow. The mean value of normoblasts averaging 13.9% before nephrectomy, decreased abruptly to 6% after the operation, and increased to 10% after 30 days (FIGURE 1).

Twenty-seven patients with acute anuria of various etiology were investigated. Blood urea levels varied from 200–600 mg percent, averaging 445 mg percent.

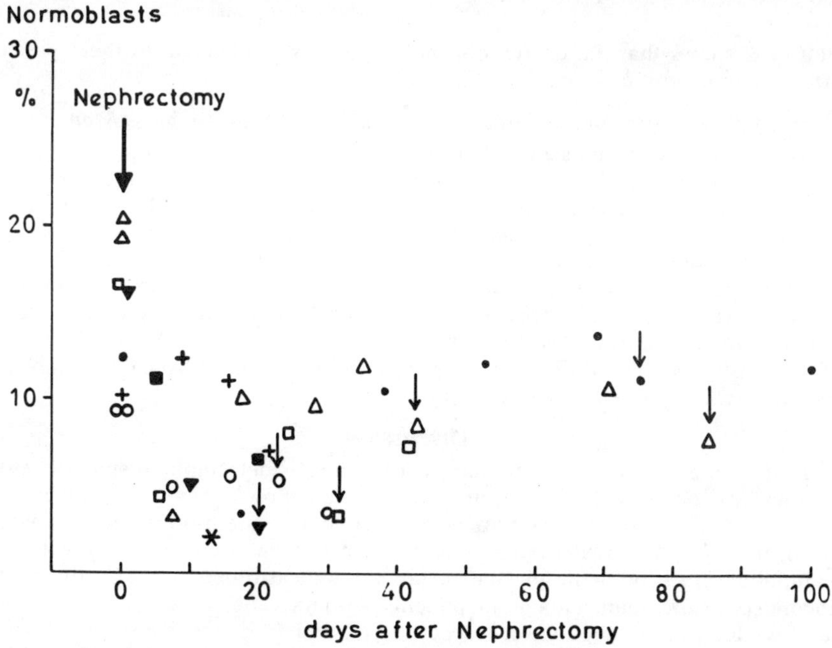

FIGURE 1. Normoblast percentage in bone marrow of anephric patients as a function of time elapsed since bilateral nephrectomy.

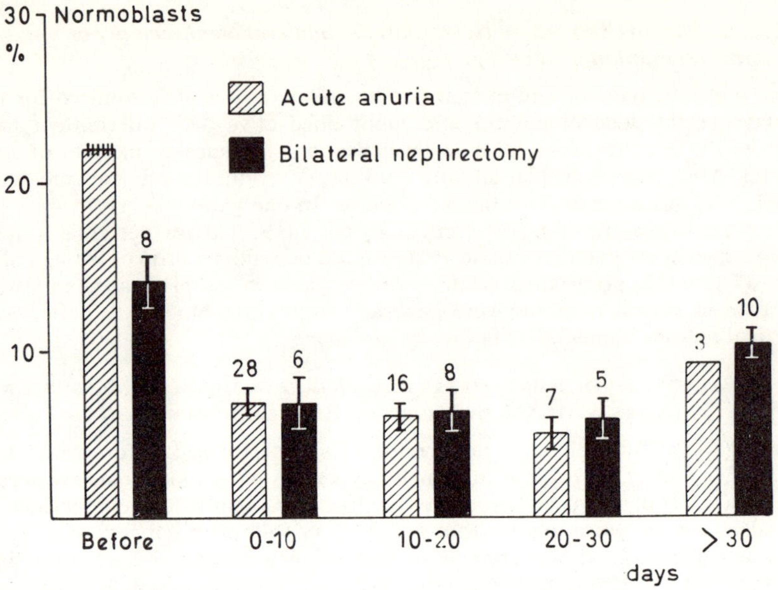

FIGURE 2. Compared effects of acute anuria and bilateral nephrectomy on normoblast percentage in the bone marrow of chronically hemodialyzed patients as a function of the time elapsed since anuria or nephrectomy. The first column represents the assumed theoretical normal value before anuria. Figures on the top indicate the number of determinations. Vertical bars represent one standard error of the mean.

FIGURE 2 shows that the decrease in normoblasts was identical in these patients after bilateral nephrectomy.

Effect of Transfusion on the Percentage of Normoblasts in Anephric Man

Normoblasts were measured before and after transfusions in five anephric patients. In one case (Bo) the observation was repeated six weeks later. The total volume transfused in two or three times amounted from 2.5 to 3.1. Normoblasts were counted from five to nine days (mean: 6.5 days) after the first, and from two to five days (mean: four days) after the last transfusion. TABLE 2 summarizes the hematological data concerning these patients. Before transfusion, red cell mass averaged 18.0 ml/kg and was increased to 27.3 ml/kg the day of the second determination of normoblasts. Normoblasts decreased from 9.2 before, to 6.7% after transfusion. The difference between these values is statistically significant: $t = 3.787; 0.02 > p > 0.01$ (Student test).

DISCUSSION

That no measurable erythropoietin plasma titer is detectable in spite of severe anemia in patients with chronic uremia has been shown previously utilizing the starved rat as bioassay animal.[6] As polycythemic mice are more sensitive towards erythropoietin than fasted rats, measurements have been repeated with this technique. Erythropoietin plasma levels were measurable in 18% of uremic anemic patients, against 84% in patients without renal failure, while the less sensitive bioassay method gave, respectively, 2 and 47% positive results (FIGURE 3). Consequently, some uremic patients at least are susceptible to respond to anemia by increased production of erythropoietin. These patients apparently

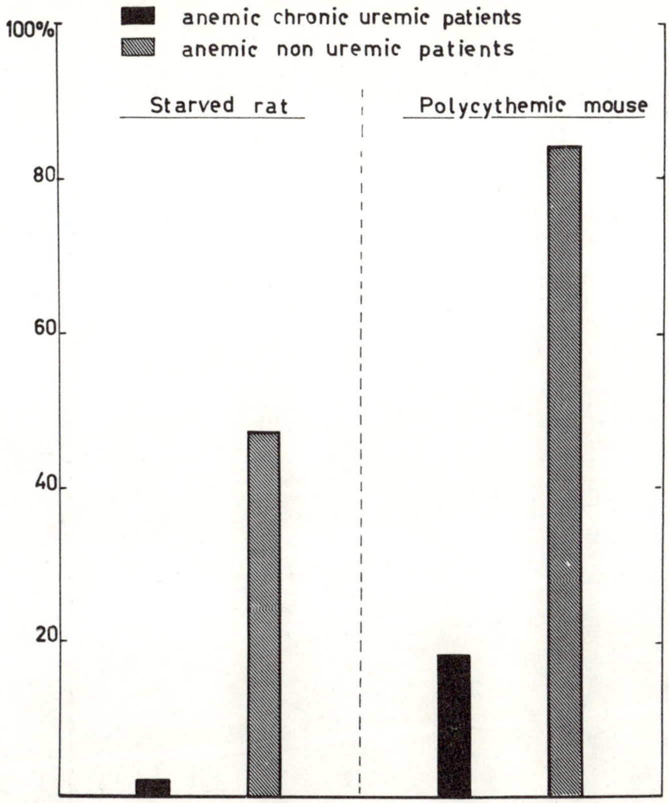

FIGURE 3. Percentage of anemic patients (with and without renal insufficiency) with measurable erythropoietin level. Comparative results with two bioassay methods.

do not differ from the others with regard to renal function or evolution of their disease. A possible dissociation between "excretory" and "erythropoietic" function of the kidney could explain the persistence of the latter in certain cases. It must be emphasized that when a selected group of 16 patients is investigated whose renal function is so severly impaired that chronic hemodialyses are necessary to keep them alive, there is no erythropoietin detectable in their plasma in spite of the intermittent correction of uremic intoxication by extrarenal epuration.

These results are identical to the data recently reported by Denny *et al.*[13] However, these authors observed increased levels of erythropoietin after renal transplantation in 10 out of 48 determinations, whereas we have detected erythropoietic activity in only one of ten determinations (TABLE 1). As these authors have already reported, erythropoietin seems unrelated to the presence of a functional transplant. The absence of erythropoietic activity found after homotransplantation could be attributed to some alteration of the renal tissue independent of its excretory function. This hypothesis is suggested by histologic abnormalities frequently observed in biopsies of transplanted kidneys even when the excretory function is satisfactory.

Although in dogs normoblasts disappear following total nephrectomy,[14] in man erythropoiesis persists as long as 100 days. Nathan *et al.*[15] reported similar ob-

TABLE 2

EFFECTS OF BLOOD TRANSFUSIONS ON ERYTHROPOIESIS OF NEPHRECTOMIZED PATIENTS

Name	Sex	Before Transfusions				After Transfusions			
		Red Cell Mass ml/kg	Hematocrit %	Hemoglobin g %	Normoblasts %	Red Cell Mass ml/kg	Hematocrit %	Hemoglobin g %	Normoblasts %
Ca	M	22.8	27	9.6	13.9	34.1	38	11.8	11.3
Fa	M	14.2	25	8.8	5.6	26.2	37	12.7	5.4
Bo	F	16.6	22	7.6	11.8	28.7	36	11.5	8.4
Du	F	22.9	31	11.8	5.0	29.4	31	10.6	3.6
Fe	M	15.7	23	7.6	8.0	21.8	30	12.1	3.4
Bo	F	15.7	20	6.7	10.8	23.7	27	9.8	7.8
Mean:		18.0	25	8.7	9.2	27.3	33	11.4	6.7

servations in patients surviving bilateral nephrectomy as long as six months. In the present study after an initial drop of normoblasts sustained for about 30 days, the percentage gradually increased to a level similar to the prenephrectomy state (FIGURE 1). In seven nonuremic patients used as controls, no significant decrease in the percentage of normoblasts was observed after different surgical procedures. Normoblasts averaged 13.9% before and 12.5% 8–18 days after operation. It is suggested that the initial drop of normoblasts could be imputable to bilateral nephrectomy, resulting in a sudden suppression of a residual production of erythropoietin by the diseased kidney. Thus, the residual erythropoiesis persistent after nephrectomy could be explained either by adaptative regulation of a "basal erythropoiesis" (independent of erythropoietin), or by the increased production of erythropoietin by the hypothetic extrarenal tissue or organ responsible for erythropoietin production outside the kidney. Accordingly, erythropoiesis persists, although reduced, after nephrectomy in rats[16] and in rabbits.[17]

The similarity of the evolution of normoblasts observed between nephrectomized and acutely anuric patients is in fact most interesting as the situation is different in both groups, for instance, concerning uremic intoxication. No humoral modification occurs in the patients submitted chronically to intermittent hemodialysis before as well as after bilateral nephrectomy, whereas acute anuria happens usually as a sudden accident in previously healthy patients with normal renal function. Consequently, it seems that the normoblastic depression observed almost immediately after acute anuria is not imputable to uremic intoxication itself.

If hemoglobin concentration is increased by transfusions in nephrectomized anemic patients, a moderate but statistically significant decrease in normoblasts percentage ensues. These results agree with the observation reported by Nathan *et al.* concerning an anephric patient who responded to acute hypoxia (cardiac tamponade) by increased reticulocytosis.[15]

It is concluded that the anephric man, contrary to the dog, is still susceptible to adaptative regulation of erythropoiesis in response to variations of hemoglobin level. Persistent regulation, although not conclusive of persistent production of erythropoietin, is however an argument in favor of this hypothesis.

Summary

Erythropoiesis has been studied in renal insufficiency and in anephric man. The erythropoietin plasma titer was slightly increased in 18% of anemic patients with chronic renal insufficiency, not measurable either in acute anuria or in hemodialyzed chronic uremic or nephrectomized patients. After renal transplantation, erythropoietic activity was detectable in only one out of seven investigated patients.

Normoblast percentage in the marrow was followed in eight anephric patients from 5 to 100 days after bilateral nephrectomy and in 27 patients with acute anuria. Identical depletion of the erythroid marrow was observed in both groups, normoblasts decreasing to 6% after anuria or bilateral nephrectomy and increasing 30 days later to 10%.

Increase in Hb level by transfusion in anephric patients was followed by a moderate but significant decrease of normoblasts in the marrow from 9.2 to 6.7%.

These data suggest that in anephric man there is a basal erythropoiesis either independent of erythropoietin, or induced by erythropoietin produced in another site than the kidney. Furthermore, some regulation of erythropoiesis seems to persist in the absence of the kidneys.

References

1. Jacobson, L. O., E. Goldwasser, W. Fried & L. Plzak. 1957. Role of the kidney in erythropoiesis. Nature **179:** 633.
2. Naets, J. P. 1958. Erythropoiesis in nephrectomized dog. Nature **181:** 1134.
3. Richet, G., D. Alagile & E. Fournier. 1954. L'érythroblastopénie aiguë de l'anurie. Presse méd. **62:** 50.
4. Naets, J. P., H. Brauman & M. Kraytman. 1960. Etude de l'érythropoïèse au cours de l'insuffisance rénale aiguë et chronique. Acta Haemat. **24:** 169.
5. Gallagher, N. I., J. M. McCarthy & R. D. Lange. 1960. Observations on erythropoietic stimulating factor (E.S.F.) in the plasma of uremic and nonuremic patients. Ann. Int. Med. **52:** 1201.
6. Naets, J. P. & A. Heuse. 1962. Measurement of erythropoietic-stimulating factor in anemic patients with or without renal disease. J. Lab. Clin. Med. **60:** 365.
7. Gurney, C. W. 1960. Erythremia in renal disease. Trans. Ass. Amer. Physicians **73:** 103.
8. Hewlett, J. S., G. C. Hoffman, D. A Senhauser & J. D. Battle. 1960. Hypernephroma with erythrocythemia. Report of a case and assay of the tumor for an erythropoietic stimulating substance. New Engl. J. Med. **262:** 1058.
9. Rosse, W. F., T. A. Waldmann & P. Cohen. 1963. Renal cysts, erythropoietin and polycythemia. Amer. J. Med. **34:** 76.
10. Donati, R. M., J. M. McCarthy, R. D. Lange & N. I. Gallagher. 1963. Erythropoiesis and neoplastic tumors. Ann. Int. Med. **58:** 47.
11. De Gowin, R. L., D. Hofstra & C. W. Gurney. 1962. A comparison of erythropoietic bioassay. Proc. Soc. Exper. Biol. Med. **110:** 48.
12. De Gowin, R. L., D. Hofstra & C. W. Gurney. 1962. The mouse with hypoxia-induced erythremia, an erythropoietin bioassay animal. J. Lab. Clin. Med. **60:** 846.
13. Denny, W. F., W. J. Flanigan & C. F. Zukoski. 1966. Serial erythropoietin studies in patients undergoing renal homotransplantation. J. Lab. Clin. Med. **67:** 386.
14. Naets, J. P. 1960. The role of the kidney in erythropoiesis. J. Clin. Invest. **39:** 102.
15. Nathan, D. G., E. Schupak, F. Stohlman, Jr. & F. Merrill. 1964. Erythropoiesis in anephric man. J. Clin. Invest. **43:** 2158.
16. Reissmann, K. R., T. Nomura, R. W. Gunn & F. Brosius. 1960. Erythropoietic response to anemia or erythropoietin injection in anemic rats with or without functioning renal tissue. Blood **16:** 1411.
17. Erslev, A. J. 1958. Erythropoietic function in uremic rabbits. Arch. Int. Med. **101:** 407.

PART IV. KINETICS OF ERYTHROPOIESIS AND SITES OF ACTION OF ERYTHROPOIETIN

RESTORATION OF STEM CELL FUNCTION AFTER IRRADIATION

D. D. Porteous* and L. G. Lajtha

Paterson Laboratories,
Christie Hospital and Holt Radium Institute,
Manchester, England

INTRODUCTION

The way in which stem cell function in the rodent returns to normal after sublethal irradiation can be studied using several different methods. These attempt to relate rate and mode of restoration to cellular changes in the hematopoietic tissues. There are two main categories into which these techniques may be divided: firstly, those employing the intact animal and secondly, those depending upon the grafting of marrow or spleen cell suspensions into heavily-irradiated recipients. Previous studies using the intact animal have made use of the polycythemic mouse (Jacobson *et al.,* 1957), the fasted mouse (Porteous *et al.,* 1963), and more recently, a method involving autorepopulation of a heavily-irradiated animal from a shielded femur (Porteous & Lajtha, 1966). Grafting studies have assessed the restorative capacity of marrow suspensions by the ability of such suspensions to form colonies in the spleens of irradiated recipient mice (Till & McCulloch, 1961). The uptake of ^{59}Fe (Hodgson, 1962a) or ^{125}IUDR Cudcowicz *et al.,* 1964). have also provided a measurement of repopulation by marrow suspensions. When any of these techniques, with either intact or grafted animals, were used to measure the radiation sensitivity of the stem cell population, results were obtained giving values for D_0 and extrapolation number which are in fairly close agreement (Gurney & Wackman, 1961; Alexanian *et al.,* 1963; Hodgson, 1962b; McCulloch and Till, 1962). However, when these techniques were used to study stem cell restoration at times after a sublethal dose of radiation, differences were seen which were dependent upon the method employed (Alexanian *et al.,* 1963; Till, 1963; Blackett *et al.,* 1964).

This paper presents recent evidence that the grafting technique gives results that are different from those using the intact animal. Further experiments which aim to elucidate this difference will also be presented.

MATERIALS AND METHODS

Animals. Male C_3H/AKR F_1 hybrid mice between 9 and 12 weeks old were used in all experiments.

Polycythemic Mice. Polycythemia was induced as previously described (Porteous *et al.,* 1965). Erythropoietin equivalent to 1 unit standard B (Bangham, 1962) was injected intraperitoneally. Forty-eight to fifty-two hours later 1 μc ^{59}Fe as ferric citrate was injected i.p. Three days later, the mice were bled out under ether anesthesia and ^{59}Fe concentration was determined on 0.2 ml samples of whole blood plated onto aluminium planchettes and counted on a scintillation counter after air drying.

Preparation of Cell Suspensions. Cell suspensions were prepared as previously described (Porteous & Lajtha, 1966).

Colony Counting. The method employed is that described by Till and McCul-

* Present address: Radiobiology Laboratory, Department of Radiobiology, State University of New York, Downstate Medical Center, Brooklyn, N. Y.

loch (1961). Heavily-irradiated recipients were injected with 10^5 cells and seven days later the animals were killed. The spleens were removed, fixed in Bouin's fluid, examined with the naked eye, and the visible colonies counted.

Autorepopulation from Shielded Femur. The technique for assessing the ability of the femur to repopulate the hematopoietic tissues was that previously described (Porteous & Lajtha, 1966).

Irradiation. All irradiations were carried out using a 300 kVp 'Resomax' operating with a half value thickness of 1.9 mm Cu at a source to surface distance of 70 cm for the 150 rad irradiations and 20 cm for the shielding studies and the lethal irradiations.

Results

Figure 1 shows that in the tests employing the erythropoietin response in polycythemic mice, LD_{50} variation after the sublethal dose and autorepopulation from a shielded femur, the pattern of restoration is similar in each test. The stem cell population as measured by these tests returns in about one week to within normal levels. Then follows a period during which responses overshoot normal levels before once more returning to preirradiation values. However, in the

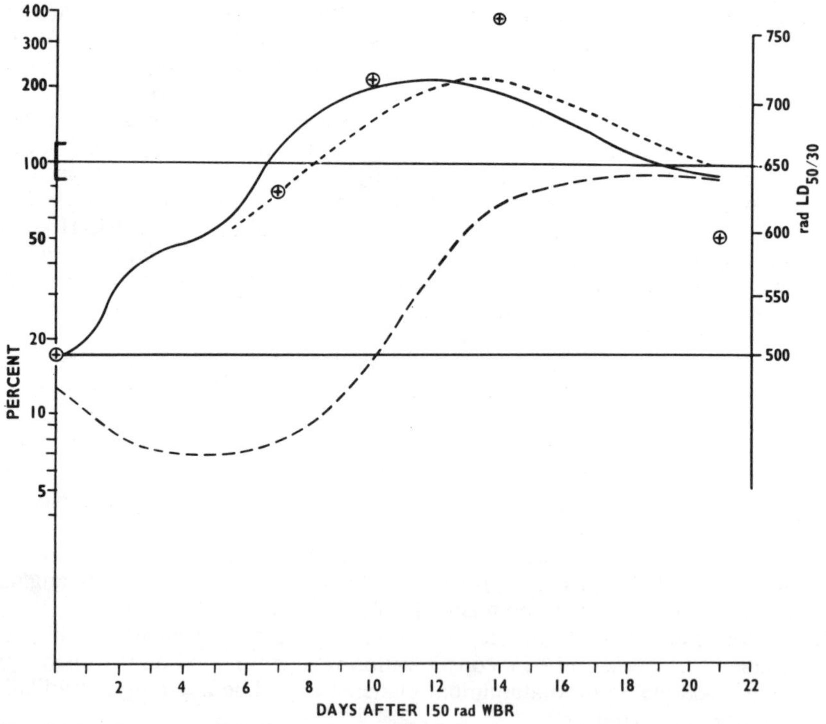

Figure 1. Four tests showing pattern of restoration following an initial dose of 150 rad whole body radiation (WBR) expressed as percentage of unirradiated animals.
———————— Values with erythropoietin dose.
– – – – – – – – – – Exorecolonizing line.
- - - - - - - - - - - - - - - - Autorepopulation line.
⊕ ⊕ ⊕ LD_{50} dose.

grafting test a different pattern was observed. Suspensions of marrow were prepared from groups of animals which were identical to those used in the tests in the intact animal. These suspensions were injected into heavily-irradiated recipients and six days later they were injected with ^{59}Fe. Uptake was measured three days later and used as an indication of the ability of the injected suspension to restore erythropoiesis in the recipient. Restoration measured was compared with that given by control suspensions. It can be seen from FIGURE 1 that the restorative ability remained below normal during the three-week period examined and no tendency to overshoot normal levels was observed.

In our studies involving femur shielding and autorepopulation, the animals received 150 rad whole body radiation (WBR) followed at different intervals by 750 rad while the femur was shielded with lead. In the grafting experiments heavily-irradiated recipients received marrow suspensions from donor mice which had received identical treatment with those that were shielded. The recipients did not, however, receive any previous 150 rad WBR. It was suggested by Blackett (personal communication) that the observed changes in the ability of the shielded femur to repopulate may be attributable to the previous 150 rad WBR. An experiment was designed to examine the effect of a dose of 150 rad WBR administered at times before the lethal irradiation and cell grafting. A plan of this experiment is shown below:

0 rad before 700 rad + 10^5 marrow cells
150 rad 3 days before 700 rad + 10^5 marrow cells
150 rad 7 days before 700 rad + 10^5 marrow cells
150 rad 14 days before 700 rad + 10^5 marrow cells

Identical groups of 12 mice each were exposed to 150 rad WBR at 3, 7 or 14 days before 700 rad. All animals were injected i.v. with the same suspension of 10^5 normal bone marrow cells. Seven days later the mean number of colonies in the spleens of each group was obtained and compared with the mean number of colonies obtained in animals given 700 rad and the same suspension, but no previous 150 rad. TABLE 1 gives the results of this experiment.

Gross examination of the colonies produced in the different groups of recipients did not reveal any difference in the size of individual colonies.

In another experiment a group of eight animals was given 150 rad seven days before 700 rad and 10^6 cells. Six days later they were given 0.5 μc ^{59}Fe and three-day incorporation was compared with that given by a comparable group which had received the same suspension but no previous 150 rad. The mean percent ^{59}Fe incorporation given by the 'conditioned' group was 29.6 ± 3.2. That given by the nonconditioned group was 20.5 ± 2.1 percent.

TABLE 1

RESULTS OF EXPERIMENT IN WHICH IDENTICAL GROUPS OF 12 MICE WERE EXPOSED TO WHOLE BODY RADIATION

'Conditioning' dose of WBR before 700 rad + Cells	Mean Number of Colonies per Spleen from 10^5 Cells
150 rad 3 days before	4.6
150 rad 7 days before	12.73
150 rad 14 days before	5.25
0 rad before	8.43

It appears from these experiments that there is indeed an effect of a previous irradiation upon the ultimate repopulation of the recipient of normal marrow cells after irradiation with 700 rad. The results from both the colony counting and ^{59}Fe incorporation experiments suggest that the 'conditioned' animals have an increased ability to accommodate the growth of cells seven days afterwards. When compared with animals not given the 'conditioning' dose, or with those given 150 rad at other times before 700 rad, it appears that the physical or physiological 'space' available to normal grafted cells is increased in some way, resulting in a higher efficiency of seeding, but apparently, not affecting the growth rate of the seeded cells.

Although changes in the final expression of grafted cells dependent upon the previous treatment of the recipient have been observed, these changes do not coincide in time with those seen in the autorepopulation assay (FIGURE 1), nor is the magnitude of this effect sufficient to explain the difference between the exo- and autografting results.

Experiments with Tritiated Thymidine ($^{3}HTdR$). In order to further elucidate the reasons for the differences observed during recovery after 150 rad, which appear to depend upon the method of assay, we have employed a technique based upon the ability of ^{3}HTdR to inhibit the growth of stem cells to S-phase. When ^{3}HTdR in large doses is incorporated into cells which are synthesizing DNA, loss of proliferative capacity follows the lethal effects of the decay of incorporated tritium. Smith *et al.,* 1962, have demonstrated that the proliferative capacity of subsequently grafted hemopoietic stem cells may be impaired by exposure to ^{3}HTdR in vivo. In their experiments 4×250 μc ^{3}HTdR was given at minus 40, minus 28, minus 16 and minus 4 hr, and a delay in granulocyte recovery was noted if a small graft was given ($< 10^4$ cells) but not if $> 10^5$ cells were grafted.

Bruce and Meeker (1965) gave six doses of 166 μc ^{3}HTdR at four-hour intervals in vivo, and found a 50 percent depression of the colony-forming ability of the hemopoietic cells of the femur. Repeating the experiments using a 20-minute in vitro incubation of cells with 200–500 ^{3}HTdR. Becker *et al.,* (1965) found no significant loss of colonizing capacity with normal marrow, a doubtfully significant effect with normal spleen, but a marked effect (about 60 percent depression) with regenerating spleen.

In three experiments with the erythropoietin test, giving a single dose of 500 μc ^{3}HTdR three to six hr before I unit of erythropoietin, we found that the response as measured with ^{59}Fe incorporation into red cells was depressed by about 70 percent. Using the same animals for grafting assay, no significant effect on the colonizing capacity of femoral marrow was found.

These results again illustrate the difference between the erythropoietin test and the exocolonizing test, and could be taken as support for the concept put forward by Bruce and McCulloch (1964) that the two techniques assay two different cell populations. An alternative explanation, however, could be that the exocolonizing assay loses a significant proportion of the cells in cycle, hence the insignificant effect of ^{3}HTdR with this test in normal steady state.

The question is far from being settled; the results presented only illustrate the outstanding problems. Experiments are in process to elucidate some of the ques-

REFERENCES

ALEXANIAN, R., D. D. PORTEOUS & L. G. LAJTHA. 1963. Stem cell kinetics after irradiation. Int. J. Rad. Biol. 7: 87–94.

BANGHAM, D. R. 1962. Biological assay and a standard for erythropoietin. *In* Erythropoiesis. L. O. Jacobson & M. Doyle, Eds. : 23–28. Grune and Stratton. London and New York.

BECKER, A. J., E. A. MCCULLOCH, L. SIMINOVITCH & J. E. TILL. 1965. The effect of differing demands for blood cell production on DNA synthesis by hemopoietic colony-forming cells of mice. Blood **26**: 296–308.

BLACKETT, N. M., P. J. ROYLANCE & K. ADAMS. 1964. Studies of the capacity of bone-marrow cells to restore erythropoiesis in heavily irradiated rats. Brit. J. Haematol. **10**: 453–467.

BRUCE, W. R. & E. A. MCCULLOCH. 1964. The effect of erythropoietic stimulation on the hemopoietic colony-forming cells of mice. Blood **23**: 216–232.

BRUCE, W. R. & B. E. MEEKER. 1965. Comparison of the sensitivity of normal haematopoietic and transplanted lymphoma colony-forming cells to tritiated thymidine. J. Nat. Cancer Inst. **34**: 849–856.

CUDKOWICZ, G., A. C. UPTON, L. H. SMITH, D. G. GOSLEE & W. L. HUGHES. 1964. An approach to the characterization of stem cells in mouse bone marrow. Ann. N. Y. Acad. Sci. **114**: 571–582.

GURNEY, C. W. & N. WACKMAN. 1961. Impairment of erythropoiesis by irradiation. Nature **190**: 1017–1018.

HODGSON, G. S. 1962a. Erythrocyte ^{59}Fe uptake as a function of bone marrow dose injected in lethally irradiated mice. Blood **19**: 460–467.

HODGSON, G. S. 1962b. Radiosensitivity of marrow cells responsible for reestablishing erythropoiesis in lethally irradiated mice. Acta Physiol. Lat. **12**: 365–369.

JACOBSON, L. O., E. GOLDWASSER, L. F. PLZAK & W. FRIED. 1957. Studies on erythropoiesis. IV. Reticulocyte response of hypophysectomized and polycythemic rodents to erythropoietin. Proc. Soc. Exp. Biol. Med. **94**: 243–249.

MCCULLOCH, E. A. & J. E. TILL. 1962. The sensitivity of cells from normal mouse bone marrow to gamma irradiation in vitro and in vivo. Radiat. Res. **16**: 822–832.

PORTEOUS, D. D., R. ALEXANIAN & L. G. LAJTHA. 1963. The fasted mouse in the study of stem-cell kinetics. Int. J. Rad. Biol. **7**: 95–100.

PORTEOUS, D. D. & L. G. LAJTHA. 1964. On stem-cell recovery after irradiation. Brit. J. Haematol. **12**: 177–188.

PORTEOUS, D. D., S. C. TSO, K. HIRASHIMA & L. G. LAJTHA. 1965. Modification of x-ray survival curves of stem-cells by different doses of erythropoietin. Nature **206**: 204–206.

SMITH, W. W., G. BRECHER, F. STOHLMAN, JR. & J. CORNFIELD. 1962. Toxicity of tritiated thymidine to bone marrow transplants. Radiat. Res. **16**: 201–207.

TILL, J. E. 1963. Quantitative aspects of radiation lethality at the cellular level. Amer. J. Roentgenol. **90**: 917–927.

TILL, J. E. & E. A. MCCULLOCH. 1961. A direct measurement of the radiation sensitivity of normal mouse bone marrow cells. Radiat. Res. **14**: 213–222.

REGULATION OF ERYTHROPOIESIS. XX. KINETICS OF RED CELL PRODUCTION*

Frederick Stohlman, Jr., Shirley Ebbe, Bernard Morse, Donald Howard and Janet Donovan

St. Elizabeth's Hospital,
Tufts Medical School
Boston, Mass.

INTRODUCTION

Since the last conference on erythropoiesis, much information has accumulated which has necessitated a revision of some of our notions as to the mechanism of red cell formation. It is still clear that the erythroid compartment is not a self-maintaining compartment, but is fed from a primitive stem cell pool. The work of Becker *et al.*[1] and Whang *et al.*[2] appeared to settle the long standing issue whether this is a unipotential or totipotential compartment. More recent evidence, however, raises the question as to whether there may not be two levels of stem cells, a more primitive totipotential stem cell compartment equivalent to the colony-forming unit of Till and McCulloch[3] and a more differentiated precursor cell for each of the identifiable hematopoietic elements. This issue is by no means settled, but data will be presented favoring the latter explanation, i.e., two levels of precursor cells. The studies on the effect of erythropoietin in the hypertransfused rodent clearly demonstrated that erythropoietin is capable of differentiating the stem cell into an identifiable erythroid precursor. The mechanism by which this is accomplished is moot and the question of whether the action of erythropoietin is confined to the stem cell or whether it may also affect differentiated cells is at present undecided. In this paper it is our purpose to present data bearing on these points. The effect of erythropoietin has been studied in normal animals and in rats in which red cell production has been perturbed by hypertransfusion and/or vincristine. Critical to these considerations are studies on megakaryocytopoiesis using tritiated thymidine. These also will be reported briefly.

METHOD AND MATERIALS

Female Sprague-Dawley rats weighing 135 to 160 g were used. When hypertransfused, washed, packed red cells were given in an amount equivalent to 3.5% of the body weight. Vincristine was given as a single i.v. injection of 0.3 mg/kg. The erythropoietin used was an alcoholic extract of human urine from a child with a congenital hypoplastic anemia. In those rats receiving thymidine, 1 μc/g of body weight of ^{3}HTdR with a specific activity of 1.9 c/mmole were given in a single injection. Bone marrow preparations were made as previously described.[4] The megakaryocytes were classified into three stages from the most immature (I) to the most mature (III) on the basis of morphologic criteria previously discussed.[4] Megakaryocyte differentials are based on the classification of 100–250 megakaryocytes and erythroid differentials on the basis of 1000 nucleated cells. The technique which we used for measuring iron incorporation has been previously detailed. Cell-size measurements were made using a Coulter model B and graphout; separation was accomplished by differential centrifugation.

* Supported in part by grants HTS–5600 and HE–07542 from the National Heart Institute.

TABLE 1

MEGAKARYOCYTE DIFFERENTIALS IN VINCRISTINE-TREATED HYPERTRANSFUSED ANIMALS*

Treatment	Time	Megakaryocyte Percent		
		Stage I	Stage II	Stage III
Control	—	18.5	25	56.5
Vincristine	1 day	11	23	66
	2 day	11	19.5	69.5
	3 day	17	22.5	60.5
	5 day	16	29	55
	8 day	11.5	21	67.5

* Days refer to the day after 0.3 mg/kg of vincristine. Stages of maturation are as described by Ebbe and Stohlman.[4] The values are based on a differential of 100 megakaryocytes. Each value refers to the average of two animals.

RESULTS

Megakaryocytopoiesis

Megakaryocyte differentials are given in TABLE 1. After flash labeling with ^{3}HTdR ~ 20% of the earliest (stage I), megakaryocytes were labeled. After two to four hr there was an increase in the labeling index at the rate of ~ 7%/hour so that after 24 hr 90–100% of the cells were labeled. Stage II and III megakaryocytes became sequentially labeled (FIGURE 1.). The mean grain count time is shown in FIGURE 2 and gave a T/2 for stage I megakaryocytes of 1.5–1.8 days. Perturbation by erythropoietin or hypertransfusion did not alter the labeling index but did change the grain count halving time FIGURE 3.[5] Hypertransfusion shortened the mean grain halving time whereas erythropoietin increased it. We feel that this represents a secondary effect. Erythropoietin by increasing red cell production increased the availability of nucleic acid breakdown products from extruded erythroid nuclei. This resulted in an increase in reutilization of ^{3}H by the megakaryocytes; this would explain the increased grain count halving time in the erythropoietin-treated group. Conversely, decreased availability of nucleic acid ^{3}H from the extruded nuclei in animals in which erythropoiesis was suppressed by hypertransfusion would account for the shortened grain count halving time. Had it been a direct effect on the megakaryocyte, one would have anticipated the reverse of that obtained, i.e., there should have been a decreased grain count halving time in the erythropoietin-treated animals and the converse in the transfused animals. From the overall megakaryocyte labeling, an index and estimate of maturation time for the entire megakaryocyte compartment could be obtained (FIGURE 4). This gives the value of ~ 60 hr for the interval after a cell differentiates to its disappearance as a recognizable bone marrow megakaryocyte. The interval from the time of injection of ^{3}HTdR to the appearance of the first labeled stage II megakaryocytes gives a minimum estimate for the transit time in the stage I compartment of ~ eight hours. The increase in percent labeling index of the stage I megakaryocytes of ~ 7%/hour gives a maximum estimate of transit time of 14 hours. In view of the fact that this is a nondividing compartment, the differential reflects the relative proportion of time in each compartment; from this and the transit time for stage I megakaryocytes, values for the stage II and III transit times can be obtained. These give ranges for the transit times of 11–19 hr for stage II and 24–42 hr for stage III. From this it can be estimated that the total maturation time is a minimum of 43 and a maximum of 75 hr and from the data in FIGURE 4 the average is about 60 hours.

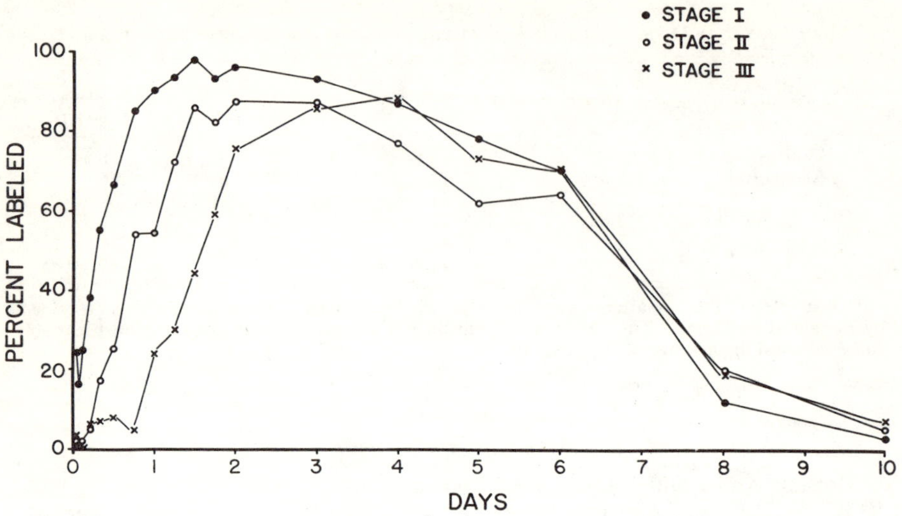

FIGURE 1. Average curves of labeling indices of rat megakaryocytes after a single injection of ^{3}HTdR. Each point is the average from two to four rats. Reprinted by courtesy of Blood.

The Effect of Erythropoietin

After five doses of erythropoietin given at 12-hour intervals, short-lived macrocytic red cells are produced in the rat.[6,7] These short-lived macrocytes were demonstrated in hypertransfused animals treated with massive doses of erythropoietin. Accordingly, it appeared of interest to study the effect of time and dose on the macrocytic response. Thirty-five units of erythropoietin were given to normal and hypertransfused animals in single and divided doses. When given to a normal animal, a macrocytic population was seen emerging after 48 hr and could be detected in the top fraction of a centrifuged column of blood (FIGURE 5). After 72 hr this fraction had developed a further complement of hemoglobin. As a result of the increased density it could no longer be clearly defined after separation by centrifugation. By contrast, when hypertransfused animals were given a single dose of ~ 35 units of erythropoietin, they developed a reticulocyte response somewhat later than the normal animal but macrocytosis could not be demonstrated. When a second dose of 35 units of erythropoietin was given to the hypertransfused animal 24 hr later, macrocytes were clearly seen (FIGURE 6). Normal animals given a second dose of erythropoietin 24 hr later continued to demonstrate macrocytes at the end of 72 hr and the degree of macrocytosis was greater than that observed after a single injection. Both the reticulocyte response and macrocytosis developed ~ 24 hr earlier in the normal than in the hypertransfused animal. It is also to be noted that the degree of macrocytosis was substantially greater in normal rats receiving erythropoietin than it was in the transfused animal.

The effect of a fractional dose of 35 units on macrocyte production in the hypertransfused animal was also evaluated. Animals received either 7 units of erythropoietin initially and 28 units in a second injection 24 hr later or the reverse. The results are shown in FIGURE 7. Pronounced macrocytosis was seen 72 hr after the fractional dose, but a single dose of 35 units was again ineffective in producing macrocytes in the hypertransfused animals. It appeared, therefore,

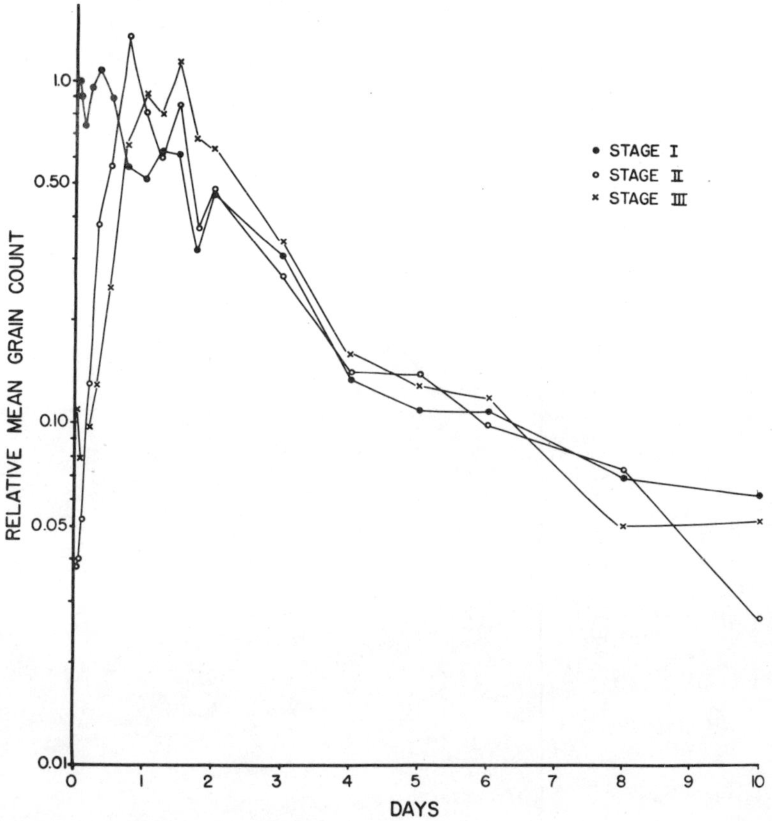

FIGURE 2. Average curve of relative mean grain counts of labeled rat megakaryocytes after a single injection of ^{3}HTdR. Each point is the average from two to four rats. Reprinted by courtesy of Blood.

that to demonstrate significant macrocytosis one needed the presence of differentiated erythroid precursors at the time of injection of erythropoietin.

The Effect of Vincristine

Vincristine is a stathmokinetic agent which profoundly affects both the erythroid and myeloid elements of the bone marrow. The megakaryocyte compartment, however, appears to be affected relatively little.[8] During the first 12 hr after administration of vincristine the bone marrow shows striking accumulation of metaphases in both erythroid and myeloid compartments. Abnormal metaphases were seen with star, imploded and exploded forms. Phagocytosis, karyorrhexis, and karyolysis were present. After 24 hr no erythroid elements were seen, but myeloid elements were present. Ana-telophase forms were not seen in the erythroid series indicating that the cells did not, as previously implied for colchicine, escape "metaphase block." Parenthetically it may be noted that in a pilot study using colchicine we did not observe ana-telophase forms in erythroid elements. However, they are occasionally seen in myeloid elements. From data on

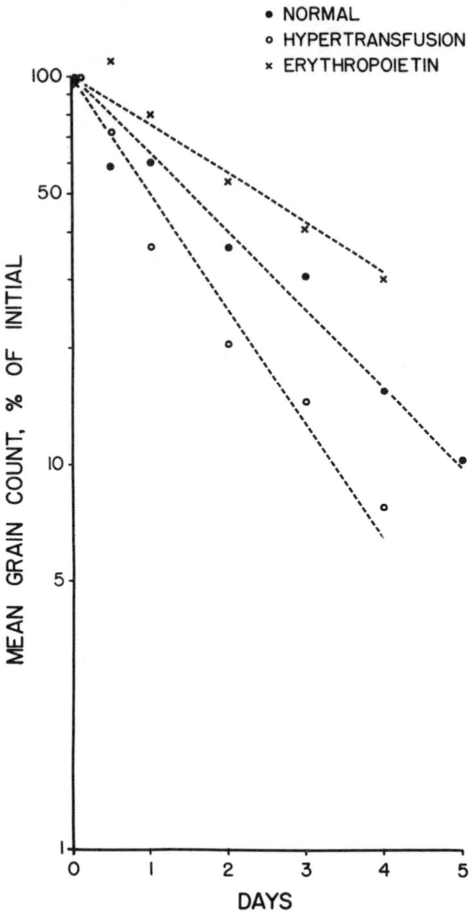

FIGURE 3. Mean grain count, expressed as percent of initial value, for labeled group I megakaryocytes after injection of ^{3}HTdR in normal (●), hypertransfused (○) and erythropoietin-treated (x) rats. Reprinted by courtesy of the Proceedings of the Society for Experimental Biology and Medicine.

metaphase accumulation it could be estimated that the generation time for erythroid elements was ~ 12 hours.

In contrast to the profound effect on myeloid and erythroid elements, there was relatively little effect on megakaryocytes. Seventeen hr after vincristine the megakaryocyte differentials were: stage I – 13–18%; stage II – 21–36%; and stage III – 51–66% as compared with control values of stage I – 16–22%, stage II – 26–33%, and stage III – 47–55%. During the subsequent ten days of study there was no significant change in the megakaryocyte differential.

The bone marrow response of the various formed elements to vincristine was also reflected in the peripheral blood counts. Absolute reticulocytopenia was observed within two days after the administration of vincristine. The platelet count, however, fell to only about 70% of control values and the nadir was reached on

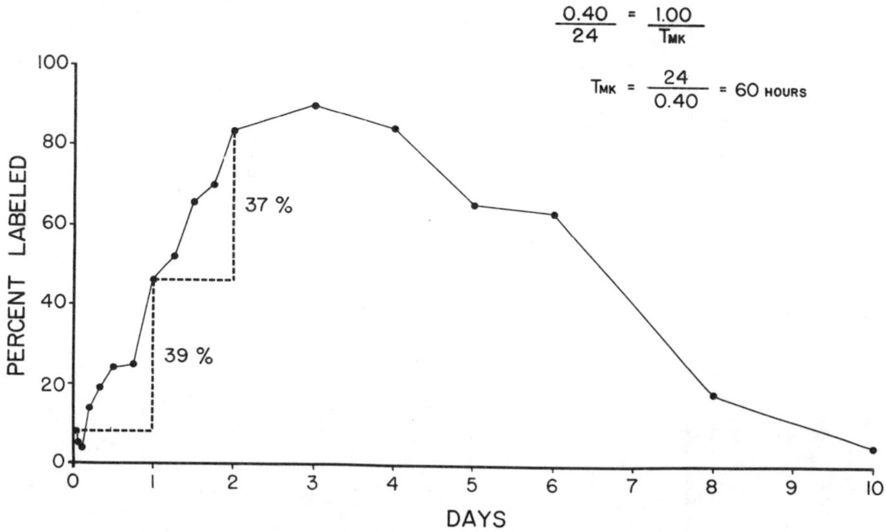

FIGURE 4. Curve of labeling index of all rat megakaryocytes after a single injection of ^{3}HTdR. Each point is the average from two to four rats. The increase of about 40 percent per day implies a total time in the megakaryocyte compartment (T_{MK}) of about 60 hours.

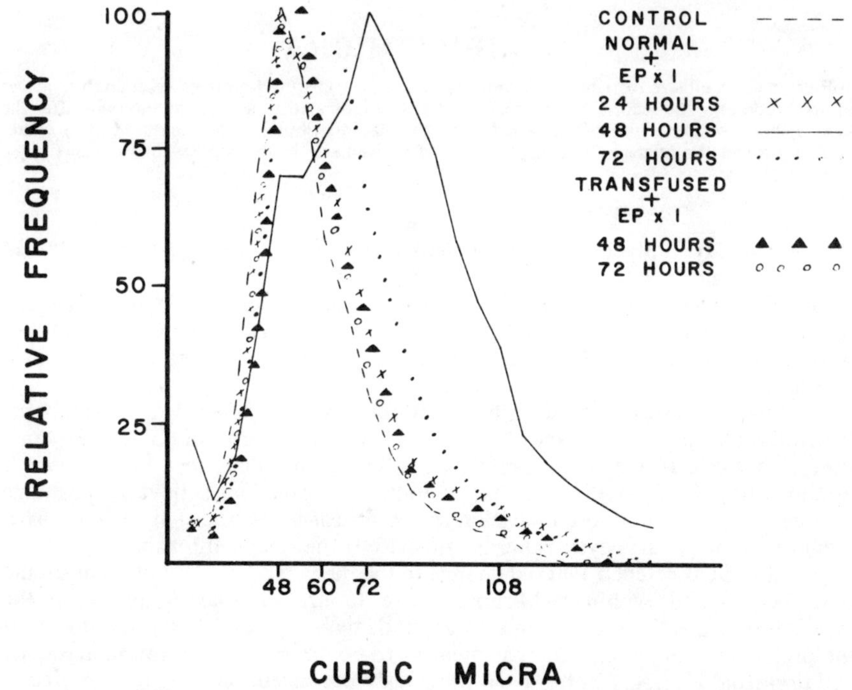

FIGURE 5. Cell size distribution from normal and transfused animals given 35 units of erythropoietin at indicated times prior to sacrifice. The plot represents the relative frequencies of cells of a given size in the top 2% of the centrifuged column of blood.

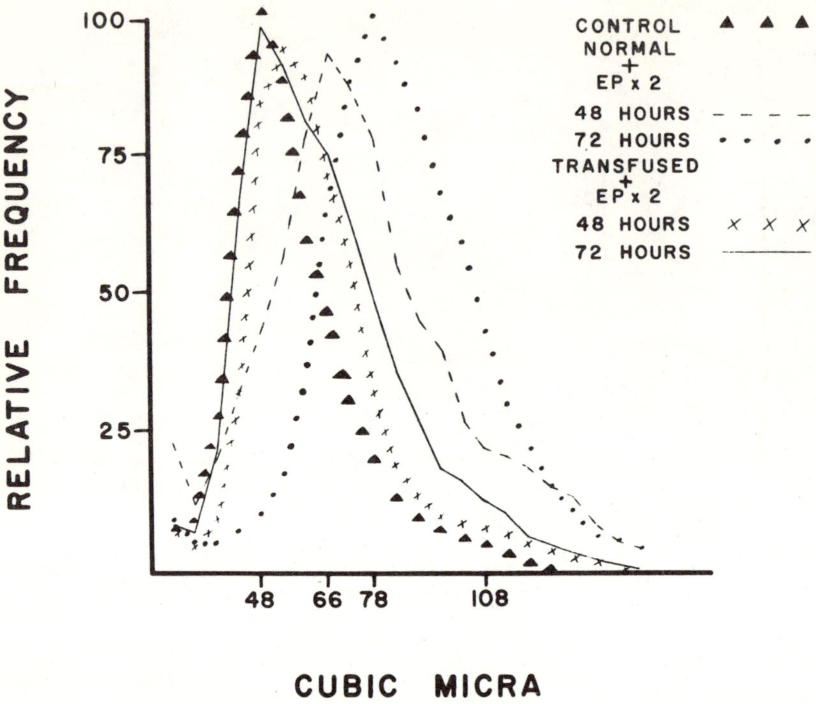

FIGURE 6. Cell size distribution in normal and hypertransfused animals receiving two doses of erythropoietin, the second 24 hr after the first. The indicated times are the intervals after the first injection of erythropoietin at which time the size distribution was measured. The values given represent the relative frequency of cells of a given size in the top 2% of the centrifuged column of blood.

the fourth day. Polychromatophilic leukocytes fell to approximately 30% of the control value.

Bone marrow recovery in the erythroid series began on the fifth day and erythroid cellularity was normal by the seventh day. There were, however, abnormal mitotic figures and multinucleated erythroid precursors still present at that time.

The question arose as to why the effect of vincristine differed so strikingly between the megakaryocytic and the erythroid series. Perhaps an obvious explanation is that one is a dividing population whereas the other to a large extent is nondividing. If this is the only explanation, one would also have to postulate that in view of the measured megakaryocyte transit times, the stem cell compartment of the megakaryocytes is hardly affected. If the stem cell for the megakaryocyte had been affected, a marked change in the megakaryocyte differential should have been noted within 8–14 hours. The failure to note a change in the megakaryocyte differential points to an undamaged precursor compartment. If the precursor or stem cell compartment were common for both megakaryocytic and erythroid elements as has been previously suggested, one might then predict that differentiation from the erythroid compartment in the vincristine-treated animal could be readily achieved by large doses of erythropoietin. To evaluate this question, studies on the response to erythropoietin of hypertransfused vincristine-treated animals were carried out.

The data are shown in FIGURES 8–10. Vincristine was given either at the time of erythropoietin or 48 hours prior to the administration of erythropoietin. In those animals receiving vincristine at the time of erythropoietin administration, differentiation of erythroid precursors was delayed. It was not seen until the third or fourth day after administration of erythropoietin. When erythropoietin was given 48 hr after vincristine, differentiation was again delayed relative to the control animals, but occurred earlier than in animals receiving vincristine and erythropoietin at the same time. It is also apparent that the degree of increase in erythroid precursors, as judged from bone marrow differentials, was somewhat greater than that which would have been predicted from the reticulocyte count or the iron incorporation. This suggests a measure of ineffective erythropoiesis and agrees with the morphologic abnormalities previously alluded to.

Discussion

During the past several years a number of models for red cell production, the mechanism of action of erythropoietin, and its relationship to the stem cell pool

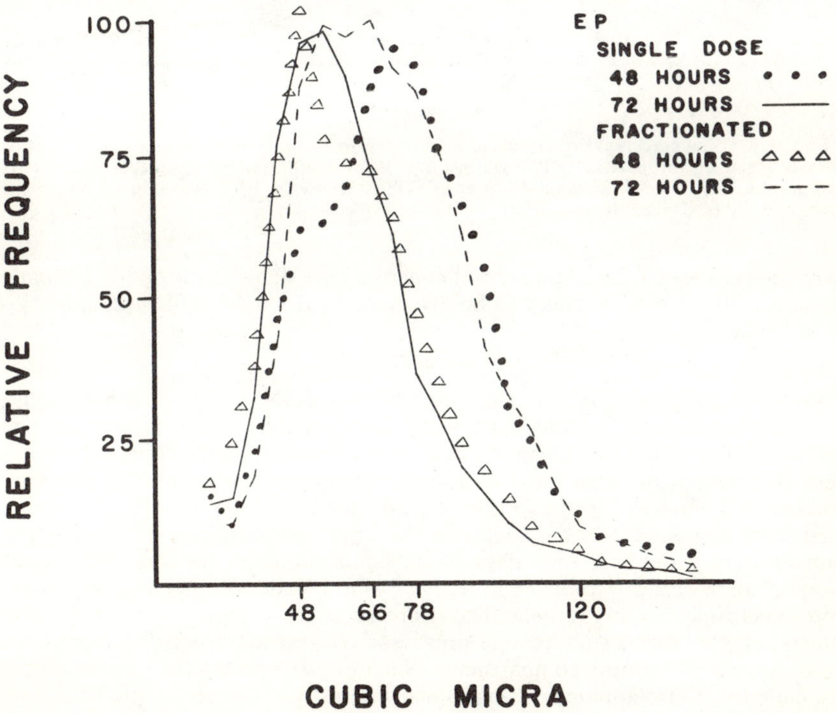

FIGURE 7. The effect of a single dose of 35 units of erythropoietin given at time 0 and fractionation of the dose and injections at time 0 and 24 hours. The hours given indicate the hours after the first injection. The values represent the relative frequency of cells of a given size in the top 2% of the centrifuged column of blood. The recipients of a single dose were normal animals and the response is similar to that in FIGURE 5. The recipients of the fractionated dose were hypertransfused animals in which macrocytes were not demonstrable after a single dose (FIGURE 5.) but were after fractionation of that dose.

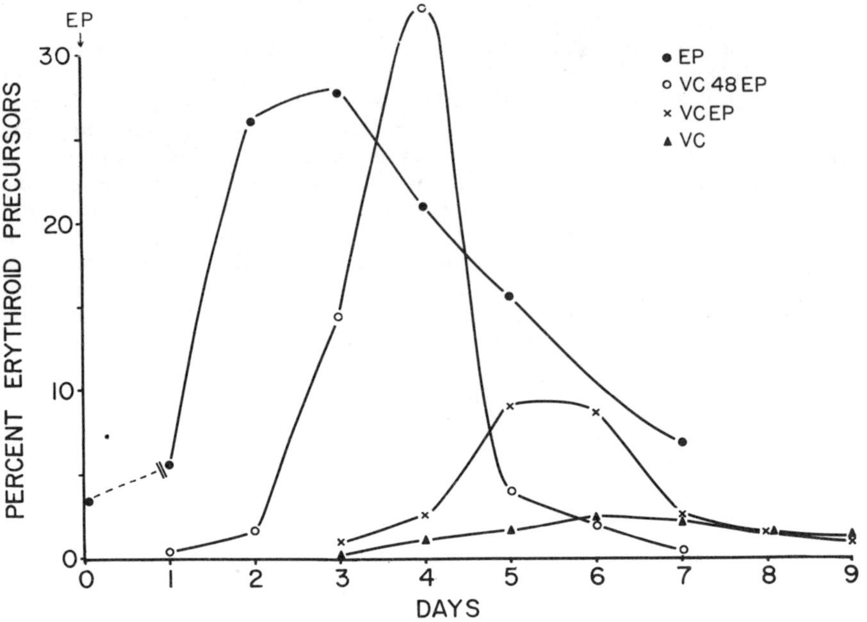

FIGURE 8. The percentage of erythroid precursors present in the marrow of hypertransfused animals given erythropoietin (EP), vincristine (VC), erythropoietin immediately after vincristine (VCEP) or erythropoietin 48 hr after vincristine (VC48EP). Reproduced by courtesy of the Journal of Clinical Investigation.

have been suggested. The data presented herein bear significantly on the evaluation of these various models and will be discussed in the light of its applicability to these models.

Stem Cell

Recently the possibility that there may be two levels of stem cells has received increasing attention.[9–11] Bruce and McCulloch[9] observed that despite increased red cell production in the spleen of mice exposed to hypoxia, the size of the splenic stem cell compartment, as judged from transplantation potential, steadily diminished after the fourth day of exposure until the termination of the study in 28 days. There also appeared to be a decrease in the colony-forming ability of the hypoxic animals during the first four days of exposure although the variability of the assay in these groups (mean 81%, range 37–137% of control) does not permit firm conclusions in this respect. The decrease in the repopulating ability of the spleen suggests that an immediate precursor compartment is being repopulated from the colony-forming compartment which in turn reduces the number of cells available for transplantation. Of particular interest was the observation that there was little change either in the number of colony-forming units or in the amount of iron incorporation by the femora. From these observations Bruce and McCulloch suggested the existence of an erythropoietin-sensitive precursor cell separate and distinct from the colony-forming cell. They did not comment on whether the erythropoietin-sensitive cell was committed to being an erythroid element or whether it still maintained totipotential characteristics.

We suggested[8,10] the schema which in modified form appears in FIGURE 11. Some of the data on which these conclusions are based have been presented. The model suggests a primitive stem cell which is capable of differentiating into erythroid, myeloid, or megakaryocytic elements. It is thought that this is the cell responsible for the transplantation phenomenon and "colony" formation. Beyond this compartment there are committed compartments that serve as the immediate precursor for the identifiable formed elements. These compartments, in large measure, may be self-supporting, but in times of severe stress, e.g. severe hemolytic anemia, feed-in from the primitive compartment may be necessary. After damage to the committed compartment, e.g. irradiation, regeneration is accomplished from the primitive precursor pool. This implies a feedback mechanism, presumably negative, between the committed and the primitive pools as well as an "inducer" for the primitive cell. The committed pool is thought to be the erythropoietin-sensitive cell for the erythroid compartment. Presumably, there are hormones analagous to erythropoietin which effect differentiation from the precursor compartments for the other formed elements of the bone marrow.

Animals receiving vincristine had a complete erythroid aplasia for a period of 72–96 hours. When hypertransfused, so that any damage would be confined to the precursor compartment, it was not possible to induce erythroid differentiation for a period of 72–96 hr after vincristine even though massive doses of erythropoietin were used. Although there was a mild decrease in peripheral platelet count of ~ 30%, the megakaryocyte compartment appeared to escape substantial injury

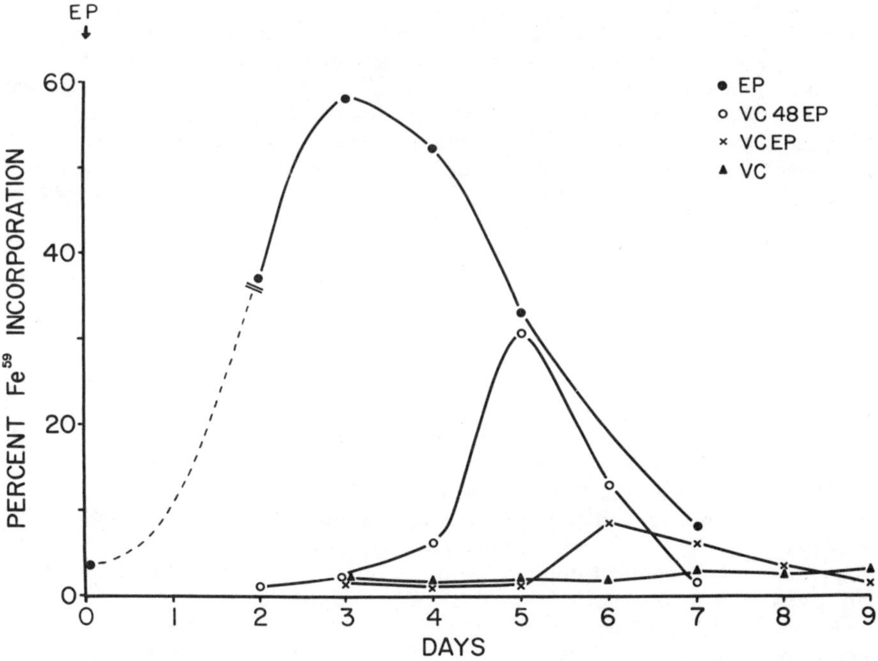

FIGURE 9. Values given represent the percent of intravenously injected iron incorporated when ^{59}Fe was given intravenously 20 hr prior to the time of sacrifice. All animals were hypertransfused five days prior to injection of vincristine (VC). Erythropoietin (EP) was given either immediately (VCEP) or 48 hr after vincristine (VC48EP).

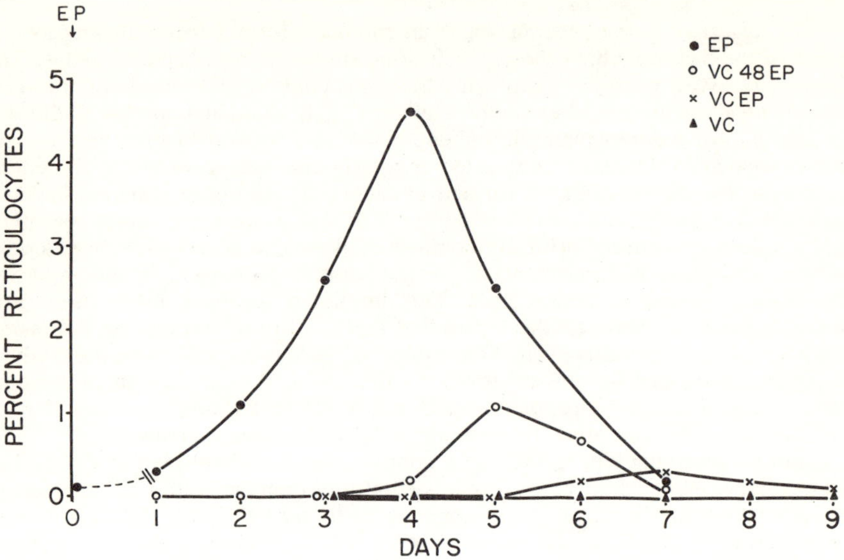

FIGURE 10. The percentage of reticulocytes in the peripheral blood of hypertransfused animals given erythropoietin (EP), vincristine (VC), erythropoietin immediately after vincristine (VCEP), or erythropoietin 48 hr after vincristine (VC48EP).

as judged from the megakaryocyte differentials and evaluation of total cellularity. From this observation together with the values for megakaryocyte transit times[4] it can be deduced that the extent of injury to the megakaryocyte precursor was significantly less than that to the erythroid immediate precursor compartment. The estimate of the total megakaryocyte transit time (FIGURE 4) is ~ 60 hr with a range of 43–72 hr, and the transit time for the stage I megakaryocyte is estimated to be between 8–14 hours. From these figures it can be seen that a significant decrease in differentiation of precursor cells into the megakaryocyte compartment would result in the depopulation of stage I megakaryocytes within a period of 8–14 hr and a substantial change in the differential at the end of this period. Within 60 hr there should have been an almost total depopulation of the entire megakaryocyte compartment. It is evident from the differentials presented that this was not the case and differentiation of precursors continued. The continued differentiation of megakaryocytes together with the depopulation of the erythroid compartment and inability to differentiate erythroid precursors can be explained by the model presented in which it is considered that there are two different precursor cells. The alternative explanation would be a biological standstill, which seems unlikely, or a selective block of erythroid differentiation. While neither of these two alternatives can be finally excluded it appears to us that the more likely explanation is that of different immediate precursor cells which, because of geometric or physiochemical differences in the membrane, have different susceptibilities to vincristine.

Porteous and Lajtha[12] and Blackett[13] have described a dichotomy between endogenous and exogenous stem cell recovery. In these studies after repeated or continuous irradiation, endogenous regeneration of erythropoiesis is maintained but colony-forming capabilities are reduced. Lajtha[14] suggests that these differences reflect the inability to transplant cells in cycle. Against such an explanation are the results of Smith *et al.*[15] using repeated high doses of ^{3}H-thymidine in vivo to establish whether stem cells are in cycle together with the subsequent study employing the in vitro thymidine suicide technic by Becker *et al.*[16] These studies suggest that normally, cells in cycle retain their transplantation potential. A model based on two levels of stem cells offers a more attractive explanation for the observations on the chronically and repeatedly irradiated animals as well as the exhaustion of stem cell potential on serial transplants described by Cudkowicz.[17] After chronic or repeated irradiation the size of the primitive compartment is reduced and the transplantation potential thereby suffers at the expense of maintaining the more differentiated compartment and endogenous hematopoiesis.

The data at hand do not permit at this time a judgment with respect to the suggestion of Brecher *et al.*[18] that dedifferentiation of the immediate precursor cell occurs as an intricate part of the regulation of cell production.

The Mechanism of Action of Erythropoietin

The observations of Alpen and Cranmore[19] and Fried *et al.*[20] clearly established the fact that erythropoietin serves to differentiate the immediate precursor cell into the recognizable or differentiated erythroid compartment. The mechanism

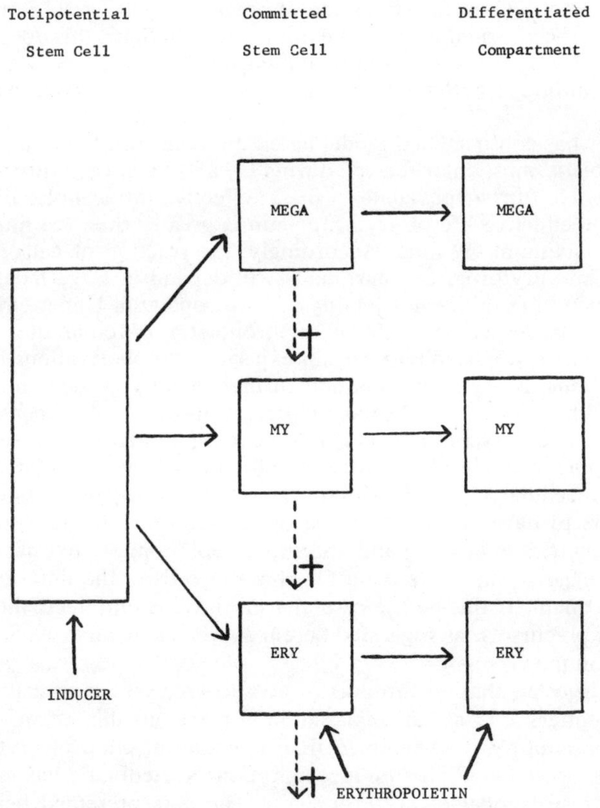

FIGURE 11. A schematic model of hematopoiesis. MEGA–megakaryocytes, ER–erythroid, MY–myeloid. Dotted arrows indicate death function.

by which this is accomplished, however, is not known. It is entirely possible that erythropoietin acts as a derepressor and thus permits messenger synthesis to direct hemoglobin formation. Studies have been reported which suggest that this may indeed be the case, but these studies are by no means conclusive. Lajtha[21] has suggested that the precursor cell in G_0 may be differentiated by erythropoietin, but that once the cell is in cycle, it is no longer available for differentiation. He further suggests that differentiation results in the triggering of other G_0 cells into cycle. From this it is clear that the bulk of precursor cells in his model must be in G_0 awaiting either differentiation or triggering into cycle. However, we have observed,[22] using continuous infusion of ^{3}H-thymidine in polycythemic animals that the precursor cells are in cycle. In these experiments, after animals were hypertransfused, a continuous infusion of ^{3}H-thymidine was initiated; after four to seven days the infusion was discontinued and 4–12 hr later a dose of erythropoietin was given. Of the pronormoblasts developing thereafter, 100% were labeled. By contrast, when a flash label of thymidine was given 4–12 hr before erythropoietin in hypertransfused animals, only 40–60% of the pronormoblasts were labeled. This would suggest that the immediate precursor cells are in continuous cycle although G_1 may be longer than estimated for other cells.

There must also be a death function. If this were not the case and differentiation did not occur, a continuous accumulation of precursor cells would result. Eventually the precursor cell would become the dominant cell. Since this does not appear to be the case, it is apparent that to maintain a steady state precursor cell in continuous cycle, although perhaps with a long G_1, it is necessary to have a death function.

Kretchmar[23] has constructed a model based on the assumption that to be effective, erythropoietin must enter the cell during G_1 and be present during a portion of the S phase. He further postulates a fixed "effective intracellular life" for erythropoietin; the effective life of erythropoietin is greater than the minimum and less than the maximum G_1 time. Accordingly, the fraction of cells that will be differentiated into erythroid compartments will depend in large measure on the length of G_1 as well as on the availability of erythropoietin. Under circumstances where G_1 exceeds the effective life of erythropoietin, differentiation would not occur. This model is applicable to certain experimental observations but appears to present an unnecessary restriction and further fails to provide an explanation for the delayed response to erythropoietin observed in the experiments presented herein. The delayed response to erythropoietin (FIGURES 8–10) suggests that either erythropoietin can be stored intracellularly or that the information imparted thereby is intracellularly stored. Moreover, as will be discussed later, erythropoietin appears to have an effect on the differentiated erythroid cell. The data of Alpen[24] using tritium labeling and microspectrophotometry to establish nucleic acid content suggests that there is no G_1 phase in cells in the differentiated erythroid compartment. If this be the case and erythropoietin affects the differentiated erythroid precursors, as suggested herein as well as by other workers, it must act in other than the G_1 phase.

Schooley suggested that erythropoietin acts to "recruit" stem cells for differentiation and offers this as an explanation for the greater effectiveness of a fractionated or multiple dose regimen than a single injection of erythropoietin. His conclusions were based on ^{59}Fe incorporation. Kretchmar[23] has incorporated this notion into his model of erythropoietin. The data presented herein on the effect of erythropoietin in inducing macrocytosis as well as the observations of Gallagher *et al.*[26] on the time-dose response curve of hypertransfused animals to erythropoietin and the studies of Hodgson[27] on starved animals would not appear to agree with this notion. The latter investigators observed that erythropoietin given to a hypertransfused animal within 24 hr after transfusion evoked a greater response than a similar dose of erythropoietin given four days after transfusion. This would appear to be best explained as the result of an effect of erythropoietin on the differentiated erythroid precursor. The studies we have reported on the comparative effect of erythropoietin in hypertransfused and normal animals with respect to the induction of macrocytosis appear to confirm such a notion. Those models which propose that erythropoietin acts only to differentiate the precursor cell, but has no effect on the differentiated cell do not provide an explanation for the above observations. The suggestion of Erslev[28] that short-lived macrocytes reflect a local metabolic deficiency does not obtain since the administration of high doses of folic acid, B_{12}, etc., does not affect the production of macrocytes, nor do the precursor cells have the maturation abnormalities characteristic of such metabolic deficiencies.

We have suggested that erythropoietin not only differentiates the precursor cell but also affects those differentiated red cells still capable of synthesizing RNA. From studies with tritiated cytidine[29] it would appear that pronormoblasts, basophilic normoblasts, and early polychromatophilic normoblasts are still capable of synthesizing RNA. The mechanism by which this erythropoietin exerts its effect is uncertain, but since the major difference between the differentiated erythroid precursor and its immediate precursor is to synthesize hemoglobin, it seemed reasonable to suggest that hemoglobin synthesis is initiated by erythropoietin and the rate of hemoglobin synthesis is governed by the availability of erythropoietin within the individual cell. From this a model shown in FIGURE 12 was constructed.[30] In this model it is suggested that erythropoietin acts as an inducer to initiate hemoglobin synthesis and further govern its rate. When a critical cytoplasmic hemoglobin concentration (CHC) is achieved, a negative feedback will be initiated which shuts off further nucleic acid synthesis. It is projected that the CHC is $\sim 20\%$. Under conditions in which there is an erythropoietin excess, e.g. from the administration of large doses of exogenous erythropoietin or as a result of severe anemia and the production of endogenous erythropoietin, the rate of hemoglobin synthesis is accelerated and not only are there additional cells differentiated into the erythroid compartment but the rate of hemoglobin synthesis is accelerated as well. The acceleration of the rate of hemoglobin synthesis in the face of a fixed generation time results in the cessation of nucleic acid synthesis at an earlier time relative to the time of differentiation than is normally the case. This in the face of a fixed generation time described by Alpen[19] and Bond [31] results in a skipped terminal division and the production of macrocytes. When the rate of hemoglobin synthesis is decreased, e.g. iron deficiency anemia where the availability of iron is a rate-limiting factor, or the interval between differentiation and the achievement of the critical CHC is prolonged, additional divisions and microcytes occur. This implies the occurrence of microcytosis prior to hypochromia, which has been demonstrated to be the case.[32,33] It also implies that in treating iron deficiency anemia macrocytes, normocytes, or microcytes may be produced depending on the dose. That this is the case has been demonstrated in both rats[34] and human beings.[35]

The data presented herein lend further confirmation to the above thesis. When erythropoietin was given to normal animals, macrocytes were seen within 48 hours. Reticulocytosis also occurred earlier than in transfused animals. If in fact erythropoietin affects the differentiated erythroid precursors, this would be an-

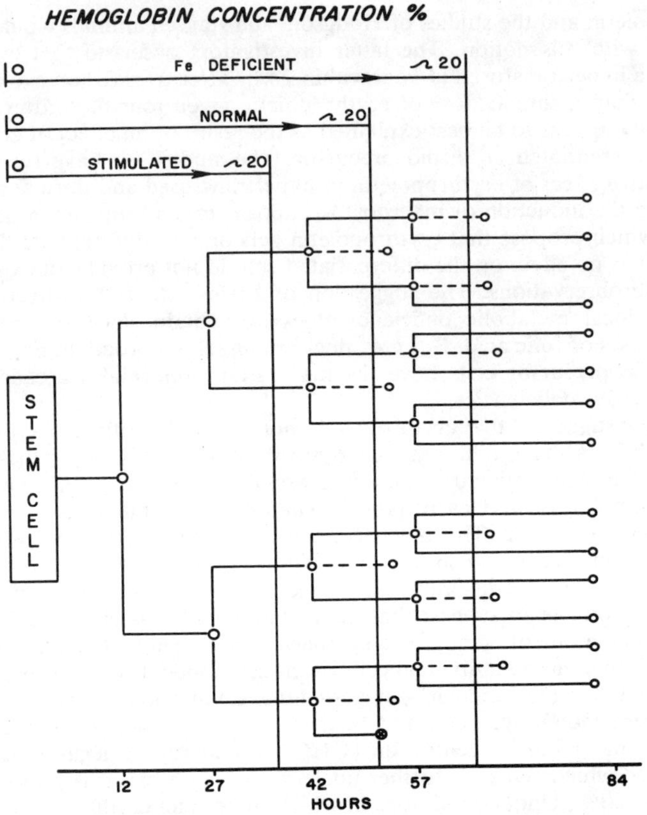

FIGURE 12. A model of the kinetics of erythropoiesis in which it is proposed that when a cytoplasmic hemoglobin concentration of ~ 20% is achieved a negative feedback is initiated which shuts off DNA synthesis and division. The average interphase time of the differentiated erythroid precursor is fixed so that changes in the rate of hemoglobin synthesis alter the numbers of division. Ineffective erythropoiesis is indicated in the lowest pathway. Reprinted by courtesy of the New York Academy of Sciences.

ticipated since the rate of hemoglobin synthesis would be increased in the pronormoblasts, basophilic normoblasts, and polychromatophilic normoblasts present at the time of injection of erythropoietin. This would lead to accelerated maturation and early release. If its effect were confined to differentiating the immediate precursor cell, then the response in terms of time and degree of macrocytosis should be the same for both normal and hypertransfused animals since the same population of cells would be affected. That this was not the case offers cogent evidence in support of the thesis that erythropoietin affects the differentiated red cell precursor. Further evidence for an effect on erythropoietin in the differentiated cell is provided by the observation that a fractionated dose proved to be more effective in inducing macrocytosis than did a single dose of erythropoietin in the hypertransfused animal.

The delayed response to erythropoietin in vincristine-treated hypertransfused animals and the difference in response to vincristine of megakaryocytes and erythroid population provide evidence for the aforementioned different immediate precursor cells. The delay in response to erythropoietin would indicate that either information imparted by erythropoietin or erythropoietin itself was stored during the period of observation of about four days. This would appear to be inconsistent with the model presented by Kretchmar.[23] At present the reason for the delay in differentiation must remain speculative but it is suggested that a certain number of cells must be present in the immediate precursor compartment before differentiation can in fact occur. This may reflect an inhibitor of differentiation either of the humoral variety, which has been suggested by a number of workers, or more likely an internal compartmental control mechanism.

Summary

Data has been presented to indicate that there is a primitive stem cell which presumably is totipotential and a more differentiated stem cell which has been referred to as the immediate precursor cell or a committed stem cell. The data presented herein would indicate that erythropoietin acts as an inducer for hemoglobin synthesis. In so doing, it can differentiate the committed immediate precursor cell but also, may accelerate the hemoglobin synthesis in the already differentiated erythroid precursor still capable of synthesizing RNA. Various models which have been suggested for the production of red cells have been discussed and a tentative model compatible with data presented herein has been described.

References

1. Becker, A. J., E. A. McCulloch & J. E. Till. 1963. Cytological demonstration of the clonal nature of spleen colonies derived from transplanted mouse marrow Cells. Nature **197:** 452.
2. Whang, J., E. Frei III, J. H. Tijo, P. P. Carbone & G. Brecher. 1963. The distribution of the Philadelphia chromosome in patients with chronic myelogenous leukemia. Blood **22:** 664.
3. Till, J. E. & E. A. McCulloch. 1961. A direct measurement of the radiation sensitivity of mouse bone marrow cells. Rad. Res. **14:** 213.
4. Ebbe, S. & F. Stohlman, Jr. 1965. Megakaryocytopoiesis in the rat. Blood **26:** 20.
5. Ebbe, S. & F. Stohlman, Jr. 1964. Effects of hypertransfusion and erythropoietin on labeling of rat megakaryocytes by tritiated thymidine. Proc. Soc. Exp. Biol. Med. **116:** 971–974.
6. Brecher, G. & F. Stohlman, Jr. 1961. Reticulocyte size and erythropoietic stimulation. Proc. Soc. Exp. Biol. Med. **107:** 887–891.
7. Stohlman, F., Jr. 1961. Humoral regulation of erythropoiesis. VII. Shortened survival of erythrocytes produced by erythropoietine or severe anemia. Proc. Soc. Exp. Biol. Med. **107:** 884–887.
8. Morse, B. S. & F. Stohlman, Jr. 1966. Regulation of erythropoiesis. XVIII. The effect of vincristine and erythropoietin on bone marrow. J. Clin. Invest. In press.
9. Bruce, W. R. & E. A. McCulloch. 1964. The effect of erythropoietic stimulation on the hemopoietic colony-forming cells of mice. Blood **23:** 216.
10. Morse, B. S., D. Howard & F. Stohlman, Jr. 1964. Vincristine effect on the stem cell. Clin. Res. Proc. **12:** 286.
11. Stohlman, F., Jr., G. Lucarelli, D. Howard, B. S. Morse & B. Leventhal. 1964. Regulation of erythropoiesis. XVI. Cytokinetic patterns in disorders of erythropoiesis. Medicine. **43:** 651.
12. Porteous, D. D. & L. G. Lajtha. 1966. On stem cell recovery after irradiation. Brit. J. Haemat. **12:** 177.
13. Blackett, N. M., J. P. Roylance & K. Adams. 1964. Studies of the capacity of bone marrow cells to restore erythropoiesis in heavily irradiated rats. Brit. J. Haemat. **10:** 453.
14. Lajtha, L. G. 1966. This Annal.
15. Smith, W. W., G. Brecher, F. Stohlman, Jr. & J. Cornfield. 1962. Toxicity of tritiated thymidine to bone marrow transplants. Rad. Res. **16:** 201.

16. BECKER, A. J., E. A. MCCULLOCH, L. SIMINOVITCH & J. E. TILL. 1965. The effect of differing demands for blood cell production on DNA synthesis by hemopoietic colony-forming cells of mice. Blood **26**: 296.
17. CUDKOWICZ, G., M. BENNETT & G. M. SHEARER. 1964. Pluripotent stem cell function of the mouse marrow "lymphocyte." Science **144**: 866.
18. BRECHER, G., W. W. SMITH & S. FRED. Personal communication.
19. ALPEN, E. L., D. CRANMORE & M. E. JOHNSTON. 1962. Early observations on the effects of blood loss. *In* Erythropoiesis. L. O. Jacobson and M. A. Doyle, Eds. : 184. Grune and Stratton. N. Y.
20. FRIED, W., L. F. PLZAK, L. O. JACOBSON & E. GOLDWASSER. 1957. Studies on erythropoiesis. III. Factors controlling erythropoietin production. Proc. Soc. Exp. Biol. Med. **94**: 237.
21. LAJTHA, L. G. 1964. Recent studies in erythroid differentiation and proliferation. Medicine **43**: 625.
22. CARMENA, A., G. LUCARELLI, D. HOWARD & F. STOHLMAN, JR. Unpublished observations.
23. KRETCHMAR, A. L. 1966. Erythropoietin: hypothesis of action tested by analog computer. Science **152**: 367.
24. ALPEN, E. L. Personal communication.
25. SCHOOLEY, J. C. 1965. Responsiveness of hematopoietic tissue to erythropoietin in relation to the time of administration and duration of action of the hormone. Blood **25**: 795.
26. GALLAGHER, N. I. & R. D. LANGE. 1960. Site of action of erythropoietin (ESF). Clin. Res. **8**: 280.
27. HODGSON, G. A. & I. ESKUCHE. Time course of effects of erythropoiesis-stimulating factor(s) on ^{59}Fe distribution. *In* Erythropoiesis. L. O. Jacobson and M. A. Doyle, Eds. Grune and Stratton. N. Y.
28. SCHUMACHER, H. R. & A. J. ERSLEV. 1965. Bone marrow kinetics. *In* Nuclear Medicine. E. Szirmai, Ed. Academic Press. N. Y. : 89.
29. FEINENDEGEN, L. E., V. P. BOND, E. P. CRONKITE & W. L. HUGHES. 1964. RNA turnover in normal rat bone marrow. Ann. N. Y. Acad. Sci. **113**: 727.
30. STOHLMAN, F., JR. 1964. Humoral regulation of erythropoiesis. XIV. A model for abnormal erythropoiesis in thalassemia. Ann. N. Y. Acad. Sci. **119**: 578–585.
31. BOND, V. P., N. ODARTCHENKO, H. COTTIER, L. E. FEINENDEGEN & E. P. CRONKITE. 1962. The kinetics of the more mature erythrocytic precursors studied with tritiated thymidine. *In* Erythropoiesis. L. O. Jacobson and M. A. Doyle, Eds. : 173. Grune and Stratton. N. Y.
32. CONRAD, M. E. & W. H. CROSBY. 1962. The natural history of iron deficiency induced by phlebotomy. Blood **20**: 173.
33. MOORES, R. R., F. STOHLMAN, JR. & G. BRECHER. 1963. Humoral regulation of erythropoiesis. XI. The pattern of response to specific therapy in iron deficiency anemia. Blood **22**: 286.
34. STOHLMAN, F., JR., D. HOWARD & A. BELAND. 1963. Humoral regulation of erythropoiesis. XII. Effect of erythropoietin and iron on cell size in iron deficiency anemia. Proc. Soc. Exp. Biol. Med. **113**: 986.
35. LEVENTHAL, B. & F. STOHLMAN, JR. 1966. Regulation of erythropoiesis. XVII. Determinants of red cell size in iron deficiency states. Pediatrics **37**: 62.

EFFECT OF POLYCYTHEMIC SERUM ON THE RATE OF RED CELL PRODUCTION*

A. J. Erslev and E. B. Thorling

Cardeza Foundation, Jefferson Medical College, Philadelphia, Pa.

The now widely accepted theory that erythropoiesis is controlled by erythropoietin is based on the assumption that a reduction in oxygen-carrying capacity of blood leads to tissue hypoxia and an increase in oxygen-carrying capacity leads to tissue hyperoxia. Since the oxygen tension must vary greatly not only from organ to organ but also within the same organ, this assumption rests primarily on theoretic calculations of oxygen supply and demand. In anemia the reduced oxygen-carrying capacity of blood and the unchanged oxygen demand must lead to a low mean capillary oxygen tension and a reduced oxygen pressure in the tissues. Increased blood flow and increased vascularity will obviously counteract this tendency but it seems unquestionable that anemias will tend to cause an overall reduction in tissue pO_2. In polycythemias the supply of oxygen is believed to be increased, leading to a lower extraction of oxygen in the capillaries and the maintenance of a high mean capillary oxygen tension and a high tissue pO_2.[1]

Recent studies of viscosity, blood flow and cardiac output have raised some doubts as to the validity of this latter conclusion.[2] When the flow of oxygen is estimated from whole blood viscosity and oxygen carrying capacity, it is found that the optimum oxygen flow occurs at hematocrits of about 45%. While this gives a hint as to the reason for our evolutionary choice of a hematocrit of 45% as "normal," it also suggests that the oxygen flow is impaired both at anemic and at polycythemic values (FIGURE 1). Impressive support for this deduction has come from animal studies in which cardiac output was measured at various normovolemic and hypervolemic hematocrits. The bell-shaped curves published by Murray *et al.,*[3] Richardson and Guyton,[4] and Weisse *et al.,*[5] depicting cell flow and systemic oxygen transport in vivo are remarkably similar to the curves in FIGURE 1. Accordingly it appears that polycythemia ought to be associated with tissue hypoxia rather than hyperoxia, making our working hypothesis on the control of red cell production untenable.

If polycythemia actually causes tissue hypoxia, it is necessary to provide an alternate explanation for the reduction in red cell production observed in mammals with transfusion polycythemia. From time to time it has been proposed that the rate of red cell production may be controlled by a physiologic inhibitor. Recently several authors have provided firm experimental support for this idea. Krzymowski and Krzymowski[6] and Whitcomb and Moore[7] have shown that plasma from hypertransfused rabbits contains an erythropoietic inhibitor, observations which are obviously of great interest for an understanding of the control of red cell production. The following studies were carried out in an attempt to confirm these reports:

Materials and Methods

Normal male New Zealand white rabbits were rendered polycythemic by an acute bleeding of 20 ml per kg with immediate replacement of 20 ml/kg of packed washed red blood cells (hematocrit 85%). The mean hematocrit of the

* This study was supported in part by grant nos. HE 6374 and HE 4612 from the United States Public Health Service.

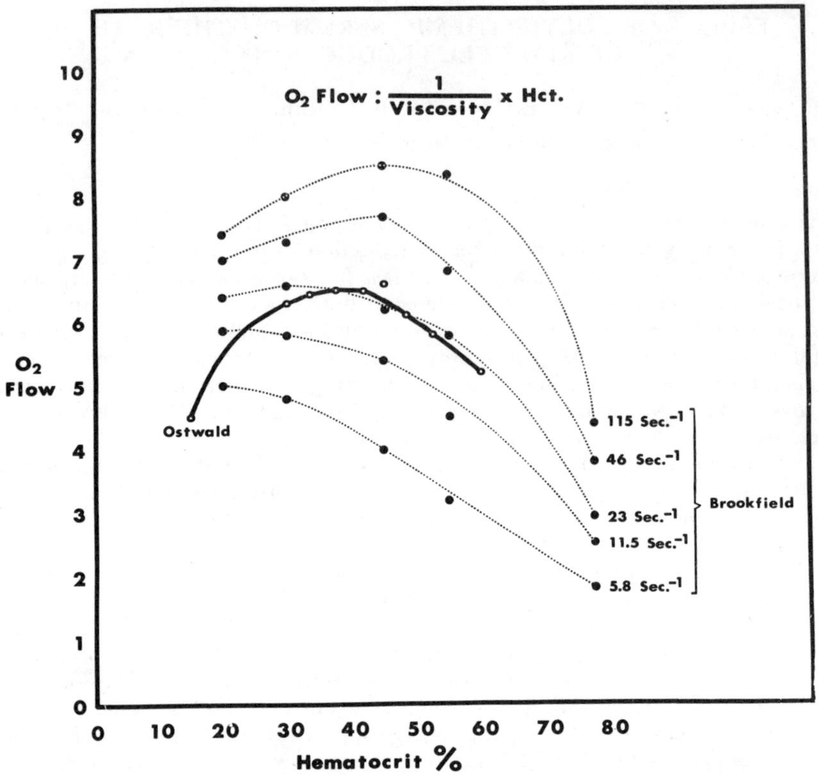

FIGURE 1. Oxygen flow calculated from viscosity and oxygen-carrying capacity of whole blood. The viscosity measurements were made either with a Brookfield cone-plate viscosimeter at varying rates of shear and with an Ostwald capillary viscosimeter at constant rates of shear.

recipients before the procedure was 42% and 48 hr later was 60%. At this point the animals were bled and the serum pooled.

Rabbit serum extract was prepared in a manner similar to the method used by Krzymowski and Krzymowski[6] and by Whitcomb and Moore.[7] Serum was acidified to a pH of 5.5 and heated to 95–100° for five minutes. A concentrated extract was obtained by perevaporation in dialyzing bags at room temperature.

Normal Swiss Webster mice and normal Sprague-Dawley rats were rendered polycythemic by intermittent exposure (16 hr a day) to 0.5 atmospheric air pressure for five weeks. The hematocrit at time of bleeding, five days after removal from the low pressure chamber, was 60–70%.

Assays for inhibitory activity were made in normal mice, in anemic rats and in starved and hypoxic rats. Reticulocyte counts and red cell iron utilization were used as measures of the rate of red cell production.

RESULTS

Assay of Rabbit Serum in Normal Mice. Whole serum obtained from normal and from polycythemic rabbits was injected i.p. into normal mice in the amount of 2 ml once a day for two days, (corresponding to a total of 200 ml serum per kg). Radioactive iron (0.5 μc ^{59}Fe) was injected i.p. 24 hr later and the 66-hour red

TABLE 1

IRON UTILIZATION: THE EFFECT OF RABBIT SERUM ADMINISTERED INTRAPERITONEALLY TO NORMAL MICE

Recipients: Normal Mice		^{59}Fe ± 66 Hour Utilization
Normal rabbit serum	2 ml × 2 i.p. (12)	23.8 ± 6.3%
Polycythemic rabbit serum	2 ml × 2 i.p. (11)	29.2 ± 13.0%

cell iron utilization was determined using an assumed blood volume of 5% of body weight. TABLE 1 shows that the iron incorporation was about the same for both groups.

Assay of Mouse and Rat Serum in Hypoxic Mice. Normal mice received 2 ml whole serum i.p. Immediately afterwards they were exposed to 0.5 atm air pressure. After 20 hr of hypoxia they were removed and 30 hr later they were given 0.5 μc ^{59}Fe i.p. and the 48-hour iron utilization determined. TABLE 2 lists the 48-hour iron utilization in the group receiving serum from normal and from polycythemic mice, and from normal and polycythemic rats. As can be seen, we have no indication that the polycythemic serum exhibited a specific inhibition on the rate of red cell production.

Assay of Unconcentrated Rabbit Serum Extract in Anemic Rats. Normal rats were bled 20 ml/kg with an immediate infusion of 20 ml/kg of either extract from normal rabbit serum or extract from polycythemic rabbit serum. The same amount of extract was administered i.v. once a day for the next three days for a total of 80 ml/kg body weight (corresponding to a total of 160 ml serum per kg). Six hours after the last infusion 0.5 μc ^{59}Fe was given i.v. and the 18-hour red cell iron utilization was determined using an assumed blood volume of 5% body weight. FIGURE 2 shows that the reticulocyte response to the initial bleeding was the same in rats receiving normal extract as in those receiving polycythemic extract. There was also no significant difference between the values for the 18-hour red cell utilization.

Assay of Rabbit Serum in Starved, Hypoxic Rats. Normal rats were deprived of food but given water ad libitum. Twenty four and 48 hr after the onset of starvation they received 20 ml/kg of serum i.p. Immediately after the first infusion they were placed at 0.5 atmospheric air pressure. After 48 hr of hypoxia they were removed from the low pressure tank, given 0.5 μc ^{59}Fe i.v. and the 18-hour red cell iron utilization was determined. FIGURE 3 shows that the polycythemic serum did not suppress the erythropoietic response to hypoxia.

Assay of Concentrated Rabbit Serum Extract in Starved Hypoxic Rats. Rabbit serum extract, concentrated five times by evaporation was tolerated reasonably well by rats when given i.p. and this extract (corresponding to about 700 ml

TABLE 2

THE EFFECT ON IRON UTILIZATION OF MOUSE AND RAT SERUM ADMINISTERED INTRAPERITONEALLY TO MICE SUBSEQUENTLY EXPOSED TO 0.5 ATMOSPHERIC AIR PRESSURE

Recipients: Hypoxic Mice		^{59}Fe ± 48 Hour Utilization
Normal mouse serum	2 ml i.p. (8)	34.9 ± 3.2%
Polycythemic mouse serum	2 ml i.p. (10)	35.7 ± 7.5%
Normal rat serum	2 ml i.p. (7)	33.6 ± 5.5%
Polycythemic rat serum	2 ml i.p. (6)	35.6 ± 4.1%

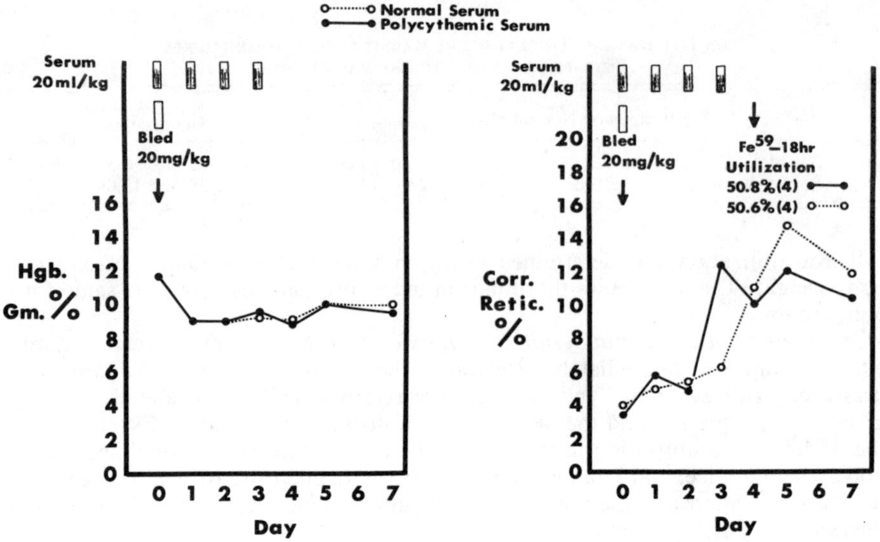

FIGURE 2. The effect of unconcentrated serum extract from normal and polycythemic rabbit on reticulocyte counts and iron utilization of four recipient rats.

serum per kg) was administered to starved hypoxic rats as in the above study. FIGURE 3 shows that even in this dose, serum extract from polycythemic rabbits did not suppress the erythropoietic response to hypoxia more than extract from normal rabbits.

DISCUSSION

In the studies reported here, serum and serum extract obtained from normal and transfused animals were assayed in mice or rats. Despite the administration of up to 200 ml of whole serum per kg of body weight to mice and up to 40 ml of whole serum per kg of body weight to rats, there was no significant difference between the rates of red cell production of animals receiving normal serum and animals receiving serum from polycythemic donors. This result appears to be at variance with the data reported by Krzymowski and Krzymowski[6] and by Whitcomb and Moore.[7] Neither of these authors tested whole serum but the amount of concentrated polycythemic serum extract claimed by Krzymowski and Krzmowski to induce an erythropoietic inhibition corresponds to a smaller amount of whole serum than that used in the present study. They reported that concentrated polycythemic rabbit serum extract derived from 8 ml of whole serum will suppress red cell production in recipient rabbits when given once a day for 10 days. The amount given to rats and claimed to produce an erythropoietic suppression corresponds to about 30 ml whole serum per kg. In the present study, 40 ml serum per kg was administered to rats without any noticeable suppressive effect.

Since considerably larger amounts of concentrated serum extract was employed by Whitcomb and Moore, serum from normal and polycythemic rabbits were extracted and concentrated according to the methods employed by these authors. Unconcentrated extract was first assayed in anemic rats in amounts corresponding to 160 ml whole serum per kg body weight. Despite being more than five times the amounts assayed by Krzymowski and Krzymowski, there was no ap-

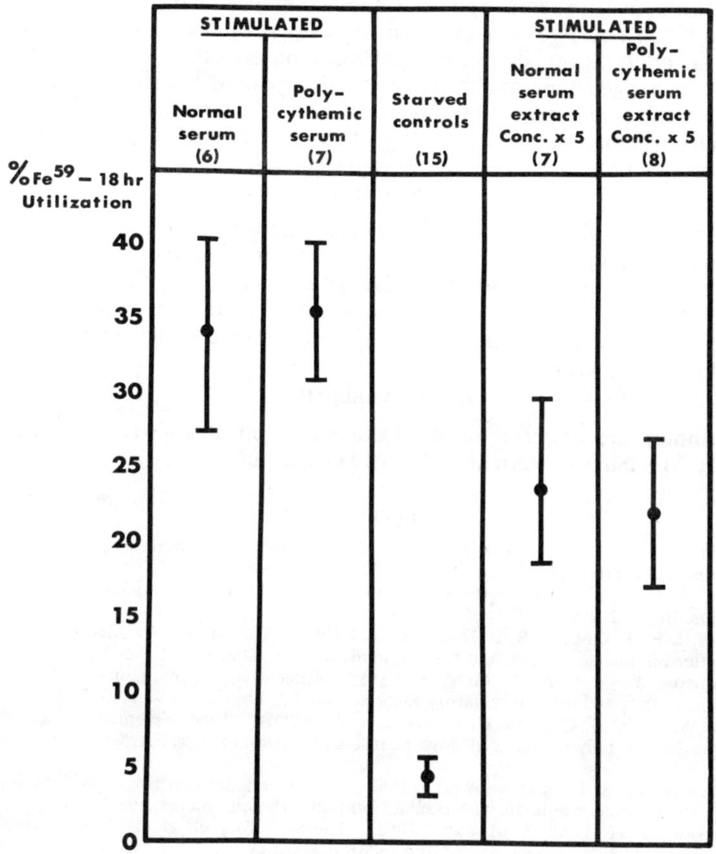

FIGURE 3. The effect of whole rabbit serum and serum extract concentrated five times on the iron utilization of starved, hypoxic rats. The rats received 3.5 ml of material i.p. on two successive days.

parent inhibiting effect of polycythemic serum extract. When this extract was concentrated by evaporation, the hypertonic extract was found to be too toxic for i.v. administration. However, when administered i.p. in hypoxic rats, they tolerated amounts corresponding to about 700 ml of serum per kg body weight. Nevertheless, even at this level there was no significant difference between the effect of concentrated extract from normal and from polycythemic donor rabbits.

Although the schedule and the preparations of the assay animals differ considerably from those used by Krzymowski and Krzymowski[6] and by Whitcomb and Moore,[7] the negative results raise grave doubts about the existence of a physiologic inhibitor of erythropoiesis in polycythemia of animals or humans.[8,9] The existence of such an inhibitor would have provided a welcome explanation for the lack of erythropoietic stimulation in transfusion polycythemia. Unfortunately, we were unable to demonstrate such an inhibitor and we are left without an explanation for the transfusion induced erythropoietic suppression. It is of course possible that the kidney with its intricate microcirculation can differentiate between anemic hypoxia caused by reduced oxygen-carrying capacity of whole blood and polycythemic hypoxia caused by decreased blood flow. On the other hand, it is also possible that our assumption of the effects of whole blood viscosity on oxygen flow to the tissues needs revision. Direct measurements of the tension of oxygen in various tissues are needed before it can be stated unequivocally whether or not red cell production is controlled by tissue hypoxia and erythropoietin.

Summary

Attempts to confirm the presence of an inhibitor of erythropoiesis in polycythemic animals has been reported. Serum and serum extracts from normal and polycythemic rabbits, rats and mice were obtained and assayed in mice and rats. Although the assay animals were made sensitive to the action of an inhibitor by being rendered anemic or hypoxic, in no instance could an erythropoietic inhibitor be demonstrated.

Acknowledgment

The authors are grateful for the valuable technical assistance of Miss Kay Cornelius, Mrs. Sharon Stern and Mrs. Aida Rodriguez.

References

1. Houston, C. S. & R. L. Riley. 1947. Perspiratory and circulatory changes during acclimatization to high altitude. Amer. J. Physiol. **149:** 565.
2. Erslev, A. J. 1966. The erythropoietic effect of hematocrit variations in normovolemic rabbits. Blood **27:** 629.
3. Murray, J. F., P. Gold & B. L. Johnson, Jr. 1963. The circulatory effects of hematocrit variations in normovolemic and hypervolemic dogs. J. Clin. Invest. **42:** 1159.
4. Richardson, T. Q. & A. C. Guyton. 1959. Effects of polycythemia and anemia on cardiac output and other circulatory factors. Amer. J. Physiol. **197:** 1167.
5. Weisse, A. B., F. M. Colton, H. Kuida & H. A. Hecht. 1964. Hemodynamic effects of normovolemic polycythemia in dogs at rest and during exercise. Amer. J. Physiol. **207:** 1361.
6. Krzymowski, T. & H. Krzymowski. 1962. Studies on the erythropoiesis-inhibiting factor in the plasma of animals with transfusion polycythemia. Blood. **19:** 38.
7. Whitcomb, W. H. & M. Z. Moore. 1965. The inhibitory effect of plasma from hypertransfused animals on erythrocyte iron incorporation in mice. J. Lab. Clin. Med. **66:** 641.
8. Reynafarje, C., J. Ramos, J. Faura & D. Villavicencio. 1964. Humoral control of erythropoietic activity in man during and after altitude exposure. Proc. Soc. Exper. Biol. Med. **116:** 649.
9. Whitcomb, W. H., M. Moore, R. Dille, L. Hummer & R. M. Bird. 1965. Erythropoietin and erythropoiesis inhibitor activity in man. J. Clin. Invest. **44:** 1110.

STUDIES ON HYPOXIA. VI. CHANGES IN LYMPHOCYTES AND TRANSITIONAL CELLS IN THE MARROW DURING THE INTENSIFICATION OF PRIMARY HYPOXIA AND REBOUND

J. M. Yoffey,* R. V. Jeffreys, D. G. Osmond, M. S. Turner, S. C. Tahsin and P. A. R. Niven

Department of Anatomy, University of Bristol, Bristol, England

Introduction

The studies now presented are the third in a group designed to investigate by quantitative methods the changes in the bone marrow during either stimulation or depression of erythropoiesis. Apart from observing the changes in erythropoiesis, it was also hoped that the experiments might help to throw light on the stem cell problem. For example, a sudden stimulus to increased erythropoiesis might make such a heavy demand on the stem cells that their numbers would appreciably diminish, while, conversely, depression of erythropoiesis could result in an accumulation of stem cells, and in either case the change might allow quantitative assessment. Stimulation of erythropoiesis has been produced by hypoxia throughout.

Our first experiments were performed at the Hochalpine Forschungsstation, Jungfraujoch, at an altitude of around 11,000 feet.[1] They were not entirely satisfactory since the work was done on a variety of animals of different ages. The second series of experiments was performed with a decompression chamber[2] at a simulated altitude of 14,000 feet.[3,4] In this second group, we investigated not only the initial response to hypoxia, which we termed primary hypoxia, but also studied (a) what we termed the period of rebound (posthypoxic polycythemia) during which erythropoiesis was greatly diminished, and (b) a second period of hypoxia following the rebound phase, which we termed secondary hypoxia.[5]

At 14,000 feet, apart from the increase in the nucleated erythroid cells of the marrow, the most notable change in primary hypoxia was a fall in the marrow lymphocytes, which just reached the conventional significance level, while during rebound in addition to the depression of erythropoiesis, there was a rise in the marrow lymphocytes, again only slightly significant. We therefore decided to investigate the effects of intensifying the hypoxia and rebound to ascertain whether the changes in the marrow lymphocytes would become accentuated.

Accordingly, animals were kept in the decompression chamber at a simulated altitude of 17,000 feet for seven days, at the end of which they were markedly polycythemic. In fact the polycythemia was still present even after seven days of rebound, and thus, the subsequent depression of erythropoiesis was more marked than in the earlier studies. Under these experimental conditions the resultant changes in the bone marrow significantly involved all three major cell groups, namely, erythroid, myeloid and lymphoid cells.

Materials and Methods

The work has been done throughout on a standard experimental animal, a male guinea pig of the Dunklin-Hartley strain weighing approximately 400 g at the termination of the experiments. This animal has been employed in our laboratory for a number of years, and a wide variety of data are available from previous experiments.[8]

* Recipient of a contribution from the Wellcome Trust.

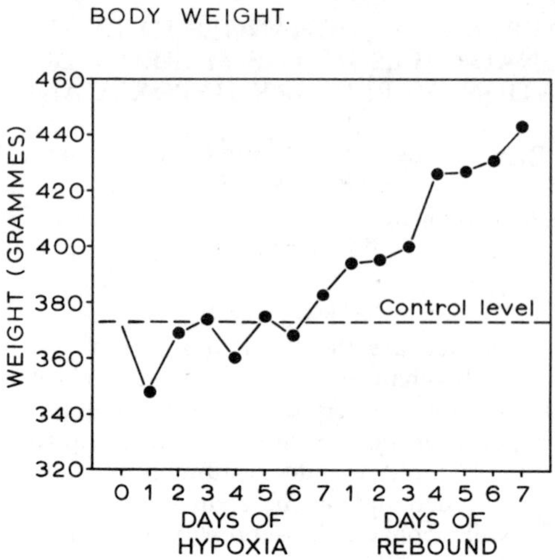

FIGURE 1. Weight changes in guinea pigs subjected to hypoxia at an altitude equivalent of 17,000 feet for seven days, and then kept in ambient air for seven days during the period of rebound. During the first six days of hypoxia, the weight fluctuates at or below the control level. During rebound the animals gain weight steadily.

Animals were placed in the decompression chamber[2] and decompressed at 4,000 fpm until a level of 17,000 feet was reached. They were removed from the chamber for a few minutes each day so that the cage could be cleaned, and then decompressed again.

Eight animals were used for each day, i.e., eight animals were placed in the decompression chamber for one day, eight for two days, eight for three days, and so on until seven days. For the study of rebound eight animals after seven days of hypoxia were kept in room air for one day, eight for two days, eight for three days, and so on until seven days. Thus a total of 56 animals experienced primary hypoxia for times ranging from 1–7 days, and 56 animals were examined during rebound also for times ranging from 1–7 days.

Blood was examined in each animal at the termination of the experiment, i.e., immediately after removal from the decompression chamber in primary hypoxia, and after the appropriate time during rebound. Blood was obtained by nicking an ear vein after first warming the ear.

The marrow was examined by a quantitative technique which has been described and critically assessed on a number of occasions.[6–8] The essence of the technique is that a known volume of marrow is placed in a known volume of serum. Mechanical agitation then breaks up the marrow and gives rise to a uniform suspension of cells which, like blood, can be examined both quantitatively and qualitatively. Blood was examined by standard hemocytometric techniques. Bhuyan's[9] method was found to give the best results for reticulocyte counting.

RESULTS

Body Weight and General Condition

FIGURE 1 presents the changes in body weight during the experimental period. For the greater part of primary hypoxia the weight either fell or returned to the starting level until a rise on the seventh day which continued throughout rebound.

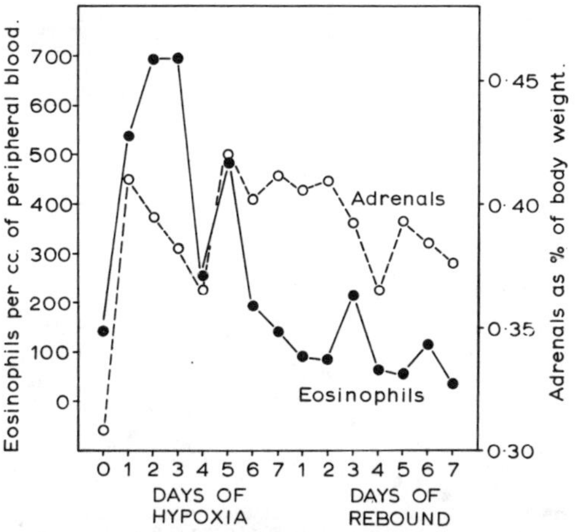

FIGURE 2. Changes during hypoxia and rebound in adrenal weight (expressed as a percentage of body weight) and the eosinophile count per cu mm of blood. The significant increase in adrenal weight suggests stress response, but the marked increase in circulating eosinophils does not seem to be in accord with this. The increase in eosinophils may be due to their expression from the marrow by the rapid proliferation of erythroid cells.

Although the animals displayed normal activity and appeared to feed well from the outset, it was felt that the failure to gain weight might be due to stress, evidence for which was sought both in the weight of the adrenals and the level of the circulating eosinophils. The increase in adrenal weight suggests a stress response although the eosinophilia does not (FIGURE 2). However, in this particular series of experiments, special eosinophile-counting techniques were not employed though data are available from another series in which they were used and these are in full accord with the present finding.[10]

Changes in the Blood

FIGURE 3 presents the changes in the hemoglobin, red blood cells and packed cell volume in the circulating blood. In all three parameters there was a highly significant rise during the seven days of primary hypoxia, and even at the end of rebound all three were significantly above control level. The blood reticulocytes (FIGURE 4) rose rapidly, reaching their peak on the fifth day, after which they diminished. The fall in the blood reticulocytes continued throughout rebound at the end of which they had almost disappeared from the blood.

Apart from the eosinophiles, there were no other significant changes in the blood leukocytes.

Changes in the Marrow

The changes in the marrow reticulocytes departed in two respects from what had been expected on the basis of earlier observations. Although they showed a significant rise during the last few days of hypoxia, they fell significantly during the first two days (FIGURE 4). Furthermore, they showed a sharp rise at the beginning of rebound, at a time when the blood reticulocytes were rapidly falling (FIGURE 4). By the seventh day of rebound, when there were hardly any reticulocytes in the blood, an appreciable number were still present in the marrow.

After fluctuating for the first four days, the total marrow count of nucleated cells fell significantly on the fifth day of hypoxia (FIGURE 5) and then appeared

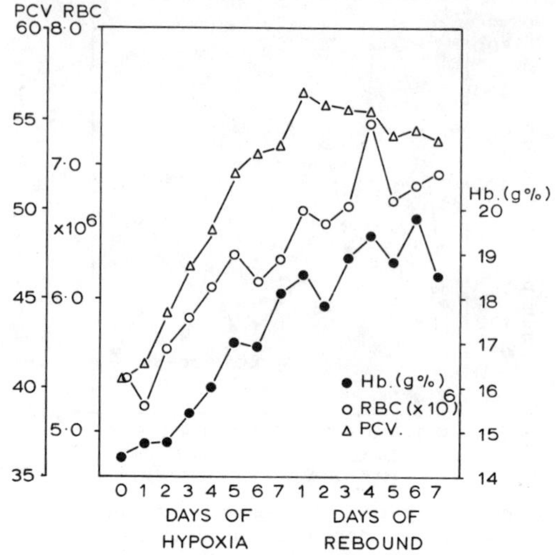

FIGURE 3. Changes in packed cell volume, hemoglobin, and red cell count during primary hypoxia and rebound. There is a definite polycythemia even after seven days of rebound.

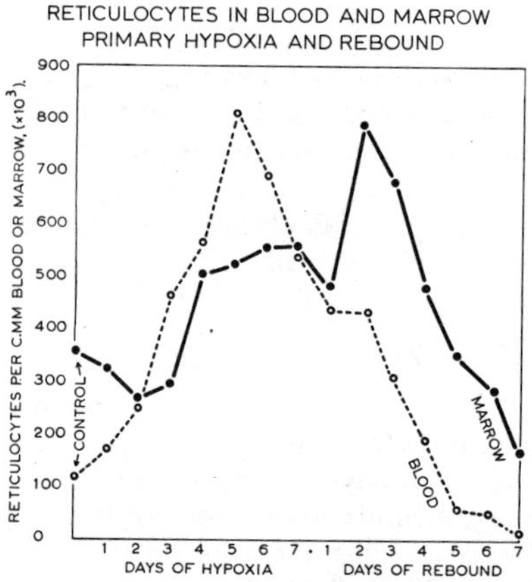

FIGURE 4. Reticulocytes per cu mm of blood and marrow during primary hypoxia and rebound. The fall in marrow reticulocytes during the first two days of hypoxia is associated with a very much greater increase in the blood reticulocytes. Since the blood volume is about 4 × that of the red marrow, the increase in the circulating reticulocytes after two days of hypoxia is about 5 × the fall in the marrow reticulocytes.

to rise again although the increase from the seventh day of hypoxia to the seventh day of rebound was not statistically significant. Analysis of the three main cell groups (FIGURE 6), namely erythroid, myeloid and lymphoid cells, showed that both the lymphoid and the myeloid cells fell during the first five days of hypoxia, while the erythroid cells, which rose rapidly during the first three days, then leveled off and also fell on the fifth day. On the fifth day of primary hypoxia, therefore, the myeloid and lymphoid cells were well below their normal level, while the erythroid cells after their initial rise were almost back to their control

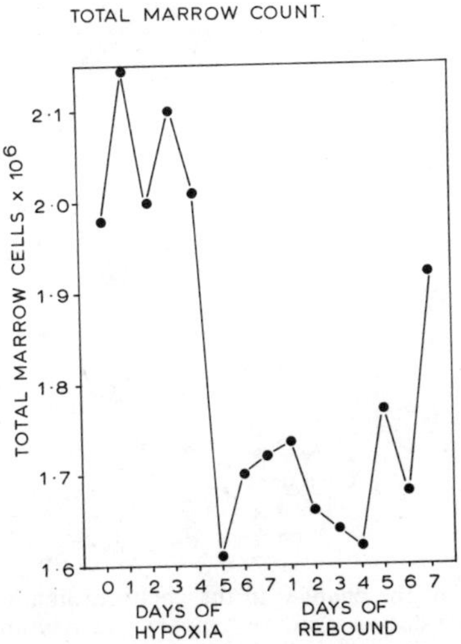

FIGURE 5. Total nucleated cells per cu mm marrow during primary hypoxia and rebound. The marked fall on the fifth day of primary hypoxia is due to a sudden leveling off of nucleated red cells at the same time as the lymphocytes and myeloid cells are also well below normal.

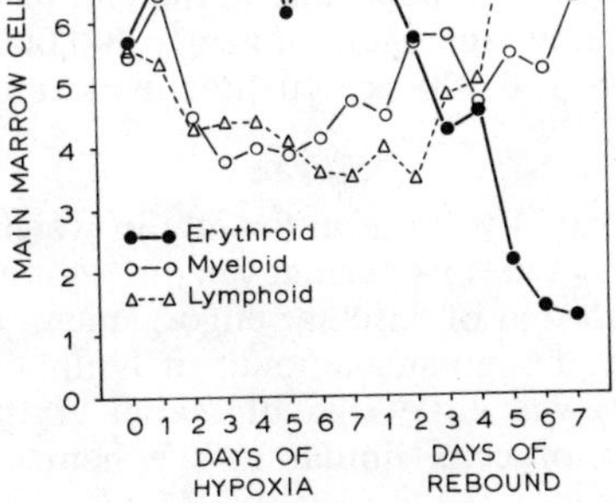

FIGURE 6. Changes (in absolute counts per cu mm marrow) of the main marrow cell groups during primary hypoxia and rebound. The nucleated erythroid cells show a marked increase during the first four days of primary hypoxia, on the last three days of which they level off, and begin to fall rapidly from the first day of rebound. The myeloid cells fall during hypoxia, and gradually return towards normal during rebound. The lymphocytes fall significantly during primary hypoxia, and from the third day of rebound rise rapidly to well above their control level.

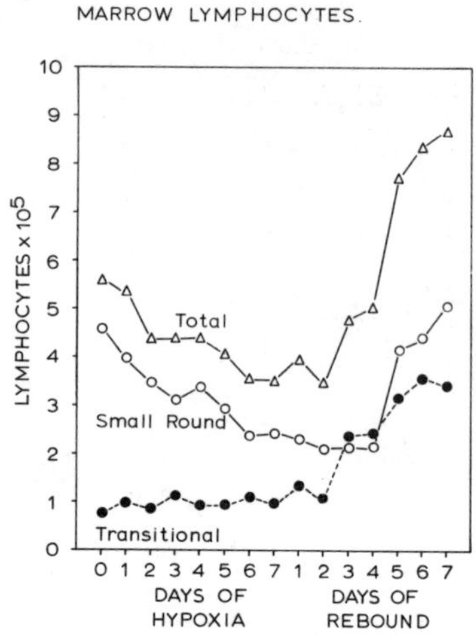

FIGURE 7. A comparison of the changes in the pachychromatic small lymphocytes ("small round") and transitional cells during primary hypoxia and rebound. During primary hypoxia it is pachychromatic small lymphocytes which fall, while the transitionals seem to be increasing slightly. During rebound there is a highly significant increase in both groups.

level. The fall in the total nucleated cell count on the fifth day is due to the coincidence of all three factors.

During rebound the nucleated erythroid cells fell to a very low level, about one fourth their number in the control animals. But they did not completely disappear. The myeloid cells returned to approximately their normal level, or slightly above it, although not significantly so. The lymphocytes rose significantly during rebound, at the end of which they were nearly double their normal numbers. When one analyzes the lymphocyte curve more fully, it becomes clear that the fall in the marrow lymphocytes during hypoxia was due primarily to a diminution in the number of the pachychromatic small lymphocytes and not of the transitional cells. The increase in the number of lymphocytes during rebound was due to an increase in both groups, and at the end of rebound the transitional cells attained the remarkably high figure of nearly 400,000 per cu mm of marrow, compared with less than 100,000 per cu mm in normal marrow (FIGURE 7).

Spleen

The spleen increased rapidly and significantly in weight, and by the sixth day of hypoxia was about four times its normal weight (FIGURE 8). Upon histological examination there was no sign of vascular engorgement, and the weight increase was due to the presence of a greater amount of lymphoid tissue and of splenic pulp. Surprisingly, there was little sign of actual erythropoiesis. There were, however, large numbers of cells similar to the hemocytoblasts seen in bone marrow.

DISCUSSION

Reticulocytes

Reticulocyte Discharge from Marrow

From FIGURE 4 it is evident that the marrow reticulocytes fell during the first two days of hypoxia, while at the same time the blood reticulocytes increased,

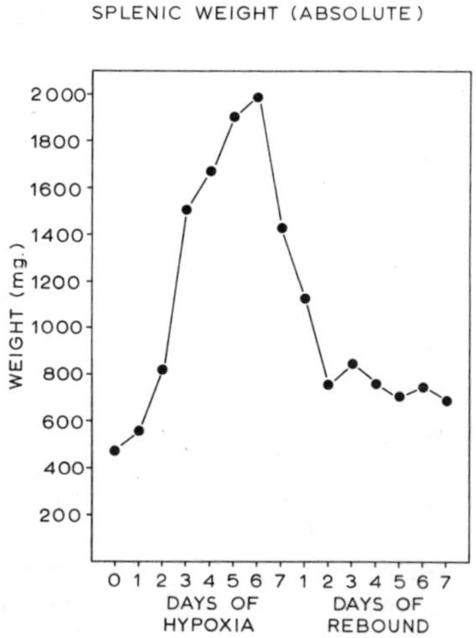

FIGURE 8. Splenic weight during primary hypoxia (17,000 feet) and rebound. The weight becomes diminished on the last day of primary hypoxia, and continues to diminish rapidly on the first two days of rebound.

both changes being significant by the second day. Moffatt *et al.*[3] did not find an initial drop in the marrow reticulocytes at 14,000 feet hypoxia, but recently Yoffey *et al.*[11] reported a fall both at 10,000 and 20,000 feet. The latter results are probably more reliable since they were based on the improved technique of Bhuyan,[9] which gives excellent staining and permanent preparations of reticulocytes. The fall in the marrow reticulocytes while those in the blood are rising seems to imply an accelerated discharge from the marrow in the first 48 hours.

The mechanism by which hypoxia increases the discharge of reticulocytes from the marrow is not known, but there is some evidence to suggest that it may be due to erythropoietin. Gordon *et al.*,[12] using the isolated perfused femur of the rat, reported a rapid stimulation of reticulocyte discharge from the marrow following the administration of erythropoietin. In intact rats, Fruhman & Fischer[13] found young Grade I reticulocytes in the blood as early as 12 hr after the injection of erythropoietin. More recently Fisher *et al.*[14] have confirmed the early discharge of reticulocytes from the marrow after erythropoietin in the isolated perfused hind limb of the rabbit, and they suggest that erythropoietin acts on the erythron at more than one point.

Stimulation of New Red Cell Formation

A comparison of the changes in the marrow reticulocytes (FIGURE 4) with those in the nucleated erythroid cells (FIGURE 6) makes it clear that the rapid increase in these cells during the first three days of hypoxia precedes the increase in marrow reticulocytes on the fourth day. This type of relationship between the nucleated erythroid cells and the reticulocytes was first noted in the Jungfrau experiments.[1] The evidence then available made it unlikely that there was any change of note in the generation time of the erythroid cells, and it was then suggested that if that were the case, the only way in which the nucleated erythroid population could increase was by feeding in new stem cells. This view was later supported by Erslev[15] Alpen & Cranmore[16] Lajtha & Oliver[17] & Jacobson *et al.*[18]

Suit *et al.*[19] suggested that an appreciable number of red cells might even mature from the "early normoblast" without intervening cell division, and if this holds good when erythropoiesis is augmented, the requirement for stem cells will be proportionately greater. The maturation of some erythrocytes from stem cells without any intervening mitoses could accelerate the process of red cell formation (*cf. ref.*[20]), in which case the fall in marrow reticulocytes during the first two days of hypoxia underestimates the number of reticulocytes actually leaving the marrow.

Reticulocyte Accumulation in the Marrow

It has already been noted that during primary hypoxia the marrow reticulocytes showed an initial fall (FIGURE 4), and the simultaneous rise in the blood reticulocytes presumably means that there is an increased discharge from the marrow. By contrast, during the first two days of rebound the marrow reticulocytes rise to a much higher level than during primary hypoxia, and yet at the same time the blood reticulocytes are falling. The most obvious interpretation is that under these circumstances newly formed reticulocytes are being retained in the marrow.

A similar sort of relationship, though to a much lesser degree, may hold good for the last day of rebound, when the number of reticulocytes in the marrow is still appreciable even though reduced somewhat below the normal level (FIGURE 4), whereas the blood reticulocytes have almost completely disappeared. It is noteworthy that despite the great depression of erythropoiesis, some reticulocytes are still present both in the marrow and in the blood. This was reported by Boycott & Oakley[21] in cases of transfusion polycythemia.

The increase in the level of the marrow reticulocytes during the first few days of rebound makes it necessary to interpret with special care the results of experiments in which there is an increased discharge of reticulocytes from the marrow. For example, Stohlman[20] gave erythropoietin to rats rendered polycythemic by blood transfusion, and found that increased numbers of reticulocytes appeared in the blood as early as 24–48 hr after the administration of erythropoietin. On the basis of this finding he concluded that he was dealing either with a shortening of generation time in the erythroid cells or with what he termed "skipped mitoses", i.e., passage from stem cells to mature erythrocyte without cell division. However, if the polycythemic animals to which he gave erythropoietin had a high level of reticulocytes in the marrow and if, as has already been suggested, erythropoietin can act on the reticulocyte end of the erythron and stimulate the discharge of reticulocytes from the marrow, then the early appearance of reticulocytes in Stohlman's experiments would permit a much simpler explanation than that which he gives and would make it unnecessary to invoke the occurrence of "skipped mitoses," although it does not, of course, eliminate the possibility of this occurrence.

The Nucleated Erythroid Cells

The Extent of Erythropoietic Stimulation

Mention has already been made of the relationship between the increase in the nucleated erythroid cells and the reticulocyte population of the marrow. This raises a further question: How far, in fact, can the nucleated red cells increase in numbers?

In the Jungfraujoch experiments, at 11,000 feet the nucleated erythroid cells rose to just over 600,000 per cu mm of marrow.[1] This actually represented about a doubling of the control level, which in the Jungfrau animals was at 310,000 per cu mm, lower than in the standard guinea pig employed in the present series.

In hypoxia at a simulated altitude of 14,000 ft[3] the nucleated red cells slightly more than doubled, rising from a control level of 407,000 ± 113,000 per cu mm to a maximum of 895,000 ± 356,000 on the second day of hypoxia.

In the present experiments about 1,000,000 nucleated erythroid cells per cu mm of marrow seems to be the maximum level attainable, and there are probably a number of factors determining this end point.

The marrow in the 400 g guinea pig is predominantly red[8] and has virtually no reserve space occupied by fatty marrow. As the marrow is contained within a rigid bony cavity, it cannot undergo a rapid increase in volume. Hudson[22] has shown that even in animals hypoxic from birth, there is very little scope for increase in the volume of red marrow. In the guinea pig and the smaller laboratory animals one deals with a low reserve marrow.[8] The position in man is different, at any rate in the adult, where according to the data of Mechanik[23] one is dealing with a high reserve marrow, in which the effective marrow volume can be doubled through the replacement of fatty by red marrow. By contrast, the position in the human fetus resembles that in the smaller laboratory animals, where one deals with a low reserve marrow[24] even below that of the standard guinea pig, at 1.4 ml per 100 g as against 1.5 ml in the guinea pig.

It follows from these considerations that in the guinea pig there is no scope for an increase in the marrow volume, and that as far as the marrow is concerned, any increase in erythropoiesis must depend upon increasing the number of erythropoietic cells. This can only occur either by the absorption of a few fat cells which are normally to be found in red marrow, or by the displacement of other marrow cells. The rise in the nucleated erythroid cells during the first few days of hypoxia is associated with a significant fall in both myeloid cells and lymphocytes (FIGURE 7). But there seems to be a point below which these other cells will not fall, and this may be responsible for the failure of the erythroid cells to increase any further. Whether or not this is true, it appears that in the guinea pig somewhere between 2x–3x is the limit of increase of the nucleated erythroid cells in the marrow. In the high reserve marrow of man, where the red marrow can virtually double its volume, the limit of increase is correspondingly greater, and should be 4x–6x. Although we do not have quantitative data on the cell content of human marrow, estimates of its regenerative capacity do in fact suggest that red cell production can be increased sixfold even though one cannot be quite sure whether some of this may be extramedullary.[25–28]

Extramedullary Erythropoiesis

Extramedullary erythropoiesis is generally thought to occur mainly in the spleen, and during hypoxia the weight of the spleen increases more than fourfold (FIGURE 8). The gain in weight is evident on the first day, and is already quite marked by the second day of hypoxia. The gain in weight appears to be due to an increase of splenic tissue, not to engorgement of blood vessels. We have been puzzled by the fact that upon histological examination there is little evidence of actual red cell formation. The most conspicuous feature is the presence of large numbers of cells which in the marrow would be termed hemocytoblasts. In the rat, Rambach *et al.*[29] have estimated, on the basis of ^{59}Fe uptake, that the spleen can be responsible for 16% of the total red cell output of the body when erythropoiesis is stimulated.

Can extramedullary erythropoiesis occur anywhere else besides the spleen? We have carefully examined the intestinal mucosa where one can quite frequently observe granulopoiesis, but we have been unable to see any sign of erythropoiesis. On occasion, a small erythropoietic island has been found in the deep cervical lymph gland, though not in the glandula mesenterica magna or in the thymus. Although it was a rare finding, the presence of erythropoietic tissue in the deep cervical lymph gland was a very striking phenomenon.[30]

However, as the erythropoiesis in this situation involves only a small number of cells, it seems unlikely that they can make a significant contribution to the need for increased red cell output. Furthermore, with erythroid as with myeloid metaplasia, the question arises as to whether one is dealing with a true metaplasia, or whether it merely represents a local proliferation of erythropoietic cells which have colonized the lymph gland from the blood stream.

Relation Between Spleen and Bone Marrow

If the spleen itself does not produce large numbers of red cells, it could still make an important contribution to the increased erythropoiesis by the production of stem cells which could then migrate through the blood stream and colonize the bone marrow. The present studies do not afford any direct evidence on this problem, which has been fully reviewed elsewhere.[8]

Myeloid Cells

Hypoxia at 17,000 feet is associated with significant lowering of the marrow granulocytes (FIGURE 6). The reason for this fall is not clear, but the fact seems undoubted. The simplest of the various possible explanations is that the granulocytes are crowded out of the marrow by the proliferating erythroid cells. If there is a common stem cell for granulocytes and erythrocytes, stem cell competition might also influence the result.

Lymphocytes and Transitional Cells

While in our earlier investigations on the effects of hypoxia the changes in the marrow lymphocytes were not very clear-cut, whether at an altitude of 11,000 feet at the Jungfrau[1] or at an altitude equivalent of 14,000 feet in the decompression chamber,[3,4] the changes in the present series of 17,000 feet were much more definite.

During the period of primary hypoxia (FIGURES 6 & 7) there is a highly significant fall in the marrow lymphocyte population. When one analyzes this fall in more detail, it is seen to occur essentially in the pachychromatic small lymphocytes ("small round" in FIGURE 7), whereas the transitional lymphocytes appear to be fairly constant. The morphology of the pachychromatic small lymphocytes and transitional cells has recently been fully described and illustrated elsewhere (see reference 31; FIGURES 1–13, and FIGURE 25), and a detailed description is not therefore required here.

During rebound, on the other hand, after a lag of two days, the lymphocyte population shows a steep rise so that by the seventh day it is more than 55% above its control level, which is regained about the fourth day of rebound. This return to the normal number is attributable both to the small lymphocytes and to the transitional cells. In fact the rise in the transitional cells precedes by two days the increase in the small lymphocytes (FIGURE 7). Furthermore, the transitional cells continue to increase so that by the seventh day of rebound they are well over 300,000 per cu mm, (FIGURE 7) as compared with well below 100,000 per cu mm in the normal animal.[7,8]

Judging from the evidence of thymidine labeling, the transitional lymphocytes must be in a state of very active proliferation. We first noted the high labeling rate in the transitional cells of guinea pig marrow some years ago[32,33] and this fact has since been repeatedly confirmed.[31,34,35]

In the present studies we have been able to confirm and amplify our earlier findings. These radio-autographic studies will be described fully elsewhere. A typical count on the seventh day of rebound shows that one hour after the administration of thymidine, out of 300 lymphocytes and transitionals, 95 were pachychromatic small lymphocytes none of which was labeled, and the remaining 205 cells were transitional lymphocytes which we grouped roughly as small medium and large. Of the small transitionals, six out of 80 were labeled, of the medium transitionals, 39 out of 86 and of the large transitionals, 30 out of 41. Taking the transitionals as a group, about 35% showed flash labeling with thymidine. This is in full accord with the findings of Osmond & Everett[34] in the guinea pig, and would suggest that the marrow lymphocytes are formed in the marrow. As against this, there is evidence that both in the rat[36] and in the dog[31] considerable numbers of lymphocytes come to the marrow from the blood stream. For the time being, therefore, we must leave open the question of the extent to which the marrow lymphocytes and transitional cells are myelogenous, hematogenous, or both.

There is however another aspect of the problem which is raised by the present experiments. The recent studies of Cudkowicz *et al.*[38,39] seem to show that the hemopoietic stem cells in mouse marrow are to be found in the lymphocyte group.[1,35] If this is so, the accumulation of lymphocytes and transitional cells during a period of erythropoietic depression could be interpreted as the accumulation of stem cells which are not being called upon to undergo erythropoietic differentiation. In fact there are two sets of changes which could be interpreted along these lines. The first is the fall in lymphocytes during the stimulation of erythropoiesis in primary hypoxia (FIGURES 6 & 7). This fall could presumably be due to a greatly increased demand for stem cells, with which the stem cell compartment cannot keep pace. The second is the reverse change, already noted, namely, the marked accumulation during erythropoietic depression. If we are not dealing here with the lowering or raising of the numbers of stem cells, the changes in the marrow lymphocytes become very difficult to explain.

How far can the accumulation of lymphocytes and transitional cells proceed? FIGURES 6 & 7 only give the changes up to the seventh day of rebound. In some further experiments which are now in progress, we have obtained marrows which on the eighth day of rebound contain over 70% lymphocytes, but with a marked drop in the transitional cells as compared with the seventh day, so that in these 8th-day marrows most of the lymphocytes are really of the pachychromatic small variety.[40]

The rise in lymphocytes and transitional cells in the marrow does not occur until the third day of rebound, i.e., 10 days after the initiation of hypoxia. In a previous communication[5] we commented on the differential response of the marrow in primary and secondary hypoxia, and noted that on the second day of secondary hypoxia, i.e., 12 days after the first hypoxic stimulation, there was a sharp rise in the marrow lymphocytes and transitionals. The experimental conditions were somewhat different, in that there were only five days' exposure to hypoxia at 14,000 feet, followed by five days of rebound and then secondary hypoxia again at 14,000 feet. In view of our present findings, it is possible that the increase in lymphocytes and transitionals during secondary hypoxia was not the result of the secondary hypoxia per se, but was merely the continuation of changes which had begun during rebound.

To what extent is there a parallel between the experimental depression of erythropoiesis by the rebound technique and the depression of erythropoiesis which occurs in some types of aplastic anemia? In one type of aplastic anemia the marrow contains an unusually large proportion of lymphocytes. Holmes & Broun[41] reported in a case of aplastic anemia that 42% of all the nucleated marrow cells were lymphocytes. Rhoads & Miller[42] in 15 cases of aplastic anemia – the so-called "hyperplastic" type – found an average count of 36.9% of what would now be termed lymphocytes though at that time they considered them to be "primitive" cells.

The transitional cell had not yet been clearly recognized as a separate entity, but it is evident that a distinctive group of cells had been seen and had given rise to some doubt in these conditions of maturation arrest. Bomford & Rhoads[43] concluded that many of the cells which Rhoads & Miller has previously regarded as "primitive" were in fact early erythroblasts. Davidson *et al.*[44] noted in cases of refractory anemia the appearance of what they termed "Q" cells, and from their description is would appear that they were looking at the type of cell we now call transitional.

It is also of interest to note that the same cellular accumulation is to be observed in cases of arrested granulocytosis. We have not yet been able to devise a satisfactory experimental model for the study of the changes following the arrest of granulopoiesis in the same way as after depression of erythropoiesis. But in the neutropenia which occurs clinically Blackburn[45] reported an accumulation of lymphocytes in the marrow during the period of neutropenia while in the recovery phase the resumption of normal granulopoiesis was accompanied by a rapid fall in the marrow lymphocytes. More recently Pisciotta *et al.*[46] have considerably amplified these findings in agranulocytosis, and have confirmed, both on the morphological appearance and on the basis of thymidine-labeling properties, the occurrence of appreciable numbers of transitional cells.

Finally, it should be pointed out that Jordan[47] was one of the earliest observers who clearly suggested that the accumulation of lymphocytes in the marrow during conditions of maturation arrest was essentially an accumulation of stem cells not undergoing differentiation.

Summary

The bone marrow of the guinea pig has been investigated quantitatively both during primary hypoxia for seven days at a simulated altitude of 17,000 feet and for an additional seven days during the subsequent period of rebound (post-hypoxic polycythemia). During primary hypoxia the marrow not only shows evidence of increased erythropoiesis, but also of a fall in granulocytes and lymphocytes. During rebound, on the other hand, erythropoiesis is depressed, granulopoiesis returns to normal, while lymphocytes and transitional cells show a striking increase to well above their normal level. The significance of these findings is discussed. The marrow during rebound provides an admirable experimental model for the study of lymphocytes and transitional cells.

Acknowledgments

It is a pleasure to acknowledge my thanks to my secretary, Miss L. Lloyd, for her assistance in the preparation of the manuscript, and to Mr. A. K. Sykes for the preparation of the Figures.

References

1. Yoffey, J. M. 1957. Cellular equilibria in the blood and blood-forming tissues. Homeostatic mechanisms. Brookhaven Symposia in Biology: No. 10, 1–30.
2. Gall, W. J., A. F. Rogers & J. M. Yoffey. 1954. A low-pressure chamber. J. Physiol. **124:** 54P.
3. Moffatt, D. J., C. Rosse, I. H. Sutherland & J. M. Yoffey. 1964a. Studies on hypoxia. I. The response of the bone marrow to primary hypoxia. Acta Anat. **58:** 26–36.
4. Moffatt, D. J., C. Rosse, I. H. Sutherland & J. M. Yoffey. 1964b. Studies on hypoxia. II. A quantitative study of changes in the bone marrow of the guinea pig during posthypoxic polycythaemia (rebound). Acta Anat. **59:** 188–197.
5. Yoffey, J. M., C. Rosse, D. J. Moffatt & I. H. Sutherland. 1965. Studies on hypoxia. III. The differential response of the bone marrow to primary and secondary hypoxia. Acta Anat. **62:** 476–488.
6. Yoffey, J. M. 1956. The mobilization and turnover times of cell populations in blood and blood-forming tissue. J. Histochem. Cytochem. **4:** 516–530.
7. Hudson, G., D. G. Osmond & P. J. Roylance. 1963. Cell populations in the bone marrow of the normal guinea pig. Acta Anat. **53:** 234–239.
8. Yoffey, J. M. 1966. Bone Marrow Reactions. Edward Arnold, London.
9. Bhuyan, R. K. 1964. A method for a permanent preparation of blood and bone-marrow reticulocytes. J. Anat. (Lond.) **98:** 300–301.
10. Hudson, G., N. C. W. Smith, R. S. Wilson & J. M. Yoffey. 1966. Eosinophil granulocytes and hypoxia. Nature. In press.
11. Yoffey, J. M., N. C. W. Smith & R. S. Wilson. 1966. Studies on hypoxia. IV. The differential haemopoietic response to moderate and severe hypoxia. Scand. J. Haematol. **3:** 186–192.
12. Gordon, A. S., J. LoBue, B. S. Dornfest & G. W. Cooper. 1962. Reticulocyte and leukocyte release from isolated perfused rat legs and femurs. Erythropoiesis. Jacobson, L. O. & Doyle, M. Eds. : 321. Grune & Stratton. N. Y.
13. Fruhman, G. & S. Fischer. 1962. The short-term effects of a single dose of erythropoietin in starved rats. Experientia **18:** 462–464.
14. Fisher, J. W., L. G. Lajtha, A. S. Buttoo & D. D. Porteous. 1965. Direct effects of erythropoietin on the bone marrow of the isolated perfused hind limb of rabbits. B. J. Haemat. **11:** 342–349.
15. Erslev, A. J. 1959. The effect of anemic anoxia on the cellular development of nucleated red cells. Blood **14:** 368–398.
16. Alpen, E. L. & D. Cranmore. 1959. Observations on the regulation of erythropoiesis and on cellular dynamics by ^{59}Fe autoradiography. *In* The Kinetics of Cellular Proliferation. F. Stohlman, Jr., Ed. : 290–300. Grune & Stratton. New York and London.
17. Lajtha, L. G. & R. Oliver. 1960. Studies on the kinetics of erythropoiesis: A model of the erythron. *In* Ciba Found. Symp. on "Haemopoiesis: Cell Production and its Regulation. G. E. W. Wolstenholme & M. O'Connor, Eds. : 289–314. J. & A. Churchill Ltd., London.
18. Jacobson, L. O., E. Goldwasser & C. W. Gurney. 1960. Transfusion-induced polycythaemic as a model for studying factors influencing erythropoiesis. *In* Ciba Found. Symp. on Haemopoiesis: Cell Production and its Regulation. G. E. W. Wolstenholme & M. O'Connor, Eds. : 423–445. J. & A. Churchill, London.
19. Suit, H. D., L. G. Lajtha, R. Oliver & F. Ellis. 1957. Studies on the ^{59}Fe Uptake by normoblasts and the failure of x-irradiation to affect uptake. Brit. J. Haemat. **3:** 165–174.
20. Stohlman, F. Jr. 1961. Humoral regulation of erythropoiesis. VI. Mechanism of action of erythropoietin in the irradiated animal. Proc. Soc. Exp. Biol. Med. **107:** 751–754.
21. Boycott, A. E. & C. L. Oakley. 1933. Regulation of marrow activity: experiments on blood transfusion and on the influence of atmospheres rich in oxygen. J. Path. Bact. **36:** 205–241.
22. Hudson, G. 1960. Volume and cellular constitution of bone marrow in guinea-pigs hypoxic from birth. Blood **16:** 1199–1204.
23. Mechanik, N. 1926. Untersuchungen über das Gewicht des Knochenmarkes des Menschen. Z. Anat. Entwicklungsgesch. **79:** 58–99.
24. Hudson, G. 1965. Bone-marrow volume in the human foetus and newborn. Brit. J. Haemat. **11:** 446–452.
25. Crosby, W. H. & J. H. Akeroyd. 1952. The limit of hemoglobin synthesis in hereditary hemolytic anemia. Am. J. Med. Sci. **13:** 273–283.
26. Dacie, J. V. & P. L. Mollison. 1943. Survival of normal erythrocytes after transfusion to patients with familial haemolytic anaemia. Lancet **i:** 550–552.

27. MOLLISON, P. L. 1947. Survival of transfused erythrocytes with special reference to cases of acquired haemolytic anaemia. Clin. Sci. **6:** 137–172.
28. HEDENSTEDT, S. 1947. Elliptocyte transfusions as a method in studies on blood destruction, blood volume and peritoneal resorption. Acta Chir. Scand. Suppl. **95:** 1–141.
29. RAMBACH, W. A., H. L. ALT & J. A. D. COOPER. 1957. The mode of action and nature of a heat stable plasma erythropoietic factor. Blood **12:** 1101–1113.
30. YOFFEY, J. M. & R. K. BHUYAN. 1964. Myeloid metaplasia in the cervical lymph gland of the normal guinea-pig. J. Anat. (Lond.) **98:** 681P.
31. YOFFEY, J. M., G. HUDSON & D. G. OSMOND. 1965. The lymphocyte in guinea-pig bone marrow. J. Anat. (Lond.) **99:** 841–860.
32. EVERETT, N. B., W. O. REINHARDT & J. M. YOFFEY. 1959. Unpublished data cited by Yoffey 1960b, p. 31.
33. YOFFEY, J. M. 1960b. The lymphomyeloid complex. *In* Ciba Found. Symp., Haemopoiesis: Cell Production and its Regulation, Wolstenholme & O'Connor, Eds. : 1–36. J. & A. Churchill. London.
34. OSMOND, D. G. & N. B. EVERETT. 1964. Radioautographic studies of bone marrow lymphocytes in vivo and in diffusion chamber cultures. Blood **23:** 1–17.
35. HARRIS, P. F., G. HAIG & J. H. KUGLER. 1963. Quantitative studies of mitoses and DNA-synthesizing cells in bone marrow and blood of guinea-pigs recovering from sublethal whole-body gamma irradiation. B. J. Haemat. **9:** 385–405.
36. BOND, V. P., L. E.. FEINENDEGEN, E. HEINZE & H. COTTIER. 1964. Distribution of transfused tritiated cytidine-labeled leukocytes and red cells in the bone marrow of normal and irradiated rats. Ann. N. Y. Acad. Sci. **113:** 1009–1019.
37. KEISER, G., H. COTTIER, N. ODARTCHENKO & V. P. BOND. 1964. Autoradiographic study on the origin and fate of small lymphoid cells in the dog bone marrow: effect of femoral artery clamping during in vivo availability of ^{3}H-thymidine. Blood **24:** 254–266.
38. CUDKOWICZ, G., A. C. UPTON, L. H. SMITH, D. G. GOSSLEE & W. L. HUGHES. 1964. An approach to the characterization of stem cells in mouse bone marrow. Ann. N. Y. Acad. Sci. **114:** 571–582.
39. CUDKOWICZ, G., M. BENNETT & G. M. SHEARER. 1964. Pluripotent stem cell function of the mouse marrow "lymphocyte." Science **144:** 866–868.
40. JONES, H. B., J. J. JONES & J. M. YOFFEY. 1967. Brit. . Haemat. In press.
41. HOLMES, W. F. & G. O. BROUN. 1932–1933. Clinical study of bone marrow by the method of sternal puncture. Proc. Soc. Exp. Biol. Med. **30:** 1306–1308.
42. RHOADS, C. P. & D. K. MILLER. 1938. Histology of the bone marrow in aplastic anemia. Arch. Path. **26:** 648–663.
43. BOMFORD, R. R. & C. P. RHOADS. 1941. Refractory anemia. I. Clinical and pathological aspects. Q. J. Med. **34:** 175–234.
44. DAVIDSON, L. S. P., L. J. DAVIS & J. INNES. 1943. Studies in refractory anaemia. I. The technique and interpretation of sternal puncture biopsies. Classification. Edinb. Med. J. **50:** 226–236.
45. BLACKBURN, E. K. 1947–8. Some observations of thiouracil neutropenia. J. Clin. Path. **1:** 295–300.
46. PISCIOTTA, A. V., A. S. SANTOS & C. KELLER. 1964. Studies on Agranulocytosis. V. Patterns of recovery from drug-induced bone marrow damage. J. Lab. Clin. Med. **63:** 445–458.
47. JORDAN, H. E. 1939. Aplastic anemia with special reference to the significance of the small lymphocytes. Arch. Path. **27:** 1–14.

SELECTIVE INHIBITION OF ERYTHROID CELL DIFFERENTIATION IN THE MOUSE BY LOW DOSES OF ACTINOMYCIN D*

Kurt R. Reissmann and Kenjiro Ito

Department of Medicine, University of Kansas Medical Center, Kansas City, Kan.

Actinomycin D has a selective cytotoxic effect on rapidly proliferating tissues. In doses approaching the LD_{50} (1200 μg/kg in mice) it is reported to cause depopulation of bone marrow, lymphoid organs and intestinal epithelium.[1] Its primary biochemical action, namely, inhibition of DNA-dependent RNA formation, is demonstrable in nonproliferating tissues as well and does not necessarily result in cell death. For instance, actinomycin has been shown to inhibit RNA and protein synthesis in normal liver without causing hepatocellular damage.[2] The drug has also been reported to inhibit reversibly the action of a number of hormones in their target tissues.[3] Hematologic effects of the drug have been studied from the viewpoint of cytotoxicity, and were reported to resemble those of ionizing radiation.[1] In our studies[4] small doses of actinomycin D† were given to mice in an attempt to dissociate its grossly destructive action from the inhibition of RNA synthesis so that the latter could be studied in regard to the development of hematopoietic cells. Daily s.c. injections of 60 μg/kg were found to be reasonably well tolerated over periods of several weeks and had the following sharply defined hematological effects (FIGURE 1): 1) cessation of erythropoiesis due to complete disappearance of erythroid marrow cells; 2) absence of demonstrable inhibition of myelo-, megakaryo-, and lymphopoiesis; 3) absolute refractoriness to erythropoietic effects of erythropoietin; and 4) reappearance of erythroid cells within 36 hr after discontinuation of the drug.

It is now widely accepted[5-7] that erythropoiesis entails a continuous flow of cells from an undifferentiated stem-cell pool towards the reticulocyte stage, and sufficient evidence has accumulated to indicate that the first step in red cell development, namely, transformation of stem cells into pronormoblasts, is induced and regulated by erythropoietin. The pronormoblasts undergo a number of successive divisions; after each division both daughter cells progress into the next maturation stage. The latter differs from the preceding stage by a smaller nuclear mass and a greater hemoglobin concentration. The proliferating stages of erythroid as well as of myeloid development are known to be sensitive against a variety of myelotoxic agents,[5] but it appeared doubtful to us that the observed selectivity of actinomycin could be attributed to differences in the rate of proliferation between erythroid and myeloid cells. Moreover, the complete absence of erythroid cells suggested a block in cell development at a stage preceding the proliferating erythroid cells. Experiments were therefore carried out to obtain more detailed information on the inhibitory action of the drug on the three principal cell stages of erythroid development, namely, 1) undifferentiated stem cells; 2) dividing erythroblasts (pronormoblasts, early normoblasts); and 3) nondividing, maturing cells (late normoblasts, reticulocytes).

The action of actinomycin on cells of classes 2 and 3 (above) was studied in mice made polycythemic by i.p. injection of isologous red cells. The hypertransfusion resulted in the well-known disappearance of erythroid marrow elements, and the mice then received a single i.v. injection of erythropoietin in order to

* Supported by UPHS grant AM 07239–03.

† Actinomycin D was kindly supplied by Dr. H. Brown of Merck, Sharp and Dohme.

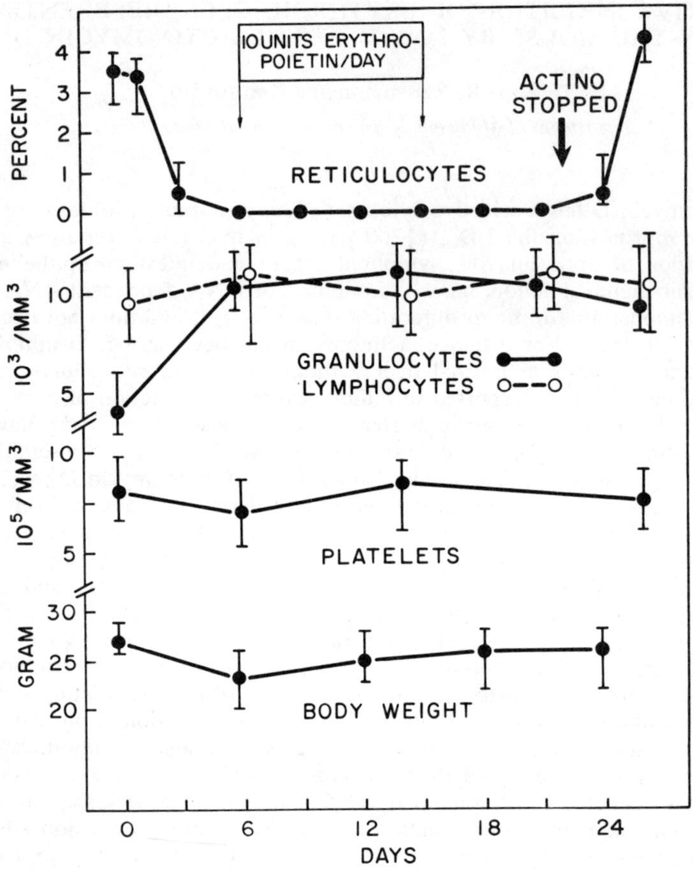

FIGURE 1. Hematologic effects of daily s.c. injections of 60 μg/kg actinomycin D in mice. (Mean and range, six mice).

induce the formation of one finite crop of pronormoblasts. These progressed during the following days as a cohort through the various stages of erythroid development as seen in TABLE 1. After 36 hr, for instance, most of the cells had reached the early normoblast stage, and after 72 hr they had progressed to the reticulocyte stage and were ready for release into the blood. The number of new red cells that were formed during this induced wave of erythropoiesis was assessed by blood reticulocyte counts (four days after erythropoietin) and by measurements of red cell ^{59}Fe incorporation (^{59}Fe was injected two days after erythropoietin, and counted in red cells 48 hr later). One group of mice received erythropoietin alone, the other five groups also received one i.v. injection of 120 μg/kg actinomycin D at a time after erythropoietin as indicated in TABLE 1. Actinomycin D has been shown to act rapidly in mammalian cells[2] and if the rapid entrance holds for erythroid cells, measurements of reticulocytes and ^{59}Fe incorporation in the drug-injected groups should provide information on its inhibitory effects upon the cell type which was predominantly present in the marrow at the time of drug injection. Injection of the drug at 36 and 48 hr had

TABLE 1

EFFECT OF ACTINOMYCIN D (120 μG I.V.) ON VARIOUS MATURATION STAGES OF A COHORT OF ERYTHROID CELLS INDUCED IN POLYCYTHEMIC MICE BY SINGLE I.V. INJECTION OF ERYTHROPOIETIN (E)

Actinomycin Injected Hrs after E	Erythroid Marrow* at Time of Actino. Injection			Effective Red Cell Formation**	
	PN	EN	LN	% ^{59}Fe Inc.	% Retic.
1	0	0	0	0.2 ± .1	0 ±0
16	3	0	0	3.0 ± 1.3	.4 ± .1
24	32	18	3	6.3 ± 0.9	.7 ± .1
36	22	58	34	14.0 ± 1.1	1.2 ± .2
48	18	69	114	14.2 ± 0.8	1.3 ± .1
No Actino.				14.9 ± 1.4	1.4 ± .2

* Per 1000 cells, PN = pronormoblasts, EN = early normoblasts, LN = late normoblasts.
** Mean and SEM, four mice.

no effect (TABLE 1), indicating that the early and late normoblasts developed normally into reticulocytes. Injection of actinomycin one hour after erythropoietin prevented the appearance of any erythroid cells, and red cell formation remained zero. Injection at 16 and 24 hr after erythropoietin markedly reduced the effective red cell formation. This is attributed in part to a decrease in differentiation of stem cells into pronormoblasts. This process continues after a single injection of erythropoietin for as long as 48 hr[8] and was undoubtedly curtailed by the injection of actinomycin at 16 and 24 hours. The rate of erythropoiesis is known to depend in first order on the rate of stem-cell differentiation. It is not possible, however, to quantitate the curtailment of the latter with regard to the observed depression of red cell formation, and an inhibitory effect of the drug on the proliferation of pronormoblasts can therefore not be excluded. Such an inhibition, however, can hardly account for the total absence of erythroid cells in the group of mice which received the drug one hour after the erythropoietin injection.

The depression of erythroid proliferation may thus contribute to the absence of erythroid elements, but the main site of inhibition must be sought in an earlier cell stage, namely, the stem cells. Their failure to develop into pronormoblasts could be due to one of two processes: 1) the drug rapidly killed stem cells and thus critically reduced the number of integer stem cells available for differentiation; or 2) it actually inhibited the process of differentiation in the stem cells. The former mechanism is generally regarded as the cause of the delay in repopulation of the marrow after large doses of ionizing radiation. In Rosenthal's experiments[9] total body irradiation of rats with 700 r caused absence of erythroid cells from the marrow during the first through tenth postirradiation day. Myeloid cells and megakaryocytes disappeared somewhat later (fourth to seventh days) but showed a similar delay in their reappearance. This delay in recovery confirms theoretical computations on stem-cell kinetics carried out by Lajtha[10] and by Kretchmar.[11] Discontinuation of the actinomycin injections in our experiments resulted in the appearance of pronormoblasts on the second day after the last injection. According to present concepts of marrow kinetics,[10] such a rapid recovery excludes a critical reduction of stem-cell number as the cause of erythroid eradication. This conclusion was further supported by the absence of cumulative effects of the drug on stem-cell response as tested by the method of Gurney *et al.*[12] One group of mice received daily injections of 60 μg/kg actinomycin from the first through 21st days, the other, one injection only on the 21st day. All animals were hypertransfused on the 17th and 18th days and were then divided into six

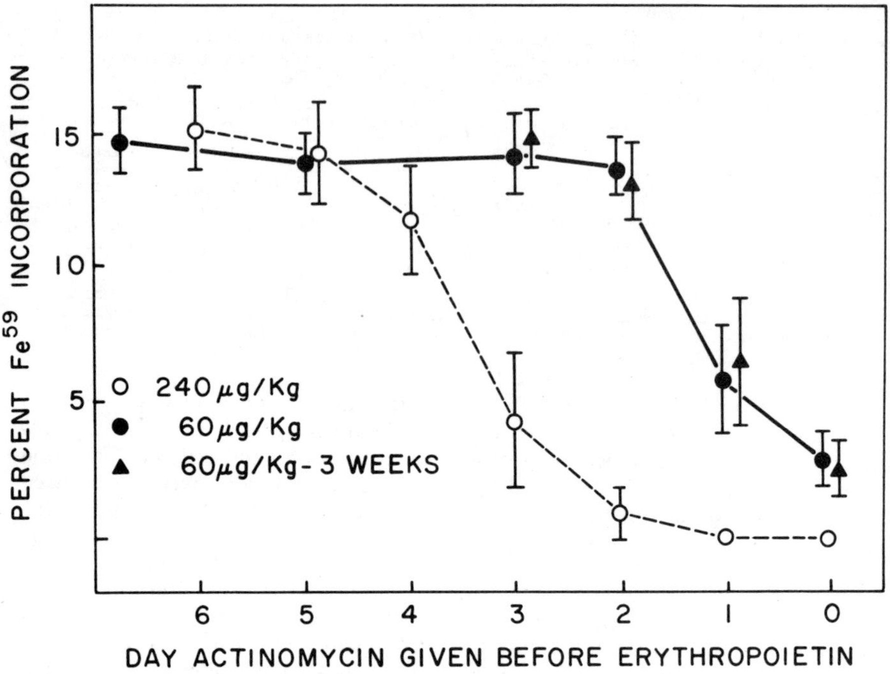

FIGURE 2. Stem-cell response in polycythemic mice after single i.v. injection of actinomycin D. Group represented by ▲ – ▲ was pretreated with 21 daily injections of 60 μg/kg. (Five mice each group, mean and SEM.)

subgroups. Each subgroup received one single injection of erythropoietin on days 0, 1, 2, 3, 4, and 5 after the last actinomycin injection, respectively. The stem-cell response, assessed by red cell ^{59}Fe incorporation (FIGURE 2) was nearly the same in the chronic and the single actinomycin injection groups, indicating that its repeated injection had not resulted in a progressive depletion of the stem-cell system.

Since stem-cell depletion or cytotoxic damage in pronormoblasts and succeeding stages cannot account for the total absence of erythroid cells, it is concluded that actinomycin inhibits the intermediate step, namely, the differentiation of stem cells into pronormoblasts. This process is normally induced by erythropoietin, and its inhibition by actinomycin is of interest with regard to the mode of action of erythropoietin in stem-cell differentiation. The stem cell has no specific functions nor can it be identified on the basis of morphological characteristics. Erythropoietin transforms this cell within 18 hr into an early pronormoblast.[8] The latter is easily recognized microscopically and its functional differentiation is strikingly demonstrated by its newly gained ability to synthesize hemoglobin. It is reasonable to assume that the genetic information relevant to protein formation in erythroid cells was repressed as long as the cell was a stem cell. With some justification erythropoietin is therefore thought to effect a derepression, and as the result the relevant genetic information is transcribed into RNA templates, thus initiating the synthesis of new proteins. There is no evidence available that erythropoietin acts as a derepressor, but our experiments indicate that the transformation of stem cells into erythroblasts depends on RNA synthesis which is highly sensitive to actinomycin inhibition. As long as this RNA synthesis was blocked, erythropoietin was completely ineffective, but the stem cell quickly regained its responsiveness to erythropoietin when drug administration was stopped. No indication of a significant depopulation of the stem-cell compartment was noted during chronic administration of the drug. If this finding can be further substantiated, it would provide additional evidence of a dissociation of actinomycin effects on mandatory versus optional programs of cellular protein synthesis.[13] Since the drug exerted its effects in the stem cell without damaging it, one must assume that it did not interfere with enzyme synthesis essential for the life of the cell. Differentiation into an erythroblast is, in contrast, an optional program and normally may never occur in a considerable percentage of the stem-cell population. It requires, in all probability, formation of a set of new RNA templates, and if this is prevented, the optional program simply does not proceed and the inducer, erythropoietin, remains ineffective.

References

1. Philips, F. S., H. S. Schwartz, S. S. Sternberg & C. T. C. Tan. 1960. The toxicity of actinomycin D. Ann. N. Y. Acad. Sci. **89:** 348.
2. Schwartz, H. S., J. E. Sodergran, M. Garofalo & S. S. Sternberg. 1965. Actinomycin D effects on nucleic acid and protein metabolism in intact and regenerating liver of rats. Cancer Res. **25:** 307.
3. Samuels, L. D. 1964. Actinomycin and its effects. New Eng. J. Med. **271:** 1252.
4. Reissmann, K. R. & Kenjiro Ito. 1966. Selective eradication of erythropoiesis by actinomycin D as the result of interference with hormonally controlled effector pathway of cell differentiation. Blood **28:** 201.
5. Lajtha, L. G. 1961. The effect of ionizing radiations and tumor-chemotherapeutic agents on the bone marrow. Progr. Biophys. **11:** 79.
6. Cronkite, E. P. 1964. Enigmas underlying study of hematopoietic cell proliferation. Fed. Proc. **23:** 649.
7. Stohlman, F. 1962. Erythropoiesis. New Eng. J. Med. **267:** 392.
8. Ito, K., J. W. Schmaus & K. R. Reissmann. 1964. Protein metabolism and erythropoiesis. III. The erythroid marrow in protein-starved rats and its response to erythropoietin. Acta Haemat. **32:** 257.
9. Rosenthal, R. L., B. I. Pickering & L. Goldschmidt. 1951. A semiquantitative study of bone marrow in rats following total body x-irradiation. Blood **6:** 600.
10. Lajtha, L. G., R. Oliver & C. W. Gurney. 1962. Kinetic model of a bone-marrow stem-cell population. Brit. J. Haemat. **8:** 442.
11. Kretchmar, A. L. 1966. Erythropoietin: Hypothesis of action tested by analog computer. Science **152:** 367.
12. Gurney, C. W., L. G. Lajtha & R. Oliver. 1962. A method for investigation of stem-cell kinetics. Brit. J. Haemat. **8:** 461.
13. Davidson, E. H., V. G. Allfrey & A. E. Mirsky. 1963. Gene expression in differentiated cells. Proc. Nat. Acad. Sci. **49:** 53.

ULTRASTRUCTURAL AND AUTORADIOGRAPHIC STUDIES OF ERYTHROPOIETIN-INDUCED RED CELL PRODUCTION*

Donald Orlic**, Albert S. Gordon and Johannes A. G. Rhodin

Department of Biology, Graduate School of Arts and Science, New York University, New York, N. Y. and Department of Anatomy, New York Medical College, New York, N. Y.

INTRODUCTION

Many aspects of hematopoiesis remain unclear, such as the chemical and structural nature of events that initiate the process of blood cell maturation. A better understanding of these early events would provide a new basis for explaining how formed elements of the blood emerge to replace aging cells and might clarify one widely held theory, i.e. the derivation of mature elements from "totipotent" stem cells. To this end, several problems of blood cell origin are dealt with in this study. The most important considerations constitute an effort to characterize the initial features of erythropoietin-induced red cell maturation.

There is little definitive information on the mode of erythropoietin action. Some investigations point to the late stages of erythroid maturation as those responsive to erythropoietin (Borsook *et al.,* 1962; Gallagher *et al.,* 1963); others to a "primitive" precursor cell as the target element (Alpen & Cranmore, 1959; Erslev, 1964). Similarly, there is considerable disagreement concerning the characteristics of the molecular changes that occur in cells during their response to this factor. Literature can be cited to support the idea that erythropoietin enhances the rate of hemoglobin synthesis (Stohlman *et al.,* 1963), that it leads to a shorter maturation period (Brecher & Stohlman, 1962), or that it initiates the process of erythroid cell differentiation (Kurtides *et al.,* 1963; Krantz & Goldwasser, 1965).

In adult mice splenic red cell production can be altered by changing the environmental or humoral conditions, e.g. lowered oxygen tensions being countered by increased erythropoiesis (Brecher & Stohlman, 1959). Conversely, when the hypoxic stimulus is removed, polycythemic mice show a markedly inhibited erythropoietic activity. In this state virtually no definitive nucleated erythroid elements are seen in the spleens. At this time such spleens are sensitive to exogenous erythropoietin and respond to a single injection by producing a cohort of erythroid elements that undergo a synchronized process of maturation. Histological preparations of splenic tissue reveal the presence of proerythroblasts 24 hr after activation, and erythroblasts at 48 hours. Peak peripheral reticulocytosis occurs between 72–96 hr, after which the erythroid wave subsides (Filmanowicz & Gurney, 1961).

The present study, undertaken to identify the morphological and chemical bases of erythropoietin-induced activity, extends our earlier autoradiographic findings (Orlic *et al.,* 1965a), which for the first time, indicated that the stem cell response to erythropoietin involves an almost immediate or simultaneous incorporation of ^{3}H-thymidine. In addition, this work provides information on the molecular and ultrastructural changes that occur during the early hours of response, as well as later stages when erythropoietin-activated transitional cells are replaced by more mature red cell elements. Identification of erythropoietin-sensitive stem cells is

* Supported by Grant 5–R01–HE03357–09 from the National Heart Institute of the National Institutes of Health, U.S.P.H.S.

** Work done during the tenure of N.I.H. fellowships (1–F1–GM–22,446–01A1 and 1–F2–HE–22,446–01).

made by autoradiographic determination of ^{3}H-thymidine and ^{3}H-uridine incorporation within minutes after an injection of erythropoietin. When observed in the cells, these nucleic acid precursors suggest the type of macromolecular synthesis that is occurring at a given time in response to the action of erythropoietin.

Materials and Methods

Adult mice of the CF-1 strain were used throughout this work. Discontinuous exposure to 0.4 atm for 200 hr during a three-week period was adequate to elevate the hematocrit to 55 percent or higher. At the onset of erythropoietic depression, three to four days following removal from the decompression chamber (Weintraub *et al.*, 1963), each polycythemic mouse received an i.v. injection of 6 units of erythropoietin† at time zero. This was followed one to two min later by a single i.v. injection of 125 μc of ^{3}H-thymidine.‡ Spleens were fixed 72 hr later. A second group of mice received erythropoietin and 30 min later, a single injection of 25 μc of ^{3}H-thymidine; spleens were fixed at 1, 2, 6 and 12 hr after erythropoietin. Other animals received 50 μc of ^{3}H-thymidine i.v., 30 min after stimulation by erythropoietin and were sacrificed at 15, 24, 48 and 72 hours. These larger doses of ^{3}H-thymidine were given to animals sacrificed at 15–72 hr after treatment in order to prevent dilution of label by cell divisions to levels too insignificant to detect.

Erythropoietically depressed control polycythemic mice were given an injection of saline followed 30 min later by 50 μc of ^{3}H-thymidine. These animals were sacrificed at one and 24 hr after saline administration and their spleens examined for labeled cells.

In another study in polycythemic mice a single i.v. injection of 125 μc of ^{3}H-uridine§ was given at 0.5, 1.5, 3.5 and 5.5 hr after erythropoietin administration. Spleens in all except two animals were fixed 30 min after ^{3}H-uridine. The spleens from the two mice that received this label at 5.5 hr were taken at 24 and 48 hr after administration of erythropoietin to test for continued presence of early incorporated ^{3}H-uridine in erythroblasts and reticulocytes.

Some spleens were fixed in 2–3 percent glutaraldehyde followed by 1 percent osmic acid (OsO_4) adjusted to pH 7.4, others only in OsO_4, but all were dehydrated in a graded series of alcohol and propylene oxide solutions and embedded in Epon 812 (Luft, 1961). Sections were prepared for light and electron microscopy by the following method. A selected area of embedded tissue was trimmed to a size just larger than one opening in a 75-mesh grid used in electron microscopy. From this area using an LKB Ultrotome, a series of single, alternate thick and thin sections was prepared. Each thick section was placed onto a glass slide and coated with Ilford K5 photographic emulsion. Thin sections were picked up on 75-mesh grids, one per grid.

Five g of Ilford K5 emulsion were diluted in 40 ml of distilled water at 45° C for 15 min (Revel & Hay, 1961). Thick sections were dipped into this solution under conditions of total darkness, dried and placed into a light-tight box provided with desiccant to reduce "background" effects. The boxes containing these slides were sealed with electrical tape and kept at 4° C for 21 days to three months. After exposure, all autoradiograms were developed in D-19 for two to five min, washed in distilled water, fixed for five min in Kodak acid fix and rinsed.

† Step IV sheep plasma erythropoietin (Armour and Co., lot K–103–124). Preparation supplied by the National Heart Institute of the National Institutes of Health, U.S.P.H.S.

‡ Sp. Act. 1.9 c/mM; Schwartz, BioResearch, Inc.

§ Sp. Act. 7.7 c/mM; New England Nuclear Corp.

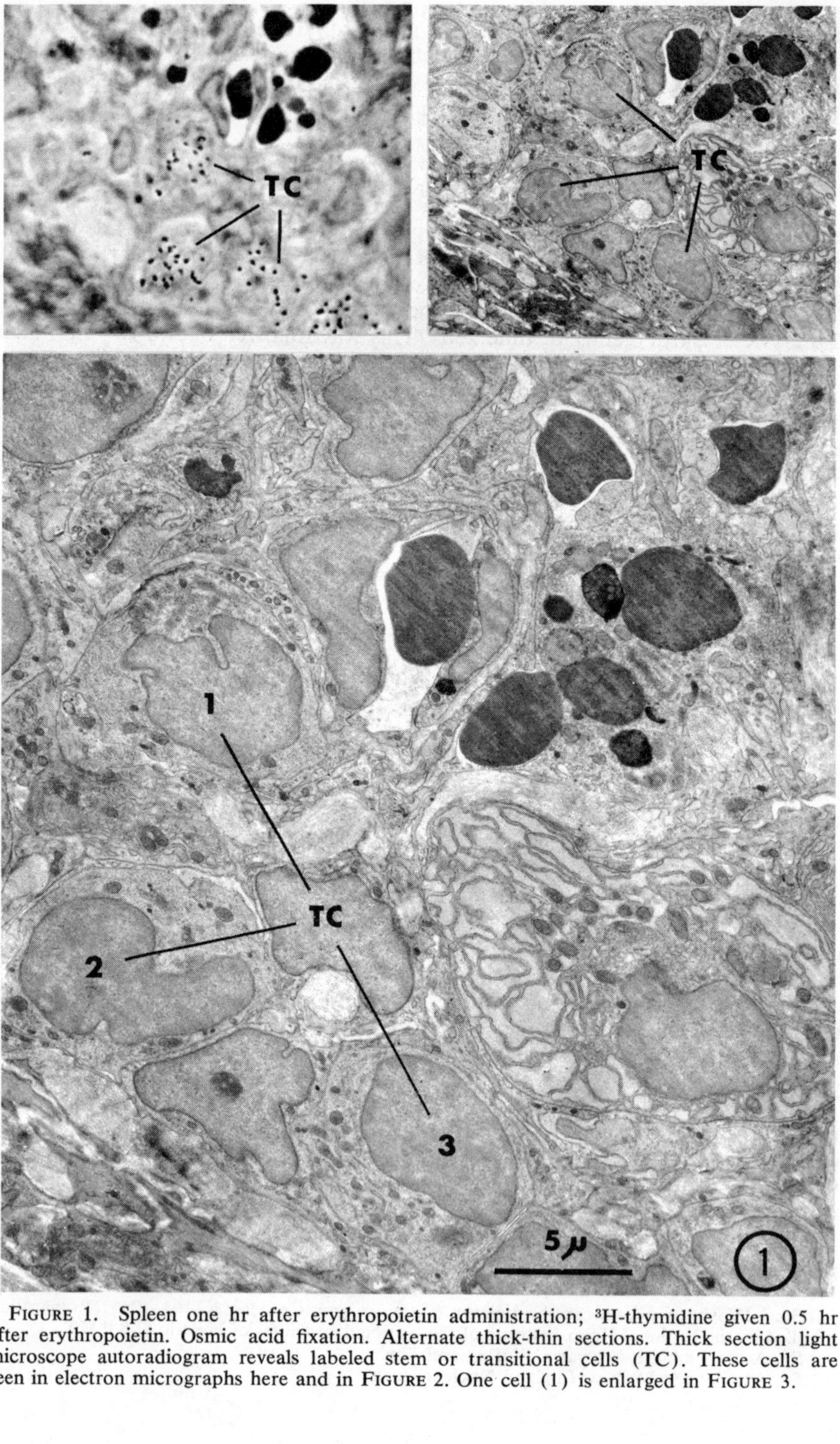

FIGURE 1. Spleen one hr after erythropoietin administration; ^{3}H-thymidine given 0.5 hr after erythropoietin. Osmic acid fixation. Alternate thick-thin sections. Thick section light microscope autoradiogram reveals labeled stem or transitional cells (TC). These cells are seen in electron micrographs here and in FIGURE 2. One cell (1) is enlarged in FIGURE 3.

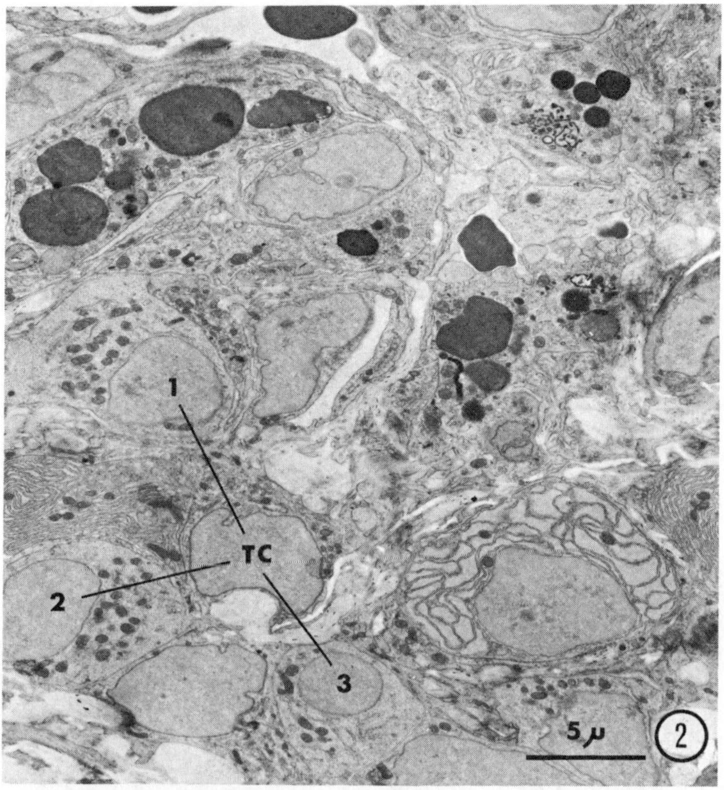

FIGURE 2. Electron micrograph of a thin section through a different level of labeled stem or transitional cells (TC) seen in FIGURE 1. One cell (1) is enlarged in FIGURE 4.

When dry, the sections were stained with toluidine blue and examined by light microscopy. Labeled cells were photographed.

The fogging problem of thin section autoradiography was, of course, not encountered in the alternate thick-thin section preparations because only the thick sections for light microscopy were coated with emulsion. The thick-section autoradiograms indicated which cells were labeled with ^{3}H-thymidine or ^{3}H-uridine; these cells were then found and photographed in alternate thin sections prepared for electron micoscopy. This task of finding the same cell was greatly simplified by one feature of the technique, that is, approximately 75 percent of the total surface area of the thin section fell within the area of one opening in the electron microscopic grid, provided the section was properly picked up, thus making orientation a relatively simple matter. Once located in the electron microscope, these cells could be readily taken to high magnifications for purposes of resolving fine structural detail.

RESULTS

Erythropoietin-sensitive cells, referred to as "stem cells," respond to erythropoietin by incorporating nucleic acid precursors, ^{3}H-thymidine and ^{3}H-uridine. At 12–24 hr and 48–72 hr of maturation these cells develop respectively into proerythroblasts and erythroblasts that show at least a portion of the original label.

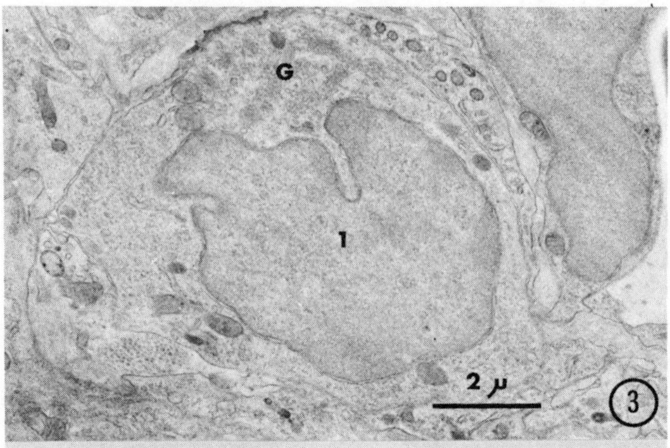

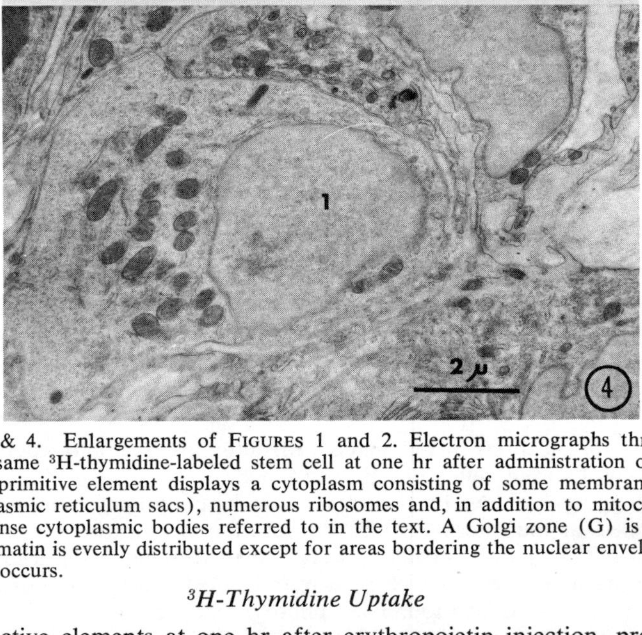

FIGURES 3 & 4. Enlargements of FIGURES 1 and 2. Electron micrographs through two levels of the same ^{3}H-thymidine-labeled stem cell at one hr after administration of erythropoietin. This primitive element displays a cytoplasm consisting of some membranous structures (endoplasmic reticulum sacs), numerous ribosomes and, in addition to mitochondria, a number of dense cytoplasmic bodies referred to in the text. A Golgi zone (G) is seen. The granular chromatin is evenly distributed except for areas bordering the nuclear envelope where some packing occurs.

^{3}H-Thymidine Uptake

Several active elements at one hr after erythropoietin injection, presumably erythropoietin-activated stem cells, are shown in FIGURES 1–4. Their nuclei occasionally reveal an irregular configuration with deep indentations like those seen in "stem cells" of another erythropoietic system (Zamboni, 1965). Small chromatin clumps at the nuclear margins interrupt an otherwise even distribution of chromatin in some stem cells. In others a higher degree of clumping is seen. The cytoplasm contains numerous ribosomes, a moderate number of mitochondria and a Golgi apparatus. Endoplasmic reticulum is sparse when present, as in later developmental stages.

Dense, sometimes homogeneous, bodies are found in the cytoplasm of these cells. They are enclosed by a single or double membrane and some contain one or more small, very dense inclusions. These bodies possibly correspond to the

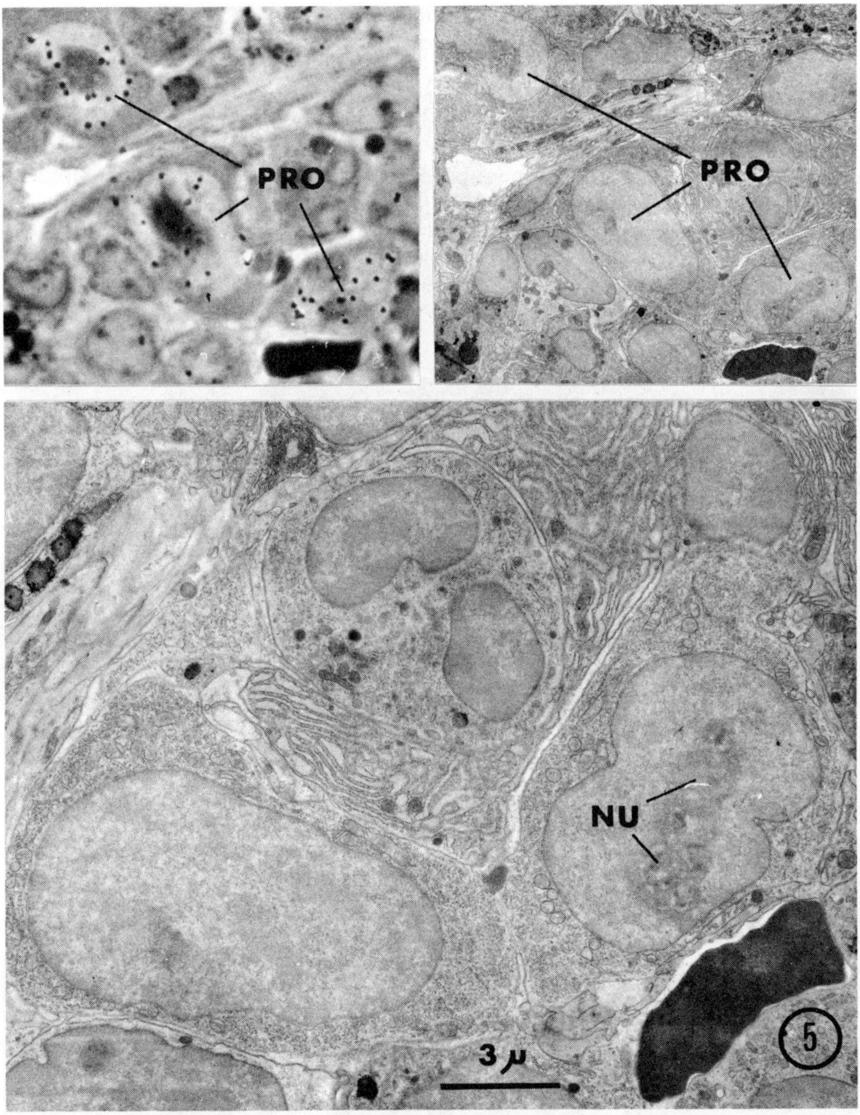

FIGURE 5. Spleen 12 hr after erythropoietin administration; ^{3}H-thymidine given 0.5 hr after erythropoietin. Osmic acid fixation. Alternate thick-thin sections. In the thick section light microscope autoradiogram, three labeled proerythroblasts (PRO) are indicated. Two are located adjacent to each other. This "pairing" suggests a cell division within 12 hr after erythropoietin activation. Nucleoli (Nu) at this time are large and numerous ribosomes and mitochondria characterize the cytoplasm.

microbodies thought to be precursor material for mitochondria in avian proerythroblasts (Benedetti & Leplus, 1958) or to lipid bodies that occur in immature blood elements of the hemopoietic islands of guinea pig yolk sac (Sorenson, 1961).

Stem cells undergo maturation and in spleens taken at 12 hr after erythropoietin activation, become morphologically distinct proerythroblasts (FIGURE 5). The latter frequently are ovoid in shape and display larger nucleoli which persist throughout proerythroblast maturation, i.e., more than 24 hours.

At six hr and more frequently, at 12 and 15 hr after erythropoietin (FIGURE 5), pairs of adjacent proerythroblasts are noted and both nuclei are labeled. This finding differs from that at one hr after activation: at this time erythropoietin-activated stem cells generally do not border one another. With continued maturation of proerythroblasts, spleens at 24 hr after erythropoietin treatment often show larger proerythroblast nests, composed of four or more cells.

A striking change occurs at 48 hr after erythropoietin is administered to polycythemic mice. Previously formed small foci of erythrogenic elements are replaced

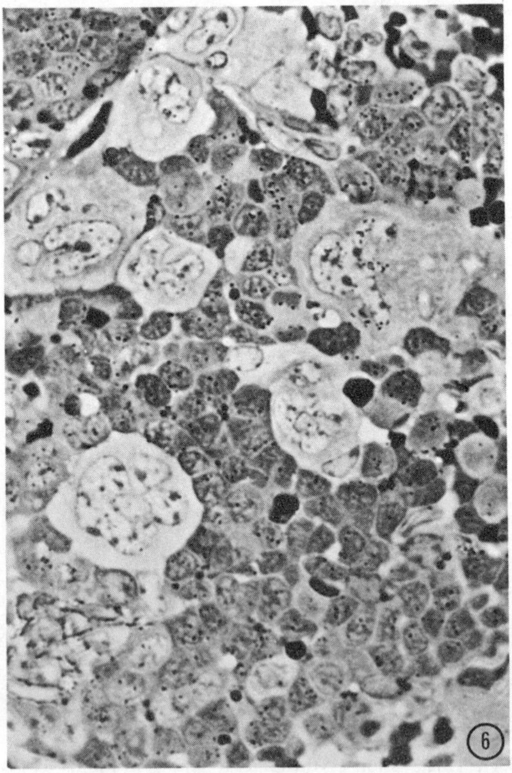

FIGURE 6. Spleen 48 hr after erythropoietin administration; ^{3}H-thymidine given 0.5 hr after erythropoietin. This light microscope autoradiogram shows closely packed erythroblasts and several megakaryocytoblasts. The number of silver grains per erythroblast is lower than the total found over proerythroblasts even though this autoradiogram was exposed four times longer and the animal given a two-fold greater dose of ^{3}H-thymidine. × 390.

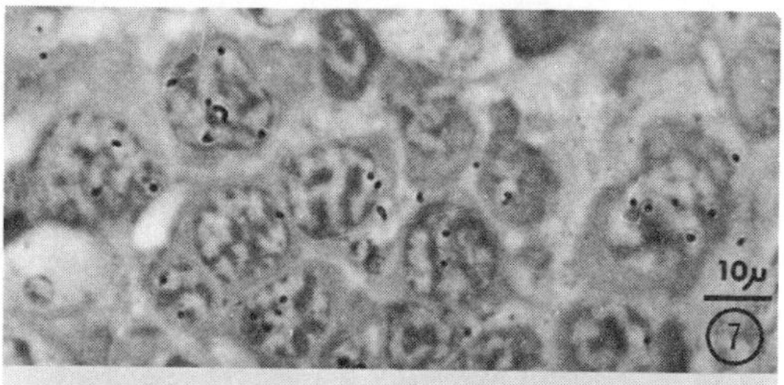

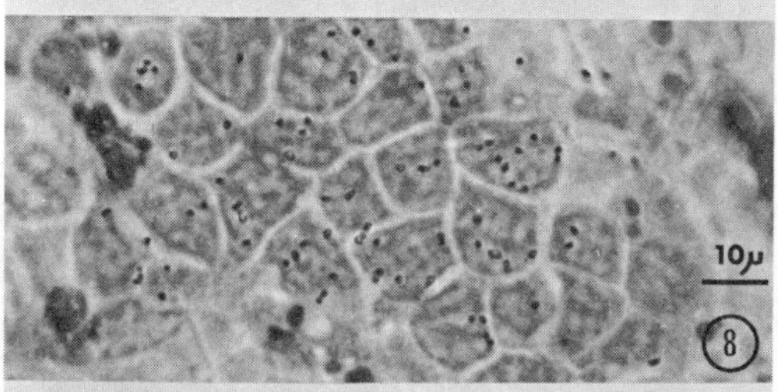

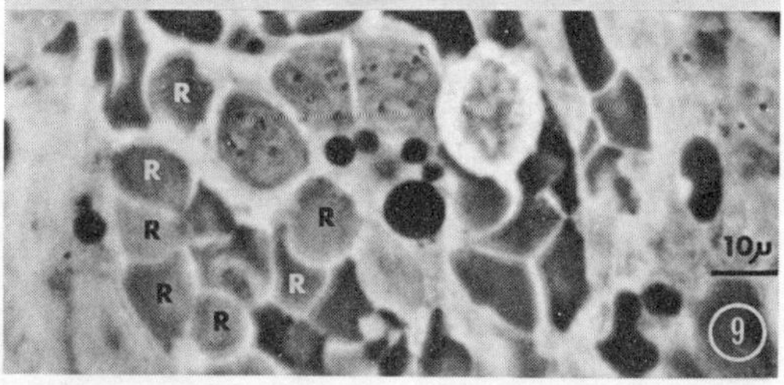

FIGURE 7. Same specimen as FIGURE 6. Nest of labeled erythroblasts seen in a light microscope autoradiogram.

FIGURE 8. ^{3}H-thymidine given one to two min after erythropoietin; spleen fixed 72 hr later. Nest of labeled erythroblasts.

FIGURE 9. Same specimen as FIGURE 8. Nest of erythroid elements composed of reticulocytes (R) and three labeled erythroblasts.

by large clusters of cells that occupy much of the area of splenic red pulp (FIGURE 6). Sections through erythroblast nests reveal as many as 18–36 closely packed cells (FIGURE 7) and although nearly every cell is labeled, they all show no more than 2–8 grains per cell. This degree of labeling is low but considerably higher than can be accounted for by background. Erythroid cell nests are still found at 72 hr after erythropoietin (FIGURE 8) and they are often composed mainly of reticulocytes (FIGURE 9).

^{3}H-Uridine Uptake

Another aspect of the present work is concerned with the initiation and duration of RNA synthesis in erythropoietin-activated stem cells. These features are revealed by erythropoietin-induced ^{3}H-uridine incorporation at increasing time intervals after an injection of erythropoietin. Thirty minutes after administration of ^{3}H-uridine, all spleens contain labeled stem cells or proerythroblasts.

The ^{3}H-uridine-labeled erythroid cells at one, two, four and six hr after erythropoietin administration are in many respects morphologically similar. Autoradiograms show ^{3}H-uridine label throughout the nuclear material in all prepara-

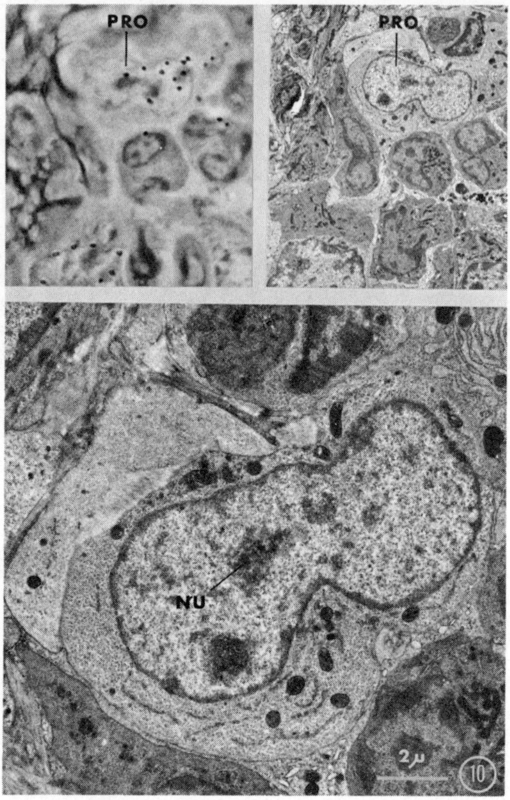

FIGURE 10. Spleen two hr after erythropoietin administration; ^{3}H-uridine given 1.5 hr after erythropoietin. Glutaraldehyde and osmic acid fixation. Alternate thick-thin sections. At higher magnification, nucleolar material (Nu) of the young proerythroblast (PRO) is resolved.

tions from one to six hr after erythropoietin administration (FIGURES 10–12). Erythropoietin-activated cells incorporating label at one to two hr possess a relatively smaller nucleolus than erythroid cells at four to six hours.

To ascertain that these early labeled cells are indeed erythroid elements requires that the period of time after labeling be extended to allow for further maturation. This depends, of course, on whether the macromolecules with incorporated ^{3}H-uridine are stable entities. Rather arbitrarily, since it is not firmly established when proerythroblast RNA synthesis for later hemoglobin production occurs, 5.5 hr after activation was selected as the time for labeling cells that would mature in 24 and 48 hours.

The ^{3}H-uridine incorporated 5.5 hr after erythropoietin stimulation is found in proerythroblasts at 24 hours. These cells, which sometimes form small erythrogenic nests, show very large nucleoli and much of the earlier incorporated ^{3}H-uridine is within the nucleus.

Several stages of erythroblast maturation are encountered 48 hr after erythropoietin activation of stem cells, and erythroblast nests at this time indicate the

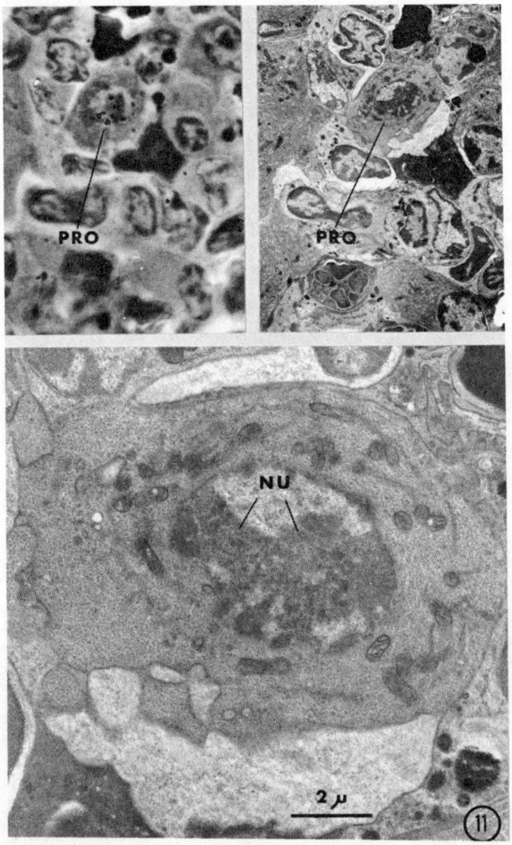

FIGURE 11. Spleen four hr after erythropoietin administration; ^{3}H-uridine given 3.5 hr after erythropoietin. Glutaraldehyde and osmic acid fixation. Alternate thick-thin sections through a proerythroblast (PRO). Silver grains lie over dense nuclear material resolved in thin section electron micrographs as the nucleolus (Nu).

continued presence of ^{3}H-uridine taken up by red cell elements 5.5 hr after activation (FIGURE 13). Both late erythroblasts and reticulocytes are labeled and in the former many grains fall over nuclei.

Nonerythroid Cell Activity

Incorporation of ^{3}H-thymidine and ^{3}H-uridine by granulocytic elements and megakaryocytoblasts occurs in both erythropoietin-treated animals and saline-injected controls. In the former numerous ^{3}H-uridine-labeled metamyelocytes are found in spleens at one to six and 24 hr after treatment. This cell type in ^{3}H-thymidine studies is labeled when observed in 24- and 48-hour specimens and at 48 hr a number of the earlier metamyelocytes are replaced by well-defined granulocytes. Tritiated-thymidine labeling occurs in megakaryocytoblasts of all preparations.

Granulocytopoiesis occurs in nests composed of cells at the same stage of maturation (FIGURE 14), and this feature is maintained throughout maturation.

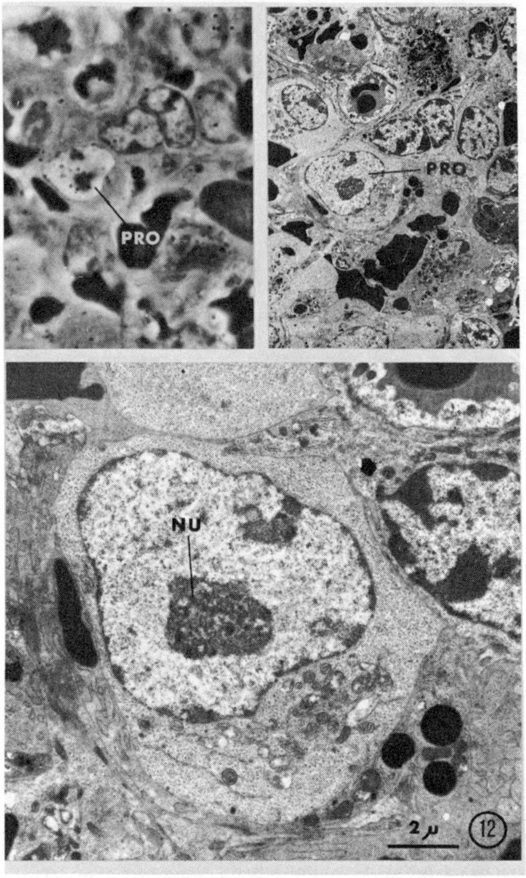

FIGURE 12. Spleen six hr after erythropoietin administration; ^{3}H-uridine given 5.5 hr after erythropoietin. Glutaraldehyde and osmic acid fixation. A labeled proerythroplast (PRO), in thick-thin sections, displays a well defined nucleolus (Nu). Mitochondria are clustered at one pole of the cell.

However, synchronous formation is not the pattern in megakaryocytopoietic nests (FIGURE 15). In addition, unlike granulocytic maturation in which all cells of a given nest are or are not labeled, a megakaryocytoblastic nest shows both labeled and unlabeled cells.

The formation of ^{3}H-thymidine-labeled granulocytic elements and continued presence of labeled megakaryocytoblasts at 48 hr after administration of erythropoietin indicates that some immature cells incorporating ^{3}H-thymidine at one hr are not erythropoietin-activated elements. Furthermore, this suggests that all formed elements are derived from a highly similar or identical cytologic compartment.

Some labeled stem cells are seen in control polycythemic mice at one hour. This finding is disturbing, particularly because the autoradiographic technique used here does not lend itself to quantitative work at the cellular level. However,

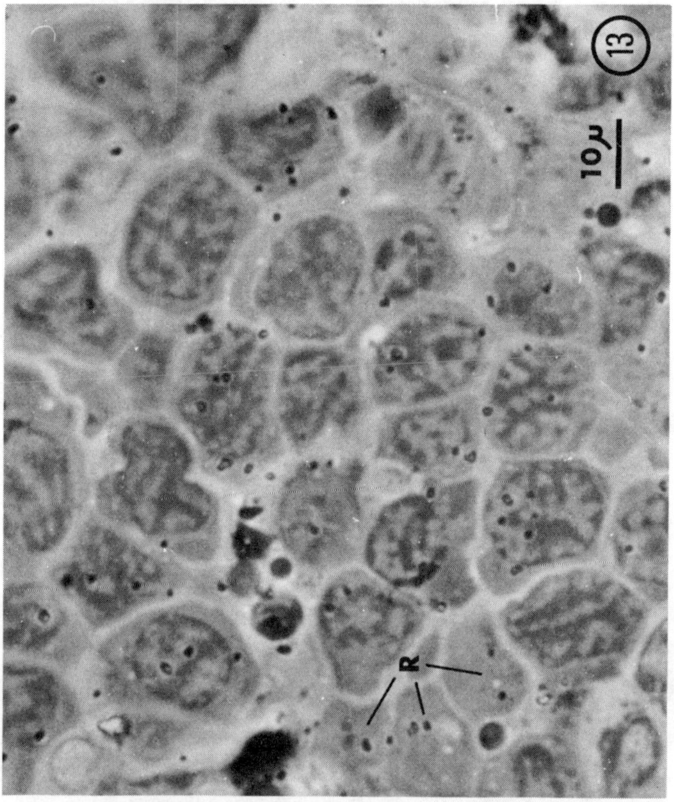

FIGURE 13. Spleen 48 hr after erythropoietin administration; ^{3}H-uridine given 5.5 hr after erythropoietin. Light microscope autoradiogram of a nest of erythroid elements. Most cells of this nest are erythroblasts. Several reticulocytes (R) are seen; each is labeled with ^{3}H-uridine originally incorporated by proerythroblasts.

a recent observation in our laboratory may lead to a clarification of the functional role of labeled stem cells in control animals. When ^{3}H-thymidine is injected 30 min before erythropoietin, simultaneously, or 30 min after the hormone, more than 85 percent of the erythroblasts that emerge 48 hr later are labeled. The percentage of labeled erythroblasts drops to less than one-half this total if the isotope is given three or five hr before or after erythropoietin. According to this, cycling stem cells in S-phase are sensitive to erythropoietin and so at least a portion of the stem cells that incorporate ^{3}H-thymidine in controls would respond to the hormone if it were available.

DISCUSSION

One aspect of this paper deals with a morphological description of hemic cells sensitive to erythropoietin. On the basis of indirect evidence, obtained by autoradiography, erythropoietin-sensitive stem cells are identified as primitive hemopoietic elements found in splenic red pulp. The ultrastructural features of these cells differ from those of elements belonging to erythrocytic and granulocytic lines.

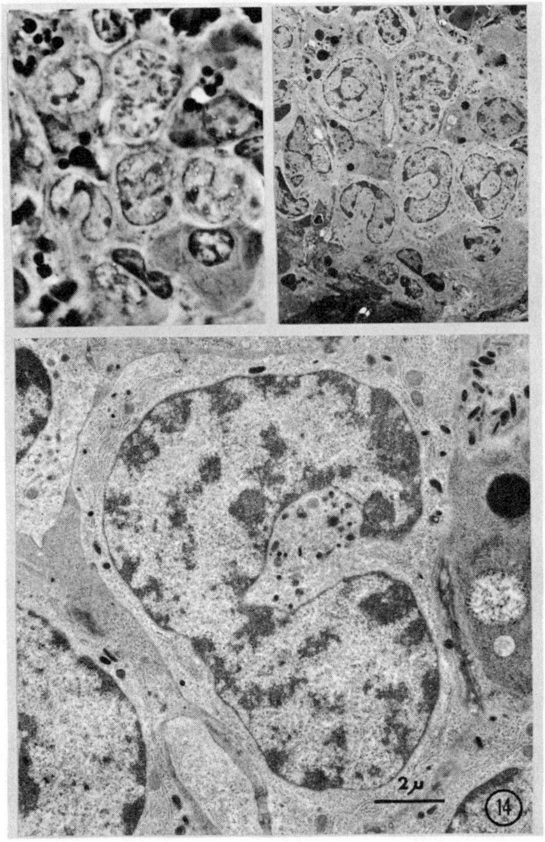

FIGURE 14. Spleen two hr after erythropoietin administration; ^{3}H-uridine given 1.5 hr after erythropoietin. Glutaraldehyde and osmic acid fixation. Alternate thick-thin sections through a nest of metamyelocytes. Silver grains, phase-negative white dots, over the nuclei indicate ^{3}H-uridine incorporation. One cell, seen at higher magnification, shows chromosomal condensation during early prophase.

A second aspect pertains to the nature of the biochemical events that transform erythropoietin-sensitive stem cells into proerythroblasts.

Erythropoietin-Induced Molecular Activity

Proerythroblasts, the earliest recognizable erythroid element, are intensely basophilic due to a high level of RNA. When lost through maturation, they are replaced by cells derived from a progenitor compartment in which specific erythroid molecular changes occur.

The present autoradiographic study does not indicate into which RNA fraction ^{3}H-uridine is incorporated at one, two, four and six hr after erythropoietin activation, but these new macromolecules may be the RNA that confers, upon maturing cells, the classically recognized basophilia of the proerythroblast.

The initial molecular response to erythropoietin is still obscure because both ^{3}H-thymidine- and ^{3}H-uridine-labeled stem cells are seen within the first hour after

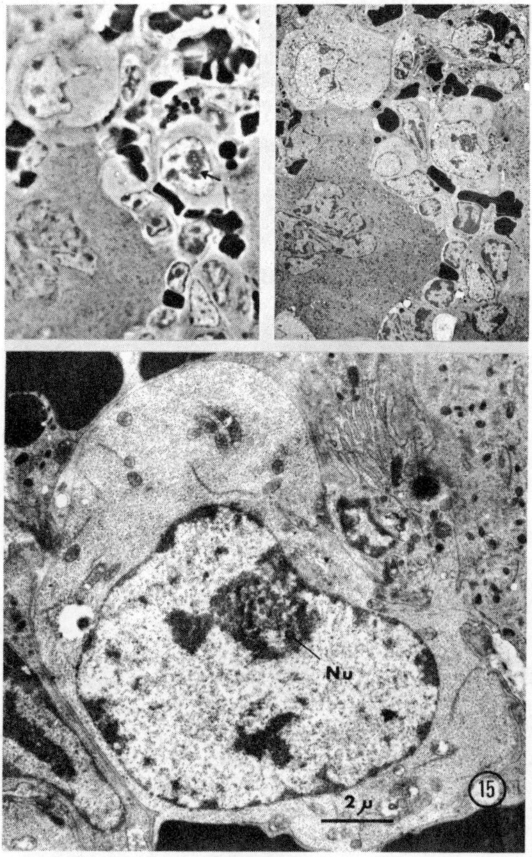

FIGURE 15. Spleen six hr after erythropoietin administration; ^{3}H-uridine given 5.5 hr after erythropoietin. Glutaraldehyde and osmic acid fixation. Alternate thick-thin sections through a nest of megakaryocytoblasts at several stages of maturity. The most immature cell displays a large nucleolus (Nu) and phase-negative silver grains are seen directly over this organelle (arrow).

erythropoietin administration. A simultaneous DNA-RNA synthesis would be in accord with patterns found in the nucleic acid systems of many mammalian cells where RNA synthesis apparently takes place during the entire cell cycle with the possible exception of the brief period from mid-prophase to mid-telophase (Prescott & Bender, 1963; Baserga & Kisieleski, 1963; Konrad, 1963).

Incorporation of ^{3}H-thymidine during the first hour indicates the onset or continuation of a DNA synthetic phase. This finding does not agree with certain in vitro studies that revealed no increased DNA synthesis for at least 9.5 hr after the addition of erythropoietin to the culture (Krantz & Goldwasser, 1965). Other recent reports also point to this factor as a differentiating agent not involved in increased ^{3}H-thymidine incorporation (Kurtides *et al.,* 1963; Erslev, 1964; Gallien-Lartigue & Goldwasser, 1965). However, it is recognized that since almost all cells of the hemopoietic system incorporate ^{3}H-thymidine, the formation of a few additional proerythroblasts engendered by erythropoietin might not result in biochemical changes significant enough to detect (Erslev, 1964).

An alternative to the hypothesis that early uptake of ^{3}H-thymidine indicates DNA replication prior to division envisions an action of erythropoietin on genic mechanisms. According to this, ^{3}H-thymidine taken up in response to erythropoietin is incorporated into new macromolecules of DNA formed during the replication of genes that participate in hemoglobin production. Replication of only a portion of the cellular DNA, as suggested here, is without precedent; therefore, it may do well to consider that this early DNA synthesis represents the S-phase for the first erythroid cell cycle.

Erythroblasts in mouse embryos require 11 hr to complete one generation (Atlas & Bond, 1965). Their DNA synthetic phase is 5.5 hr long and the post-synthetic gap lasts about 1.0 hour. The remaining time is divided between a 1.0-hour mitotic period and a 3.5-hour presynthetic gap. These figures relate to events in cells with uninterrupted cycles. It may be, however, that sensitive stem cells are at the completed end of the presynthetic gap, or in S-phase, and upon activation show a period of DNA synthesis. This sequence of events would lead to a cell division less than 7 hr after activation. Such a scheme could explain the occurrence of adjacent labeled proerythroblasts at 12 hr after erythropoietin administration. This seems probable since in another system division of a single ^{3}H-thymidine-labeled cell yields a pair of labeled cells that tend to remain adjacent (Pelc, 1964).

Continued uptake of ^{3}H-uridine at two, four and six hr following erythropoietin treatment further establishes that both types of nucleic acids are synthesized early. Large nucleoli are often seen as early as four hr after erythropoietin administration and remain a constant feature to beyond 24 hr of maturation. Most ^{3}H-uridine at two to six hr after erythropoietin is still within nuclei 30 min after administration of the label, but silver grains are also seen over the cytoplasm, possibly indicating transit after incorporation into nuclear RNA. This would agree with work, done on avian and mammalian cells in vitro, which shows all ^{3}H-uridine in the nucleus for the first 15 min with passage of some label into the cytoplasm after this period (Taylor, 1960a; Fraser, 1964).

The large nucleoli of proerythroblasts disappear when basophilic erythroblasts emerge (Orlic *et al.,* 1965b). Cells in this stage contain all the informational RNA needed to carry on hemoglobin production, which is not concluded until after nuclear extrusion and reticulocyte maturation are completed. Young reticulocytes contain ribosomal clusters and electron microscope preparations indicate that strands of messenger-RNA, for directing hemoglobin synthesis, are an inclusive part of these polysomes (Warner *et al.,* 1962). No RNA is synthesized by reticulocytes from rat blood under in vitro conditions (Marks *et al.,* 1962; Pinheiro *et al.,* 1963). Their ribosomal and messenger-RNA must therefore be stable entities.

In the present work ^{3}H-uridine is found in erythroblasts observed 48 hr after erythropoietin administration. Grains over nuclei may indicate either nuclear RNA involved in synthesis of hemoglobin (O'Brien, 1960; Schjeide *et al.,* 1964) or, simply, cytoplasmic material trapped during the previous mitosis. In either event, this finding indicates that ^{3}H-uridine taken up by the cell at 5.5 hr after activation is incorporated into a stable entity still present 42 hr later. This entity would seem to be an RNA fraction. Many reticulocytes emerge at 48 hr containing ^{3}H-uridine. Reticulocytes do not show label, however, in the ^{3}H-thymidine study; hence, if any ^{3}H-uridine is converted to ^{3}H-thymidine and incorporated into DNA, at least a portion of the original ^{3}H-uridine should persist as RNA in reticulocytes. A second study now underway in our laboratory further establishes this point. When ^{14}C-uridine was injected into mice and DNA and RNA fractions obtained from splenic homogenates, ^{14}C was recovered only in RNA fractions (Peets & Gordon, unpublished).

The quantity of ^{3}H-uridine per erythroblast and reticulocyte is considerably lower than the original total incorporated six hr after stem cell activation despite a three-to-four-fold longer exposure time for the 48-hour preparations. Less labeled RNA in late erythroblasts may result either from degradation during hemoglobin synthesis, a decrease in the total number of ribosomes and in the size of polysomes that constitute features of maturation (Rifkind *et al.,* 1964), or from mechanical features of maturation that involve decreasing cell volume and a halving of all macromolecules with each successive division. If unequal sharing of labeled materials occurs at each cell division, it is conceivable that some late erythroblasts may contain quantities of isotope too insignificant to detect.

Similarly, quantities of ^{3}H-thymidine in proerythroblasts were greater than in erythroblasts even when mice exhibiting the latter cells were given higher original doses and their autoradiograms exposed for longer times. Replication of DNA and its distribution to each daughter cell may serve as a basis to explain this finding. While passing through the erythron a cell divides three to four times (Lajtha, 1962) thus diluting the original complement of labeled DNA by a factor of 8–16. Furthermore, ^{3}H-thymidine may be available for as little as 1–15 min (Rubini *et al.,* 1960) and since chromosomal duplication is asynchronous and very limited early in the DNA synthetic phase (Taylor, 1960b; German, 1964), perhaps only early duplicating chromosomes contain incorporated label. If so, this small number of labeled chromosomes could be segregated in such a way that some erythroblasts would contain no label. An additional or alternative mechanism may work to reduce labeled DNA levels in this system. Microspectrophotometric studies indicate a less than interphase value in extruded erythroblast nuclei (Grasso *et al.,* 1963) and it is suggested that a large DNA loss occurs just before cells reach the polychromatophilic stage of maturation (Borsook, 1964).

A schematic summary is presented to show the fate of early incorporated nucleic acid precursors during erythroid maturation leading to the formation of reticulocytes (FIGURE 16).

Summary

An electron microscopic study was made of the wave of red cell formation induced by erythropoietin in the spleens of hypoxia-induced polycythemic mice, initially exhibiting markedly inhibited erythropoiesis. Identification of newly activated erythropoietin-sensitive stem cells depended upon thick section autoradiographic localization of labeled nucleic acid precursors that were incorporated by primitive cells responding to the action of the hormone at time intervals of one to two min to six hr after its administration. The same cells were then found in alternate thin sections prepared for electron microscopy, their fate during maturation followed, and ultrastructural features noted.

Within one hour after an injection of erythropoietin, stem cells became labeled with both ^{3}H-thymidine and ^{3}H-uridine. Erythropoietin-sensitive stem cells displayed numerous ribosomes, sparse endoplasmic reticulum, mitochondria and in some instances a well developed Golgi apparatus. Chromatin either was arranged in dense masses or was evenly distributed with only slight packing along the nuclear border. Little nucleolar material was seen prior to four hr but from 4–12

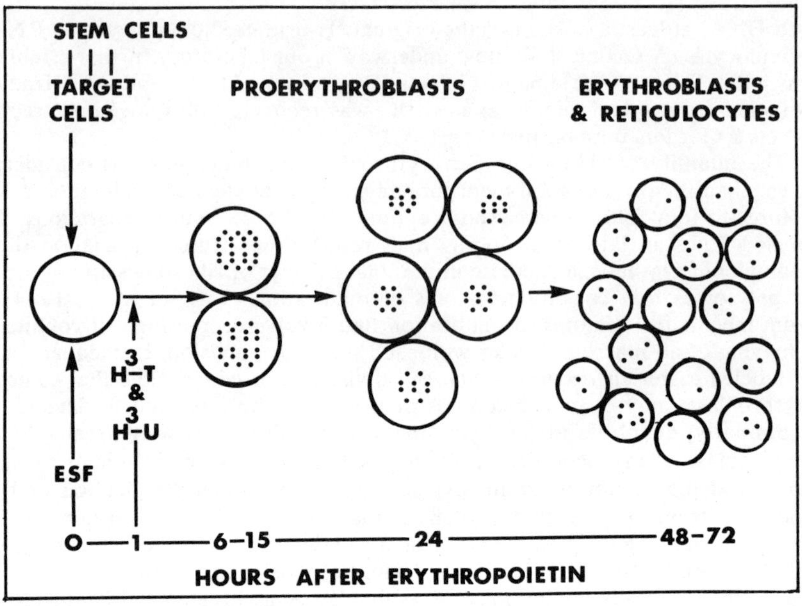

FIGURE 16. This scheme summarizes some of the findings reported in this paper. It is not known whether erythropoietin-sensitive elements are stem cells or erythroid transitional cells (target cells for erythropoietin may be immature elements previously committed to the red cell line). The incorporation of ^{3}H-nucleic acid precursors is represented by black dots (silver grains) over cells of the erythroid series. Both ^{3}H-thymidine and ^{3}H-uridine are incorporated within one hr after administration of erythropoietin, and ^{3}H-uridine uptake continues at 1.5, 3.5 and 5.5 hours. The autoradiographic study did not include quantitation of labeled nucleic acid levels but even after much longer exposures (three months) erythroblast autoradiograms indicated greatly reduced numbers of silver grains per cell compared with the total found in proerythroblast autoradiograms exposed for shorter times (three to four weeks). This dilution of label appears to occur through cell division.

hr after activation large nucleoli formed. These remained prominent throughout proerythroblast maturation.

Levels of early incorporated isotopes were diluted during erythroid cell maturation and, by 48 hr after erythropoietin administration, radioactive materials originally incorporated by perhaps as few as one to four proerythroblasts were distributed to cells of erythroid nests totalling 18–36 erythroblasts.

In conclusion, we have established by electron microscopy and autoradiography that erythropoietin activation of stem cells is associated with DNA synthesis and have identified the ^{3}H-thymidine-labeled stem elements that give rise to labeled proerythroblasts and erythroblasts during the ensuing wave of erythropoiesis.

REFERENCES

ALPEN, E. L. & D. CRANMORE. 1959. Observations on the regulation of erythropoiesis and on cellular dynamics by ^{59}Fe autoradiography. *In* The Kinetics of Cellular Proliferation. F. Stohlman, Jr., Ed. : 290–300. Grune & Stratton. New York, N. Y.

ATLAS, M. & V. P. BOND. 1965. The cell generation cycle of the eleven-day mouse embryo. J. Cell Biol. **26:** 19–24.

BASERGA, R. & W. E. KISIELESKI. 1963. Autobiographies of cells. Sci. Amer. **209:** 103–110.

BENEDETTI, L. E. & R. LEPLUS. 1958. Cytologie de l'érythroblastose aviaire. Etude au microscope électronique. Rev. Hematol. **13:** 199–230.

BORSOOK, H. 1964. A picture of erythropoiesis at the combined morphologic and molecular levels. Blood **24**: 202–207.

BORSOOK, H., J. B. LINGREL, J. L. SCARO & R. L. MILLETTE. 1962. Synthesis of haemoglobin in relation to the maturation of erythroid cells. Nature **196**: 347–350.

BRECHER, G. & F. STOHLMAN, JR. 1959. Humoral factors in erythropoiesis. *In* Progress in Hematology, vol. II. L. M. Tocantins, Ed. : 110–132. Grune & Stratton. New York, N. Y.

BRECHER, G. & F. STOHLMAN, JR. 1962. The macrocytic response to erythropoietin stimulation. *In* Erythropoiesis. L. O. Jacobson and M. Doyle, Eds. : 216–221. Grune & Stratton. New York, N. Y.

ERSLEV, A. J. 1964. Erythropoietin in vitro. II. Effect on "stem cells." Blood **24**: 331–342.

FILMANOWICZ, E. & C. W. GURNEY. 1961. Studies on erythropoiesis. XVI. The response to a single dose of erythropoietin in the polycythemic mouse. J. Lab. Clin. Med. **57**: 65–72.

FRASER, R. C. 1964. Autoradiographic analysis of DNA and RNA synthesis in the red blood cells of developing chick embryo. Exp. Cell Res. **33**: 473–480.

GALLAGHER, N. I., G. L. SEIFERT, J. L. CALLINAN, A. A. MAES & R. D. LANGE. 1963. Influence of erythropoietin on erythropoiesis in polycythemic rats. J. Lab. Clin. Med. **61**: 258–265.

GALLIEN-LARTIGUE, O. & E. GOLDWASSER. 1965. On the mechanism of erythropoietin-induced differentiation. I. The effects of specific inhibitors on hemoglobin synthesis. Biochim. Biophys. Acta **103**: 319–324.

GERMAN, J. 1964. The pattern of DNA synthesis in the chromosomes of human blood cells. J. Cell Biol. **20**: 37–55.

GRASSO, J. A., J. W. WOODWARD & H. SWIFT. 1963. Cytochemical studies on nucleic acids and proteins in erythrocytic development. Proc. Nat. Acad. Sci. **50**: 134–140.

KONRAD, C. G. 1963. Protein synthesis and RNA synthesis during mitosis in animal cells. J. Cell Biol. **19**: 267–277.

KRANTZ, S. B. & E. GOLDWASSER. 1965. On the mechanism of erythropoietin-induced differentiation. II. The effect on RNA synthesis. Biochim. Biophys. Acta **103**: 325–332.

KURTIDES, E. S., W. A. RAMBACH, H. L. ALT & J. C. WURSTER. 1963. Effect of erythropoietin on tritiated thymidine incorporation by the rat spleen. J. Lab. Clin. Med. **61**: 23–33.

LAJTHA, L. G. 1962. Stem cell kinetics and erythropoietin. *In* Erythropoiesis. L. O. Jacobson and M. Doyle, Eds. : 140–150. Grune & Stratton. New York, N. Y.

LUFT, J. H. 1961. Improvements in epoxy resin embedding methods. J. Biophys. Biochem. Cytol. **9**: 409–414.

MARKS, P. A., E. R. BURKA & D. SCHLESSINGER. 1962. Protein synthesis in erythroid cells. I. Reticulocyte ribosomes active in stimulating amino acid incorporation. Proc. Nat. Acad. Sci. **48**: 2163–2171.

O'BRIEN, B. R. A. 1960. The presence of hemoglobin within the nucleus of the embryonic chick erythroblast. Exp. Cell Res. **21**: 226–228.

ORLIC, D., A. S. GORDON & J. A. G. RHODIN. 1965a. Electron microscopic and autoradiographic studies of erythropoietin-induced erythropoiesis. Blood **26**: 884 (abstract).

ORLIC, D., A. S. GORDON & J. A. G. RHODIN. 1965b. An ultrastructural study of erythropoietin-induced red cell formation in mouse spleen. J. Ultrastruct. Res. **13**: 516–542.

PELC, S. R. 1964. Labeling of DNA and cell division in so-called nondividing tissues. J. Cell Biol. **22**: 21–28.

PINHEIRO, P., C. P. LEBLOND & B. DROZ. 1963. Synthetic capacity of reticulocytes as shown by radioautography after incubation with labeled precursors of protein or RNA. Exp. Cell Res. **31**: 517–537.

PRESCOTT, D. M. & M. A. BENDER. 1963. Synthesis and behavior of nuclear proteins during the cell life cycle. J. Cell Comp. Physiol. **62** (suppl. 1) : 175–194.

REVEL, J. P. & E. D. HAY. 1961. Autoradiographic localization of DNA synthesis in a specific ultrastructural component of the interphase nucleus. Exp. Cell Res. **25**: 474–480.

RIFKIND, R. A., D. DANNON & P. A. MARKS. 1964. Alterations in polysomes during erythroid cell maturation. J. Cell Biol. **22**: 599–611.

RUBINI, J. R., E. P. CRONKITE, V. P. BOND & T. M. FLIEDNER. 1960. The metabolism and fate of tritiated thymidine in man. J. Clin. Invest. **39**: 909–918.

SCHJEIDE, O. A., R. G. MCCANDLESS & R. J. MUNN. 1964. Relationships between hematin synthesis and morphological structures in adult and fetal red cells. Growth **28**: 29–39.

SORENSON, G. D. 1961. An electron microscopic study of hematopoiesis in the yolk sac. Lab. Invest. **10**: 178–193.

STOHLMAN, JR. F., D. HOWARD & A. BELAND. 1963. Humoral regulation of erythropoiesis. XII. Effect of erythropoietin and iron on cell size in iron deficiency anemia. Proc. Soc. Exp. Biol. Med. **113:** 986–988.

TAYLOR, J. H. 1960a. Nucleic acid synthesis in relation to the cell division cycle. Ann. N. Y. Acad. Sci. **90:** 409–421.

TAYLOR, J. H. 1960b. Asynchronous duplication of chromosomes in cultured cells of Chinese Hamster. J. Biophys. Biochem. Cytol. **7:** 455–464.

WARNER, J. R., A. RICH & C. E. HALL. 1962. Electron microscope studies of ribosomal clusters synthesizing hemoglobin. Science **138:** 1399–1403.

WEINTRAUB, A. H., A. S. GORDON & J. F. CAMISCOLI. 1963. Use of the hypoxia-induced polycythemic mouse in the assay and standardization of erythropoietin. J. Lab. Clin. Med. **62:** 743–752.

ZAMBONI, L. 1965. Electron microscopic studies of blood embryogenesis in humans. II. The hemopoietic activity in the fetal liver. J. Ultrastruct. Res. **12:** 525–541.

THE INCREASED DOSE-RESPONSE OF ESF AFTER ESF STIMULATION*

Jan Fogh

Department of Nuclear Medicine, Rigshospitalet, Copenhagen, Denmark

Erythropoietin (ESF) can only be measured by its biologic effect. The action of ESF has not been fully elucidated and therefore, any unexpected observation of the effect of ESF should be investigated in order to gain more information on its mode of action.

Fractionated administration of an ESF-dose substantially increases the dose-response. Generally two or more injections of the ESF-material are administered in order to increase the sensitivity of the ESF-bioassay in animals whose erythropoiesis has been suppressed. The effect of fractionated administration of ESF in the erythremic-mouse-assay is demonstrated in FIGURE 1. The results confirm earlier observations, (Reichlin & Harrington, 1960; Gurney *et al.*, 1961; Schooley & Garcia, 1962; Gallagher *et al.*, 1963; and Fogh, 1966. This phenomenon of fractionated administration of ESF has been studied in details at the Department of Nuclear Medicine, Rigshospitalet, Copenhagen.

Methods

Human erythropoietin from a patient with aplastic anemia was obtained from 20 1 of urine. The urine was dialyzed in Visking tubings (27/32) for 20 hr against tap water and for four hr against distilled water. The urine in the dialysis-tubing was concentrated over a period of 24 hr at room temperature to 1/10 of its original volume. The concentration was effected by the draft from an electrical fan. The inspissate was redialyzed against distilled water for half an hour in order to redissolve any material adherent to the membrane. The concentrated urine was filtered (S & S filter no. 589, white ribbon), freeze-dried and finally redissolved in 250 ml saline. By comparing the dose-response in a series of four dilutions to that of erythropoietin standard B (ESB),† it was found that the final urine concentrate contained 20 i.u. per ml. Female St/Eh mice six to eight weeks old were used for the assay. Each test group contained five to ten mice. Erythremia was induced by exposure to carbon monoxide hypoxia (Fogh, 1966). Erythropoietin was administered i.p. in volumes not exceeding 0.5 ml per injection. 1 μc of ^{59}Fe-citrate was given i.v. to the animals not earlier than the seventh day after the hypoxic period. Sixty-six hours after injection of the tracer, blood was sampled for determination of the ^{59}Fe incorporation into red cells. Those results obtained from mice whose final hematocrit proved to be less than 55% were discarded (Fogh, 1966). The results are given as the middle observation for each test group (Dean & Dixon, 1951). When dealing with more than 10 observations, the results are given as a mean value ± the standard deviation $\left(SD = \sqrt{\frac{\Sigma(\bar{a}-a)^2}{n-1}} \right)$ The standard deviation of the difference between the results in two groups (A and B) was calculated according to the formula $SD_{diff} = \sqrt{SD_A^2 + SD_B^2}$.

* This investigation was supported by a grant from Statens Almindelige Videnskabsfond.

† ESB was kindly supplied by the Dept. of Biological Standards Medical Research Council, Mill Hill, London.

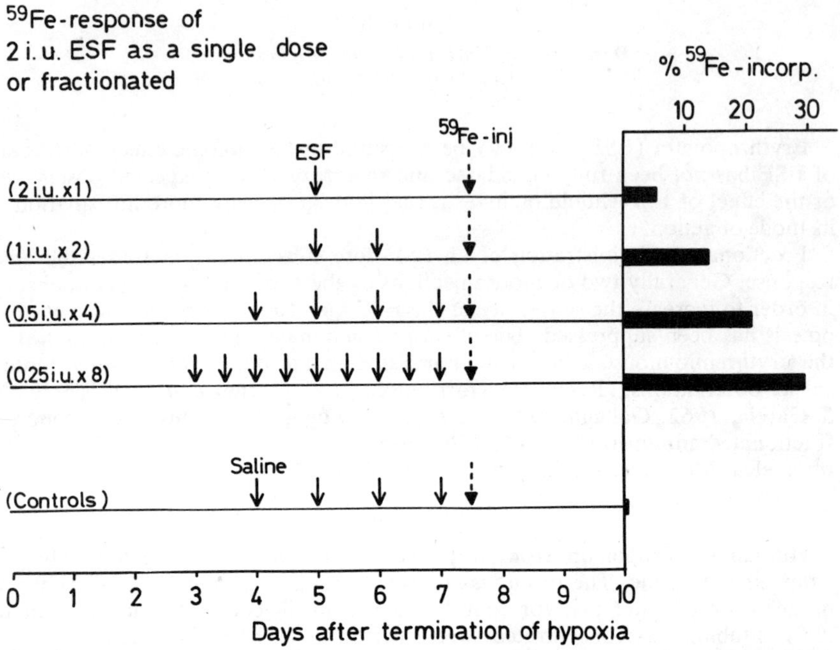

FIGURE 1. Each horizontal line represents a group of erythremic mice. The arrows indicate injections. The time of the injections can be read on the abscissa. The horizontal bars show the percentage of ^{59}Fe incorporated into the red cells.

Results

In a series of experiments conducted at our laboratory the discrete effect of two consecutive ESF- injections has been studied. The test mice were distributed in four groups A, B, C and S. Three groups of mice were given injections of ESF. Group A received a single injection of 1 i.u. on the sixth day after termination of the hypoxia, group B two injections of 1 i.u. – one on the sixth and one on the seventh day. Group C received a single injection of 1 i.u. on the seventh day. The mice in group S were controls and were injected with saline. All animals received ^{59}Fe on the eighth day and the incorporation into the red cells was determined 66 hr later. The results are shown in FIGURE 2. As expected the values obtained in group B, which received two doses each of 1 i.u., was larger than in groups A and C, both of which received one unit only. When the response in group B originating from the first of the two injections, (which must correspond to the result obtained in group A) is subtracted from the total response in group B, the difference (B − A) can be ascribed to the second injection. This difference was significantly greater than the results obtained in group C. The experiment shows that the effect of ESF on the incorporation of ^{59}Fe is enhanced in animals previously stimulated by exogenous ESF. This observation explains the increased dose-response obtained by fractionated administration of ESF.

In the latter experiment the interval between the first and the second ESF-injection was one day. In another set of experiments the interval between the first and second injection was extended to two, three, four and five days, respectively. The first injection of ESF was not given before the eighth day following the hypoxic period when the spontaneous erythropoiesis had ceased completely. In the experiments in which the interval between the two ESF-injections was four and five days, it was necessary to give the animals a transfusion of washed and packed homologous red cells two days prior to the first ESF-injection in order to maintain the hematocrit value above 55%. The results of these studies are demonstrated in the lower part of FIGURE 3. The interval between the two injections of ESF is shown on the abscissa. The ordinate shows the percentage of ^{59}Fe incorporated into the red cells due to the second ESF-dose. The shaded area represents the mean value ± SD of the results obtained with a similar dose in 33 animals not previously stimulated with exogenous ESF (corresponding to group C in FIGURE 2). Since the response of the second ESF-dose is calculated as a difference between the middle value obtained in two groups of mice (group B and A), the spread is conspicuous. This is indicated by the vertical lines in the Figure. The data show that the increased dose-response lasts up to four days after a previous ESF-stimulation. On the third and fourth day the response decreases and five days after preliminary stimulation the dose-response does not differ from that obtained in previously untreated animals.

Since the response in these experiments was measured by the incorporation of ^{59}Fe into the red cells, the present observation of an increased response in mice previously stimulated by ESF could be due to the effect of ESF on the turnover of iron in the test animals. The serum iron concentration of the erythremic mice

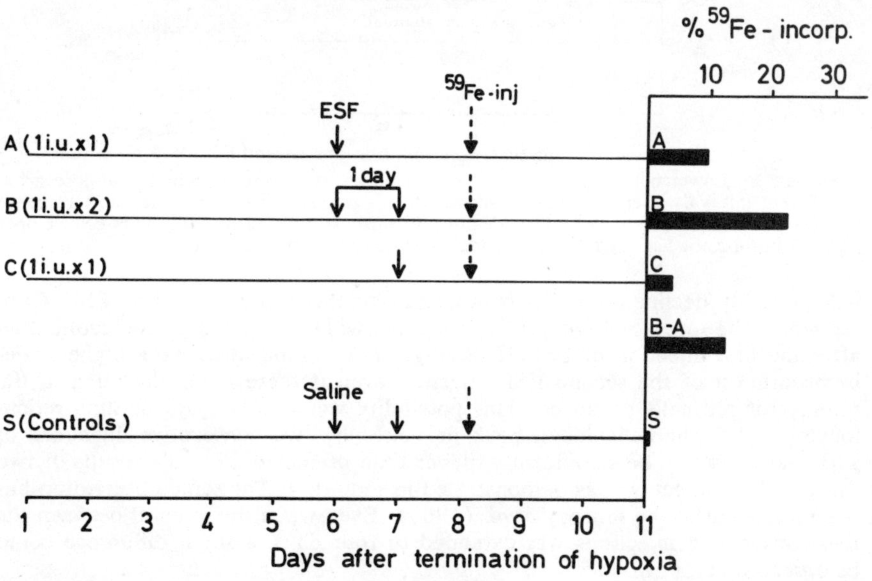

FIGURE 2. Potentiated ESF-effect in erythremic mice one day after a previous ESF-stimulation (see text). (B-A) represents the estimated response in group B due to the second ESF-injection.

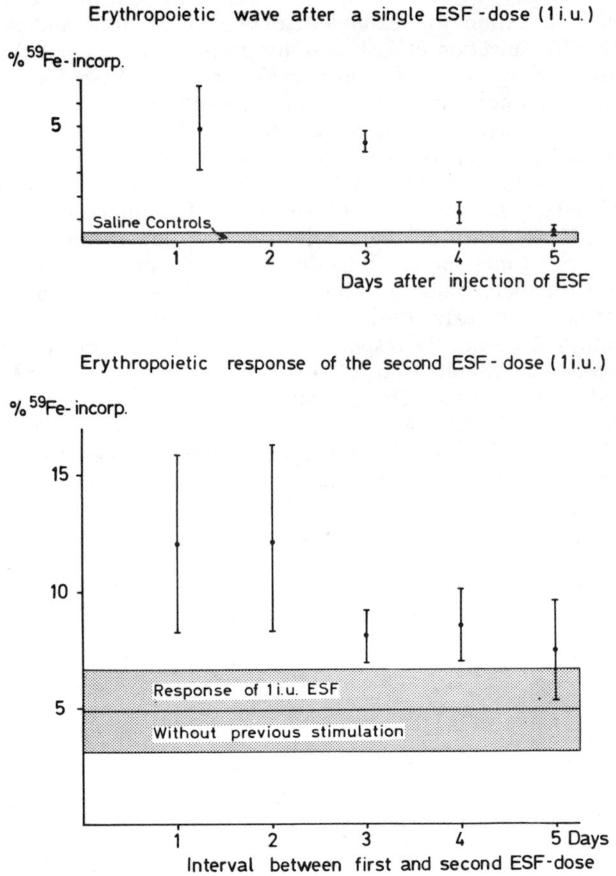

FIGURE 3. Lower part: The "discrete" (estimated) response to a second ESF-dose given at different intervals after the first ESF-dose. The shaded area represents the mean response (±SD) of the same ESF-dose in 33 mice not previously stimulated by exogenous ESF. Upper part: Erythropoietic activity following a single ESF-dose (see text for details).

will probably decline when the hemoglobin synthesis is activated by ESF. Consequently, the specific activity of ^{59}Fe in serum will be higher after the second than after the first injection of ESF. This might conceivably provoke a higher ^{59}Fe-incorporation of the second ESF-injection even if there is no alteration in the number of red cells produced. This possibility was checked by counting reticulocytes daily. The reticulocyte-peak provoked by two consecutive injections of ESF was shown to be significantly higher than predicted from the results of two "single" ESF-injections, as demonstrated in FIGURE 4. The same observation has been made earlier by Gurney *et al.* (1961). Even when the interval between the two consecutive injections was extended to four days, a slight difference could be observed (FIGURE 5).

The cause of the increased response to ESF after previous stimulation with ESF is unknown. It has previously been suggested (Fogh, 1966) that the response to ESF depends not only on the ESF-dose but also on the number of ESF-sensitive cells available. This hypothesis is in agreement with observations made by Schooley (1965) that ESF in doses ranging from 0.25–4.0 i.u. stimulate erythropoiesis to the same extent when allowed to act for only six hours. If this concept is correct, the increased response to the second ESF-dose could be due to an increase in the number of ESF-sensitive cells induced by the first dose. Furthermore it appears that the increase in number of ESF-sensitive cells occurs within 24 hr after stimulation with ESF and lasts for about four days.

The problem as to the nature of the ESF-sensitive cell has not been definitely solved. It is generally accepted that ESF acts by stimulating the differentiation of stem cells into the red cell series. In addition, some authors believe that ESF acts directly on the nucleated red cells. In the present study the response to the first ESF-dose must originate from an effect on the stem cells since no nucleated red cells were present in the marrow of the erythremic mice seven days after termination of the hypoxic period. At the time of the second ESF-injection, however, nucleated red cells from the erythropoietic wave provoked by the first injection would be present in the marrow, and the increased response observed could be due to an action of ESF on these cells.

In order to study whether the increased response to the second ESF-injection was correlated to the presence of erythropoietic activity in the marrow originating from the first ESF-injection, a fifth group of erythremic mice (group D) was included in the series of experiments already mentioned. As shown in FIGURE 6, this group D received an ESF-dose of 1 i.u. at the same time the first ESF-injection was given in group B, but at the time of the second ESF-injection in group B,

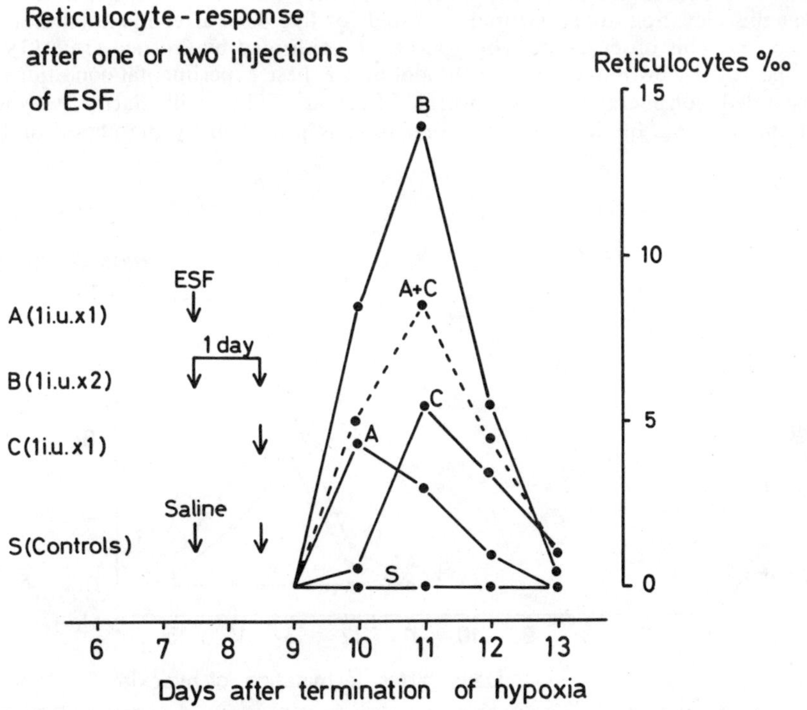

FIGURE 4. Reticulocyte counts in erythremic mice following one (A and C) or two (B) ESF-injections with an interval of one day.

the mice in group D were injected with ^{59}Fe. Under these circumstances the response obtained in group D would indicate the magnitude of the erythropoietic activity at the time when the second ESF-dose was administered. Since the response of group D was significantly larger than the response of nonstimulated erythremic mice (group S), it can be concluded that the erythropoietic activity provoked by the first ESF-injection did not cease three days later. Consequently, nucleated red cells will be present in the marrow at the time of the second ESF-injection if the interval between the two consecutive stimulations in group B is three days.

The progression of the erythropoietic wave provoked by a single ESF-dose of 1 i.u. is shown at the top of FIGURE 3. A fairly good correlation was found between the increased response to the second ESF-dose and the extent of erythropoietic activity due to the first dose, estimated by studies similar to those shown in FIGURE 6, group D. This correlation does not prove that the increased response of the second ESF-dose depends on the presence of erythropoietic activity in the marrow, or that the nucleated red cells are sensitive to ESF. The observed phenomenon might be due solely to the interaction between ESF and the stem cell pool.

During recent years methods for investigation of stem cell kinetics have been developed. Alexania *et al.* (1963) have studied the recovery of stem cell response to ESF in irradiated polycythemic mice. They found, that the response became normal by the seventh day after irradiation but then rose above normal and remained elevated for the next ten days. An approximate two-fold increase above the control level was measured at approximately the 12th day. It is noteworthy that this elevation above normal persisted for five days after maximal elevation occurred. This observation, which has been confirmed by Gurney *et al.* (1965), supports the view that the stem cell pool under these experimental conditions had expanded considerably above normal. Further studies will clarify whether a similar increase of the stem cell population is provoked by the action of ESF.

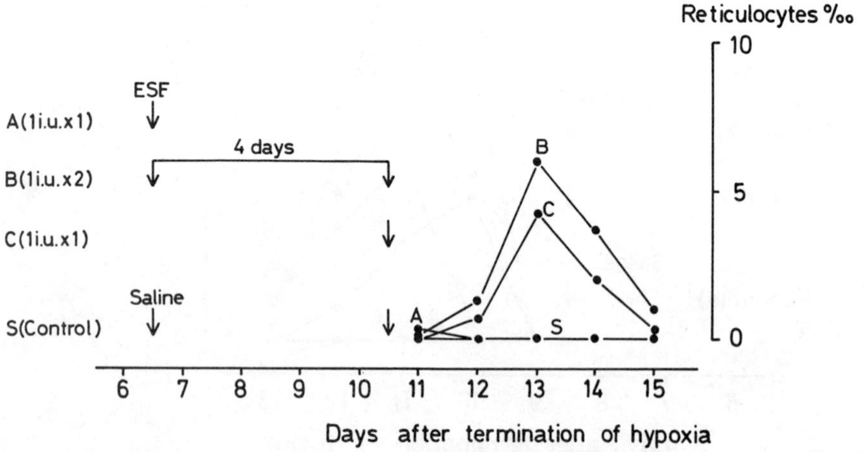

FIGURE 5. Reticulocyte counts in erythremic mice following one or two ESF-injections with an interval of four days.

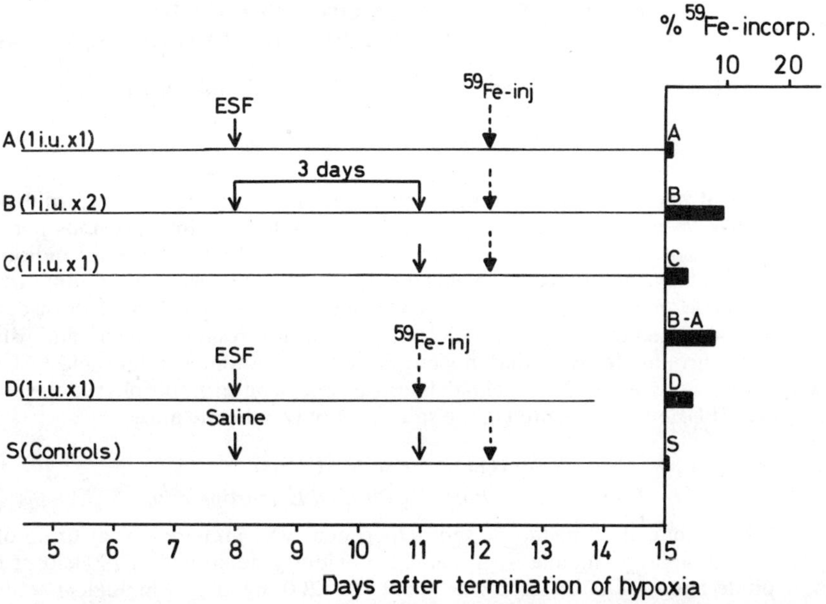

FIGURE 6. Potentiated ESF-effect in erythremic mice three days after a previous ESF-stimulation. The erythropoietic activity in group B originating from the first ESF-injection is estimated at the time of the second ESF-injection by the response in group D (see text for details).

Summary

The effect of ESF on the ^{59}Fe-incorporation into the red cells of polycythemic mice is substantially greater when the dose is given in fractions. It has been demonstrated that this phenomenon is due to an increased dose-response in mice previously stimulated by ESF. The increased dose-response can be demonstrated up to four days after a previous ESF-stimulation. During these four days the response declines towards the response in polycythemic animals which have not previously been stimulated with exogenous ESF. A rather good correlation was found between the duration of the increased response and the presence of nucleated hemoglobin-synthesizing cells in the marrow. No conclusions can be drawn from these experiments as to the nature of the ESF-sensitive cells.

References

ALEXANIA, R., D. D. PORTEOUS & L. G. LAJTHA. 1963. Int. J. Radiat. Biol. **7**(1): 87.

DEAN, R. B. & W. J. DIXON. 1951. Analyt. Chemist. **23**: 636.

FOGH, JAN. 1966. Scand. J. Clin. Lab. Invest. **18**: 33.

GALLAGHER, N. I., G. L. SEIFERT, J. L. CALLINAN, A. A. MAES & R. D. LANGE. 1963. J. Lab. Clin. Med. **61**: 258.

GURNEY, C. W., N. WACKMAN & E. FILMANOWICZ. 1961. Blood **17**: 531.

GURNEY, C. W., D. HOFSTRA & A. MANGALIK. 1965. Report from Argonne Cancer Research Hospital (A.C.R.H.) **23**: 21.

REICHLIN, M. & W. J. HARRINGTON. 1960. Blood **16**: 1298.

SCHOOLEY, J. C. & J. F. GARCIA. 1962. Proc. Soc. Exp. Biol. Med. **109**: 325.

SCHOOLEY, J. C. 1965. Blood **25**: 795.

ENZYMATIC STUDIES ON ERYTHROID DIFFERENTIATION AND PROLIFERATION*

Kiku Nakao, Shigeru Sassa, Osamu Wada and Fumimaro Takaku

The Third Department of Internal Medicine, Faculty of Medicine, University of Tokyo, Tokyo, Japan

Action of erythropoietin leading to stem cell differentiation to erythroid precursors has been demonstrated by several investigators.[1-4] In a previous paper,[5] we carried out experiments showing an increased RNA synthesis, radioiron uptake, and heme synthesis in the spleens of polycythemic mice after administration of erythropoietin. The present experiment has been performed to discover the enzyme of heme synthesis, which is first induced in response to an administration of erythropoietin. With that in view, activity of δ-aminolevulinic acid (ALA) synthetase, δ-aminolevulinic acid dehydrase, and iron-protoporphyrin-chelating enzyme (IPCE) was measured in the spleens of polycythemic mice.

Materials and Methods

Preparation of Partially Purified Erythropoietin

Erythropoietin used in the present experiment was prepared from urine of a patient with aplastic anemia by a method previously described.[5] The yield of the precipitate from 1 liter of urine was about 180–200 mg and its biological activity was 1–3 cobalt unit per mg by the method of starved rat assay.[6]

Method of Hypertransfusion

All the animals used in the present study were ddO mice, which were inbred in the Research Institute of Infectious Disease in Tokyo. They were maintained on a Purina chow diet made by the Oriental Solid Food Company in Tokyo. Mice were made polycythemic by being transfused i.p. with 1 ml of 80 percent saline suspension of isologous red cells for two days. They were given erythropoietin injection on the sixth day after the second transfusion. On the 8th, 12th, 24th, 28th, 52nd and 100th hr following the erythropoietin injection, the mice were sacrificed and enzyme activities in the spleen were assayed.

Enzyme Preparations

The spleen was removed immediately after sacrifice, crushed, and suspended in 5 ml of cooled isologous plasma. This suspension was passed through a fine mesh. Nucleated cell counting and preparation of smears of the cell suspension were carried out first. Cells were then washed twice with cold buffered saline (0.01 M Na_2HPO_4 NaH_2PO_4–0.154 M NaCl) at 4° C. The packed cells were lysed by adding 2 vol of cold water and stirring thoroughly. After exactly four min isotonicity was restored by the addition of solid KCl (1.15 g per dl of added water). After centrifugation at 6000 g at 0° C for 30 min ALA dehydrase activity was measured in the supernatant fluid. The residue was washed four to five times with cold 0.154 M KCl-2 mM KH_2PO_4 K_2HPO_4 (pH 7.4) until the washings were free of hemoglobin. The packed residue was suspended in 1 ml of the above potassium phosphate buffer (pH 7.4). All small lumps or clots were removed. The suspended residue was used to determine the activity of ALA synthetase and iron-protoporphyrin-chelating enzyme (IPCE).

* This investigation was supported in part by I.A.E.A. grant no. 385/RB.

Determination of δ-Aminolevulinic Acid (ALA) Synthetase Activity

ALA synthetase activity was measured in a standard assay mixture containing glycine, 50 μmole; α-ketoglutarate, 3 μmole; potassium phosphate buffer (pH 7.4), 25 μmole; $MgCl_2$ 2 μmole; EDTA 1 μmole; pyridoxal phosphate, 0.2 μmole; coenzyme A, 0.25 μmole; enzyme, 0.2 ml and water to give a final volume of 0.5 ml. Incubations were carried out at 38° C in unstoppered glass tubes that were shaken 100 times per minute. After incubation, 1 ml of cold 5 percent trichloracetic acid was added. The 5 percent TCA supernatant (1.0 ml) was mixed with 1 ml of 1 M sodium acetate buffer (pH 4.5)–acetylacetone (one-tenth of the buffer). The mixture was heated at 100° C. for 15 min and cooled to room temperature. ALA content of the mixture was estimated according to the method of Granick and Urata.[7]

Determination of δ-Aminolevulinic Acid (ALA) Dehydrase Activity

ALA dehydrase was assayed by the method of Gibson *et al.*,[8] using 0.2 ml of the supernatant of the spleen hemolysate.

Determination of Iron-Protoporphyrin-Chelating Enzyme (IPCE) Activity

IPCE activity was assayed by the method of Nishida and Labbe.[9] A mixture containing protoporphyrin IX 0.02 μmole; $^{59}FeSO_4$, 0.02 μmole (0.1 μc); tris (pH 8.0), 100 μmole; GSH, 40 μmole; enzyme, 0.4 ml, and water to give a final volume of 1 ml was incubated under nitrogen for two hr at 38° C.

TABLE 1

ACTIVITY OF δ-AMINOLEVULINIC ACID SYNTHETASE IN THE SPLEENS OF HYPERTRANSFUSED MICE AFTER ERYTHROPOIETIN INJECTION

Group No.	Hours after Erythropoietin Injection	No. of Mice	Ht. % (Mean)	ALA Synthetase Activity mμmole ALA/2 hr 38° C/10⁸ Cells
1	control	5	71.8	0
2	8	5	67.4	1.12
3	12	5	76.6	1.22
4	24	5	74.1	2.23
5	28	5	68.8	2.31
6	52	5	68.8	4.55
7	100	5	72.2	1.08

Results

As shown in TABLE 1 and FIGURE 1, ALA synthetase activity was not demonstrable in the residual fraction (containing mitochondria) of the polycythemic mouse spleen, whereas normal mouse spleen had an ALA synthetase activity of 2.48 mμmole ALA formed/two hr, 38° C/10^8 nucleated cells. When the polycythemic mice were injected with 6 cobalt unit of urinary erythropoietin, ALA synthetase activity was shown to appear on the eighth hour after injection. The activity increased thereafter reaching a maximum on the 52nd hour, and followed by a decrease.

This appearance of ALA synthetase activity following an injection of erythropoietin was completely blocked by a previous administration of 200 μg/kg of Actinomycin D. When Actinomycin D was injected six hr after an administration of erythropoietin, however, its effect was not observed (FIGURE 2).

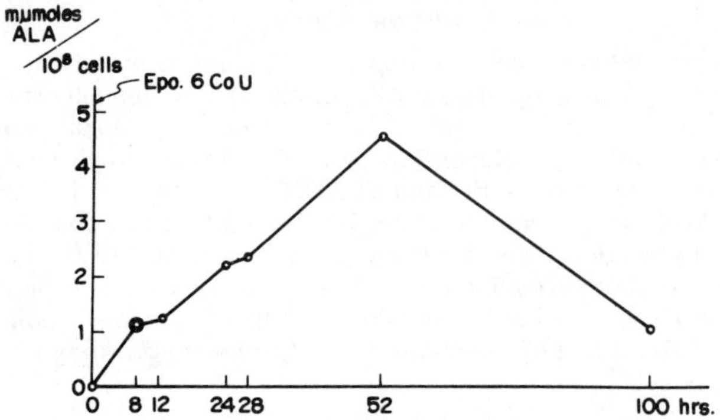

FIGURE 1. ALA-synthetase activity in the spleens of polycythemic mice after erythropoietin injection. Each point in the figure represents the ALA-synthetase activity of the spleens collected from five polycythemic mice at the indicated intervals after an erythropoietin injection.

TABLE 2

ACTIVITY OF δ-AMINOLEVULINIC ACID DEHYDRASE IN THE SPLEENS OF HYPERTRANSFUSED MICE AFTER ERYTHROPOIETIN INJECTION

Group No.	Hours after Erythropoietin Injection	No. of Mice	Ht. % (Mean)	ALA Dehydrase Activity mμmoles PBG/1 hr 38° C/10^8 Cells
1	control	5	71.8	7.5
2	8	5	67.4	7.4
3	12	5	76.6	9.0
4	24	5	74.1	16.4
5	28	5	68.8	23.1
6	52	5	68.8	94.0
7	100	5	72.2	19.6

The supernatant fraction of lysed spleen cells of hypertransfused mice showed an activity of 7.5 mμmole PBG formed/one hr, 38° C/10^8 nucleated cells. The activity of ALA dehydrase remained unchanged for eight hr after erythropoietin injection. The activity started to increase on the 12th hour. The maximal activity was reached on the 52nd hr after erythropoietin injection (TABLE 2).

The activity of IPCE, which was not demonstrated in the spleens of polycythemic mice, first started to increase on the 28th hr after administration of erythropoietin (TABLE 3).

DISCUSSION

ALA-synthetase has been regarded as a key enzyme in heme synthesis.[10] A rapid appearance of ALA-synthetase activity after an erythropoietin injection demonstrated in the present paper is considered to indicate an intimate relationship between the erythropoietin-induced stem cell differentiation and the appearance of the ALA-synthetase activity.

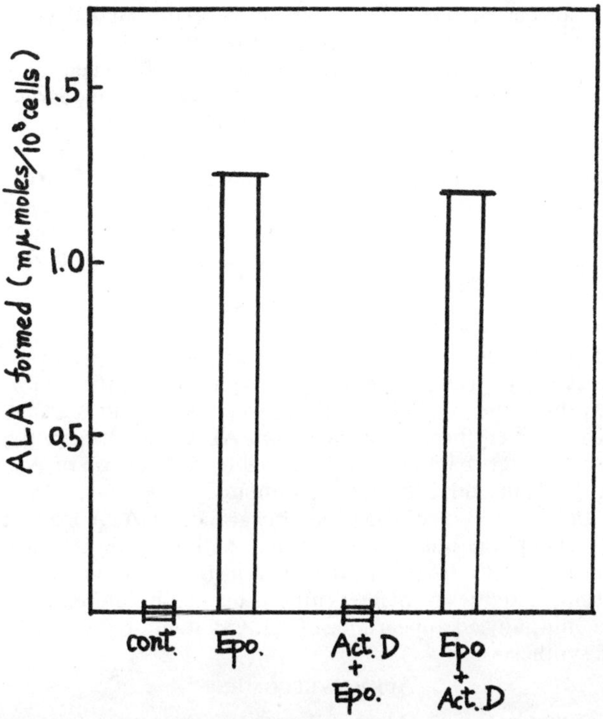

FIGURE 2. ALA-synthetase activity in the spleens of polycythemic mice after erythropoietin injection. Columns in the Figure show (from the left to the right): (1) no injection of erythropoietin; (2) injection of 6 cobalt units of erythropoietin; (3) injection of 200 μg/kg of Actinomycin D before the injection of the erythropoietin; (4) injection of 200 μg/kg of Actinomycin D six hr after the injection of the erythropoietin.

TABLE 3

ACTIVITY OF IRON-PROTOPORPHYRIN-CHELATING ENZYME IN THE SPLEENS OF HYPERTRANSFUSED MICE AFTER ERYTHROPOIETIN INJECTION

Group No.	Hours after Erythropoietin Injection	No. of Mice	Ht. % (Mean)	IPCE Activity cpm/mg Hemin/10^8 Cells
1	control	5	71.8	76.8
2	8	5	67.4	82.0
3	28	5	68.8	202
4	52	5	68.8	1869
5	100	5	72.2	542

This appearance of the ALA-synthetase was completely blocked by the previous administration of Actinomycin D. On the contrary, when Actinomycin D was injected six hr after an erythropoietin injection, it did not have this inhibitory effect. These results also support the above suggestion on the relationship between the ALA-synthetase activity and the stem cell differentiation.

Successive appearances of ALA-dehydrase and IPCE activity were demonstrated after an injection of erythropoietin. ALA-dehydrase activity, which was present in the spleens of hypertransfused mice before an EP injection, is considered to be derived mainly from circulating red cells.

Exogenous erythropoietin has been reported to be cleared rapidly from the general circulation.[11] Therefore, it is felt that the appearance of ALA-dehydrase and IPCE may not need the existence of erythropoietin.

It is tempting to speculate that the erythropoietin acts as derepressor on the repressed hemoglobin synthesis in undifferentiated stem cells. One of the enzymes appearing first as a result of the de-repression could be the ALA-synthetase. Stem cells thus differentiated by erythropoietin could continue hemoglobin synthesis by successive de-repression of the enzymatic process pertaining to the hemoglobin synthesis.

Summary

To study the process of erythroid differentiation, the occurrence of ALA synthetase, ALA dehydrase, and iron-protoporphyrin-chelating enzyme (IPCE), the enzymes in the heme synthetic pathway were assayed in the spleen of hypertransfused mice after erythropoietin injection. ALA synthetase activity appeared on the eighth hour after the injection, followed by an increase of ALA dehydrase and IPCE on the 12th and 28th hour. Actinomycin D, when administered with erythropoietin, completely abolished the appearance of ALA synthetase activity. The inhibitory effect was not observed when Actinomycin D was administered six hr after erythropoietin injection. It is demonstrated in our present paper that a series of enzyme activities of heme synthesis occurs in differentiating stem cells, and erythropoietin-induced appearance of ALA synthetase is dependent on DNA-directed RNA synthesis.

Acknowledgment

The authors thank Dr. G. Urata, the National Institute of Public Health, Tokyo, Japan, for his kind advice during the course of this work.

References

1. Jacobson, L. O., E. Goldwasser, L. F. Plzak & W. Fried. 1957. Proc. Soc. Exp. Biol. Med. **94:** 243.
2. Alpen, E. L. & D. Cranmore. 1957. *In* The Kinetics of Cellular Proliferation. F. S. Stohlman, Jr., Ed. : 290. Grune and Stratton. New York, N. Y.
3. Erslev, A. J. 1959. Blood **14:** 386.
4. Lajtha, L. G. & R. Oliver. 1960. *In* CIBA Foundation Symposia on Hemopoiesis. G. E. W. Wolstenholme and M. O'Connor, Eds. : 289. J. and A. Churchill. London.
5. Nakao, K., F. Takaku, S. Fujioka & S. Sassa. 1966. Blood **27:** 537.
6. Fried, W., L. F. Plzak & L. O. Jacobson. 1957. Proc. Soc. Exp. Biol. Med. **94:** 237.
7. Granick, S. & G. Urata. 1963. J. Biol. Chem. **238:** 821.
8. Gibson, K. D., A. Neuberger & J. J. Scott. 1955. Biochem. J. **61:** 618.
9. Nishida, G. & R. F. Labbe. 1959. Biochim. Biophys. Acta **31:** 519.
10. Granick, S. & R. D. Levere. 1964. *In* Progress in Hematology. Vol. IV. C. V. Moore and E. B. Brown, Eds. : Grune and Stratton. New York and London.
11. Weintraub, A. H., A. S. Gordon, E. L. Becker, J. F. Camiscoli & J. Contrara. 1963. Blood **22:** 808.

THE PARTICIPATION OF SPLEEN AND BONE MARROW IN THE RECOVERY OF MICE AFTER SUPPRESSION OF ERYTHROPOIESIS BY ACTINOMYCIN D*

José L. Scaro

Institute of High Altitude Biology, National University of Tucuman, San Salvador de Jujuy, Argentina

The course of the erythropoietic suppression by actinomycin D in female mice was studied after a large dose of the antibiotic, 0.4 μg/g. i.v.[1] Each of the following observations is based on 20–50 mice. Forty-eight hours after actinomycin the spleen was devoid of differentiated elements except for a few pronormoblasts. A large cohort of pronormoblasts reappeared at 72–96 hours. Changes in spleen weight and in its ^{59}Fe uptake capacity (measured three hr after tracer administration) followed a similar pattern. From 48 to 72 hr the ^{59}Fe incorporation by the spleen was completely abolished. An increase in spleen weight slightly preceded the resumption of ^{59}Fe incorporation capacity. At 96 to 120 hr a complete line of erythroid precursors was again present in the spleen, which then showed a typical picture of hyperplasia. At the same time the ^{59}Fe uptake in the spleen reached a value significantly above normal.

In unmanipulated control mice the three-hour ^{59}Fe incorporation in bone marrow is about twice that of the spleen. After actinomycin it declined in 48 hr, but at its lowest point it still retained about one-fourth its normal capacity to take up ^{59}Fe. While the recovery in bone marrow follows chronologically the same pattern as that of the spleen, its magnitude of response is significantly lower and does not reach normal values even at 120 hours. Splenectomy did not substantially modify this pattern of bone marrow response.

* This work was supported in part by a grant from the National Council of Scientific and Technical Investigation, Argentina.

Reference

1. Keighley, G. & P. H. Lowy. 1966. Blood **27**: 637.

CHANGES IN THE ERYTHROPOIETIN-RESPONSIVE CELL AFTER EXPOSURE TO IRRADIATION*

George Hodgson and Irma Eskuche

Facultad de Ciencias, Universidad de Chile, Santiago, Chile

The main effect of erythropoietin (EP) is to induce the differentiation of stem cells into recognizable erythrocyte precursors.[1,2] It has been postulated that the erythropoietin-responsive cell population is a type II B[3] with a major random fraction of cells in Go (state of rest). Cells in Go can either differentiate or be triggered into cell cycle G_1–S–G_2 and subsequently undergo mitosis.[4] The differentiating cells enter a period of limited growth, going through a few cycles before ending up as a cell incapable of further division.[4] The in vitro study of synchronized mammalian cell population shows that there are marked changes in radiosensitivity during cell cycle.[5] Observations of the effects of radiation on the capacity to respond to EP might thus shed some light as to which part of the cycle the cells respond to EP. If they could respond at any time during Go, then, assuming radiosensitivity is invariant during this phase, ionizing radiation should produce similar effects when given at different times prior to EP. If, on the other hand, response could only occur for a fixed time soon after mitosis, the increase in radiosensitivity at mitosis should be observed. Useful additional information on the characteristics of the EP-responsive stage may be obtained by comparing the results of irradiation with the effects of colchicine and actinomycin D, known to block mitosis[6] and DNA-dependent RNA synthesis,[7] respectively.

Effects of Ionizing Radiation on the Response to Erythropoietin

FIGURE 1 shows the effects of irradiation of 100 and 200 r ^{137}Cs (6 r/min) on the response of fasted rats to 20 units EP.[8] A clear-cut maximum in radiosensitivity is seen when irradiation is given about four hr before EP. This maximum could be interpreted as occurring four hr before cells become responsive to EP. After this, maximum radiosensitivity drops rapidly to a minimum which lasts for about six hr, then increases again to a new maximum at 16 hours. From this moment on, radiosensitivity drops constantly. Studies of the effects of ^{137}Cs irradiation on the response of normal rats to EP show the same pattern of change in radiosensitivity.[9] A study of the effects of 150 r of 250 kv x-rays (120 r/min) on the response to EP of plethoric mice (TABLE 1) shows that similar changes of radiosensitivity occur in this assay system. However, the depression produced by x-rays given 24 hr prior to EP is greater than that observed in γ-irradiated fasted rats while that produced 24 hr after EP is less.

The difference in radiosensitivity observed when irradiation is given four hr before EP and four hr after could be the result of changes in D_{37}, or a change in the shoulder of the "survival" curve, or a combination of these two mechanisms. When irradiation is given before EP, varying EP dose has no effect on the shape of the "survival" curve (FIGURE 2, a & b). The D_{37} for nonfasted rats, 137 r (FIGURE 2, a), however, is greater than that of fasted animals, 87 r (FIGURE 2, b). When irradiation is given after EP, "survival" increases with EP dose (FIGURE 2, c & d). In nonfasted rats injected with 20 units EP prior to irradiation the "survival" curve shows a shoulder and an increase in D_{37} from 137 to 260 r (FIGURE

* Supported in part by AEC grant NYO–AT(30–1)–2488–5.

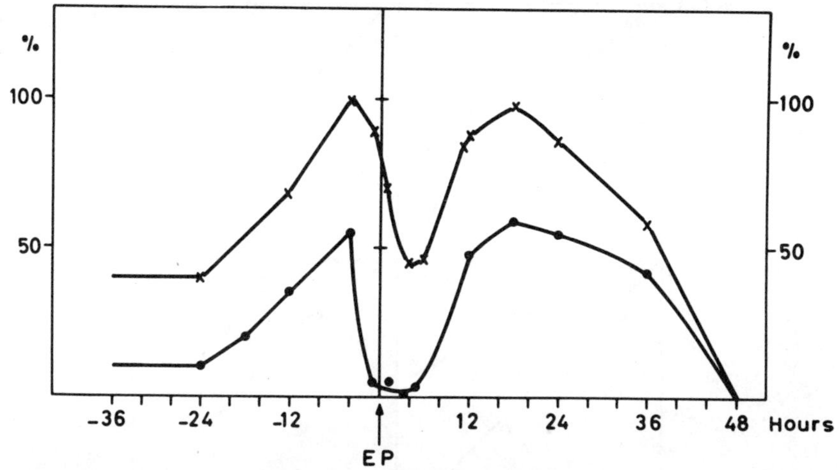

FIGURE 1. Effects of γ irradiation (6 r/min, ●——● 100 r, x——x 200 r) on response of fasted rats to EP. Total fast four days. EP injected after two days. ^{59}Fe at end of fourth day.[8]

$$\text{Ordinate: } \frac{IUER_o - IUER_x}{IUER_o} \times 100$$

Abscissa: Time of irradiation in relation to EP injection.
o = Nonirradiated.
x = Irradiated.
IUER = iron uptake erythroid tissue.

2, c). Survival curves for fasted rats injected with EP prior to irradiation show a greater D_{37}, 137 r, than that for preirradiated fasted animals. Increase of EP dose from 5 to 20 units enlarges the shoulder. The changes observed in the "survival" curves for erythropoiesis in rats injected with exogenous EP prior to irradiation are similar to those obtained in rats irradiated with high endogenous levels of EP.[10] The most sensitive animals are those with lowest endogenous levels at the moment of irradiation as transfused mice[10] and the fasted rats of this communication.

The marked difference in radiobiological behavior described above probably reflects different mechanisms. Cells hit by irradiation after coming in contact with EP may or may not express their response to EP, depending on the dose of the latter. At higher doses of EP the fraction of cells which go through the skipped division pathway increases and thus the chance of dying at mitosis decreases.[11]

TABLE 1

UPTAKE OF ^{59}Fe IN RBC PER ML OF BLOOD IN TRANSFUSED B10.H-2[d] • THREE-MONTH-OLD MICE*

Time of Irradiation in Relation to EP Injection								EP	Control
−24	−4	−1	+4	+8	+16	+25	+33 hr.	5 U	
1.85 ±0.3	0.52 ±0.06	1.4 0.2	4.4 0.1	1.0 ±0.1	5.1 0.5	5.6 ±0.8	4.8 ±0.8	11.6 ± 0.7	0.26 ±0.03

* Heart blood hematocrit > 60%. EP 5 units, injected five days after first transfusion; ^{59}Fe injected 48 hr later, bled 24 hr post-tracer injection. Note: In all experiments presented in this paper a pool of native plasma 9 units EP/ml obtained from phenylhydrazine-treated irradiated rats was used as the EP-containing preparation.

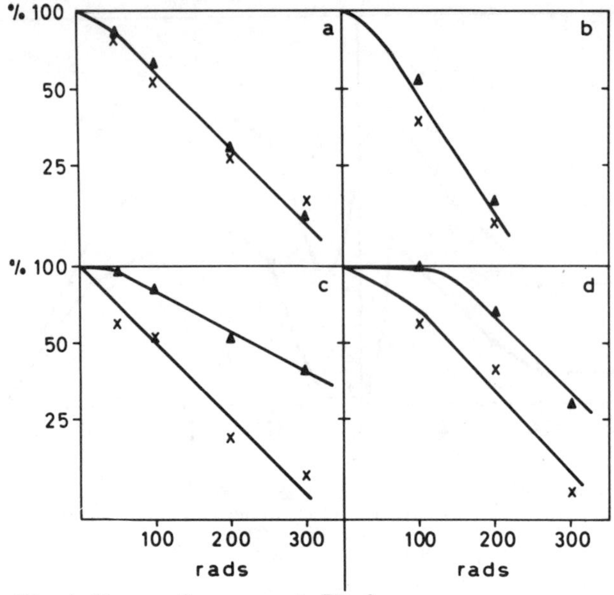

FIGURE 2. "Survival" curves for response to EP of:
a) Normal rats (x——x) and normal rats injected with 20 units EP (▲——▲) four hr after irradiation.
b) Fasted rats injected with 5 units (x——x) and 20 units EP (▲——▲) four hr after irradiation.
c) Normal rats (x——x) and normal rats injected with 20 units EP (▲——▲) six hr prior to irradiation.
d) Fasted rats injected with 5 (x——x) and 20 units EP (▲——▲) four hr prior to irradiation.

$$\text{Ordinate: } \frac{\text{I U E R}_x}{\text{I U E R}_o}\ 100$$

Abbreviations as in FIGURE 1.

If this explanation is valid, it suggests that EP-responsive cells, hit by irradiation four hr prior to EP, can either lose or retain their capacity to respond to EP and that those cells that retain the capacity are not exposed to death at subsequent divisions. Thus, going through the skipped division pathway would be of no advantage to them.

*Effect of Actinomycin D**

Actinomycin D blocks DNA-dependent RNA synthesis.[7] It is known that the earliest detectable effect of EP in rat marrow[12,13] and in the plethoric mouse spleen[14] is an increased uptake of labeled precursors into rapidly labeled RNA. Study of the effects of this drug on the response to EP could contribute useful information for analyzing the early events that occur after a stem cell is triggered into differentiation. The dose of the drug which we have chosen to use is one (0.01 μg/g) that has no effect on rapidly labeled RNA synthesis of resting liver[15] and yet is able to prevent the rise in rapidly labeled RNA synthesis and RNA polymerase activity that follows partial hepatectomy.[15] Dactinomycin® in doses of 0.016 μg/g also interferes with the entry of ascitic cells into DNA synthesis

* Kindly supplied by Merck Sharp and Dhome, Research Laboratories, Rahway, N. J. under the name Dactinomycin®.

without affecting the synthesis of those already in S phase.[15] FIGURE 3 shows the sensitivity to Dactinomycin, in doses of 0.01 μg/g i.p. once an hour for four hr, of the erythropoietic response (^{59}Fe uptake by spleen) of plethoric mice injected with 5 units EP. Sensitivity of Dactinomycin is maximum from 0–8 hr after EP injection, then diminishes sharply on either side. When the dose of Dactinomycin is raised to 0.016 μg/g, no response to EP is seen when the drug is injected from 0–8 hr after EP. The EP-responsive cell thus enters a period of extreme sensitivity to actinomycin at a time when it is least sensitive to ionizing radiation. Thus suggests that RNA synthesis triggered by EP is not an especially radiosensitive process. One may speculate that this RNA synthesis is related to the transformation of a stem cell into a proerythroblast; perhaps the newly-formed RNA may act as a depressor[17] of that segment of the genome concerned with the differentiation process. It seems probable, however, from the present results, that Dactinomycin in these doses does not interfere with synthesis of m-RNA for hemoglobin, since synthesis of this protein does not start until about 24 hr after of EP injection[18] at which time Dactinomycin does not affect the response.

Effects of Colchicine

We have observed (unpublished results) that colchicine in the doses of 2 mg/kg produces marked toxic effects in fasted rats (loss of weight, listlessness, anemia, increased erythrocyte sedimentation), and completely suppresses the

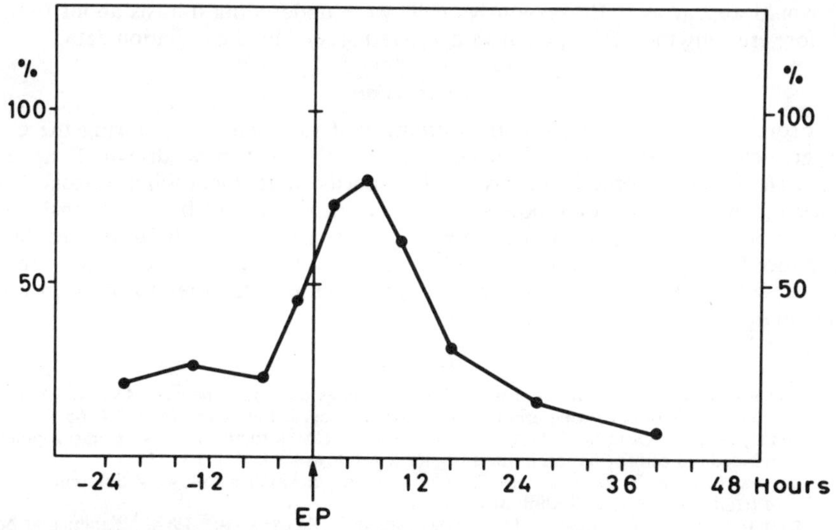

FIGURE 3. Effects of Dactinomycin 0.01 μg/g × 4, once an hour i.p. on the response of RBC-transfused mice to 5 units EP.

Ordinate: $\dfrac{S^{59}Fe_o - S^{59}Fe_A}{S^{59}Fe_o} \times 100$

Abscissa: Time of actinomycin injection in relation to that of EP injection. The time corresponds to the midpoint of the period of Dactinomycin injection.

$S^{59}FE$ = ^{59}Fe uptake by spleen measured two hr after tracer injection. Tracer injected 48 hr after EP.

● = No actinomycin.

A = Actinomycin treated.

TABLE 2

EFFECT OF COLCHICINE ON ^{59}Fe UPTAKE BY CIRCULATING RBC OF FASTED RATS THREE HR AFTER TRACER INJECTION*

Dose of Colchicine	Time of Colchicine in Relation to EP				EP	Control
	−24	−4	+4	+24 hr	20 U	
0.1 mg/kg	23.4 ± 0.6	16.8 ± 1.0	23.5 1.5	21.8 ± 1.1		
0.25 mg/kg	18.4 ± 0.6	13.9 ± 1.9	19.7 0.7	15.8 ± 2.1	23.7 ± 0.7	0.35 ±0.03
0.50 mg/kg	2.6 ± 0.6	11.0 1.5	17.0 ± 0.8	2.0 ± 0.26		

* Experimental set up as in reference no 8; colchicine given at indicated intervals prior to or after 20 units EP.

response to EP when given either at 24 and four hr before or four and 24 hr after. However, when colchicine is injected in a dose of 0.25 mg/kg, which, dissolved in its volume of distribution, would give a concentration of about 0.5 μg/ml, a clear depression of the response is obtained when injection is carried out at four hr before but not four hr after EP (See TABLE 2). It is conceivable that at this low dosage, mitotic block is the most important action of the drug.[19] If this is so, it would appear as if EP-responsive cells were undergoing mitosis about four hr before entering the EP-responsive stage, as suggested by the radiation data.

Conclusions

From the data presented, and assuming that radiosensitivity during the cycle is greatest at mitosis, the following tentative picture can be drawn. It appears as if stem cells become responsive to EP shortly after undergoing mitosis. Once they reach this stage, they become relatively radioresistant but very sensitive to Dactinomycin. This period lasts about eight hr, after which the proerythroblasts produced would be about to enter a radiosensitive phase preparatory to S.[5] Increased DNA synthesis is known to begin about 16 hr after EP both in rats[20] and in mice.[14]

References

1. FILMANOWICZ, E. & C. W. GURNEY. 1961. Studies on erythropoiesis. XVI. Response to a single dose of erythropoietin in polycythemic mice. J. Lab. Clin. Med. **57:** 65.
2. ORLIC, D., A. S. GORDON & J. A. RHODIN. 1965. Ultrastructural study of erythropoietin-induced red cell formation in mouse spleen. J. Ultrastruct. Res. **13:** 513.
3. LAJTHA, L. G. & R. OLIVER. 1962. Cell population kinetics following different regimes of irradiation. Brit. J. Radiol. **35:** 131.
4. LAJTHA, L. G., C. W. GILBERT, D. D. PORTEOUS & R. ALEXANIAN. 1964. Kinetics of bone marrow stem cell population. Ann. N. Y. Acad. Sci. **113:** 742.
5. TERASIMA, T. & L. J. TOLMACH. 1963. Variation in several responses of Hela cells to x-irradiation during the division cycle. Biophys. J. **3:** 11.
6. DUSTIN, P. 1959. The quantitative estimation of mitotic growth in the rat by the stathmokinetic (colchicine) method. *In* Kinetics of Cellular Proliferation. F. Stohlman, Ed. : 150. Grune and Stratton. N. Y.
7. REICH, E., R. M. FRANKLIN, A. J. SHATKIN & E. L. TATUM. 1962. Action of actinomycin D on animal cells and virus. Proc. Nat. Acad. Sci. **48:** 1238.
8. ESKUCHE, I. & G. HODGSON. 1965. Effect of gamma irradiation on response of fasted rats to erythropoietin. Proc. Soc. Exper. Biol. Med. **119:** 1102.

9. Eskuche, I. & G. Hodgson. 1966. Effect of gamma irradiation on the response of non-fasted rats to erythropoietin. Proc. Soc. Exper. Biol. Med. **112**: 440.
10. Eskuche, I. & G. Hodgson. 1965. Radiosensitivity of erythropoiesis as a function of its activity. Proc. Vth. Interamerican Symposium on Peaceful Applications of Nuclear Energy. Pan American Union, Washington, D. C. : 163.
11. Porteous, D. D., S. T. Hirashima & L. G. Lajtha. 1965. Modification of x-ray survival curves of stem cells by different doses of erythropoietin. Nature **206**: 204.
12. Krantz, S. & E. Goldwasser. 1965. The mechanisms of erythropoietin-induced differentiation. II. Effect on RNA synthesis. Biochim. Biophys. Acta **103**: 325.
13. Pieber-Perretta, M., W. Rudolph, M. Perretta & G. Hodgson. 1965. Effect of erythropoietin on ^{14}C-Formate incorporation into rat bone marrow RNA. Biochim. Biophys. Acta **95**: 360.
14. Hodgson, G. 1967. Synthesis of RNA and DNA at various intervals after erythropoietin injection in transfused mice. Proc. Soc. Exper. Biol. Med. **124**: 1045.
15. Lieberman, I., P. Kane & J. Short. 1965. The portal vein and the control of liver ribonucleic acid metabolism. Biol. Chem. **240**: 3140.
16. Baserga, R. R., R. D. Estensen & R. O. Petersen. 1965. Inhibition of DNA synthesis in Ehrlich ascitic cells by actinomycin D. II. The presynthetic block in cell cycle. Proc. Nat. Acad. Sci. **54**: 1141.
17. Frenster, J. H. 1965. The control of RNA synthesis within interphase chromatin. Blood **26**: 865.
18. Murialdo, H. & G. Hodgson. 1964. Síntesis de Hem y Globina en bazo de ratón policitémico después de la inyección de eritropoyetina. Proc. VI Congress Lat. Amer. Physiol. Soc. Editorial Universitaria, Santiago, Chile. : 112.
19. Puck, T. T. 1964. The studies of the life cycle of mammalian cells. Cold Spring Harbour Symposia. Quant. Biol. **29**: 167.
20. Kurtides, E. E., W. S. Rambach, H. Alt & J. C. Wurster. 1963. The effect of erythropoietin on tritiated thymidinc uptake by rat spleen. J. Lab. Clin. Med. **61**: 23.

HUMORAL EFFECTS ON MARROW CELL DIFFERENTIATION

Donald R. Korst and Janet Quirk

Department of Medicine, Madison General Hospital and University of Wisconsin Medical School, Madison, Wis.

The differentiation of the marrow stem cells into distinct cell lines appears to be determined at least in part, if not solely, by humoral regulator or stimulator systems (Jacobson, 1962). Whether a single multipotential cell or several types of stem cells are responsible is undetermined. It does appear fairly well established that a cell of the lymphoid reticuloendothelial system (RES) present in the bone marrow space or spleen will differentiate into hematopoietic tissue. The cell has morphologic characteristics of a lymphocyte with dense chromatin nucleus, deeply basophilic cytoplasm and a striking ability to concentrate tritiated thymidine in the blood or in the hypoplastic marrow following irradiation or drug injury (Gordon, 1959; Jacobson, 1960; Lange, 1964; Linman, 1960; Stohlman, 1959; & Thomas, 1965).

The purpose of the experiment has been to study the effects of drug or x-ray depression of marrow stem cells in the mouse by measuring responsiveness to stimulation by erythropoietin or a leukocytosis-inducing factor(LIF).

Erythropoietin Preparation and Assay

A human urine extract source of erythropoietin was prepared by E. D. Nicolaides, Department of Chemistry, Parke, Davis Research Laboratories, using the method of Winkert and Gordon. Urine was collected in 24-hour periods with 10 ml phenol per 2 l plastic bottle, pooled, a frozen (Winkert, 1961). The patient is a 48-year-old white male with paroxysmal cold hemoglobinuria due to a macroglobulin whose mean hematocrit has been 20 to 25%. He did not receive transfusions or specific therapy during the time of urine collection and an occasional urine contained hemoglobin. The urine protein was precipitated with 80% ethanol at $-15°$ C overnight, spun down, and dialyzed at 4° C before freeze-drying. The crude material was then run through a DEAE cellulose column at 4° C in .05 M sodium phosphate buffer at pH 7.4 to absorb erythropoietin. The active material was then eluted from the column with phosphate buffer plus 0.13 NaCl at 4° C at pH 7.4. The final material was then dialyzed and freeze-dried. Up to 200 mg of crude protein material was recovered in 1 liter of urine, 1 g of which yielded up to 140 mg of material with erythropoietin activity of 3.6 units/mg.

The erythropoietin was assayed in 10-week-old male white stock Ha/ICR mice (A. R. Schmidt, Madison) that had been rendered polycythemic either by hypertransfusion of autologous cells or by two weeks' exposure to 0.4 atm in a hypobaric chamber (Gurney, 1963). Hematocrits were between 60 to 70% when used and the reticulocytes were down to 0.1 to 0.2% by five days after removal from the chamber. Erythropoietin was injected i.p. each day for two days and radioiron (1 μc = 0.14 μg) given i.p. eight hr later. Forty hr later the mouse was bled by open heart puncture and three 0.3 ml aliquots counted for radioiron activity, a hematocrit, and a wet preparation slide for reticulocyte counting. Results were expressed as the mean and one standard deviation of groups of five mice for each determination. Each assay contained a saline control group and an erythropoietin standard control group. The standards used were a human urine extract provided by Dr. M. Cotes of the British Research Council (specific activity 1 unit/1.48 mg dry weight or 10 units/ampule) as Standard B or phenylhydrazine anemic sheep plasma extract (Standard A–Armour, University of Chicago–specific activity 22 units/mg), and a human urine extract provided by Dr. R. Lange (specific activity 2.5 units/mg). These values were determined by our laboratory assay method.

Studies were also carried out in the fasted mouse system suggested by Porteous *et al.* (1963). This method is to observe the endogenous erythropoietin response in the mouse following restoration of food after a fasting period sufficient to stop erythropoiesis.

Reticulocyte counting was facilitated by using acridine-orange staining of fresh wet erythrocytes, counting a field of cells under dark-field or bright light and then counting the same field under ultra-blue fluorescence (Vander, 1963). We believe this method provides an accuracy of $\pm$ 0.1% and the normal human reticulocyte level is 2.0%, the normal mouse, 4.0%, and the polycythemic mouse, 0.2%.

Spleen Colony Method

Inbred strain dd/s mice (A. R. Schmidt, Madison, female, age 12 weeks) maintained *Pseudomonas*-free were irradiated in groups of 12 to a total body dose of 750 r through a cone in the standard large field of a General Electric Maxitron 300. The methods used are modifications of Till and McCullouch (1964) and of Lewis and Trobaugh (1964). Twenty-four mice were used in each experiment. Syngeneic bone marrow from four femora of nonirradiated mice was placed in Hank's solution so that 0.25 ml contained 100,000 nucleated cells. This was injected into the tail veins of the irradiated mice within several hours after exposure (Lewis, 1964; McCulloch, 1960; Till, 1961). About 50% of these mice survived for nine days when they were sacrificed and the femur marrow removed for microscopic films. Films were also made of blood and imprints of liver and spleen and prepared with Wright's stain. In three-fourths of the mice the spleen contained up to 15 discreet pinhead colonies that could be snipped free and imprinted on a glass slide. Mice with one spleen colony or less were rejected.

Autoradiographs were performed by taping the imprint slides to a thin piece of black paper or aluminized mylar and this placed against the sensitive surface of Polaroid 410 (10,000 speed) film for 24 hours. The mice had been given 15 μc of ^{59}Fe two hr prior to sacrifice so that there would be maximum uptake of iron in the erythroid areas of the spleen hematopoietic colonies.

Leukocytosis-inducing factor (LIF) was prepared by gavaging the peritoneal space of the rat with 25 or 10 ml solution of 0.1 ml Piromen (Baxter–Pseudomonas polysaccharide) diluted to 1000 ml sterile 0.9% saline for human use (Fruhman 1960; & Gordon 1960). This was done three times daily for three days so that about eight to ten billion leukocytes were removed. The serum of the rat was then frozen and used in 0.5 ml aliquots. In the normal mouse given erythropoietin or normal rat serum the total white blood count is 5000 $\pm$ 1000 cells/mm^3 thousand at hourly intervals up to 24 hours. Mice given 1.0 ml of LIF serum developed PMN leukocytosis to 16,000 cells/mm^3 maximum at four hr and sustained at 24 hours.

Erythropoietin Assay

The reproducibility of the assay methods in our laboratory was satisfactory but it was always necessary to include a control group of saline and one that received a known erythropoietin standard substance (Gurney, 1960). We believe that the simultaneous use of reticulocyte counting as well as radioiron turnover added

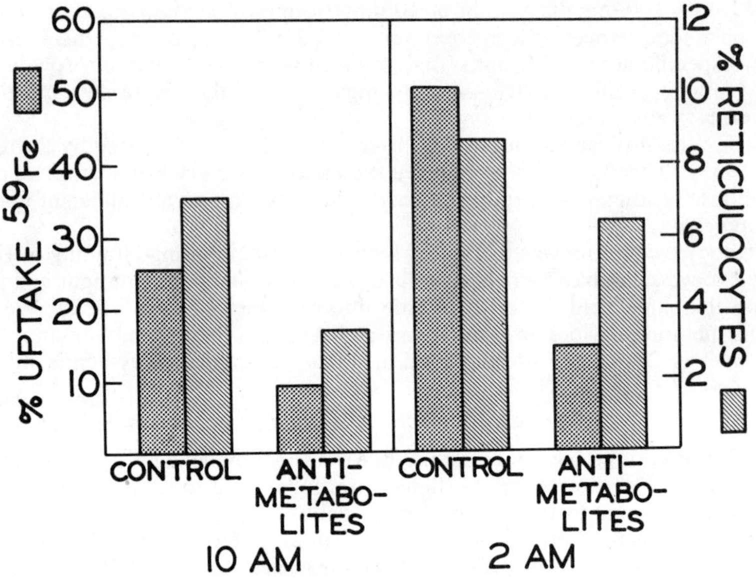

FIGURE 1. The influence of circadian (diurnal) rhythm on bone marrow mitotic activity during normal variation (control 10 AM and 2 AM) and the effect of antimetabolite drug depression. The relative marrow depression is the same at the low mitosis time (10 AM) and at the maximum mitosis time (2 AM). However, the absolute depression is different at different times for the same drug dose.

to the reliability of the assay. The results correlated very well with relative differences of activity of various sources of erythropoietin.

In the normal mouse there is a sharp reticulocytosis maximum at two hr following a single dose of erythropoietin. We believe this represents a release phenomenon. In the polycythemic mouse the rise is gradual to a maximum at three days and represents the effect of the increased stem cell erythroid differentiation (Gurney, 1961). Correlation between relative reticulocyte rise and radioiron uptake increase seemed better in the transfusion-induced polycythemic mice but the difference was probably not significant.

Careful attention must be paid to the time of injection and the time of taking blood specimens because of the influence of circadian or diurnal rhythms in mice and rats (Clark, 1965: Mauer, 1965). The effect of a given dose of stimulator or marrow-depressing drugs may have a different absolute effect depending on the time of injection (FIGURE 1). The relative effect is similar but the absolute effect is different because there may be varying numbers of cells in mitosis depending on the circadian rhythm. It seems likely that the stimulating or the cytotoxic depressant act at the stem cell level during the synthesis period before mitosis.

The Parke, Davis material (PD) was assayed against the British Research Council Standard B (BRC-B) (FIGURES 2 & 3). These studies indicated that the best extract was X77B with an activity of 3.6 units/mg dry weight (TABLE 1). It is of interest that 2.0 mg of PDX77B produced a response nine times that of PDX45 but at a 10 mg dose the response was only four times greater, suggesting either the presence of some inhibitor in the crude material or that an optimum response was in effect. The inhibitor contamination seems more likely. Extraction

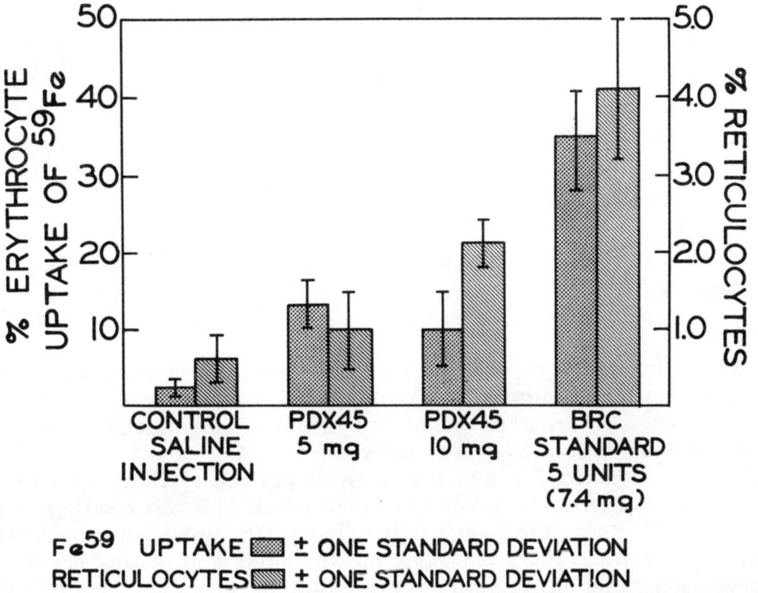

FIGURE 2. The erythropoietin assay comparing a human urine extract (PDX45) with the British Research Council Standard B. Each group represents eight polycythemic mice out of hypobaric chamber five days. Two injections of test material given i.p. a day apart.

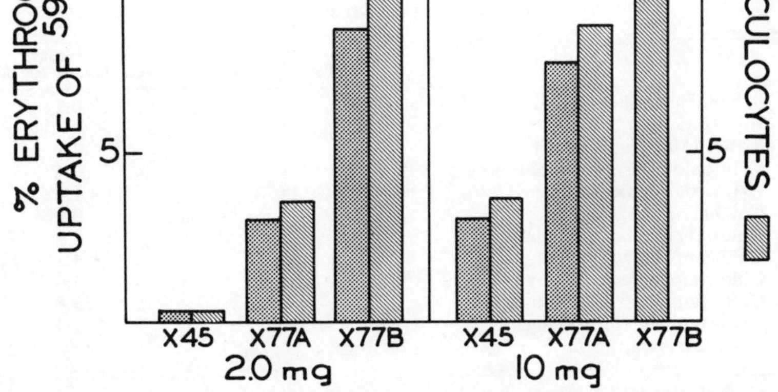

FIGURE 3. Erythropoietin assay in the hypobaric chamber polycythemic mouse comparing a further purified extract of human urine (PDX77).

TABLE 1

COMPARISON OF ACTIVITY OF ERYTHROPOIETINS

Material	Source	Specific Activity Cobalt Units/mg Protein
Standard A	Sheep serum	22 units/mg
Standard B	Human urine	10 units/amp 0.68 units/mg
Dr. Lange's lab	Urine extract	2.5 units/mg
PDX45	Human urine	0.4 units/mg
PDX77A	Human urine	1.2 units/mg
PDX77B	Human urine	3.6 units/mg

of erythropoietin from urine seems to vary from one urine collection to another. This observation has been noted by Gurney in this conference. Large scale erythropoietin extraction programs might best seek anemic animal sera or human urine collection under controlled conditions.

It has been suggested that administration of purified erythropoietin extracts bound with normal serum would enhance their effect. This was investigated with PDX45 and did not result in significantly different ^{59}Fe uptake or reticulocytosis than when the extract was given alone i.p. Inhibitors and plasma effects must also depend somewhat on the purity of the erythropoietin (Gardner, 1966; Whitcomb, 1965).

Studies of this type emphasize the necessity of using standardized erythropoietin materials and the increased accuracy obtained by the simultaneous counting of reticulocytes 72 hr after the first dose of erythropoietin and 48 hr after the second dose plus measurement of blood radioactivity 40 hr after ^{59}Fe injection. Some slight increase in iron or reticulocyte values might be obtained by extending the time of bleeding to three or four days rather than two days after the last dose of erythropoietin. However, the data obtained here seem to be equally significant at either time.

TABLE 2

ATTEMPTS TO BLOCK STEM CELL DIFFERENTIATION RESPONSE TO ERYTHROPOIETIC STIMULUS*

	Percent ^{59}Fe Uptake	Percent Reticulocyte Response
Saline control	5	0.5
Erythropoietin	31	3.2
X-ray, 150 r (total body)	1	0.3
Cytotoxic drugs, maximum dose	1	0.4
Cytotoxic drugs, ½ dose	15	1.4
Colchicine, 1.65 mg/k	5	0.5
Chloramphenicol, 360 mg/k	23	2.1
Chloramphenicol, 800 mg/k	30	4.2
Chloramphenicol, 1000 mg/k	31	3.6
Chloramphenicol, 1300 mg/k	30	3.8
Chloramphenicol, 800 mg/k + cytotoxic ½ dose	17	1.4

* Assays performed in both the hypobaric chamber polycythemic mouse given exogenous erythropoietin and in the fasted mouse given food and tested at time of maximum endogenous erythropoietin response.

Marrow Stem Cell Differentiation

The radioiron and reticulocyte response to a given dose of a known and standardized batch of erythropoietin extract is reproducible in controlled experiments to a degree that one can measure the blocking or depressing effect of drugs or x-ray. The same method has more recently been used to measure the erythropoietin inhibitory action of certain sera. Almost complete inhibition of erythropoietin response is effected by administration of colchicine, x-ray, or antimetabolites (cyclophosphamide, methotrexate and 5-fluorouracil) injected 24 hr prior to the first dose of erythropoietin. The animals own response to endogenous erythropoietin can be measured in the refed starved animal and the effect of depression can be ascertained by administering drugs or x-ray just prior to the refeeding time. Both of these methods were used to obtain the data in TABLE 2.

The degree of depression by a drug can be assayed by this method as shown by the lesser ^{59}Fe and reticulocyte depression in the half maximum-tolerated dose of antimetabolites compared to the full dose. Varying doses of chloramphenicol were studied because in humans it has been postulated that erythropoiesis may be inhibited at a somewhat different stage of stem cell differentiation than antimetabolites. If chloramphenicol inhibits RNA formation in the erythrocytic cells after differentiation has been determined, then there should be no effect on erythropoietin action, assuming that erythropoietin acts at the earliest level of the stem cell differentiation. There was no evidence of inhibition of erythropoietin by chloramphenicol up to doses of 1300 mg/k and doses above this resulted in death of the animal. There was no additive inhibitory effect of half doses of antimetabolites plus chloramphenicol (TABLE 2).

Following total body irradiation animals were divided into two groups: those that received syngeneic marrow transplants (x-ray+x-plant or x-x groups), and those that received x-ray but no bone marrow (x-ray+o or x-o group). Animals of each group were sacrificed daily and tissue cytology done on blood, marrow, spleen and liver. Prior labeling of the marrow cells of the x-plant was carried out with ^{51}Cr (Na chromate) to determine the distribution in the grafted mouse. At fifteen min after i.v. injection of the labeled cells, it was found that 20% of the cells were in the blood, spleen and marrow.

Cytologic studies of the x-x and x-o groups revealed general cell death and destruction during the first five days with evidence of new RES activity at the fifth to eighth days. The control x-o groups uniformly all died by the seventh or eighth day without evidence of marrow cell regeneration. However, this group did show good evidence of liver cell regeneration. The changes in blood by the eighth or ninth day were the same in both x-x and x-o groups and then in the x-x group a distinct lymphocyte increase followed by return of all normal blood

TABLE 3

THE INFLUENCE OF HUMORAL STIMULATION ON SPLEEN COLONY DIFFERENTIATION IN POSTRADIATION MICE GIVEN SYNGENEIC MARROW TRANSPLANT

	Colonies	Erythroid Colony	Myeloid Colony	Mixed Myeloid-Erythroid Colony	Animals
Noninjected control	286	34%	31%	35%	26
Erythropoietin-injected	90	55	24	21	11
Leukocytosis-inducing factor	23	26	48	26	5

cells by the tenth to 12th days. The spleen changes in the x-o groups showed some RES activity by the fifth day but no marrow cell growth prior to death on the seventh to ninth days. The x-x group spleen imprints showed the same early RES changes but by the seventh to ninth days, colonies of marrow cell growth associated with increased cellularity of lymph and R-E cells appeared.

The bone marrow changes in both groups were decreased cellularity maximum at the fifth day and evidence of R-E cell hyperplasia with basket cells, nuclear debris and undifferentiated primitive cells. Only in the x-x group at the seventh to tenth days was there evidence of increasing marrow cell differentiation and this was well correlated with those animals who survived beyond nine days. Marrow regeneration seemed to lag slightly behind spleen colony development but in general the regeneration seemed to be occurring simultaneously in the entire blood organ.

Careful study of the cytology of the spleen colonies revealed that the majority of cells in the small, early or single colonies were of RES and lymphoid variety with a scattering of erythroid or myeloid differentiation. Only very early colonies were composed solely of RES tissue and all late colonies had some evidence of differentiation. Earlier experiments, where animals had received transplants composed of 200,000 nucleated cells, such a rapid and widespread regeneration of hematopoietic tissue occurred that specific colonies could not be counted or studied independently. The use of 100,000 marrow cells in the x-plant in our experiments was convenient to work with and gave an average of 11 colonies per x-x group mouse. However, at this amount of marrow x-plant only about

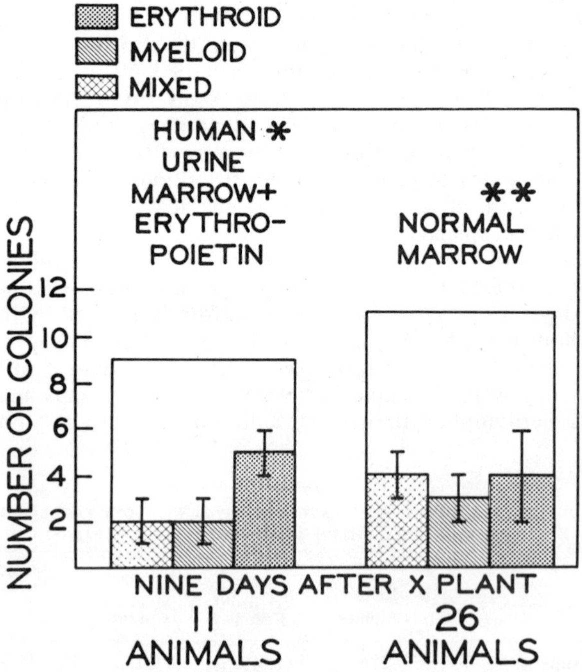

FIGURE 4. Humoral influence of erythropoietin on the differentiation pattern of spleen colonies in the lethally irradiated mouse given a syngeneic marrow transplant. The normal animals either received no injection or were given normal mouse plasma.* Marrow + human urine erythropoietin;** normal serum + marrow.

1964). The bone marrow appears to be at least 10 to 13 times as potent a source of CFU than the spleen and perhaps 36 times that of blood cells (Smith, 1966; Vos, 1966). As spleen colonies form, new cells are also developing simultaneously in the marrow and also may develop in a transplanted spleen, suggesting that only certain tissue beds are capable of supporting stem cell differentiation and growth (Wolf, 1966). Influence of the erythroid differentiation pattern, the size, and the number of erythroid colonies may be related to dose of erythropoietin administered and may be more readily influenced in a plethoric mouse (O'Grady, 1966). Our experiments were carried out in mice with hematocrits in the normal range.

It has been postulated that for a marrow x-plant to produce visible modules, there must be a doubling in size every 13 hr for eight and one-half days (Bush, 1965). This would suggest that there are an ample number of cells being influenced into a clone of differentiation at all times during marrow regeneration and that there must be a production of many new stem cells. Sublethal irradiation to mice femurs, followed by a lethal dose eight days later (except for shielding of one femur), suggests that there were increased numbers of stem cells stimulated and that a humoral regulation of stem cell population had occurred (Gurney, 1965). Whether these observations are due to specific stimulators or to reduction of specific inhibitors has not been answered to date.

Our observations would suggest that spleen colonies in the x-ray x-plant mice may not represent a clone of marrow cells, but a rapidly regenerating nodule of marrow type stem cells influenced to erythroid or myeloid differentiation purely on a random basis depending on concentration of the humoral regulator substance. The proper fertile moment of the stem cell to differentiate and the transient nature of the humoral regulator suggest that rapid regeneration of marrow tissue may be a biologic function of increased levels of humoral regulators (or removal of inhibitors) plus a rapid proliferation of fertile stem cells. Models of stem cell differentiation for erythropoiesis include a more primitive compartment of stem cells feeding the erythroid pool (Stohlman, 1962), and the ability of the erythroid pool to provide a rapid new cell by shunting or bypassing the usual dividing pool (Lajtha, 1955). Such a rapidly regenerating pool of stem cells must provide a feedback mechanism perhaps by release of an inhibitor from differentiated erythroid cells (Lajtha, 1962).

The spleen colony studies and our ability to alter differentiation patterns suggest that the clusters of stem cells are pluripotential and not predestined to be only erythroid- or myeloid-determined (Gurney, 1962). Bone marrow cells and, to a lesser degree, spleen cells may contain a type of stem cell capable of being derepressed by humoral regulators to form bone marrow cells. It would follow that a specific site of action of the humoral regulator would be to stimulate or allow formation of specific new messenger RNA (Gallien-Latigue, 1965, Krantz, 1965). The diverse potential of the single stem cell or primitive cell is also suggested by the observation that a single cell or germinal center may produce several immunoglobulins (Mellors, 1963). It is probable that the pool of regenerating stem cells may contain cells that are capable of differentiation but in an unresponsive state. This would be analogous to the observation of immunologic responsiveness of sublethal x-rayed rats to specific agglutinin production (Feldman, 1963), and that according to the "elective" theory (Medewar, 1960), every cell is genetically predetermined to form every type of antibody. One could postulate that some marrow stem cells in an unresponsive state could be stimulated or directed to differentiation along a specific cell line.

A plausible hypothesis would be that marrow cell humoral regulators act primarily to stimulate or derepress a specific type of marrow or spleen stem cell to develop along erythroid, myeloid or megakaryocyte cell lines. This same stimulation would also necessarily include a stimulus for the stem cell to reproduce itself.

A purely secondary function of humoral regulators might be to shorten the G_1 phase of already differentiated cells in order to accelerate erythropoiesis (Kretchmar, 1966). The new population of regenerating stem cells may be more sensitive to humoral regulation, or perhaps, temporarily, there are more stem cells during regeneration. It is also quite probable that there is a transient overproduction of marrow stem cells, which results in an overproduction of erythroid and myeloid cells before the feedback or inhibitor mechanisms are restored. As a protection against too much erythroid or myeloid overproduction, there are many ineffective cells produced, such as basket cells and poorly differentiated cells that probably are quite short-lived.

Conclusions

A human urine extract of erythropoietin (PDX77B) has been used with a potency of 3.6 units/mg. Simultaneous ^{59}Fe uptake and acridine-orange fluorescence of reticulocytes in polycythemic mice correlate well with various erythropoietin sources and are relatively reproducible but still require control of saline and control of an erythropoietin standard.

Studies of blocking stem cell differentiation or of spleen colony differentiation in the irradiated syngeneic marrow-transplanted mouse suggest that the primary effect of humoral regulation is at the stem cell level. This primary stimulus appears to provide more stem cells that are randomly differentiated depending on humoral regulation; a secondary effect of the stimulus may be to accelerate an increased production along normal pathways perhaps by shortened cell cycles.

References

BECKER, A. J., E. A. MCCULLOCH & J. E. TILL. 1963. Cytological demonstration of the clonal nature of spleen colonies derived from transplanted mouse marrow cells. Nature **197:** 452.

BIERMAN, H. R. 1964. Leucopoiesis in health and disease. Ann. N. Y. Acad. Sci. **113:** 511.

BOGGS, D. R., J. C. MARSH & G. E. CARTWRIGHT. 1966. Humoral regulation of neutrophil release from bone marrow. Amer. Soc. Clin. Invest. : 16.

BUSH, R. S. & W. R. BRUCE. 1965. The radiation sensitivity of a transplanted murine lymphoma as determined by two different assay methods. Radiat. Res. **25:** 503–513.

CLARK, R. H. & D. R. KORST. 1965. Diurnal variation in bone marrow mitoses and reticulocytes. Clin. Res. **13:** 411.

COTES, P. M. & D. R. BANGHAM. 1961. Nature **191:** 1065.

COTES, M. 1966. Studies on a human urine extract erythropoietin standard B. Personnel communications. To be published in 1966 Bulletin of World Health Organization.

DELMONTE, L. & R. A. LIEBELT. 1965. Granulocytosis-promoting extract of mouse tumor tissue: partial purification. Science **148:** 521–523.

DELMONTE, L., A. G. LIEBELT & R. A. LIEBEL. 1966. Granulopoiesis and thrombopoiesis in mice bearing transplanted mammary cancer. Cancer Res. **26:** 149–159.

FELDMAN, M., A. GLOBERSON & D. NACHTIGAL. 1963. The reactivation of the immuno response in immunologically suppressed animals. *In* Conceptual Advances in Immunology and Oncology. : 427–448. Harper & Row. New York.

FRUHMAN, G. F. 1960. Neutrophil mobilization into peritoneal fluid. Ann. N. Y. Acad. Sci. : 1753–1760.

GALLIEN-LARTIGUE, O. & E. GOLDWASSER. 1965. On the mechanism of erythropoietin-inducing differentiation. II. Effect on RNA synthesis. Biochem. Biophys. Acta **103:** 324.

GALLIEN-LARTIGUE, O. & E. GOLDWASSER. 1965. On the mechanism of erythropoietin-induced differentiation. I. The effects of specific inhibitors on hemoglobin synthesis. Biochem. Biophys. Acta **103:** 319.

GARNER, E. C., S. WRIGHT, J. P. LEWIS & R. R. MOORES. 1966. Erythropietin potentiation by serum proteins. A.S.C.I. Proceedings of the Amer. Soc. Clin. Invest. : 39.

GORDON, A. S. 1959. Hematopoietic mechanisms. Ann. N. Y. Acad. Sci. **77**: 407–820.

GORDON, A. S., R. O. NERI, C. D. SIEGEL, B. S. DORNFEST, E. S. HANDER, J. LOBUE & M. EISLER. 1960. Evidence for a circulating leucocytosis-inducing factor (LIF). AGTA Haematologicia. 23–32.

GORDON, A. S., E. S. HANDLER, C. D. SIEGEL, B. S. DORNFEST & J. LOBUE. 1964. Plasma factors influencing leukocyte release in rats. Ann. N. Y. Acad. Sci. **113**: 766–789.

GURNEY, C. W. & C. PAN. 1960. Studies on erythropoiesis. XIII. A comparison of methods of bioassay of erythropoietin in human plasma. J. Lab. Med. **55**: 67–72.

GURNEY, C. W., N. WACKMAN & E. FILMANOWICZ. 1961. Studies on erythropoiesis. XIII. Some quantitative aspects of the erythropietic response to erythropoietin. Blood **17**: 531-546.

GURNEY, C. W., L. G. LAJTHA & R. OLIVER. 1962. A method for investigation of stem-cell kinetics. Brit. J. Haemat. **8**: 461.

GURNEY, C. W. 1963. Effect of radiation on the mouse stem cell compartment in vivo. Perspect. Biol. Med. **VI**: 233–245.

GURNEY, C. W. & W. FRIED. 1965. The regulation of numbers of primitive hemopoietic cells. Proc. Nat. Acad. Sci. **54**: 1148–1153.

HARRIS, P. F., V. MENKIN & J. M. YOFFEY. 1956. The action of leukocytosis-promoting factor on the blood and bone marrow of the guinea pig. Blood **11**: 243–249.

JACOBSON, L. O., C. W. GURNEY & E GOLDWASSER. 1960. The control of erythropoiesis advances in internal medicine. Dock & Snalper, Eds. **10**: 297.

JACOBSON, L. O. & M. DOYLE. 1962. Erythropoiesis. Grune & Stratton. New York & London.

KRANTZ, S. B. & E. GOLDWASSER. 1965. On the mechanism of erythropoietin-inducing differentiation. II. Effect on RNA synthesis. Biochem. Biophys. Acta **103**: 324.

KRETCHMAR, A. L. 1966. Erythropoietin: Hypothesis of action tested by analog computer. Science **152**: 367–369.

LAJTHA, L. G., R. OLIVER & C. W. GURNEY. 1962. Kinetic model of a bone-marrow stem cell population. Brit. J. Haemat. **8**: 442.

LANGE, R. D. & V. PAVLOVIC-KENTERA. 1964. "Erythropoietin" in Progress in Hematology. Vol. IV. Moore, C. V. & E. B. Brown, Eds. Grune & Stratton. New York.

LINMAN, J. W. & F. W. BETHEL. 1960. Factors controlling erythropoiesis. Charles C. Thomas. Springfield, Ill.

LEWIS, J. P., M. P. FARNES, M. ALBALA & F. E. TROBAUGH, JR. 1964. Transplantation potential of fresh and stored hematopoietic tissue as estimated by standard in vitro techniques. Ann. N. Y. Acad. Sci. **114**: 601–716.

LEWIS, J. P. & F. E. TROBAUGH, JR. 1964. Marrow transplantation: Spleen colonization as a model for the study of the quantitative effect of freezing on the basic repopulating unit. Proc. 9th Congress Int. Soc. Blood Transf., Mexico, : 274–280.

MAUER, A. M. 1964. Diurnal variaton of proliferative activity in the human bone marrow. Blood **2**: 1.

MCCULLOCH, E. A. & J. E. TILL. 1960. The radiation sensitivity of normal mouse bone marrow cells, determined by quantitative marrow transplantation into irradiated mice. Radiat. Res. **13**: 115–125.

MCCULLOCH, E. A. & J. E. TILL. 1962. The sensitivity of cells from normal mouse bone marrow to gamma radiation in vitro and in vivo. Radiat. Res. **16**: 822–832.

MCCULLOCH, E. A. & J. E. TILL. 1964. Proliferation of hemopoietic colony-forming cells transplanted into irradiated mice. Radiat. Res. **22**: 383–397.

MEDEWAR, P. B. 1960. Theories of immunological tolerance. Ciba Foundation Symposium on Cellular Aspects of Immunity. Little, Brown & Co. Boston.

MELLORS, R. C. & L. KORNGOLD. 1963. The cellular origin of human immunoglobulins. J. Exp. Med. **118**: 387.

MENKIN, V. & M. A. KADISH. 1942. Presence of the leukocytosis-promoting factor in the circulating blood. Arch. Path. **33**: 193–197.

O'GRADY, L. F., J. P. LEWIS, R. LANGE & F. E. TROBAUGH, JR. 1966. Factors influencing differentiation of transplanted hematopoietic tissue. Exper. Hematol. **9**: 77–80.

O'GRADY, L. F., J. P. LEWIS, R. D. LANGE & F. E. TROBAUGH, JR. 1966. The role of erythropoietin in establishing a hematopoietic graft. Amer. Soc. Clin. Invest.

PORTEOUS, D. D., R. ALEXANIAN & L. R. LAJTHA. 1963. The fasted mouse in the study of bone marrow stem-cell genetics. Int. J. Rad. Biol. **7**: 195.

SMITH, L. H. & S. D. PHILLIPS. 1966. Relative erythropoietic competence of isologous bone marrow cells, spleen cells, peripheral leucocytes and peritoneal fluid cells. Exper. Hematol. **9**: 86–88.

STOHLMAN, F., JR. 1959. The Kinetics of Cellular Proliferation. Grune & Stratton. New York.

STOHLMAN, F., JR. 1962. Regulation of erythropoiesis. Trans. N. Y. Acad. Sci. **24**: 312.

TILL, J. E. & E. A. MCCULLOCH. 1961. A direct measurement of the radiation sensitivity of normal mouse bone marrow cells. Radiat. Res. **14**: 213–222.

TILL, J. E. & E. A. MCCULLOCH. 1964. Repair processes in irradiated mouse hematopoietic tissue. Ann. N. Y. Acad. Sci. **114**: 115–125.

THOMAS, E. D., T. M. FLIEDNER, D. THOMAS & E. P. CRONKITE. 1965. The problem of the stem cell: Observations in dogs following nitrogen mustard. J. Lab. Clin. Med. **54**: 704-803.

VANDER, J. B., C. A. HARRIS & R. E. ELLIS. 1963. Reticulocyte counts by means of fluorescence microscopy. J. Lab. Clin. Med. **62**: 132–140.

VOS, O. 1966. Mortality of radiation chimeras in relation to the number of transplanted bone marrow and lymph node cells. J. Nat. Cancer Inst. **36**: 431–443.

WHITCOMB, W. H. & M. Z. MOORE 1965. The inhibitory effect of plasma from hypertransfused animals or erythrocyte iron incorporation in mice. J. Lab. Clin. Med. **66**: 641–651.

WINKERT, J., A. S. GORDON & F. WINKERT. 1961. Purification and physiologic effects of human urinary erythropoietin. Trans. N. Y. Acad. Sci. **24**: 135–139.

WOLF, N. S. & J. J. TRENTIN. 1966. Fate of hemopoietic colony forming units present in intravenously injected suspensions of bone marrow. Fed. Proc. : 601. Abstr.

EFFECT OF ERYTHROPOIETIN ON RETICULOCYTE RELEASE FROM THE ISOLATED PERFUSED RAT SPLEEN*

Burton S. Dornfest, George W. Cooper and Albert S. Gordon

Department of Anatomy, State University of New York, Downstate Medical Center, Brooklyn, N. Y., and Departments of Biology, New York University and The City College of the City University of New York, New York, N. Y.

Erythropoietin (ESF) has been previously shown to stimulate the discharge of reticulocytes from bone marrow contained within isolated perfused hind limbs of the rat[1] and the rabbit.[2] The present study was undertaken to determine whether ESF has a similar effect on reticulocyte release from the isolated perfused rat spleen.[3] In the untreated animal, the number of reticulocytes in the rat spleen is reported to be significantly higher than that in the peripheral blood.[4,5] The rat spleen, although not normally a site of red blood cell production, can, under appropriate stimulation, become an active erythropoietic organ.[6–8] Spleens used for perfusion were obtained from rats rendered anemic by bleeding to insure that sufficient numbers of reticulocytes were available so that a response to erythropoietin could be readily detected. Moreover, since the purpose of the investigation was to determine and compare the effect of ESF on reticulocyte release from the spleen with that observed in the bone marrow, it seemed desirable that erythrogenic spleens be used since the bone marrow is an active erythropoietic site.

Materials and Methods

Male rats of a modified Sprague-Dawley strain weighing 325–375 g were used in all phases of the investigation. Spleen perfusions were accomplished by introducing small diameter polyethylene cannulas into the splenic artery and vein through incisions made in the aorta and hepatic portal vein. Subsequent to cannulation the spleens were removed and placed in a 37° C moist chamber. The operative procedure used for isolating the spleens is described in detail elsewhere.[3] The perfusion apparatus employed (see FIGURE 1) is a modification of that used previously in bone marrow perfuson studies.[1,9] A mechanical shaker maintained the perfusate cellular elements suspended in the blood reservoir in place of the magnetic stirrer used in the earlier bone marrow investigation. A peristaltic action-type pump** perfused 50–60 ml of isologous leukocyte-depleted heparinized blood (only 30–100 white cells per cu mm) through the isolated spleens at rates of 0.2–0.3 ml/min. Leukocyte-depleted blood was used since the centrifugation procedure employed for depleting blood of leukocytes also lowered the reticulocyte values in the perfusate (see TABLE 1). Detection of both reticulocytes and leukocytes released from the spleen into the venous effluent was thus facilitated. Spleens were perfused for periods of up to four hr and once blood was passed through the spleen, it was collected and not recirculated. Samples were taken periodically to determine the percentage and absolute numbers of cells in the perfusate. Reticulocytes were identified from blood smears treated with new methylene blue. Reticulocyte percentage was obtained by counting a minimum of 3,000 red blood cells, 1500 on each of two prepared slides.

Spleens used for perfusion were obtained from rats that had been bled by cardiac puncture on each of two consecutive days and sacrificed either 72 or 96 hr

* Supported by grants AM09321–02 (B.S.D.) and HE 03357–09 (A.S.G.) from the National Institutes of Health.

** Harvard Apparatus Company, Dover, Mass.

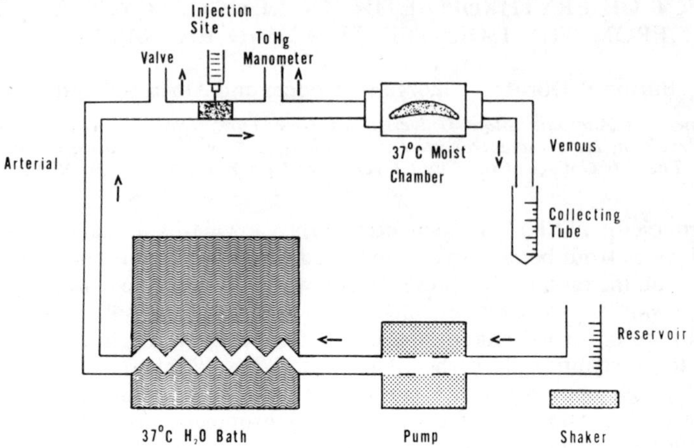

FIGURE 1. Schematic diagram of perfusion apparatus.

after the initial bleeding. A total of 8–10 ml of blood was removed from each animal. In two cases, spleens were obtained from nonbled animals. The rats were injected i.p. with 3 μc ^{59}Fe chloride (specific activity 11.5–15.8 mc per mg) 22 to 24 hr prior to sacrifice to label the spleen reticulocytes. Periodically, samples were taken from the blood passed through the spleen and counted in a well-type scintillation counter, as both cellular and plasma fractions, to determine the release of labeled cells. The cellular fractions were washed three times with isotonic saline prior to counting.

In the first group of five experiments (group I, chronic exposure), 21 units of Step 3 sheep plasma ESF† in 0.2 ml sterile isotonic saline were added to the blood reservoir in four perfusions. In a fifth experiment an equivalent amount of 6.3 mg of sheep plasma glycoprotein prepared from normal plasma by the three-step procedure of Goldwasser and White[10] was added as a control in place of the active fraction. This preparation assayed in the plethoric mouse,[11] showed no erythropoietic activity. In order to determine reaction time to the test materials introduced accurately, they were brought rapidly to the spleen by opening a valve to draw off the perfusate in the arterial tubing (see FIGURE 1). The pre-existing arterial pressure and flow rate through the spleen was maintained during this procedure. In a second group of seven experiments (group II, acute exposure), 10 units of ESF in 0.1 ml sterile isotonic saline was injected in five cases through the arterial tubing immediately proximal to the arterial cannula. In two other experiments an equivalent amount of 3 mg of inactive plasma glycoprotein was administered by the same route. In both groups I and II the test materials were added following the first hr of perfusion. The terms "chronic" and "acute" are used in reference to the duration of exposure of the spleen to ESF. In the chronic group, after the first hr, the spleens were continuously perfused with ESF. The total amount in the perfusate, based on the blood volume of a 350 g rat, was equivalent to approximately 7 units. In the acute group, 10 units of ESF in approximately 1 ml of perfusate was administered and was probably washed rapidly out of the spleen by the perfusate. In two experiments, one from group I

† Armour Pharmaceuticals, Lot K147192, kindly supplied by the National Heart Institute of the National Institutes of Health.

TABLE 1
EFFECT OF ESF ON RETICULOCYTE RELEASE FROM ISOLATED PERFUSED SPLEENS

Expt. No. and Treatment	Hrs. Sacrificed after Initial Bleeding	Percent Retics. in Reservoir (Arterial) Blood	Percent Retics. in Effluent (Venous) Blood						
			Before Addition of ESF or Inactive Glycoprotein		After Addition of ESF or Inactive Glycoprotein				
			15 Min	30 Min	1st Hr	2nd Hr	3rd Hr	4th Hr	After Epinephrine† Addition
I. Chronic (Reservoir)									
A. ESF									
1	72	1.40	2.80	2.30	1.64	0.85	0.88		
4	72	1.50	2.80	2.20	1.82	1.04	0.75	0.98**	1.60
6	72	0.19	3.00	2.10	1.45	1.09	0.87		
7	96	1.00	2.10	1.95	1.76	1.35			
B. Glycoprotein									
2	72	1.90	1.60	1.45	1.02	0.92	0.68		
II. Acute (injected)									
A. ESF									
8	Nonbled	0.48	0.77	0.67	0.60	0.45	0.47		
9*	Nonbled	3.04	1.63	1.99	2.01	1.79	2.52	2.26	
10	72	0.57	1.09	0.83	0.84	0.56	0.40	0.44**	1.56
15	72	1.40	1.20	1.08	1.02	1.12			
16	96	0.90	2.54	2.34	2.06	1.45	1.08		
B. Glycoprotein									
13	96	1.10	2.80	2.05	1.66	1.09	1.35	1.67	
14	96	0.75	1.40	1.30	1.06	1.29	1.70		
III. No materials added									
5	72	1.53	1.79	1.48	1.10	0.41	0.35		
11	72	0.78	1.71	1.51	1.06	0.64	0.56		
12	96	0.33	1.96	1.85	1.39	0.75			

* In experiment 9 leukocyte-intact blood perfusate was used.

** These counts were made after the first three hr and 45 min of perfusion.

† The absolute number of reticulocytes was markedly increased following epinephrine addition as evidenced by the increased number of red blood cells in the venous effluent (see FIGURE 2).

(experiment 4) and the second from group II (experiment 10), 1 γ of epinephrine in o.1 ml isotonic saline was added to the perfusates three hr and 45 min after initiation of perfusion by injection through the arterial tubing. In a third group of three control experiments (group III) no test materials were added.

At the end of each experiment the spleen was fixed in 10% formalin and following standard histological procedure, stained with hematoxylin and eosin.

Results

Maintenance of physiological integrity under perfusion conditions was noted in these studies and, as reported elsewhere,[3] by the ability of the spleen to: (1) consume oxygen, as evidenced by the dark red color of the venous effluent (indicating low oxyhemoglobin content) in contrast to the bright red coloration of the blood in the arterial cannula; (2) utilize glucose; (3) respond preferentially to vasoactive agents; and (4) phagocytize damaged erythrocytes. No architectural distortion of the histology of the perfused spleens was evident from examination of histological sections.

TABLE 1 (groups I, II) indicates that neither the addition of ESF nor the inactive plasma glycoprotein increased, or induced any appreciable rise in the percentage of reticulocytes in the venous blood over values recorded during the initial hour of perfusion prior to their addition. However, a nonspecific action may be exerted by glycoprotein since the reticulocyte values after the addition of either the active or inactive fractions were higher than those in group III where glycoprotein was not added. Little or no radioactivity was found in the plasma fraction of the perfusate. No significant alteration was discernible in the pattern of cellular radioiron counts in the venous blood following the addition of ESF (FIGURE 2) or the inactive protein when compared to control experiments in which these test materials were not introduced. A direct relation was found to exist between the radioactivity in the venous effluent and the numbers of reticulocytes and nucleated cells (leukocytes and probably early erythroid cells) discharged from the spleen (see FIGURE 1). The ^{59}Fe activity in the venous effluent showed a nearly exponential fall in radioactivity with time.

The percentage of reticulocytes present in the venous effluent varied among experiments. In most cases, with the exception of two experiments (experiments 8 & 9), in whch spleens were obtained from nonbled rats, the percentage of reticulocytes in the venous effluent during the first hr of perfusion was greater than in the reservoir blood (TABLE 1). This was particularly true for the first 15 to 30 min of perfusion. During the second to fourth hr the percentages of reticulocytes in the venous effluents were less than during the first hour. Quantitation of the release of reticulocytes was complicated by the possibility that reticulocytes initially present in the arterial blood were trapped in the spleen.[12] An estimate of the maximum number of reticulocytes released from the spleen during a four-hour period was about 1.5 billion. In two experiments (experiments 4 & 10), addition of epinephrine at the end of the fourth hr of perfusion markedly increased the concentration of ^{59}Fe-labeled cells, reticulocytes and probably nucleated erythroid cells, in the venous effluent. Addition of epinephrine demonstrated that in spite of the prior release, labeled cells were still retained in the spleen after four hr of perfusion. This was also indicated, based on values for nonperfused control spleens, by finding 40 to 60% of the radioiron activity present prior to perfusion in the perfused spleen at the end of the experiment. Epinephrine also resulted in an elevated red blood cell count and a decrease in flow rate. The number of mature red blood cells in the perfusate, which

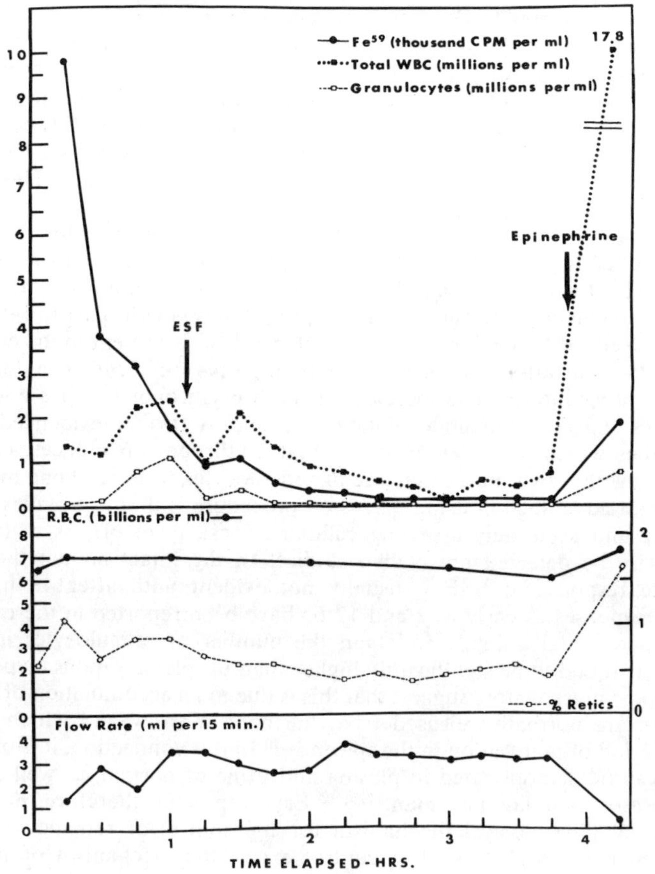

FIGURE 2. Pattern in a representative experiment (no. 10) of cellular levels and radioiron activity in initially leukocyte-depleted nonradioiron-containing blood perfused through an isolated spleen. Each point represents an assessment of the venous effluent for the parameters indicated. Arrows indicate addition of test materials.

averaged between 6 and 7 million per cu mm, otherwise remained relatively constant. A representative pattern of cell release and response to epinephrine is shown in FIGURE 1 (experiment 10). The number of nucleated cells released from the spleens of bled rats varied considerably among the individual experiments. During a standard three-hour experiment 35 to 65 million cells were discharged of which 5% were granulocytes and approximately 60 to 70% resembled small lymphocytes. Many cells were difficult to classify and approximately 5 to 15% of the cells released resembled late normoblasts. The pattern of leukocyte release from isolated perfused spleens of nonanemic rats has been reported elsewhere.[3]

Discussion

The present study indicates that sheep plasma ESF does not induce reticulocyte release from the isolated perfused rat spleen. This is in contradistinction to the stimulatory influence reported on reticulocyte release from isolated perfused rat and rabbit bone marrow.[1,2] One can only speculate on the mechanism of action of this short-term ESF effect on bone marrow reticulocytes and on its lack of influence in the spleen. An appreciation of the problem can best be obtained by first briefly reviewing the literature that prompted our perfusion investigations. Jandl[5] has reported that the rat spleen, not normally a site of erythropoiesis, contains significantly increased numbers of reticulocytes as early as 24 hr after a single bleeding (8.0% as compared to 3.8% in the untreated rat). This increase can best be explained on the basis of sequestration in the spleen of reticulocytes released from the bone marrow since 24 hr is not sufficient time for splenic stem cells to produce reticulocytes. In the same study, the distribution of ^{59}Fe in the 24-hour bled rat showed a reciprocal relation between femoral marrow ^{59}Fe (a decrease) and splenic ^{59}Fe (an increase), presumably due in part to reticulocyte migration.[5] Related to the findings is the fact that ESF is present in the circulating blood at 1 to 24 hr after a single bleeding in amounts sufficient to be detected by most assay procedures.[13] The increases in both erythropoietin titer and splenic reticulocytes suggest a possible relationship. This is further evidenced by perfusion studies which have demonstrated that erythropoietin induces, either immediately or within two hr, a discharge of reticulocytes from the bone marrow.[1,2] An important advantage in using perfusion procedure is that it provides a means for directly and accurately assessing cellular release from organs which might not otherwise be detected by in vivo studies. In the intact animal the earliest reticulocyte response to ESF is usually not evident until after 48 hours.[14-16] However, responses as early as 2 and 12 hr have been reported in the rat.[17,18] In normal experimental animals and man the number of reticulocytes in splenic pulp blood is found to be significantly higher than in splenic venous or peripheral blood.[4,5] Some investigators suggest that this is due to an accumulation of reticulocytes which are normally released from the bone marrow and which undergo a further period of maturation in the spleen.[12,19] In this connection, it is of interest that ESF can be demonstrated in plasma and urine of normal, as well as of hypoxic laboratory animals and man.[11,20-22] Erythropoietin, therefore, may represent a normal physiological mechanism for the control of reticulocyte release from the bone marrow. If such a control exists, the mechanism of its action remains to be elucidated. A probable explanation may be that the factor alters some characteristic of the reticulocyte, such as the adhesiveness,[23] or the electrokinetic properties.[24] It is conceivable that alterations of these properties, which are known to undergo changes as the cell matures,[23,24] are prerequisites for reticulocyte release. Jandl[5] suggested that the adhesiveness characteristic of immature red cells may be due to the presence of transferrin, or an immunologically similar substance, on the cell membrane. One might speculate that ESF, perhaps by mobilizing iron bound to transferrin for hemoglobin production in the immature red cell, alters the cell membrane adhesiveness.

In the perfusion studies, the finding that ESF will stimulate reticulocyte release from the bone marrow but not from the spleen could be due to inherent differences in these tissues for sequestering cells. The absence of an ESF effect on reticulocyte release from the normal and the erythrogenic spleen could be explained on the basis of the acknowledged splenic ability to trap and sequester immature red cells selectively. Assuming that the reticulocytes produced in the bone marrow and in the erythrogenic spleen have identical characteristics, reticulocyte release from the spleen need not occur in response to ESF if the cells are immediately arrested in the splenic parenchyma. That a reticulocytosis is usually not evident in the intact animal until after 48 hr[14-16] is undoubtedly a reflection of the time required for stem cells in the bone marrow and spleen to produce sufficient numbers of reticulocytes. In the rat and perhaps in other species, the spleen seems limited to the number of reticulocytes it can retain, which would contribute indirectly to the peripheral reticulocytosis reported at 48 hours. No more than approximately 2 percent of newly released red cells, a very small fraction of the total, was found to be arrested in the spleens of bled rats at any one time.[5] The addition of ESF to the isolated perfused spleen would have no relation to the arresting capacity of the spleen for reticulocytes, since no new reticulocytes could be produced under its stimulus during the short duration of the experiment. The percentage of reticulocytes in venous effluents collected from erythrogenic, but not normal, spleens was considerably higher during the first 15–30 min of perfusion than the percentage in the arterial (reservoir) blood. Since the bled rats had a pronounced peripheral reticulocytosis, the increase in the venous effluent could be at least partially attributed to the "washing out" of peripheral reticulocytes that were circulating through that organ when the animal was sacrificed. This would be a reflection of the limited capacity of the spleen for arresting reticulocytes. In the bone marrow perfusion studies, an initial "washing out" of reticulocytes was not evident.[1] That reticulocytes were present in the erythrogenic spleen after three to four hr of perfusion was demonstrated when the addition of epinephrine to the perfusate markedly elevated the venous concentration of these cells.

Alternative explanations for the absence of an ESF effect on reticulocyte release from the erythrogenic spleen that might be (1) a sufficient number of reticulocytes are not available so that a response to the factor could be detected, although this seems precluded by the response to epinephrine, or (2) the spleen inactivates the factor. Another possibility is that the factor "conditions" the spleen to retain reticulocytes, which has some basis on the finding that a smaller percentage of reticulocytes are retained in the spleen of the normal rather than the bled rat.[5]

A pharmacological effect of the ESF tested and the possibility that the results obtained in the current spleen perfusion and the earlier bone marrow studies are associated with some nonspecific impurity in the preparations cannot be excluded. In this connection, a rapid reticulocytosis can accompany heart failure[25] or be induced by procedures such as air encephalography.[26] The relation of such responses to the observed short-term effects of ESF on reticulocyte release from the bone marrow is obscure.

In conclusion, no discernible difference was evident between the effect of the inactive glycoprotein or sheep plasma ESF on reticulocyte release from the perfused spleen. Neither the inactive nor active glycoprotein was found to increase reticulocyte values in the perfusate above the levels present prior to their addition. An attempt has been made to assess and relate the current results with the short-term effect of ESF on reticulocyte release observed in bone marrow perfusion studies. In this regard, proposals are offered as to the possible action of ESF in relation to reticulocyte retention and release.

References

1. Gordon, A. S., J. LoBue, B. S. Dornfest & G. W. Cooper. 1962. Reticulocyte and leukocyte release from isolated perfused rat legs and femurs. *In* Erythropoiesis. L. O. Jacobson, Ed. Grune & Stratton. New York, N. Y.
2. Fisher, J. W., G. Lajtha, A. S. Buttoo & D. D. Porteous. 1965. Direct effects of erythropoietin on the bone marrow of the isolated perfused hind limbs of rabbits. Brit. J. Haem. **11:** 342.

3. DORNFEST, B. S. & S. J. PILIERO. 1966. Mechanisms of leukocyte production and release: VII. Factors influencing leukocyte release from isolated perfused rat spleens, with special reference to the effects of vasoactive agents. J. Lab. Clin. Med. **68:** 577.
4. BERENDES, M. 1959. Th proportion of reticulocytes in the erythrocytes of the spleen as compared with those of circulating blood, with special reference to hemolytic states. Blood **14:** 558.
5. JANDL, J. H. 1960. Th agglutination and sequestration of immature red cells. J. Lab. Clin. Med. **55:** 663.
6. RAMBACH, W. A., J. A. D. COOPER & H. L. ALT. 1953. Nucleic acid metabolism of the bone marrow and spleen in the rat: the effect of x-ray and the effect of hypoxia, U.S.A.F. Air Univ. School of Aviation Medicine, project number: 21–3501–0001, report numbers 1 and 2.
7. GURNEY, C. W., N. WACKMAN & E. FILMANOWICZ. 1961. Studies on erythropoiesis: XVII. Some quantitative aspects of the erythropoietic response to erythropoietin. Blood **17:** 531.
8. KURTIDES, E. S., W. A. RAMBACH, H. L. ALT & J. C. WURSTER. 1963. Effect of erythropoietin on tritiated thymidine incorporation by the rat spleen. J. Lab. Clin. Med. **61:** 23.
9. DORNFEST, B. S., J. LOBUE, E. S. HANDLER, A. S. GORDON & H. QUASTLER. 1962. Mechanisms of leukocyte production and release: II. Factors influencing leukocyte release from isolated perfused rat legs. J. Lab. Clin. Med. **60:** 777.
10. GOLDWASSER, E., W. F. WHITE & K. B. TAYLOR. 1962. Further purification of sheep plasma erythropoietin. Biochim. Biophys. Acta **64:** 487.
11. MIRAND, E. A., A. H. WEINTRAUB, A. S. GORDON, T. C. PRENTICE & J. T. GRACE, JR. 1965. Erythropoietic activity of untreated and deproteinized normal human plasma. Proc. Soc. Exp. Biol. Med. **118:** 823.
12. CROSBY, W. H. 1963. Hyposplenism: an inquiry into normal functions of the spleen. Ann. Rev. Med. **14:** 349.
13. GORDON, A. S. 1959. Hemopoietine. Physiol. Reviews **39:** 1.
14. GALLAGHER, N. I. & R. D. LANGE. 1960. Site of action of erythropoietin. Clin. Res. **8:** 280.
15. FILIMANOWICZ, E. & C. W. GURNEY. 1961. Studies on erythropoiesis. XVI. Response to a single dose of erythropoietin in polycythemic mice. J. Lab. Clin. Med. **57:** 65.
16. STOHLMAN, JR. F. 1961. Humoral regulation of erythropoiesis. VI. Mechanism of action of erythropoietine in the irradiated animal. Proc. Soc. Exp. Biol. Med. **107:** 741.
17. WINKERT, J., A. S. GORDON & E. WINKERT. 1961. Purification and physiological effects of human urinary erythropoietin. Trans. N. Y. Acad. Sci. **24:** 135.
18. FRUHMAN, G. J. & S. FISCHER. 1962. The short-term effects of a single dose of erythropoietin on reticulocytes in starved rats. Separatum Exper. **18:** 1.
19. AMOROSI, E. L. 1965. Hypersplenism. Seminars in hematology **2:** 249.
20. REICHLIN, M. & W. J. HARRINGTON. 1960. Studies on erythropoietin. I. Demonstration of erythropoietin in normal plasma. Blood **16:** 1298.
21. FINNE, P. H. 1965. Erythropoietin in concentrates of urine from healthy persons. Brit. Med. J. **1:** 697.
22. MANN, D. L., M. L. SITES, R. M. DONATI & N. I. GALLAGHER. 1965. Erythropoietic-stimulating activity during the first ninety days of life. Proc. Soc. Exp. Biol. Med. **118:** 212.
23. KEY, J. A. 1921. Studies on erythrocytes with special reference to reticulum, polychromatophilia and mitochondria. Arch. Int. Med. **28:** 511.
24. DOLJANSKI, F. & N. SCHULMAN. 1964. Electrokinetic properties of cells in growth processes: II. The size distribution and electrophoretic mobilities of the maturing rat red blood cell. Exp. Cell Res. **36:** 605.
25. GERKE, O. 1935. Das Verhalten der roten Blutkorperchen, Insbesondere der Retikulocyten in 1,000 m Seehohe. Ztschr. Klin. Med. **128:** 630.
26. ISTAMANOWA, T. & CHUDOROSCHEWA. 1930. Uber die Wirkung des Adrenalins auf das rote Blutbild. Ztschr. Ges. Exper. Med. **71:** 212.

ERYTHROPOIETIN AND ERYTHROPOIESIS IN ISOLATED PERFUSED HIND LEGS OF RATS: A PRELIMINARY STUDY*

Joseph LoBue, Francis C. Monette, James F. Camiscoli, Albert S. Gordon and Po-Chuen Chan

Department of Biology, Graduate School of Arts and Science, New York University, New York, N. Y.

This paper presents preliminary data relating to the mechanism(s) by which erythropoietin (ESF) produces significant increases in absolute numbers of marrow erythroblasts in short-term, isolated hind leg perfusions. This apparent direct effect of ESF has been demonstrated repeatedly in perfusion studies performed in rats[1–3] and dogs.[4]

The rationale of the experimental approach used for these experiments is illustrated in FIGURE 1. Rat hind legs were perfused with blood containing ESF. The legs were obtained from rats whose marrow erythroid precursors were "tagged" prior to perfusion by injections of ^{55}radioiron (^{55}Fe). It was assumed that if the ESF induced erythroblastosis during these perfusions, it would most likely be due to either (1) cell division of preexisting erythroblasts; (2) differentiation, during perfusion, of nonerythroid cells into recognizable erythroblasts; or (3) mobilization and redistribution of erythroid marrow from preperfusion locations not readily accessible to sampling (e.g. metaphyseal, epiphyseal marrow) to the more available diaphyseal marrow region. Since the erythroid marrow was prelabeled with ^{55}Fe prior to perfusion, some insight into the underlying mechanisms of ESF action was anticipated. This was because ^{55}Fe, due to its low energy emissions (6 kev Roentgen rays and 5–6.5 kev Auger electrons), could be utilized for high resolution autoradiography.[5] Hence, if cell division had occurred during the ESF-perfusion, a decrease in grain count should have been detected when nonperfused leg marrow autoradiograms were compared to those of perfused marrow. On the other hand, if there had been a stimulation of differentiation, a decrease in the proportions of labeled erythroblasts (labeling index) should have resulted due to influx of originally nonerythroid, and hence non-^{55}Fe-labeled, cells into the erythroid compartment, with no decrease in grain count expected. Finally, if a redistribution of marrow red cell precursors had occurred during ESF-perfusion, no change in labeling profile should have occurred since this would have involved a shifting of erythroid marrow already tagged prior to perfusion.

Materials and Methods

Hind Leg Perfusion Technique. This procedure has been described in detail by Gordon *et al.*[2] and Dornfest *et al.*[6] Following anesthesia and heparinization, the rat's right leg was amputated at the level of the acetabulum. The femoral diaphyseal marrow of this nonperfused ("control") leg was quantified[7,8] and served as the standard for comparison of effects of perfusion. The left leg was then perfused through a cannula inserted into the iliac artery, and the effluent perfusate collected from the cannulated inferior vena cava. After initiation of perfusion, the leg was isolated from the rest of the carcass by amputation. The isolated hind leg and perfusate were maintained at 37° C.

* Supported by grant 5–R01–HE03357–09 from the National Heart Institute of the National Institutes of Health, U.S.P.H.S.

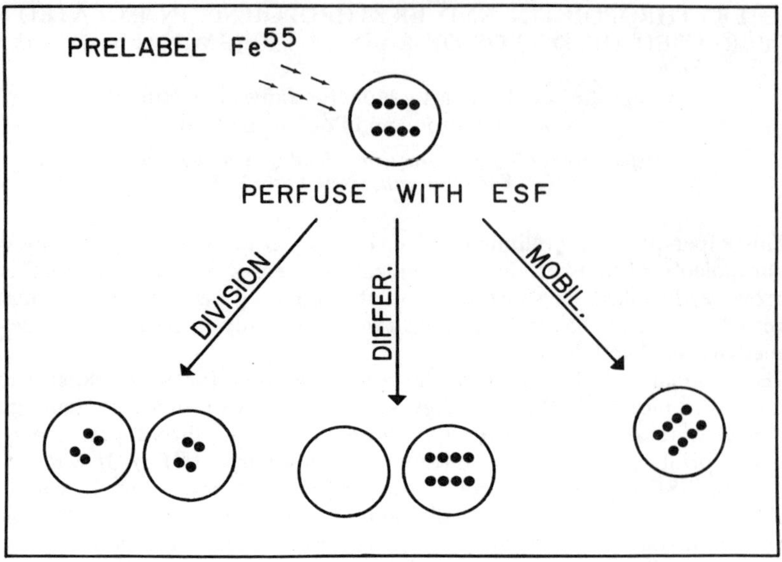

FIGURE 1. Diagram illustrating the experimental design. Circles indicate erythroblasts; black dots within circles schematize autographic grains. Abbreviations: DIFFER. refers to differentiation; MOBIL. refers to mobilization or redistribution. See text for detailed explanation.

In the present study, two hind legs were perfused for 3.5 hr with recirculated, reoxygenated whole blood containing 0.3 units of Step III sheep plasma ESF** per ml of perfusate. In experiment 1, 85 ml of perfusate was recirculated at a rate of 1.5–2.2 ml per min and in experiment 2, 100 ml was recirculated at 1.8–2.5 ml per min. The rats used for perfusion (250–290 g Long-Evans males) were injected i.p. with 24 μc ^{55}Fe (Sp. Act. 2 mc per mg Fe, obtained from the Radiochemical Centre, Amersham, England) 24 hr prior to perfusion. The heparinized whole blood used for perfusions was collected from ether-anesthetized Long-Evans female rats via abdominal aortic puncture.

^{55}Fe Autoradiography. Femoral marrow from control (i.e., nonperfused, contralateral legs) and perfused legs was quantified, and smears made for autoradiography. All smears were fixed in methanol, prestained with benzidine to differentiate hemoglobin-containing erythroid precursors,[8] dipped in Kodak NTB-2 nuclear track liquid emulsion and exposed in light-proof boxes for 42 days at 5° C. Following photographic processing, the smears were counterstained with Giemsa stain using the procedure of Monette *et al.*[9] A typical ^{55}Fe autoradiogram is shown in FIGURE 2. As can be seen, the autoradiographic resolution is comparable to that obtained with tritium.

Determination of background fogging was made from examinations of 33 photomicrographs of ^{55}Fe autoradiograms taken at random using Polaroid 46-L projection film. After removing all images of marrow cells from the photomicrographs by careful excision with a scalpel, the number of background grains in each photograph was tallied and the total area represented determined by relating

** Armour and Co., lot K–147–137. Preparation supplied by the National Heart Institute of the National Institutes of Health, U.S.P.H.S.

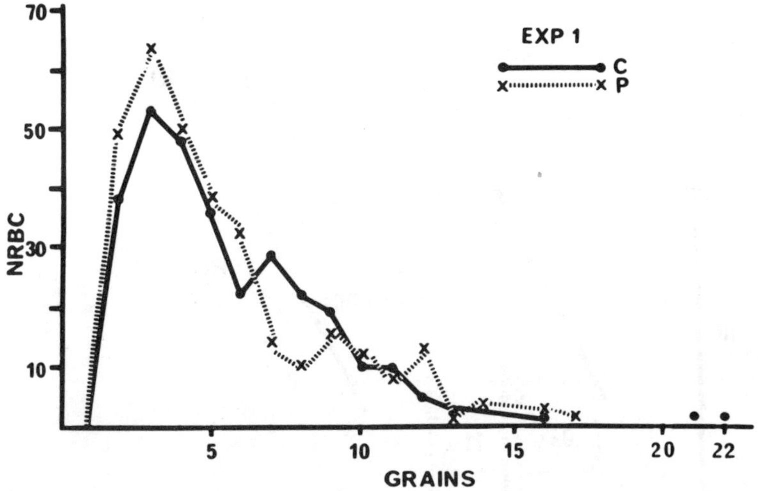

FIGURE 4*a*. Perfusion experiment 1(EXP. 1). ^{55}Fe erythroblast grain count distributions for control(C) and perfused(P) leg marrows. Ordinate: numbers of erythroblasts(NRBC) per 500 cells; abscissa: numbers of autographic grains per cell. Each curve was corrected for background as described in the text.

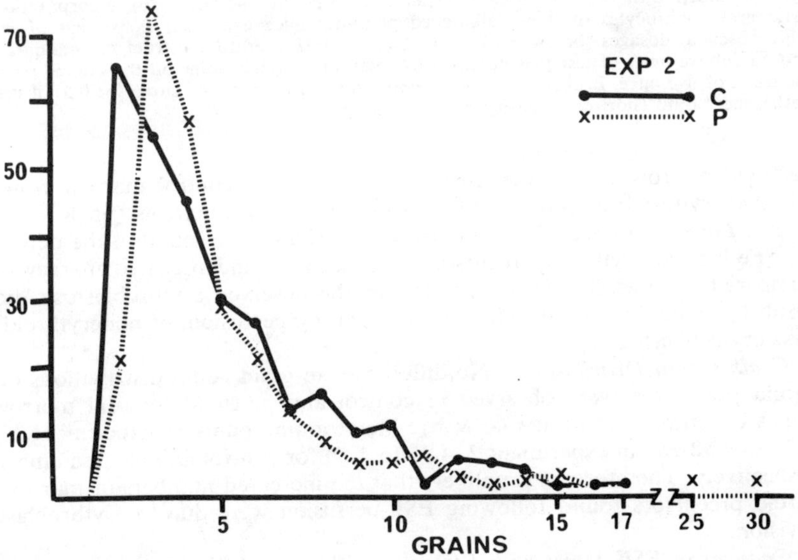

FIGURE 4*b*. Perfusion experiment 2(EXP. 2). ^{55}Fe erythroblast grain count distributions for control(C) and perfused(P) leg marrows. Ordinate: numbers of erythroblasts(NRBC) per 500 cells; abscissa: numbers of autographic grains per cell. Each curve was corrected for background as described in the text.

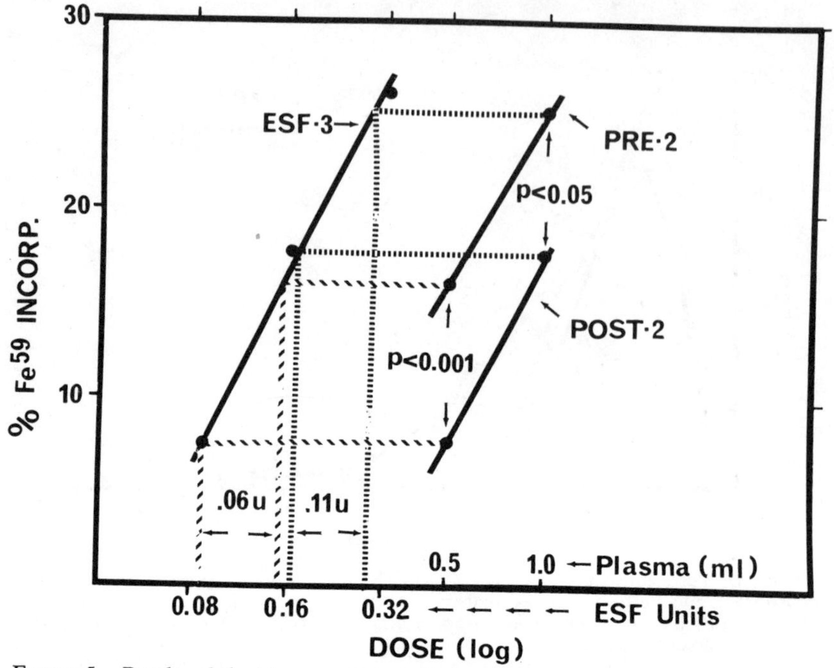

FIGURE 5. Results of the bioassay of preperfusion (PRE–2) and postperfusion (POST–2) plasma samples for ESF activity in perfusion experiment 2. Also shown is the log dose-response curve obtained with the ESF Step III standard. Ordinate: 48-hour ^{59}Fe incorporation into peripheral erythrocytes of hypoxia-induced plethoric mice expressed as percent of injected ^{59}Fe. Abscissa: dosages (below line) of the Step III ESF used to construct the standard curve and ml (above line) of test plasma given to assay mice. Each point on the curves represents the mean of five mice. Broken lines shown extrapolation to standard curve for 0.5 ml (oblique dash) and 1.0 ml (horizontal dash) plasma samples.

perfused marrow (47% increase). In experiment 2 control marrow contained 430,000 erythroblasts compared to 710,000 in perfused marrow (65% increase).

^{55}Fe-Labeling Indices. No significant alterations were found in the percentage of ^{55}Fe-labeled erythroid precursors when control and perfused marrows were compared (FIGURE 3). This suggests that the observed erythroblastosis did not result from stimulation of differentiation, during perfusion, of nonerythroid cells into erythroblasts.

Grain Count Distributions. No differences in grain count distributions of erythroid precursors were observed in control and perfused femoral marrows in either experiment (FIGURES 4a & b). Mean grain counts in experiment 1 were 4.77 to 4.52 and in experiment 2, 4.95 to 4.86 for control and perfused marrows, respectively. Therefore, it is unlikely that the increased numbers of marrow erythroid precursors found following ESF-perfusion were due to erythroblast cell division.

Changes in ESF Titers with Perfusion. When the ESF levels in postperfusion plasma samples were compared to the preperfusion values, statistically significant decreases in the amounts of ESF were found following both perfusions. The data obtained in experiment 2 are given in FIGURE 5. Similar results were obtained in experiment 1. Extrapolating the pre- and postperfusion assay data to the ESF Step III standard curve, a decrease of about 0.1 units of ESF per ml of perfusate plasma was noted for both the 0.5 ml and 1.0 ml dosages used in the plethoric mouse assay employed. Extending this analysis further, in perfusion experiment 2, 57 ml of plasma (43% hematocrit × 100 ml of whole blood perfusate) initially containing 17 units of the ESF was determined to have only 11.4 units remaining after perfusion through the isolated hind leg. This represented a decrease of 34 percent. Similar calculations for experiment 1 also indicated a 34 percent decrease in plasma ESF content. No reduction in ESF values was noted when whole blood containing 0.3 units of the ESF per ml plasma was incubated at 37° C for 3.5 hours. The observed decrease in the ESF levels following perfusion may be indicative of erythroid marrow utilization or metabolic degradation.

Discussion

Perfusion of isolated rat hind legs with whole blood containing ESF resulted in a pronounced erythroblastosis in perfused femoral marrow, thus confirming previous observations.[1–3] The data obtained in this preliminary study suggest that this phenomenon was not the result of either erythroblastic proliferation or enhanced erythroid differentiation since no concomitant changes in ^{55}Fe grain count or labeling indices occurred. Fisher *et al.*,[11] studying the effects of the ESF in isolated perfused hind legs of rabbits prelabeled with ^{59}Fe, noted a decrease in ^{59}Fe grain counts after five hr of ESF perfusion but no significant increases in the relative concentration of marrow erythroblasts. They interpreted these findings as follows: "Even though our grain count data are suggestive of a direct effect of erythropoietin on late erythroid cells, we do not feel that they prove or disprove the concept of extra cell divisions caused by erythropoietin." A direct effect of the ESF on erythroblast proliferation has been reported by Matoth and Kaufmann[12] in in vitro culture studies.

The failure to find an altered labeling profile in the present studies are tentatively interpreted to indicate that the ESF (or an undefined principle associated with it) may have induced a redistribution of erythroid marrow from loci not quantified by our techniques (epiphyseal, metaphyseal marrow) to the femoral diaphyseal marrow. Such a shifting would be detected as an increase in erythroblast concentration. Large numbers of erythroblasts, which might be available for mobilization, are known to be contained in epiphyseal regions of rat femurs.[8] The manner in which the ESF might invoke a redistribution of this kind is speculative. That this may be one action of the ESF is suggested by the findings of Gordon *et al.*[13] in isolated femur perfusions. In these studies, ESF induced a rapid release of reticulocytes and normoblasts into the perfusate. It may be that marrow erythroid relocation and delivery into the circulation are related and even sequential events both dependent upon a rapid transposition of erythroblasts from extravascular (cordal) to vascular (sinal) locations. A unified concept of ESF action at this level would require the existence of a functional relationship between vascular and extravascular marrow compartments that are responsive to the ESF. A system of this kind, under the influence of factors regulating hemopoiesis, has been postulated by Weiss.[14]

Results of the bioassay of pre- and postperfusion plasma samples for ESF content clearly indicated a decreased activity following 3.5 hr of perfusion. These data suggest that the hormone was utilized by the perfused erythroid marrows. Although metabolic fates other than marrow utilization cannot be ruled out, these findings nevertheless, support Stohlman's[15] data on utilization of endogenous ESF in normal and irradiated posthypoxic rats. They are also in accord with experiments of Matoth and Kaufmann,[12] which suggest uptake of erythropoietin by erythroblasts. On the other hand, the results are not in harmony with those of Naets and Wittek[16] who found that clearance of endogenous plasma ESF in nephrectomized dogs was independent of the numbers of marrow erythroblasts present.

Fisher *et al.*[11] observed no changes in perfusate ESF levels in their rabbit perfusion studies. However, although they noted marked reticulocyte release, no increase in marrow erythroblasts was evident and this may account for the different results obtained.

Summary

Isolated hind legs of rats, prelabeled with ^{55}Fe, were perfused for 3.5 hr with whole blood containing erythropoietin (ESF). Although the ESF induced an increase in the absolute numbers of erythroblasts in perfused leg femoral marrow, no changes in ^{55}Fe-labeling indices or erythroid grain counts were observed when autoradiograms prepared from nonperfused leg marrows were compared to those from perfused leg marrows. It was therefore tentatively concluded that the ESF did not evoke its effect by increasing erythroblast proliferation (which would reduce the grain counts) or erythroblast differentiation (which would decrease labeling indices). It is concluded that the ESF may act by causing erythroblast redistribution from loci not accessible to routine quantitation (epiphyses, metaphyses) to diaphyses. This would cause an apparent but not actual increase in total marrow erythroblast numbers.

A significant decrease in perfusate ESF titers was noted during perfusion. This suggested utilization of the ESF by the erythroid marrow, but degradation of ESF not directly related to marrow metabolism cannot at present be excluded.

References

1. Kuna, S., A. S. Gordon, B. S. Morse, F. B. Lane, III & H. A. Charipper. 1959. Bone marrow function in perfused isolated hind legs of rats. Am. J. Physiol. **196:** 769–774.
2. Gordon, A. S., J. Winkert, B. S. Dornfest & C. D. Siegel. 1959. Studies on the actions and properties of the circulating erythropoietic-stimulating factor. Ann. N. Y. Acad. Sci. **77:** 650–676.
3. Gordon, A. S., J. W. Winkert, B. S. Dornfest, J. LoBue & A. Crusco. 1959. Properties of the urinary erythropoietic-stimulating factor (ESF). *In* The Kinetics of Cellular Proliferation. F. Stohlman, Jr., Ed. : 332–343. Grune & Stratton. New York, N. Y.
4. Fisher, J. W., B. L. Roh, C. Couch & W. O. Nightingale. 1964. Influence of cobalt, sheep erythropoietin and several hormones on erythropoiesis in bone marrows of isolated perfused hind legs of dogs. Blood **23:** 87–98.
5. Forberg, S., E. Odeblad, R. Soremark & S. Ullberg. 1964. Autoradiography with isotopes emitting internal conversion electrons and Auger electrons. Acta Radiologica **2:** 241–262.
6. Dornfest, B. S., J. LoBue, E. S. Handler, A. S. Gordon & H. Quastler. 1962. Mechanisms of leukocyte production and release. II. Factors influencing leukocyte release from isolated perfused rat legs. J. Lab. Clin. Med. **60:** 777–787.
7. Fruhman, G. J. & A. S. Gordon. 1955. Quantitative effects of corticosterone on rat bone marrow. Proc. Soc. Exp. Biol. Med. **88:** 130–131.
8. LoBue, J., B. S. Dornfest, A. S. Gordon, J. Hurst & H. Quastler. 1963. Marrow distribution in rat femurs determined by cell enumeration and ^{59}Fe-labeling. Proc. Soc. Exp. Biol. Med. **112:** 1058–1062.
9. Monette, F. C., J. LoBue, A. S. Gordon & P. C. Chan. 1965. Erythropoiesis in transfusion-induced polycythemic rats studied in ^{3}H-thymidine autoradiography. Proc. Soc. Exp. Biol. Med. **119:** 445–449.

10. GORDON, A. S., E. A. MIRAND, J. WENIG, R. KATZ & E. ZANJANI. 1967. Mechanisms of steroid hormone action in erythropoiesis. This Annal.
11. FISHER, J. W., L. G. LAJTHA, A. S. BUTTOO & D. D. PORTEOUS. 1965. Direct effects of erythropoietin on the bone marrow of the isolated perfused hind limbs of rabbits. Brit. J. Haemat. **11**: 342–349.
12. MATOTH, Y. & L. KAUFMANN. 1962. Mitotic activity in vitro of erythroblasts previously exposed to erythropoietin. Blood **20**: 165–172.
13. GORDON, A. S., J. LOBUE, B. S. DORNFEST & G. W. COOPER. 1962. Reticulocyte and leukocyte release from isolated perfused rat legs and femurs. *In* Erythropoiesis. L. O. Jacobson & M. Doyle, Eds. : 321–327. Grune & Stratton. New York, N. Y.
14. WEISS, L. 1965. The structure of bone marrow. Functional interrelationships of vascular and hematopoietic compartments in experimental hemolytic anemia: an electron microscopic study. J. Morphol. **117**: 467–537.
15. STOHLMAN, F., JR. 1959. Observations on the physiology of erythropoietin and its role in the regulation of red cell production. Ann. N. Y. Acad. Sci. **77**: 710–724.
16. NAETS, J. P. & M. WITTEK. 1965. Effect of erythroid hyperplasia on utilization of erythropoietin. Nature **206**: 726–727.

PART V. IMMUNOLOGICAL STUDIES ON ERYTHROPOIETIN

A SUMMARY OF SOME STUDIES ON ERYTHROPOIESIS USING ANTI-ERYTHROPOIETIN IMMUNE SERUM*

John C. Schooley, Joseph F. Garcia, Linda N. Cantor and Virginia W. Havens
Donner Laboratory and the Lawrence Radiation Laboratory, University of California, Berkeley, Calif.

Several years ago Schooley and Garcia[1] demonstrated that serum obtained from some rabbits immunized with human urinary erythropoietin could neutralize the biological effects of erythropoietin. Lange *et al.*[2] confirmed this observation and produced immune serum after immunization with sheep plasma erythropoietin. The present paper summarizes various studies from this laboratory on the preparation and properties of the anti-erythropoietin serum and some examples of the usefulness of this immune serum in investigations of the physiology of erythropoiesis.

Preparation of the Immune Serum

Young male New Zealand rabbits of about 5–6 lb have been immunized with concentrates of human urine containing erythropoietin (ESF) by various schedules.[3] Immune sera having the highest titers have generally been obtained after immunization with alum-precipitated human urinary ESF but this method of immunization requires rather large amounts of ESF. We have utilized the following immunization schedule with fair success. Multiple s.c. injections at weekly intervals were made of about 2 ml of a 1:1 mixture of complete Freund's adjuvant and 10 mg of human urinary ESF in saline (about 200 cobalt units). Some rabbits have detectable anti-erythropoietin (anti-ESF) titers after three or four weeks, i.e., after the injection of 30 mg or 600 cobalt units of ESF. The time of harvesting serum from immunized rabbits, regardless of the schedule of immunization used, is critical. We have previously noted[3] that rabbits having high anti-ESF titers were anemic and it was demonstrated that the immune serum could neutralize rabbit ESF.[4] However, if the rabbit becomes too severely anemic as a result of neutralization of its own ESF, a marked increase in ESF production is triggered which is more than sufficient to combine with the antibody produced as a result of the immunization. Some rabbits have been observed to alternate between periods of detectable antibody production and periods of excessive production of endogenous ESF. Therefore, it is important to follow the hematocrit and reticulocyte levels of immunized rabbits and harvest the immune serum when these parameters just begin to become depressed.

It is important to realize that some sera containing anti-ESF as tested in polycythemic mice are toxic if injected in the larger amounts necessary for experiments with nonpolycythemic mice. Such toxicity often disappears if the sera are stored frozen for several months. Also of practical significance is the observation that many rabbits will produce very low-titer anti-ESF that is impossible to use in most experiments. In such cases isolation and subsequent concentration of the γ-globulin yield a more potent antibody preparation.

Garcia and Schooley[4] previously demonstrated that the biological activity of

* Supported in part by the United States Atomic Energy Commission and in part by Cancer Research Funds of the University of California.

erythropoietins found in serum or plasma of mice, rats, sheep, humans, and rabbits can be neutralized by anti-ESF obtained from rabbits immunized with human urinary ESF. Other investigators have shown that the erythropoietic activity of renal cyst fluid[5,6] as well as cerebellar hemangioblastoma cyst fluid[5] is neutralized by anti-ESF. It is evident that the erythropoietins obtained from these different sources are similar. Of interest is the fact that in one immunized rabbit the cyclic relationship between anti-ESF and ESF levels was evident during the early stages of immunization but not after prolonged immunization. Serum obtained from this rabbit after prolonged immunization when the rabbit was not anemic was able to neutralize human and sheep ESF but not rabbit ESF.[7] This suggests that although the erythropoietins of different animals are similar, they are not necessarily identical.

The fact that in most rabbits a severe anemia results as a consequence of immunization with human urinary ESF suggests that an autoimmune state has been experimentally produced. Similar autoimmune inhibitions of erythropoiesis undoubtedly occur clinically. Jepson and Lowenstein have recently[8] presented evidence for an inhibitor of erythropoiesis in patients with erythroblastopenia which exhibits a biological behavior similar to that of antisera against ESF.

Properties of the Immune Serum

Injection of anti-ESF into polycythemic mice at the same time as injection of exogenous ESF completely prevents an erythropoietic response. Injection of anti-ESF into polycythemic mice one or two days after the initiation of a wave of erythropoiesis by injection of ESF has little or no effect on the magnitude of the erythropoietic response.[3] The magnitude of the erythropoietic response depends upon the dose of ESF injected and the time of anti-ESF injection.[3] Injections of antisera against ceruloplasmin, transferrin, orosomucoid, α_1-acid glycoproteins, human urinary proteins, bovine serum albumin, bovine growth hormone, hog renin, and sheep interstitial cell-stimulating hormone do not inhibit the erythropoietic response of polycythemic mice to injections of ESF. The neutralizing ability of anti-ESF sera was not affected by absorption with kidney, spleen, or liver of normal, polycythemic, cobalt or phenylhydrazine-injected, mice, nor with normal mouse serum, nor with human urinary proteins. The addition to anti-ESF of ESF previously inactivated by acid hydrolysis only slightly decreased the subsequent ability of the anti-ESF to combine with biologically active ESF. Biologically active ESF is the *only* one of all the proteins that have thus far been used which blocks the neutralizing ability of anti-ESF.[3]

The neutralizing ability of the immune serum is associated with the γ-globulins.[3] Electrophoresis in agar and immunodiffusion studies of the purified γ-globulin using goat anti-rabbit γ-globulin have recently confirmed the purity of the isolated γ-globulin. Studies of fractions of the immune serum prepared by ultracentrifugation in sucrose gradients indicate that the neutralizing ability of the immune serum is associated with the 19S γ-globulins.

Further evidence of the importance of γ-globulin in the neutralization reaction was obtained in the following experiment. The amount of goat anti-rabbit γ-globulin (goat ARGG) required for maximum precipitation of the γ-globulin in one anti-ESF preparation was determined. The amount of that anti-ESF required to neutralize a given amount of ESF was determined by bioassay since no precipitate results from the reaction between ESF and anti-ESF. Equal aliquots of ESF, anti-ESF or normal rabbit serum, and goat ARGG were mixed in different sequences. In the first sample, ESF and anti-ESF were mixed, incubated overnight, and then goat ARGG was added; in the second sample, anti-ESF was replaced by normal rabbit serum. In the third sample, the goat ARGG was added to the anti-ESF, incubated overnight, and then the ESF was added. The precipitates formed after the goat ARGG additions were removed by centrifugation and the erythropoietic activity of the supernatant was determined, after suitable dilutions, in hypertransfused polycythemic mice by procedures previously described.[3] The results, as shown in TABLE 1, indicate that if the γ-globulin of the immune serum

TABLE 1

PERCENT ^{59}FE UPTAKE (72 HR) IN RBC OF POLYCYTHEMIC MICE

Sample		Percent ^{59}Fe Uptake (72 Hrs) in RBC of Polycythemic Mice
1	(ESF + Anti-ESF) + Goat ARGG	0.25 ± 0.08*
2	(ESF + Normal Rabbit Serum) + Goat ARGG	5.25 ± 0.62
3	(Anti-ESF + Goat ARGG) + ESF	7.61 ± 0.96
4	Normal Rabbit Serum	0.13 ± 0.01

* Standard error of the mean.

is removed by precipitation with goat ARGG prior to the addition of ESF, no neutralization of the ESF occurs. Since ESF is neutralized if the goat ARGG is added after the mixing of anti-ESF and ESF, the neutralization reaction must have occurred prior to the addition of the goat ARGG. This shows that although the evidence for neutralization requires an in vivo biological assay system, the actual combination between ESF and anti-ESF can occur in vitro. These experiments all support the view that the neutralization of ESF by anti-ESF is the result of an antigen-antibody reaction.

The availability of this immune serum provides a potent tool for investigating many problems of the regulation of erythropoiesis and stem cell kinetics. In the second portion of this paper we will briefly describe various published and unpublished experiments of Schooley, Cantor and Havens using anti-ESF.

Erythropoiesis in Normal Adult Mice

We have previously emphasized that injections of adequate amounts of anti-ESF into normal mice can essentially abolish erythropoiesis although granulocytopoiesis and megakaryocytopoiesis are little affected.[9] In FIGURE 1, a section of the spleen of an anti-ESF injected mouse (B) is compared with a section of the spleen of a mouse injected with normal rabbit serum (A). Sections of the bone marrow from the same mice are shown in FIGURE 2. The mice were injected s.c. with 0.25 ml of either of the two sera daily for four days and killed on the fifth day. It is obvious that nucleated erythroid cells have been virtually eliminated in the anti-ESF injected mice (B of FIGURES 1 & 2). This observation seems to us to be the best currently available evidence that ESF is necessary for the normal regulation of erythropoiesis even though its presence cannot be demonstrated in the blood of normal mice by current assay procedures.

Erythropoiesis in Testosterone-Injected Polycythemic Mice

The injection of testosterone into the polycythemic mouse is followed by a wave of erythropoietic activity observable several days later than that caused by injection of ESF.[10] It has been further demonstrated by several groups of investig-

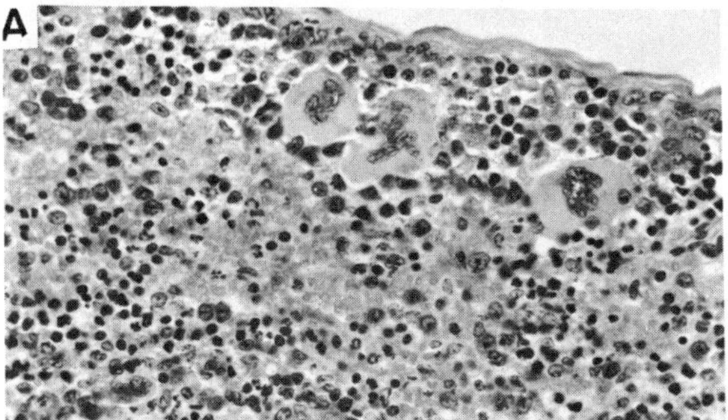

FIGURE 1. A comparison of sections of spleens of normal mice (A) injected with normal rabbit serum and (B) injected with anti-erythropoietin.

ators[11–14] that plasma taken from several animal species after injections of testosterone stimulates erythropoiesis in the polycythemic mouse. This stimulation has been generally assumed to be due to the presence of ESF in the plasma taken from the testosterone-injected animals. However, as Fried and Gurney[13] have stated, it is equally possible that a metabolic product of testosterone is responsible for the stimulation. Schooley[15] has recently shown that the injection of anti-ESF completely abolishes the erythropoietic response observed in the polycythemic mouse after testosterone injections. These results support the view that the erythropoietic stimulation resulting from testosterone injection is mediated by the production of ESF.

Erythropoiesis in WW^v Mutant Mice

Russell *et al.*[16] have studied extensively the W-series mutant mouse which suffers from a severe inherited macrocytic anemia that is well established at birth. The fact that transplants of hemopoietic tissue from normal ww mice can restore erythropoiesis in WW^v mice indicates that the genetic defect in the WW^v mouse occurs in the hematopoietic cells themselves.[16] McCulloch *et al.*[17] presented

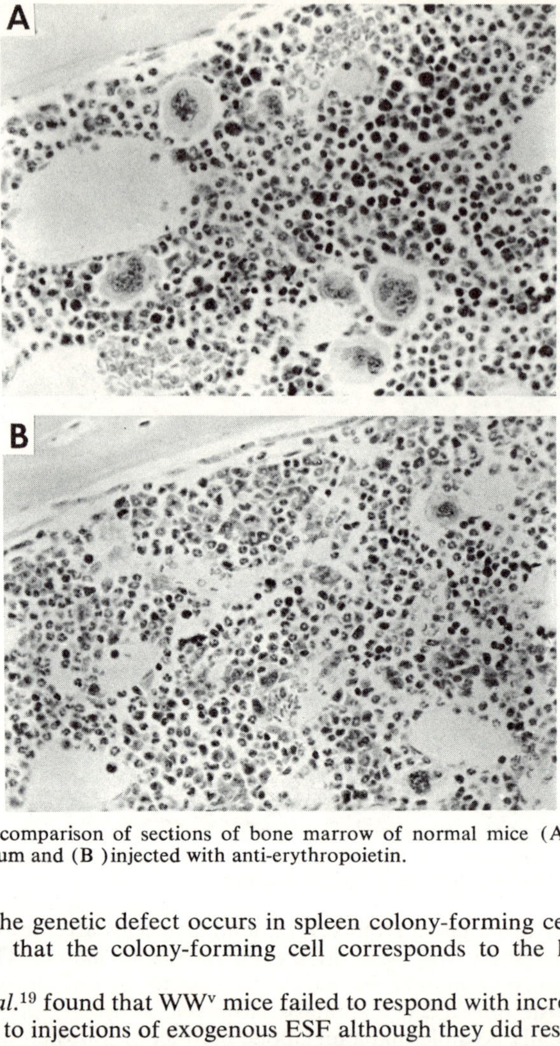

FIGURE 2. A comparison of sections of bone marrow of normal mice (A) injected with normal rabbit serum and (B) injected with anti-erythropoietin.

evidence that the genetic defect occurs in spleen colony-forming cells; other evidence suggests that the colony-forming cell corresponds to the hematopoietic stem cell.[18]

Keighley *et al.*[19] found that WW^v mice failed to respond with increased erythropoietic activity to injections of exogenous ESF although they did respond erythropoietically when exposed to simulated altitude. It was therefore of interest to study the role of ESF in the regulation of erythropoiesis in WW^v mice using anti-ESF.

Male mice of the WW^v and normal ww genotype, four to five months of age, obtained from the Roscoe B. Jackson Memorial Laboratory, Bar Harbor, Maine, were injected i.p. with 0.25 ml of anti-ESF or normal rabbit serum daily for four consecutive days. On the fifth day, 0.5 μc of ^{59}Fe as iron citrate (specific activity approximately 10 μc/mg) was injected i.v., and 24 hr later blood was taken by cardiac puncture. A measured amount of blood was washed with saline and the ^{59}Fe uptake determined. The ^{59}Fe uptake is given as the percent of ^{59}Fe in the calculated blood volume; the blood volume was assumed to be 5.5% of the body weight, according to the data of Keighley *et al.*[19] Hematocrits were measured and smears of the bone marrow made. The percentage of reticulocytes in the peripheral blood and the percentage of erythroid cells present in the marrow were determined.

The results are shown in TABLE 2. A marked decrease in the hematocrits of the WW^v mice injected with anti-ESF was observed, as well as a decrease in percentage of erythroid cells in the bone marrow, number of reticulocytes in the peripheral blood, and ^{59}Fe uptake in the peripheral blood. We conclude that erythropoiesis in the WW^v mouse, as in the normal mouse, is regulated by ESF. Keighley has also demonstrated some inhibition of erythropoiesis after injections of anti-ESF.[20]

In a similar experiment spleens from WW^v mice injected for four consecutive days with anti-ESF or normal rabbit serum were removed, pooled by sex, and a single cell suspension was prepared in medium 858. The spleen suspension was diluted with the medium to 20×10^6 cells/ml, and 0.5 ml (10^7 cells) was injected into heavily irradiated host ww, Ww, or W^vw mice of the same sex as the donor. The number of macroscopically visible colonies on the spleen was determined 10 days after irradiation and transplantation. The total colony-forming cells from WW^v mice injected with normal rabbit serum was 1.36 ± 0.31 per 10^7 cells in 44 recipient mice and from WW^v mice injected with anti-ESF was 2.13 ± 0.37 per 10^7 cells in 47 recipients. The total number of colony formers in the spleens of these mice is less than 1% of that observed in nonmutant mice. Thus, in agreement with McCulloch *et al.*,[17] we found very few colony formers in the spleens of the WW^v mice. Interestingly, the suppression of erythropoiesis for this period of time in these WW^v mice did not significantly change the number of colony formers per spleen.

Erythropoiesis in Normal Mice Exposed to Simulated Altitude

During acclimatization to altitude a marked increase in the red cell volume occurs and increased levels of ESF are found in the blood soon after exposure to altitude. The effect of anti-ESF on the erythropoietic response of female C_3H mice, five to six weeks of age, exposed to a simulated altitude was investigated. Two groups of six mice each were placed in an altitude chamber at a simulated altitude of 18,000 feet for five days. The altitude chamber was returned daily to normal atmospheric pressure for approximately 15 min and one of the groups of mice was injected i.p. with 0.25 ml of anti-ESF each day for five days. Another

TABLE 2

EFFECT OF ANTI-ERYTHROPOIETIN ON ERYTHROPOIESIS IN WW^v AND ww MICE

	WW^v		ww	
	NRS	Anti-ESF	NRS	Anti-ESF
Weight (g)	35.3 ± 1.29*	34.8 ± 0.88	33.6 ± 0.37	33.7 ± 0.77
Hematocrit (%)	37.1 ± 0.40	31.1 ± 0.94	44.4 ± 0.72	40.4 ± 0.63
24-Hour ^{59}Fe uptake (%)	37.7 ± 1.74	0.63 ± 0.21	40.0 ± 1.58	0.38 ± 0.06
Erythroid cells in marrow (%)	12.2 ± 0.82	< 0.4	12.5 ± 0.84	< 0.4
Reticulocytes in blood (%)	4.12 ± 0.31	< 0.00	2.54 ± 0.11	< 0.00

* Standard error of the mean.

group of mice, not exposed to altitude, was used as a control. ^{59}Fe was injected i.v. on the fourth day of exposure to altitude and 24 hr later blood was obtained by cardiac puncture. A measured amount of blood was washed with saline and the ^{59}Fe uptake determined. The ^{59}Fe uptake is given as the percent ^{59}Fe in the blood volume; the blood volume was assumed to be 5.5% of the body weight. Hematocrits were measured and the percentage of reticulocytes in the blood was determined. The spleens of the mice from each group were pooled and a single cell suspension was prepared using a modified Eagle's medium without calcium. The total number of nucleated cells per spleen was determined and the suspension was injected, after suitable dilution, into heavily irradiated isologous mice. Smears of the injected spleen cell suspension were examined for the presence of erythroid cells. The total number of spleen colonies was determined 10 days after transplantation; the total number of colony-forming cells per spleen was then calculated; the results are shown in TABLE 3.

It is evident both on the basis of ^{59}Fe uptake and from the reticulocyte levels that a marked stimulation of erythropoiesis occurred in mice following exposure to simulated altitude as compared to the nonhypoxic mice. This erythropoietic stimulation did not occur in hypoxic mice injected with anti-ESF. In fact, the erythropoietic response in these animals was almost 75% lower than in the normal nonhypoxic animals, but it was not decreased to the extent that one would observe in nonhypoxic mice injected with the same amount of anti-ESF. Presumably, this is due to the fact that the amount of anti-ESF injected was not sufficient to neutralize all of the ESF produced as a result of the hypoxic exposure.

The changes in the total number of colony-forming cells in the spleens of hypoxic mice and hypoxic mice injected with anti-ESF compared to the spleens of normal mice is of particular interest because of the current concepts of the interrelationship between colony-forming cells and erythropoietin-sensitive cells. Bruce and McCulloch[21] observed a progressive decrease in the total number of colony-forming cells in the spleens of mice exposed to hypoxia, but no decrease in the colony-forming cells in the marrow. They interpreted their results as indicating that ESF did not act directly on the colony-forming cell. Schooley[22] observed that the overall doubling time of colony-forming cells after transplantation

TABLE 3

EFFECT OF ANTI-ERYTHROPOIETIN ON ERYTHROPOIESIS AND ON THE CONTENT OF COLONY-FORMING CELLS IN THE SPLEENS OF HYPOXIC MICE

		Hypoxic for five Days	
	Control—Nonhypoxic	Non-Injected	Anti-ESF Injected
Weight (g)	20.3 ± 0.31*	18.5 ± 0.41	16.9 ± 0.69
Hematocrit (%)	40.5 ± 0.43	51.2 ± 0.99	39.4 ± 0.71
24-Hour ^{59}Fe Uptake (%)	22.5 ± 0.94	43.8 ± 0.57	4.97 ± 1.12
Reticulocytes (%)	4.56 ± 0.87	17.2 ± 1.00	1.24 ± 0.33
Cells/Spleen	182 × 10⁶	313 × 10⁶	144 × 10⁶
CFU/Spleen	5366 ± 300	3100 ± 393	1111 ± 100
% Decrease		42%	79%

* Standard error of the mean.

into heavily irradiated polycythemic mice was not altered by the injection of exogenous ESF. In addition, it was found that the daily injection of ESF into polycythemic hosts did not decrease the total number of spleen colonies observable on the host spleen 10 days after transplantation from the levels found in the non-ESF-injected control mice.

The changes in the total number of cells and colony formers in the spleens of polycythemic host mice following heavy irradiation and transplantation with 2×10^6 bone marrow cells was compared in ESF and non-ESF injected mice.[23] This inoculum of bone marrow contained 420 colony formers. In both groups four days after transplantation there were 250 colony formers detected in the spleen and by the sixth day there were 1000. However, during this same time interval there was an increase of about 30×10^6 nucleated cells in the spleens of the mice given erythropoietin whereas there was only a slight increase in the number of nucleated cells in the spleens of the mice receiving no ESF. Differential counts of the nucleated cells in the ESF-injected mice indicated that at least 25×10^6 erythroid cells were produced in the spleens in this two-day interval. What was the source of these erythroid cells? Assuming a generation time of eight hr, it would be impossible to produce the numbers of nucleated erythroid cells found in the spleen even if all the colony formers in the mouse, not only in the spleen but in the rest of the body as well, were stimulated to differentiate into erythroid cells. It is obvious that if all the colony formers were stimulated to differentiate, the replication of colony formers themselves should either be abolished or markedly inhibited, and yet the growth curve indicates a significant increase in colony formers in the spleen during this time of increased production of nucleated erythroid cells. These observations suggest that the nucleated erythroid cells produced during this two-day interval are not the result of the action of ESF directly on colony-forming cells, but, rather, the result of the action of ESF on much larger numbers of erythropoietin-sensitive cells present either in the bone marrow at the time of transplantation and/or produced from colony-forming cells during the first four days after transplantation. This possibility, i.e., that many of the colony-forming cells which initially settle in the spleen after transplantation become ESF-sensitive cells, may explain both the initial decrease and the lag observed before the transplanted colony-forming cells enter an exponential stage of growth. Therefore, it is concluded, in agreement with Bruce and McCulloch,[21] that ESF does not act directly upon the colony-forming cell, but upon some ESF-sensitive progeny of the colony-forming cell. The presence of this pool of cells sensitive to differentiating agents could explain the observation that colony-forming cells, or stem cells, can maintain themselves even when differentiating pressures are markedly increased.

If the above interpretations are valid, numerous questions arise regarding the properties of the progeny of colony-forming cells that are capable of responding to differentiating agents such as ESF. What regulates the movement of colony-forming cells into ESF-sensitive cells? What is the size of the ESF-sensitive pool of cells? Are all of the ESF-sensitive cells actually able to respond to ESF at any one time? Are ESF-sensitive cells continuously derived from colony-forming cells in the absence of ESF? If so, what is the fate of these cells? Does the pool of ESF-sensitive cells increase exclusively by the movement of colony-forming cells into ESF-sensitive cells or are ESF-sensitive cells capable of a limited proliferative capacity? Do ESF-sensitive cells simply die if not triggered within some limited time period to differentiate? Is the radiation sensitivity of ESF-sensitive cells different from that of colony-forming cells? Are ESF-sensitive cells pluripotential, i.e., can they also upon appropriate stimulation differentiate into granulocytic, megakaryocytic, or perhaps even lymphoid, cells? Can ESF-sensitive cells, after transplantation into heavily irradiated hosts, settle in the spleen, proliferate, and give rise to macroscopic spleen colonies? The answers to these questions are of considerable importance in interpreting experiments on the colony-forming cell. Some experimental data is available which allows reasonable speculation on at least some of these questions.

Utilizing the technique of injecting ESF into polycythemic mice and limiting the time of action by subsequent neutralization with anti-ESF, Schooley[24] has presented evidence suggesting that the ESF-sensitive cell is able to respond to ESF only during some limited period of its individual life cycle.

The fact that mice kept polycythemic for one month do not have an increased response to ESF compared to the response observed when the same dose of ESF is injected into mice kept polycythemic for one week suggests that large numbers of ESF-sensitive cells do not accumulate in the absence of erythropoietic stimulation (unpublished observations). We have observed that the total number of colony formers in the spleens of polycythemic mice is consistently higher than in nonpolycythemic mice, which suggests that the movement of colony formers into ESF-sensitive cells is decreased in polycythemic mice where ESF stimulation is minimal, and therefore, there are increased numbers of colony-forming cells.

After five days of exposure to hypoxic conditions the total number of colony formers in the spleens of mice injected wtih anti-ESF decreased by about 80% of normal as compared to about a 40% decrease in the control hypoxic mice (see TABLE 3). This suggests that in the hypoxic mouse the colony-forming population is stimulated to replace the ESF-sensitive cells which have matured in response to increased ESF production, and the colony-forming cell pool is therefore depleted. An even greater decrease in the colony-forming population occurs when the ESF in hypoxic mice is neutralized by anti-ESF, indicating that it is not the presence of increased levels of ESF which regulates the movement of colony-forming cells into ESF-sensitive cells, but that either hypoxia or some agent other than ESF produced as a result of the hypoxic condition is responsible for the regulation. It seems unlikely that the size of the ESF-sensitive cell pool itself is involved in this regulation since a considerable increase in the size of the pool should occur in the hypoxic mice injected with anti-ESF unless the cells' life cycle is very short.

There is some evidence suggesting that the ESF-sensitive cell is itself capable of division. The number of endogenous spleen colonies in a group of heavily irradiated mice was three to four times greater than normal if the mice were exposed to hypoxia after irradiation. The number in the normal mice was 1.23 ±

TABLE 4

EFFECT OF ANTI-ERYTHROPOIETIN ON ERYTHROPOIESIS IN NEWBORN RATS

	Control-Uninjected	Anti-ESF-Injected
No. of rats	14	18
Weight (g)	11.0 ± 0.25*	10.6 ± 0.19
Hematocrit (%)	30.2 ± 0.48	17.2 ± 0.48
24-Hour ^{59}Fe uptake (%)	51.0 ± 2.64	3.77 ± 0.47

* Standard error of the mean.

0.39 as compared to the hypoxic value of 4.67 ± 1.20. Since the total number of colony-forming cells which can be extracted from the spleens of hypoxic mice is decreased from normal, as shown in TABLE 3, it is rather surprising to find that in hypoxic mice the number of observable endogenous spleen colonies is increased over control nonhypoxic mice. These data suggest that some ESF-sensitive cells survive the irradiation and proliferate sufficiently to give rise to a detectable spleen colony. Bruce and McCulloch[17] found that the number of endogenous colonies in mice irradiated after a 10-day exposure to hypoxia was significantly less than that found in nonhypoxic controls. We suggest that in their experiments the available pool of ESF-sensitive cells is extremely low at the time of irradiation because of the previous hypoxic exposure and therefore, very few ESF-sensitive cells are present to produce colonies. The colonies that are observed are presumably derived from colony-forming cells.

On the basis of mature cell types in any given colony, numerous investigators have classified colonies as exclusively one cell type or as mixtures of granulocytic, erythroid, or megakaryocytic cells. We find after the transplantation of normal bone marrow cells that about 60% of the colonies can be classified as exclusively erythroid. It is our impression, however, that following the transplantation of regenerating hematopoietic tissue, almost all of the colonies are mixed. We have studied the cellular composition of spleen colonies in heavily irradiated polycythemic mice on the 10th day after transplantation of bone marrow when ESF has been injected on either the eighth or ninth day, and have observed that foci of as many as 20,000 erythroid cells are found within obvious granulocytic colonies as well as in areas beneath the splenic capsule where no other mature hematopoietic cells are present. The possibility that ESF-sensitive cells themselves have a proliferative capacity sufficient to form distinct colonies may explain the observed cellular compositions.

The failure of some accumulations of cells within the spleen to become granulocytic or megakaryocytic in the absence of ESF[23] and the observations that other accumulations of cells within granulocytic colonies can become erythroid in the presence of ESF[23] suggests that the ESF-sensitive cell is only capable of stimulation into the erythroid series, i.e., it is not a pluripotential cell. This view would propose that the colony-forming cell is a pluripotential cell that gives rise to progeny that are unipotential. If this interpretation is correct, the speculations concerning the behavior of ESF-sensitive cells would apply equally to cells capable of differentiation into the granulocytic and megakaryocytic series.

To summarize, we feel on the basis of the evidence presented above that it is probable that not all of the colonies observed on the surface of the spleen are derived directly from colony-forming cells, but some colonies are derived from cells which are sensitive to differentiating agents and have a limited proliferative capacity adequate to give a detectable colony. Thus, a rigorous definition of a colony derived from a colony-forming cell should perhaps include the requirements: (1) the colony is mixed and/or (2) retransplantation of the colony gives rise to mixed colonies.

Erythropoiesis in Mice after 200 r Irradiation

Temporal changes in the precursor cell populations which give rise to spleen colonies and which respond to ESF were measured in polycythemic mice before and at various times after 200 r whole-body ^{60}Co irradiation.[22] The results are shown in FIGURE 3. Immediately after irradiation the responsiveness of the mice to the i.v. injection of one cobalt unit of ESF was depressed to about 75% of normal; by the fifth day after irradiation the response approached normal and during the 9th to 12th days the response was slightly above normal. These data of ESF sensitivity essentially agree with the data of Alexanian *et al.*,[25] Gurney *et al.*,[26] and Gurney.[27] The total number of spleen colony formers in the spleen and femurs was depressed to about 20–30 percent of normal; this depression continued for at least 13 days after irradiation. The number of colony formers in the spleen by the 15th day after irradiation increased to about four times the normal level; the marrow colony formers by the 20th day increased to but did not rise above the normal level. Till[28] has reported that the recovery of colony-forming cells in the marrow after 155 r follows a pattern similar to that shown above, and he has also indicated that following 400 r, the colony formers in the spleen recover much more rapidly than we have shown after 200 r. Therefore, the increased responsiveness of these irradiated mice to ESF occurs at a time when the number of colony formers in the spleen and bone marrow is far below normal and no greater than that observed immediately after irradiation when the response to ESF is very low. Blackett *et al.*[29] have also observed that the recovery of erythropoiesis in rats irradiated with 200 r occurs before the recovery of the repopulating ability of the marrow. This repopulating ability is presumably a measure of the

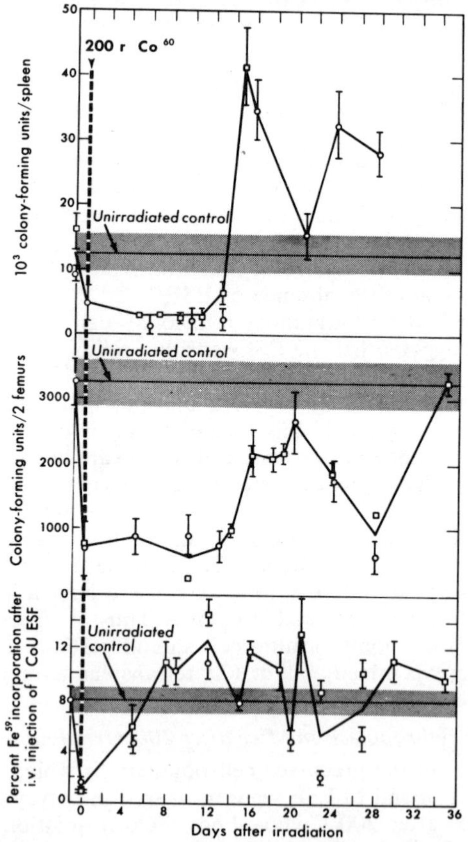

FIGURE 3. A comparison as a function of time of erythropoietin sensitivity and colony-forming cells in the bone marrow and spleens of polycythemic mice irradiated with 200 r whole body ^{60}Co gamma rays. Standard errors of the mean are shown.

number of stem cells (or by definition, colony-forming cells) in the recovering bone marrow. Other data[22] using the mitotic poison, vinblastine, according to the technique of Becker,[30] show that a large proportion of the colony-forming cells are actively dividing soon after exposure to 200 r. Since the number of colony formers does not increase at this time, it seems probable that the colony-forming cells immediately move into a population of cells sensitive to ESF or other differentiating agents.

If one cobalt unit of ESF is injected into a polycythemic mouse and six hr later enough antibody against ESF is injected in the mouse to neutralize all the ESF which has not acted, a small but measurable erythropoietic response occurs. During the 9th to 12th days after 200 r irradiation, if ESF acts in the polycythemic mouse for only six hr, an erythropoietic response of about four times that observed in the nonirradiated polycythemic mouse occurs, as shown in FIGURE 4. These results suggest that four times the number of ESF-sensitive cells exist in the irradiated polycythemic mouse at this time than in a nonirradiated polycythemic mouse. It is unlikely that these ESF-sensitive cells could have been produced by division of the available colony-forming cells or ESF-sensitive cells in six hours.

Erythropoiesis in the Newborn Rat

Jacobson *et al.* observed several years ago[31] that transfusion of a pregnant mouse resulted in suppression of erythropoiesis in the mother but not in the fetuses. Schooley and Giger (unpublished observations) confirmed Jacobson's observations and in addition, found that after injection of anti-ESF into pregnant mice, erythropoiesis was significantly suppressed in the mother and in some but not all of the fetuses.

The effect of anti-ESF on the erythropoiesis of newborn rats was investigated.

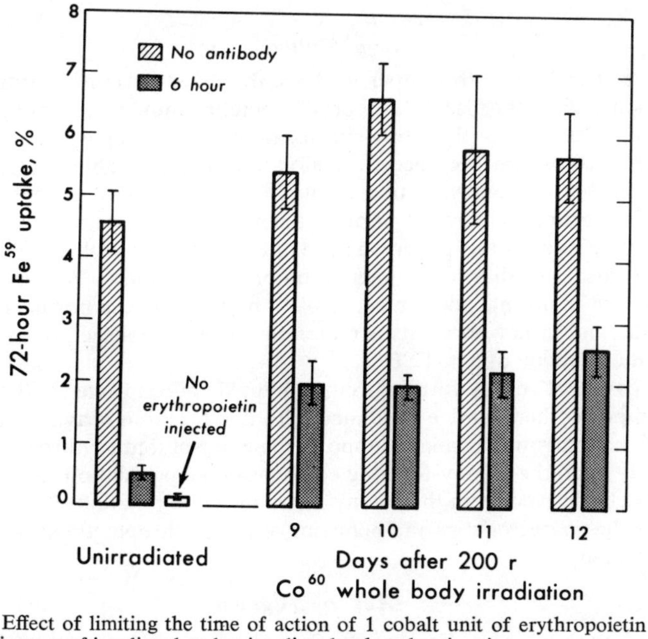

FIGURE 4. Effect of limiting the time of action of 1 cobalt unit of erythropoietin to six hr on the responsiveness of irradiated and unirradiated polycythemic mice.

Several litters of rats were used; half of each litter received injections of 0.1 ml of anti-ESF each morning and evening for six days. On the fifth day after birth 0.5 μc ^{59}Fe was injected i.p. and 24 hr later blood was taken by cardiac puncture. The ^{59}Fe uptakes were determined and the results expressed as the percentage of the injected ^{59}Fe in the blood volume; the blood volume was assumed to be 7% of the body weight according to the data of Garcia.[32] Hematocrits were measured; smears of the femoral marrow were made, and the spleen and liver fixed in Bouin's fixative for histological examination. The results are shown in TABLE 4. It is evident that a marked suppression of erythropoiesis on the basis of ^{59}Fe uptake occurred. Nucleated erythroid cells were rarely observed in the spleen and bone marrow, and the erythropoietic foci present in the livers of the control mice were absent in the anti-ESF injected mice. Very few reticulocytes with well-developed reticulum were observed in the anti-ESF-injected animals.

The erythropoietic activity of 1 ml of plasma obtained from five-day-old rats was assayed in the polycythemic mouse. The percent ^{59}Fe uptake in the assay mice was 0.54 ± 0.05, compared to 0.11 ± 0.01 when adult rat serum was injected. This difference is highly significant ($P < 0.001$), indicating that detectable amounts of ESF occur in the newborn rat.

Lucarelli *et al.*[33] have recently demonstrated that erythropoiesis is little affected by nephrectomy in newborn rats. They concluded that erythropoiesis in the newborn rat is controlled independently of a renally produced ESF. Our experiments with newborn rats indicate that ESF does control erythropoiesis at this age, but they provide no information about the organ producing the hormone. The inhibition of biological activity of ESF in both newborn and adult animals by anti-ESF does not necessarily indicate that the entire ESF molecule is identical at the two ages but does suggest that identical sites are involved in the neutralization reaction.

Summary

In the first section of this paper we have discussed current information on the preparation and properties of anti-erythropoietin immune serum and presented new evidence indicating that the neutralization of erythropoietin by the immune serum depends on the presence of γ-globulin. The available evidence supports the concept that the neutralization of the biological activity of erythropoietin by the immune serum is the result of an antigen-antibody reaction.

In the remainder of this paper we have illustrated the usefulness of anti-erythropoietin in various studies on the regulation of erythropoiesis. We have shown that erythropoiesis in normal adult mice, in WW^v mutant mice, in normal mice exposed to hypoxia, and in newborn rats is either completely abolished or markedly inhibited by the injection of anti-ESF.

The behavior of colony-forming cells in hypoxic mice injected with anti-erythropoietin in polycythemic mice irradiated with 200 r, and in heavily irradiated mice given a bone marrow transplant supports the concept that erythropoietin does not act directly upon the colony-forming cell but upon a population of erythropoietin-sensitive cells derived from the colony-forming cell population. Some speculations regarding the characteristics and behavior of the erythropoietin-sensitive cell have been presented.

Acknowledgment

We wish to thank Mrs. Caroline N. Schooley for taking the photomicrographs.

References

1. SCHOOLEY, J. C. & J. F. GARCIA. 1962. Immunochemical studies of human urinary erythropoietin. Proc. Soc. Exp. Biol. Med. **109:** 325–328.
2. LANGE, R. D., E. GARDNER, JR., C.-S. WRIGHT & N. I. GALLAGHER. 1964. Neutralization of the biological activity of erythropoietin by immune sera. Brit. J. Haematol. **10:** 69–74.
3. SCHOOLEY, J. C. & J. F. GARCIA. 1965. Some properties of serum obtained from rabbits immunized with human urinary erythropoietin. Blood **25:** 204–217.
4. GARCIA, J. F. & J. C. SCHOOLEY. 1963. Immunological neutralization of various erythropoietins. Proc. Soc. Exp. Biol. Med. **112:** 712–714.
5. ROSSE, W. F. & T. A. WALDMANN. 1964. A comparison of some physical and chemical properties of erythropoiesis-stimulating factors from different sources. Blood **24:** 739–749.
6. VAN DYKE, D. Personal communication.
7. GARCIA, J. F. In preparation.
8. JEPSON, J. H. & L. LOWENSTEIN. 1966. Inhibition of erythropoiesis by a factor present in the plasma of patients with erythroblastopenia. Blood **27:** 425–434.
9. SCHOOLEY, J. C. & J. F. GARCIA. 1962. Immunologic studies on the mechanism of action of erythropoietin. Proc. Soc. Exp. Biol. Med. **110:** 636–641.
10. FRIED, W., R. DEGOWIN & C. W. GURNEY. 1964. Erythropoietic effect of testosterone in the polycythemic mouse. Proc. Soc. Exp. Biol. Med. **117:** 839–842.
11. FRIED, W. & C. W. GURNEY. 1965. Use of mild plethora to demonstrate an erythropoietic effect from small amounts of androgens. Proc. Soc. Exp. Biol. Med. **120:** 519–521.
12. JANDA, W. E., W. FRIED & C. W. GURNEY. 1965. Combined effect of cobalt and testosterone on erythropoiesis. Proc. Soc. Exp. Biol. Med. **120:** 443–446.
13. FRIED, W. & C. W. GURNEY. 1965. Erythropoietic effect of plasma from mice receiving testosterone. Nature **206:** 1160–1161.
14. MIRAND, E. A., A. S. GORDON & J. WENIG. 1965. Mechanism of testosterone action in erythropoiesis. Nature **206:** 270–272.
15. SCHOOLEY, J. C. 1966. Inhibition of erythropoietic stimulation by testosterone in polycythemic mice receiving anti-erythropoietin. Proc. Soc. Exp. Biol. Med. **122:** 402–403.
16. RUSSELL, E. S. 1963. Problems and potentialities in the study of genic action in the mouse. *In* Methodology in Mammalian Genetics. W. J. Burdette, Ed. : 217–232. Holden-Day, Inc. San Francisco, Calif.
17. MCCULLOCH, E. A., L. SIMINOVITCH & J. E. TILL. 1964. Spleen colony formation in anemic mice of genotype WW^v. Science **144:** 844–846.
18. MCCULLOCH, E. A., J. E. TILL & L. SIMINOVITCH. 1965. Host-cell interactions in mice bearing isologous hemopoietic grafts. *In* La Greffe des Cellules Hématopoïétiques Allogéniques. G. Mathé, J.-L. Amiel & L. Schwarzenburg, Eds. : 61–71. Editions du Centre National de la Recherche Scientifique. Paris.
19. KEIGHLEY, G., E. S. RUSSELL & P. H. LOWY. 1962. Response of normal and genetically anaemic mice to erythropoietic stimuli. Brit. J. Haematol. **8:** 429–441.
20. KEIGHLEY, G. Personal communication.
21. BRUCE, W. R. & E. A. MCCULLOCH. 1964. The effect of erythropoietic stimulation on the hemopoietic colony-forming cells of mice. Blood **23:** 216–232.
22. SCHOOLEY, J. C., L. N. CANTOR & V. W. HAVENS. 1966. Relationship between growth of colony-forming cells and erythropoietin-sensitive cells in mice irradiated with 200 r of ^{60}Co gamma rays. Exptl. Haematol. **9:** 55–56 (abstr.).
23. SCHOOLEY, J. C. 1966. The effect of erythropoietin on the growth and development of spleen colony-forming cells. J. Cell. Physiol. **68:** 249–262.
24. SCHOOLEY, J. C. Responsiveness of hematopoietic tissue to erythropoietin in relation to the time of administration and duration of action of the hormone. Blood **25:** 795–808.
25. ALEXANIAN, R., D. D. PORTEOUS & L. G. LAJTHA. 1963. Stem cell kinetics after irradiation. Int. J. Rad. Biol. **7:** 87–94.
26. GURNEY, C. W., L. G. LAJTHA & R. OLIVER. 1962. A method for investigation of stem-cell kinetics. Brit. J. Haematol. **8:** 461–466.
27. GURNEY, C. W. 1963. Effect of radiation on the mouse stem cell compartment in vivo. Perspect. Biol. Med. **6:** 233–245.
28. TILL, J. E. 1963. Quantitative aspects of radiation lethality at the cellular level. Amer. J. Roentgenol. **90:** 917–927.
29. BLACKETT, N. M., P. J. ROYLANCE & K. ADAMS. 1964. Studies of the capacity of bone-marrow cells to restore erythropoiesis in heavily irradiated rats. Brit. J. Haematol. **10:** 453–467.

30. Becker, A. J. 1964. A radiobiological study of murine hemopoietic stem cells. Thesis, University of Toronto, Ontario, Canada.
31. Jacobson, L. O., E. K. Marks & E. O. Gaston. 1959. Studies on erythropoiesis. XII. The effect of transfusion-induced polycythemia in the mother on the fetus. Blood **14**: 644–653.
32. Garcia, J. F. 1957. Changes in blood, plasma and red cell volume in the male rat, as a function of age. Amer. J. Physiol. **190**: 19–24.
33. Lucarelli, G., D. Howard & F. Stohlman, Jr. 1964. Regulation of erythropoiesis. XV. Neonatal erythropoiesis and the effect of nephrectomy. J. Clin. Invest. **43**: 2195–2203.

APPLICATION OF ERYTHROPOIETIN ANTISERA TO STUDIES OF ERYTHROPOIESIS*

Robert D. Lange, Lois F. O'Grady, Jerry P. Lewis and Frank E. Trobaugh, Jr.

University of Tennessee Memorial Research Center, Knoxville, Tenn. and The Section of Hematology, Presbyterian-St. Luke's Hospital, The University of Illinois, Chicago, Ill.

INTRODUCTION

The development of antiserum to erythropoietin provides a new tool for the study of the action of this hormone, its site of formation, and its target cell, as well as for the development of an immunoassay. This paper describes some of the immunologic properties of erythropoietin antiserum, reports the results of in vivo and in vitro studies of its effect on erythropoiesis, and discusses problems associated with its production.

METHODS AND MATERIALS

Production of Antisera. Antisera to erythropoietin were produced by two methods. Antiserum to sheep plasma erythropoietin (SPE) was prepared by injecting rabbits s.c. with sheep plasma suspended in complete Freund's adjuvant. One ml of the antigen-adjuvant mixture containing 11.6 mg of protein was injected s.c. once weekly for four weeks. Rabbits were first bled one week after the last injection; further injections were followed at appropriate intervals by additional serum collections. Contaminating antibodies were absorbed by serum obtained from sheep which had been made polycythemic.

Antiserum to human urinary erythropoietin (HUE) was prepared by injecting rabbits with alum precipitates of a crude extract of urine obtained from a patient with refractory anemia according to the method of Kabat and Mayer.[1] The suspension contained 1.5 mg of protein per ml. The first injection was s.c. while all others were i.v., given three times weekly by the following schedule: three injections of 1.0 ml; three of 1.5 ml; four of 2.0 ml; four of 3.0 ml and two of 5.0 ml. One week after the last injection the animals were bled. Later, immunized animals were injected i.v. with 2.0 ml booster doses of the same suspension and bled after one week. Contaminating antibodies were absorbed from the anti-HUE with either normal human serum or serum obtained from a patient with polycythemia.

Immunologic Tests. Ouchterlony gel diffusion studies and immunoelectrophoresis were performed by standard methods.[2,3]

Cutaneous passive anaphylaxis was tested in guinea pigs by the method of Campbell *et al.*[4] The back of a guinea pig was shaved and injected i.d. with 0.1 ml of unabsorbed antiserum, 0.1 ml of absorbed antiserum or 0.1 ml of normal saline. Six hr later the guinea pig was challenged by a 1 ml i.v. injection of saline and Evan's blue which contained either 0.04 ml of normal human serum or 0.45–0.9 mg of concentrated erythropoietin. The reaction was considered positive if blue color appeared at the skin site of antiserum injection.

Erythropoietin Assay. Erythropoietin was assayed indirectly by measuring the incorporation of radioiron into the red blood cells of polycythemic mice.[5]

* Investigations supported in part by U.S.P.H.S. research grant no. HE 10567–01 and N.S.F. grant no. GB 4818 to the University of Tennessee and research grant no. C–4144 from the National Cancer Institute, U.S.P.H.S., and by a grant from the American Cancer Society, Inc. Illinois Division to the Presbyterian-St. Luke's Hospital.

Neutralization Studies. In vitro tests for the neutralization of erythropoietin were conducted using suspension cultures of rabbit bone marrow. Bone marrow of white, female, New Zealand rabbits was spooned into 37° C Hanks' solution, the cells dispersed by forcing the suspension through 16-, 20-, and 26-gauge needles, and the suspension adjusted to contain approximately 10,000 nucleated cells per mm^3 in Eagle's minimum essential media. Two ml of the cell suspension, 0.3 ml of autologous serum previously incubated for 30 min with 0.03 μc of ^{59}Fe citrate, and test materials usually not exceeding 0.3 ml were placed in 50 ml Erlenmyer flasks; 500 units of penicillin, 750 μg of streptomycin, and 1500 units of mycostatin were then added. The flasks were tightly stoppered and placed in a shaking incubator for 45 hours. The cell suspensions were then centrifuged; the cells were washed with saline, resuspended, and their radioactivity measured in a well scintillation counter. The iron incorporated by samples incubated with autologous serum at 37° C was taken as the 100% value. The amount of iron absorbed to the cell membranes was estimated from suspensions maintained at 4° C. The effect on iron incorporation of added erythropoietin* and/or antiserum to erythropoietin was compared to these values.

In vivo tests for neutralization of erythropoietin were performed by mixing graded doses of antiserum with a known amount of erythropoietin and assaying the mixture for erythropoietin activity in plethoric mice.

In Vivo Hematopoietic Colony Studies. Other in vivo studies observed the effect of antiserum and erythropoietin on the development of hematopoietic colonies in the spleens of mice.

Assay Animals. CAF_1/Cum 13–14-week-old female mice were used throughout. They were housed in groups of six in disposable plastic cages and received food** and chlorinated water (1 ml of sodium hypochlorite to one gallon of tap water) ad lib.

Description of Irradiation. In groups of six, mice were irradiated with a total dose of 750 ± 40 r at the rate of 76 r per minute. This dosage was given in a vertical beam from a Westinghouse x-ray machine at: 200 KVP, 18 ma 50 cm distance, 0.5 mm copper and 1 mm aluminum—HVL, 1 mm copper, open field.

Preparation and Injection of Cells. Marrow cells were obtained from the femurs of isologous mice. The marrow plug was flushed out of the femur cavity with one ml of Hanks' solution using a 22-gauge needle. A cellular suspension was made from the marrow plug by aspirating and injecting it repeatedly in and out of the same syringe. The cellular concentration of the suspension was determined in a hemocytometer and dilutions prepared so that 15,000 cells were contained in 0.5 ml of suspension. Each injection was given into a tail vein using a tuberculin syringe and a one-inch 27-gauge needle. Prior to injection the animals were warmed under an infrared lamp in order to induce vascular dilatation. All test suspensions were prepared less than four hr prior to administration and all animals were injected less than five hr after irradiation.

Study I: Effect of Hypertransfusion. Test animals were hypertransfused three and two days prior to irradiation with either 1 ml or 2 ml of blood. This resulted in a mean hematocrit on the day of sacrifice of 47.7 and 57.5%, respectively. The mean hematocrit of the control group on the day of sacrifice was 38.7%. All animals were then transplanted with 15,000 isologous cells prepared as described above.

* The sheep plasma erythropoietin used in these studies was obtained through the Hematology Study Section of the National Institutes of Health.

** Purina Mouse Breeder Chow, Ralston Purina Company, St. Louis, Mo.

Eight days later the animals were sacrificed; their spleens were removed, fixed in buffered formalin, and serially sectioned at 4 μ. Every 20th section was then mounted and stained with hematoxylin and eosin. The slides were read by three independent observers, and the size and morphologic type of each colony were recorded on an outline drawn of the spleen sections. Colonies were described as erythroid, granulocytic, megakaryocytic, or mixed. Colonies designated as mixed were those which contained two or more cellular elements regardless of the relative numbers; for example, a granulocytic or erythroid colony with one megakaryocyte was designated as mixed.

To derive the volume of an erythroid colony, each microscopic section of a colony was projected at a set and known magnification and the area determined by planimetry. The volume was then calculated from the formula:

$$\text{Vol (mm}^3) = \frac{\begin{matrix}\text{planimetric} \\ \text{vernier units}\end{matrix} \times \begin{matrix}\text{thickness} \\ \text{of section}\end{matrix} \times F \times C}{(\text{magnification})^2}$$

where C is a conversion factor showing the relation of mm^2 to vernier units and F shows the relation of number of sections mounted to total number of sections cut.

Study II: Exogenous Erythropoietin. Test animals were transfused three and two days before irradiation with 2 ml of blood, an amount sufficient to block formation of erythroid colonies. The animals were then irradiated, injected with 15,000 isologous marrow cells, and immediately given the first of eight daily i.p. injections of erythropoietin. The erythropoietin was obtained from the urine of a patient with refractory anemia concentrated by column chromatography[6] and standardized against erythropoietin standard B.† The mice were then divided into seven groups; the mice of each group received one of the following daily doses of erythropoietin: 0, 0.01, 0.02, 0.04, 0.08, 0.16, or 0.32 unit. On the eighth day the spleens were removed and processed as described above.

Study III: Antisera to Erythropoietin. Nontransfused mice were irradiated and injected with 15,000 bone marrow cells. Absorbed anti-HUE, prepared as described above, was suspended in Hanks' solution, and appropriate dilutions were made so that mice could be injected i.v. with either 0.3 or 0.6 ml of antiserum for eight days following irradiation. The animals were then sacrificed and the spleen sections prepared.

Results

Immunological Tests

The ability of anti-HUE to neutralize the biological activity of erythropoietin extracted from human urine is shown in FIGURE 1. It should be noted that the addition of antiserum reduced the in vivo incorporation of iron to the value found in animals injected with saline. Previous experiments have shown that antiserum after absorption with normal human serum retained the ability to neutralize the biologic activity of erythropoietin. In one experiment saline-injected animals incorporated 0.21% of the injected radioiron; mice injected with 0.4 unit erythropoietin, 6.05%; and mice injected with 0.2 unit erythropoietin plus 0.1 ml absorbed anti-HUE, 0.28%, a value similar to that found in saline controls.

Unabsorbed anti-HUE reacted with a concentrated erythropoietin solution by the formation of multiple precipitin lines when tested by immunoelectrophoresis

† Furnished by the Medical Research Council, National Institute for Medical Research, London, England.

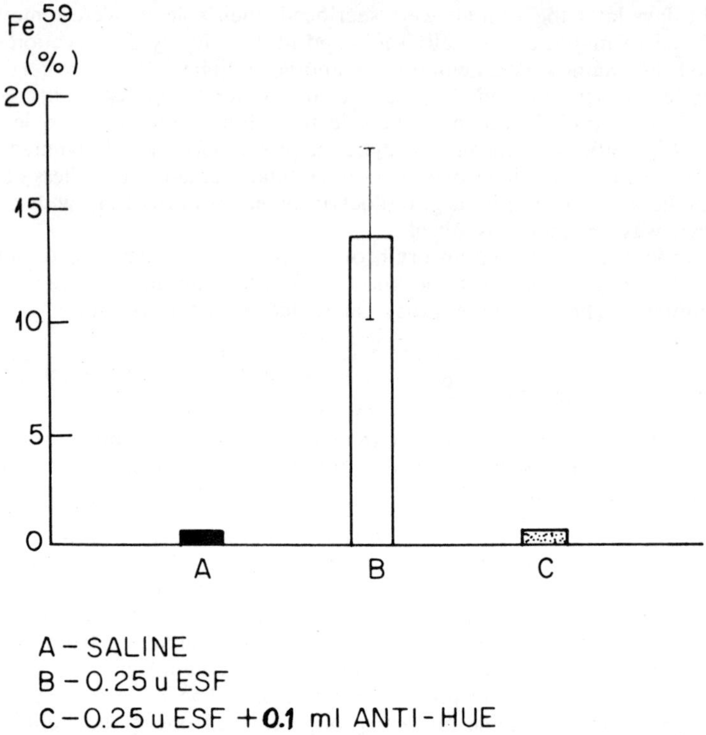

FIGURE 1. Effect of anti-HUE on RBC ^{59}Fe incorporation in polycythemic mice injected with 0.25 unit of erythropoietin.

or Ouchterlony gel diffusion. After absorption of the anti-HUE with normal human serum, no precipitin lines were found.

When tested by cutaneous passive anaphylaxis in the guinea pig, unabsorbed HUE reacted to both normal human serum and concentrated human urinary erythropoietin (FIGURE 2). The absorbed antiserum did not react with normal human serum but did react with the concentrated erythropoietin.

In Vitro Neutralization Studies

FIGURE 3 contrasts the results of in vitro experiments in which anti-SPE was added at the start of incubation of the suspension culture with those in which the antiserum was added 21 hr later. It should be noted that when erythropoietin was added (Column C), the iron incorporation of the suspension was increased. Addition of anti-SPE at the start of the incubation period completely blocked the incorporation of iron. If the anti-SPE was added after 21 hr of incubation, there was little effect on the 45-hour iron incorporation by the bone marrow cells.

In Vivo Hematopoietic Colony Studies

Study I. In studying the ability of hypertransfusion to suppress erythropoiesis, 400 hematopoietic colonies were analyzed; the results are shown in FIGURE 4. With increasing degrees of plethora there was a decrease in size and in number of

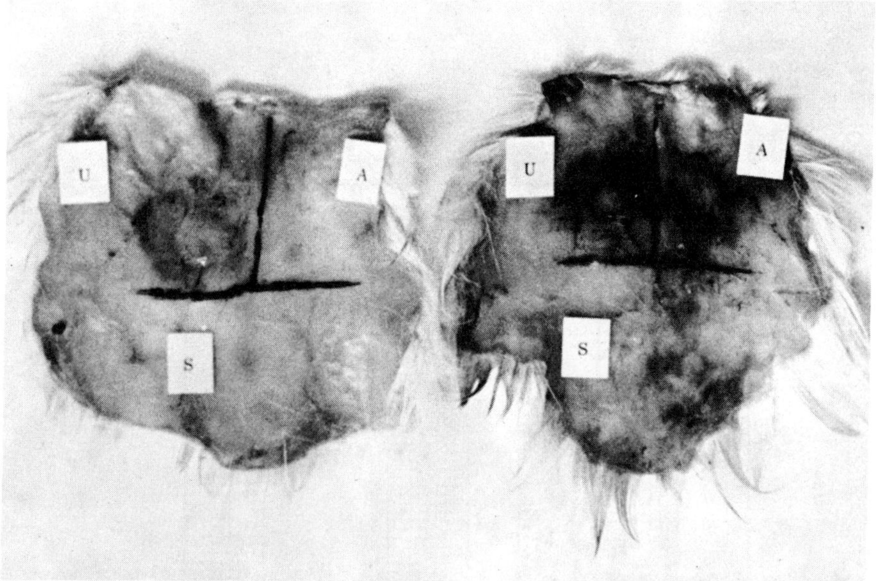

FIGURE 2. Cutaneous passive anaphylaxis. A—absorbed anti-HUE; U—unabsorbed anti-HUE; S—saline.. Animal on left challenged with 0.04 ml normal human serum and animal on right with human urinary erythropoietin (0.32 mg protein/ml injected material).

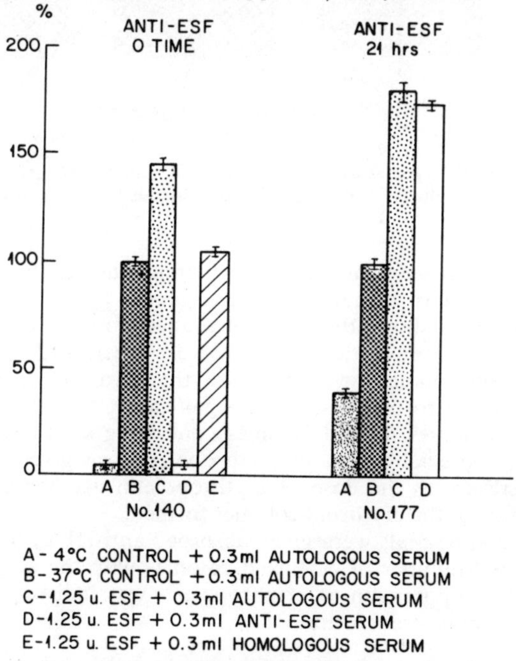

FIGURE 3. Effect of sheep plasma erythropoietin (ESF) and anti-SPE on the 45-hour radioiron incorporation in rabbit bone marrow suspension culture. 37° C with autologous serum is taken as 100% value. Anti-SPE added at the start of incubation and after 21 hr incubation.

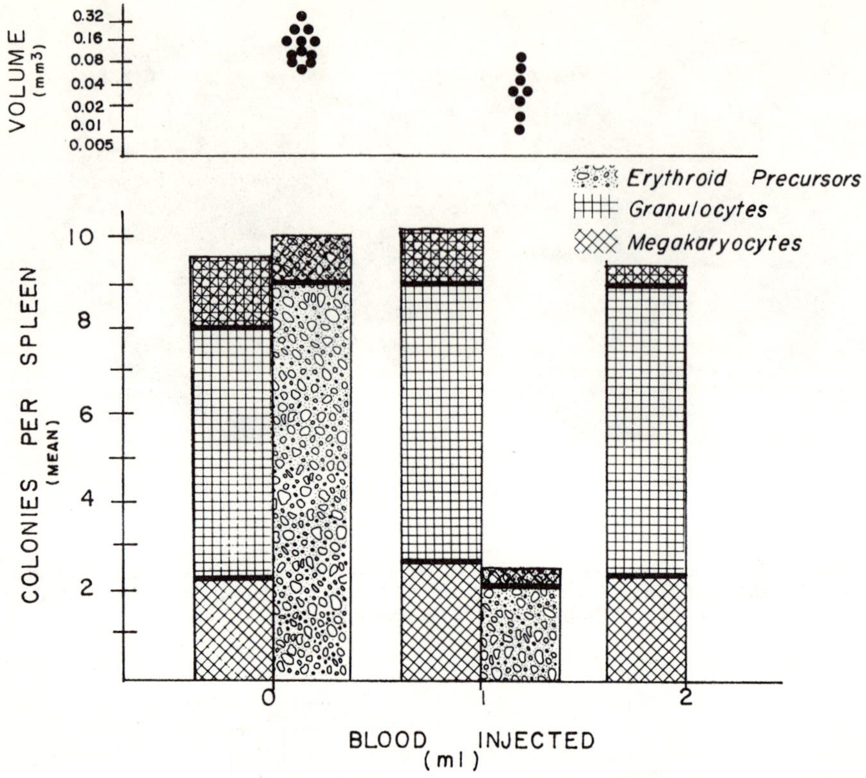

FIGURE 4. Effect of hypertransfusion on size and number of hematopoietic colonies in spleens of CAF_1 female mice injected with 15,000 isologous bone marrow cells following 750 r irradiation.

erythroid colonies. In the range of polycythemia studied, there was no apparent effect on granulocytic or megakaryocytic colonies.

Study II. FIGURE 5 shows the effect of graded doses of erythropoietin on the number and cellular composition of colonies in spleens of hypertransfused mice. As the dose of erythropoietin was increased, there was an increase in the number of erythroid colonies formed without a significant effect on the granulocytic or megakaryocytic colonies. Mixed colonies containing erythroid elements did not appear until an appreciable dose of erythropoietin was given. In addition to this numerical difference, as the dose of erythropoietin was increased there was an increase in the size of the erythroid colonies formed.

Study III. When animals were given absorbed anti-HUE, there was a decrease in the volume and number of erythroid colonies with the addition of antiserum (FIGURE 6). This suppression of erythropoiesis was indistinguishable from that produced by mild hypertransfusion.

DISCUSSION

Although attempts in our laboratory to produce antisera to erythropoietin in guinea pigs and sheep have been unsuccessful, in ours and other laboratories

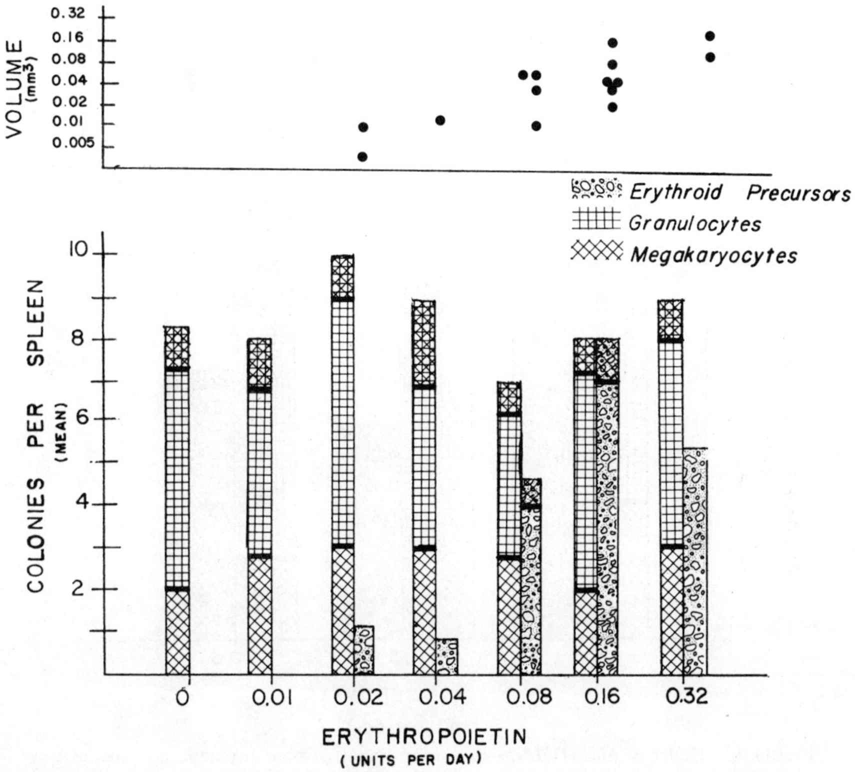

FIGURE 5. Effect of graded doses of erythropoietin (HUE) on size and cellular composition of spleen colonies in hypertransfused irradiated mice injected with 15,000 isologous bone marrow cells.

rabbits have been immunized to erythropoietin obtained from human urine,[7–9] sheep plasma[10-12] and human plasma (HPE).[13] These antisera have been produced either by the use of alum-precipitated material or by the incorporation of erythropoietin into complete Freund's adjuvant, the routes of antigen administration and dosage schedule having varied with each laboratory.

The low level of antigenicity of erythropoietin leads to problems with the production of antisera. A suitable antiserum is produced only in approximately one-third of the rabbits immunized,[14,15] and with the development of neutralizing antibodies some of the immunized animals develop anemia.[15] Another problem is the low titer that is usually produced. Schooley and Garcia[15] have been able to produce an anti-HUE that neutralized the equivalent of 0.59 units of erythropoietin in a 1:10 dilution but the antisera had no neutralizing effect at a 1:100 dilution. In our laboratory we have found it necessary to use 0.6 ml of absorbed antisera to neutralize 1.2 units of erythropoietin. We have previously reported that 0.0625 units of erythropoietin inhibited the hemagglutination of tanned red blood cells when a 1:8000 dilution of an absorbed anti-SPE was used.[10]

Other problems associated with producing the antisera are the consequence of the lack of pure erythropoietin. Since partially purified extracts of erythropoietin are utilized for immunization, the resulting antisera frequently contain contamin-

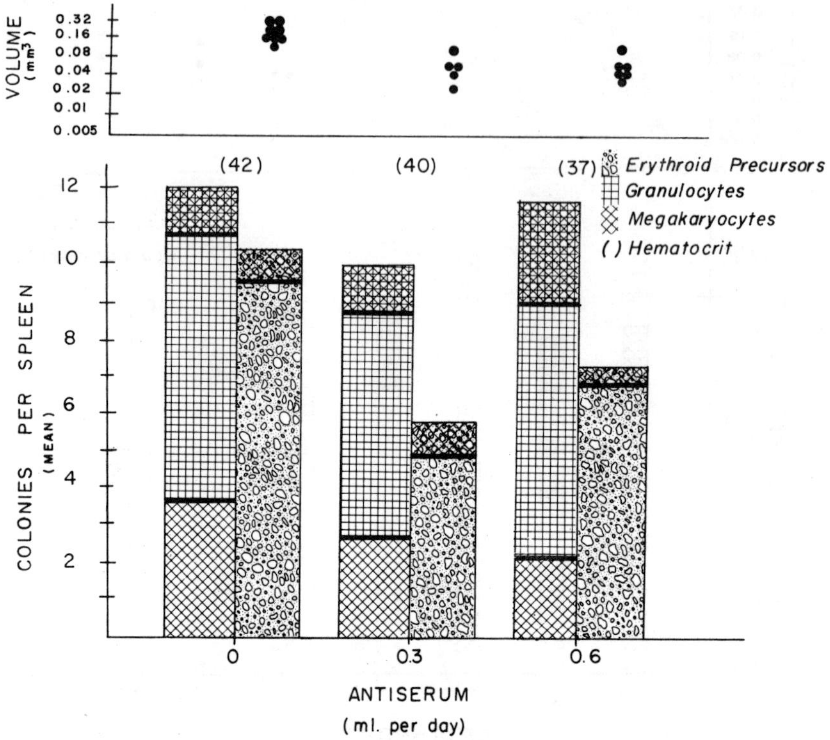

FIGURE 6. Effect of anti-HUE on size and number of hematopoietic colonies in spleens of nontransfused mice irradiated and injected with 15,000 isologous bone marrow cells.

ating antibodies to other proteins found in plasma or urine, and visible precipitates may result when unabsorbed antisera are mixed with human serum or concentrated erythropoietin. Multiple lines may also be found if unabsorbed antiserum is tested for precipitin by Ouchterlony gel diffusion or immunoelectrophoresis. However, after absorption with sera containing little or no erythropoietin, either a single line[11,13] or no precipitin lines are found[15] even though the absorbed antisera have retained their ability to neutralize the biologic activity of erythropoietin. The lack of these precipitin lines on gel diffusion or immunoelectrophoresis indicates that the antibodies to erythropoietin are of the nonprecipitating variety.

Cutaneous passive anaphylaxis represents another sensitive method of testing the purity of the antisera. With this test one can determine the amount of polycythemic, uremic, or normal serum needed to absorb contaminating antibodies. Unabsorbed antiserum will react to the challenge of normal human serum. After absorption, the antiserum no longer reacts with the normal human serum, but will still react when challenged with concentrated erythropoietin.

The neutralizing ability of the antisera can be demonstrated by several procedures. Anti-HUE and anti-HPE have been shown to depress erythropoiesis in intact mice[16] and rats,[13] as measured by the incorporation of radioiron into red blood cells. The bone marrows of such animals morphologically demonstrate their almost complete lack of erythroid elements.

A more commonly used test to demonstrate the neutralizing ability is to add antiserum to erythropoietin in vitro and then to test for erythropoietin activity in polycythemic mice or starved rats. As reported here and elsewhere,[7–13] antiserum under these circumstances can completely block the erythropoietic-stimulating activity of erythropoietin and may be used to test for species specificity. For example, an anti-HUE has been shown to block erythropoietin from mice, rats, rabbits, and sheep[17] and an anti-HPE was found to cross-react with rabbit and rat erythropoietin.[13] However, another anti-HUE did not block the action of erythropoietin produced in a Japanese quail[18] although this same antiserum blocked the erythropoietin activity found in the serum of patients with aplastic anemia or hypoxic erythrocytosis and the activity in renal cyst fluid or in extracts of cerebellar hemangioblastomas found in patients with erythrocytosis.[8] These studies suggest that erythropoietin from mammalian sources share common antigenic determinants and are similar if not identical.

Optimally absorbed anti-HUE has been found to fix complement up to a titer of 1:16.[9] Schooley and Garcia found that heating an anti-HUE for 30 min at 56° C did not alter the neutralizing effect.[15] However, as they pointed out, since the test for neutralizing ability was carried out in vivo, the effect of complement could not be assessed.

The antisera are useful in studying the kinetics of erythropoiesis since antiserum can limit the availability of a stimulating dose of erythropoietin. Schooley demonstrated that different doses of erythropoietin caused approximately the same red blood cell ^{59}Fe incorporation when the injection of antiserum limited the action of the hormone to six hours.[19] In earlier studies he and Garcia found that anti-HUE had no effect on the magnitude of erythropoietic response when injected into polycythemic mice 24 to 44 hr after initiation of a wave of erythropoiesis.[16] Injections of the serum one hour before or at the same time that erythropoietin was administered completely abolished the erythropoietic response. As reported in this paper, anti-HUE has been used to demonstrate an effect on erythroid colony formation in the spleens of mice lethally irradiated and then injected with 15,000 bone marrow cells. The injection of small amounts of anti-HUE caused a definite decrease in the size of the developing erythroid colonies. The present report and other studies[20–22] indicate that the formation of erythroid colonies in spleens of irradiated mice is blocked by hypertransfusing mice and that this block can be overcome by administration of exogenous erythropoietin.[21,23] It seems probable, therefore, that by using larger doses of anti-HUE, the formation of erythroid colonies in the mouse spleen can be completely blocked by an appropriate antiserum. Studies utilizing larger amounts of antiserum are in progress.

Just as antiserum to erythropoietin blocks the action of erythropoietin in vivo, so can the action of erythropoietin be blocked in vitro. When antiserum is added to a bone marrow suspension at the start of incubation, the increased iron incorporation due to erythropoietin, as well as the iron incorporation caused by factors present in normal serum, is blocked.[24] Whether these factors present in normal serum represent endogenous erythropoietin remain to be elucidated. One could hypothesize that the antisera prevent enzyme induction and thus prevent erythroid differentiation, or possibly that the effect of the antiserum at the cell membrane level is to prevent the transfer of iron to the developing and maturing cells. These problems await future investigation.

It had been hoped that antisera could be utilized in studies of the site of formation of erythropoietin and for development of an immunoassay. In early studies we used the indirect fluorescent antibody technique of Mellors to demonstrate a decrease in fluorescence of kidney sections when specific antiserum was absorbed with polycythemic serum.[10] Fisher *et al.*[11] showed that the glomerular tuft of sheep kidneys stained with fluorescein-labeled anti-SPE prepared in rabbits, suggesting these tufts as the site of formation of erythropoietin. With similar techniques, Baum *et al.*[12] found staining in the peripheral cells of all glomeruli in the kidneys of bled sheep, but found no staining in the kidneys or other organs of normal sheep or rats.

These studies of fluorescent localization and immunoassay have been hampered by the impurity of the erythropoietin. As a consequence the antiserum must be absorbed, but there is no assurance that all of the contaminating antibodies, especially the nonprecipitating variety, have been removed. Similar difficulties are present in attempting to develop an immunoassay since it is necessary to start with a relatively pure antigen to label and the techniques for separating the free from the bound form of the antigen are cumbersome. However, such systems have been developed for the assay of insulin,[25] glucagon,[26] growth hormone,[27] and other smaller molecular weight hormones.[28,29] Whether or not the systems will work for erythropoietin and its antiserum remains a problem for the future.

Summary

Antiserum has been produced which blocks the normal iron incorporation induced by erythropoietin and which, after all precipitating antibodies have been absorbed, is still capable of producing cutaneous passive anaphylaxis in the guinea pig. In vitro studies have shown that this antiserum blocks iron incorporation by bone marrow cells. To study its effect in vivo, its ability to reduce erythropoietin activity has been compared to that of hypertransfusion. Increasing plethora reduces the size and number of erythroid colonies in the spleens of mice irradiated and transplanted with marrow. With sufficient plethora, no erythroid elements are found; this effect, however, is reversible by the administration of exogenous erythropoietin. In nonhypertransfused mice the injection of the antiserum also effects a decrease in the size and number of the colonies.

Acknowledgments

The authors wish to acknowledge the advice and help of the following investigators who participated in some of the experiments reported: Drs. E. Gardner, V. Pavlovic-Kentera, Jasper P. Lewis, C.-S. Wright and N. I. Gallagher. We also wish to thank Drs. A. I. Chernoff, T. P. McDonald and P. A. McFate for their helpful reviews of the manuscript.

References

1. Kabat, E. A. & M. M. Mayer. 1964. *In* Experimental Immunochemistry. : 871. Charles C. Thomas. Springfield, Ill.
2. Ouchterlony, O. 1958. Diffusion-in-gel methods for immunological analysis. Prog. Allergy. **5**: 1–78.
3. Scheidegger, J. J. 1965. Une microméthode de l'immunoélectrophorèse. Intern. Arch. Allergy Appl. Immunol. **7**: 103–110.
4. Campbell, D. H., J. S. Garvey, N. E. Cremer & D. H. Sussdorf. 1964. *In* Methods in Immunology. : 216–217. W. A. Benjamin, Inc. New York.
5. Pavlović-Kentera, V., D. P. Hall, C. Bragassa & R. D. Lange. 1965. Unilateral renal hypoxia and production of erythropoietin. J. Lab. Clin. Med. **65**: 577–588.
6. Lewis, J. P., D. A. Alford, J. H. Rathjen, Jr. & R. D. Lange. 1965. Preparation of human urine concentrate for erythropoietin studies. J. Lab. Clin. Med. **66**: 987–993.
7. Schooley, J. C. & J. F. Garcia. 1962. Immunochemical studies of human urinary erythropoietin. Proc. Soc. Exp. Biol. Med. **109**: 325–328.
8. Rosse, W. F. & T. A. Waldmann. 1964. A comparison of some physical and chemical properties of erythropoiesis-stimulating factors from different sources. Blood **24**: 739–749.

9. LANGE, R. D., V. PAVLOVIĆ-KENTERA, E. GARDNER & J. P. LEWIS. 1964. Antisera to human urinary erythropoietin. Characterization and in vitro effect. Abstracts X Cong. Intern. Soc. Hemat. Abs. M 18.
10. LANGE, R. D., E. GARDNER, C.-S. WRIGHT & N. I. GALLAGHER. 1962. Neutralization of the biologic activity of erythropoietin by immune sera. Proc. IX Cong. Intern. Soc. Hemat. **3:** 135–141.
11. FISHER, J. W., G. TAYLOR & D. D. PORTEOUS. 1965. Localization of erythropoietin in glomeruli of sheep kidney by fluorescent antibody technique. Nature **205:** 611–612.
12. BAUM, J., W. SUKI & E. P. FRENKEL. 1965. Localization of erythropoietin in the kidney by immunofluorescence. Clin. Res. **13:** 68 (Abstr.).
13. GOUDSMIT, R. & P. G. L. C. KRUGERS DAGNEAUX. 1964. Immunological studies of erythropoietin. Abstracts X. Cong. Intern. Soc. Hemat. Abs. M 19.
14. LANGE, R. D., E. GARDNER, JR., C.-S. WRIGHT & N. I. GALLAGHER. 1964. Neutralization of the biological activity of erythropoietin by immune sera. Brit. J. Haematol. **10:** 69–74.
15. SCHOOLEY, J. C. & J. F. GARCIA. 1965. Some properties of serum obtained from rabbits immunized with human urinary erythropoietin. Blood **25:** 204–217.
16. SCHOOLEY, J. C. & J. F. GARCIA. 1962. Immunologic studies on the mechanism of action of erythropoietin. Proc. Soc. Exp. Biol. Med. **110:** 636–641.
17. GARCIA, J. F. & J. C. SCHOOLEY. 1963. Immunological neutralization of various erythropoietins. Proc. Soc. Exp. Biol. Med. **112:** 712–714.
18. ROSSE, W. F. & T. A. WALDMANN. 1966. Factors controlling erythropoiesis in birds. Blood **27:** 654–661.
19. SCHOOLEY, J. C. 1965. Responsiveness of hematopoietic tissue to erythropoietin in relation to the time of administration and duration of action of the hormone. Blood **25:** 795–808.
20. LIRON, M. & M. FELDMAN. 1965. The specific suppression of the differentiation of erythroid clones in polycythemic animals. Transplantation **3:** 509–516.
21. CURRY, J., J. TRENTIN & N. WOLF. 1964. Control of spleen colony histology by erythropoietin, cobalt and hypertransfusion. Exp. Hemat. **7:** 80 (Abstr.)
22. SCHOOLEY, J. C. 1964. Studies on the regulation of erythropoiesis in spleen colonies. Exp. Hemat. **7:** 79 (Abs.).
23. BLEIBERG, I., M. LIRON & M. FELDMAN. 1965. Reversion by erythropoietin of the suppression of erythroid clones caused by transfusion-induced polycythemia. Transplantation **3:** 706–710.
24. PAVLOVÍC-KENTERA, V., R. D. LANGE, J. P. LEWIS & E. GARDNER, JR. 1965. Effect of erythropoietin and antisera to erythropoietin on the in vitro ^{59}Fe incorporation by rabbit bone marrow cells. Jugoslov. Physiol. Pharmacol. Acta **1:** 15–27.
25. BERSON, S. A., R. S. YALOW, A. BAUMAN, M. A. ROTHSCHILD & K. NEWERLY. 1956. Insulin-^{131}I metabolism in human subjects: Demonstration of insulin binding globulin in the circulation of insulin treated subjects. J. Clin. Invest. **35:** 170–190.
26. UNGER, R. H., A. M. EISENTRAUT, M. S. MCCALL, S. KELLER, H. C. LANZ & L. L. MADISON. 1959. Glucagon antibodies and their use for immunoassay for glucagon. Proc. Soc. Exp. Biol. Med. **102:** 621–623.
27. UTIGER, R. D., M. L. PARKER & W. H. DAUGHADAY. 1962. Studies on human growth hormone I. A radioimmunoassay for human growth hormone. J. Clin. Invest. **41:** 254–261.
28. BERSON, S. A., R. S. YALOW, G. D. AURBACH & J. T. POTTS, JR. 1963. Immunoassay of bovine and human parathyroid hormone. Proc. Nat. Acad. Sci. **49:** 613–617.
29. FELBER, J. P. 1963. ACTH antibodies and their use for a radioimmunoassay for ACTH. Experientia **19:** 227–229.

SOME OBSERVATIONS ON THE LOCALIZATION OF ERYTHROPOIETIN

Eugene P. Frenkel, Wadi Suki and John Baum

Department of Internal Medicine of The University of Texas Southwestern Medical School, Dallas, Tex.

In order to seek direct evidence for the renal localization of erythropoietin and attempt to identify precisely its site of production, an immunofluorescent study was performed.[1] Antibody was produced in rabbits to partially purified sheep erythropoietin, the Immunoglobulin G separated and then fluoresceinated and the antierythropoietin activity was absorbed from the fluoresceinated IgG.[2] Immune staining was performed on cryostat, air-dried tissue sections. Blocking studies were done by treatment of the tissue sections with unfluoresceinated antierythropoietin prior to staining with the fluoresceinated material.

Specific staining was not identified in any tissues obtained from normal sheep nor from any tissues other than kidney in the anemic sheep. Where significant anemia was induced with peripheral hematocrits below 20 vol. percent, specific staining was noted in virtually every glomerulus. FIGURE 1 demonstrates one such glomerulus with the staining that characteristically involved the periphery of the glomerulus in a crescent-like pattern. Under oil immersion bright fluorescent granules were noted in the cytoplasm of the stained cells. No staining of the tubular or juxtaglomerular region was noted. This fluorescence was eliminated by absorption with normal sheep serum and by blocking with unfluoresceinated antierythropoietin. In addition, controls with rabbit anti-sheep globulin failed to reveal this pattern of tissue staining.

The specific immune staining of the peripheral portions of virtually all of the glomeruli in the kidney of an appropriately anemic sheep strongly suggests the presence of erythropoietin in the kidney with very specific localization to the glomeruli. Such staining suggests this portion of the glomerulus as a site of production of the erythropoietin but does not rule out the possibility that this area serves as storage for erythropoietin. This latter possibility seems unlikely since staining was identified only with profound anemia. Similarly, it is unlikely that the identifiable stained sites are precursor forms of erythropoietin.

In conclusion, these immunofluorescent studies suggest that the peripheral portion of the sheep glomerulus is the site of production of erythropoietin.

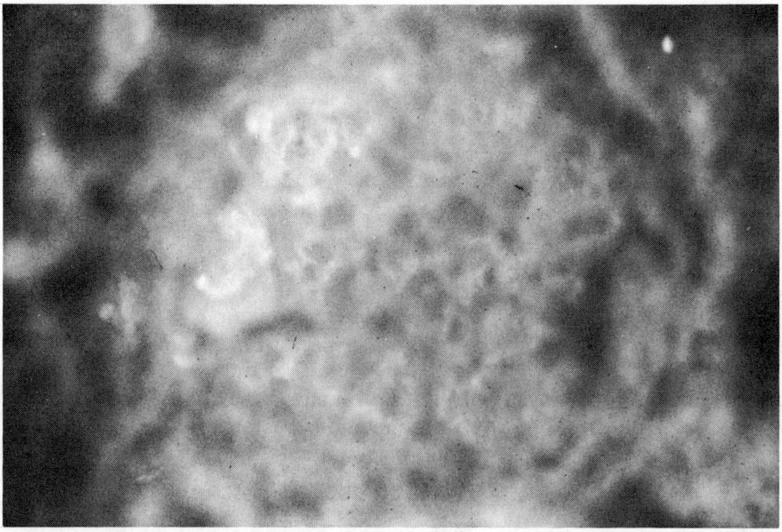

FIGURE 1. Crescent-shaped bright fluorescence of the peripheral border of the glomerulus of an anemic sheep kidney stained with fluoresceinated rabbit anti-sheep erythropoietin Immunoglobulin G.

REFERENCES

1. BAUM, J., W. SUKI & E. P. FRENKEL. 1965. Localization of erythropoietin in the kidney by immunofluorescence. Clin. Res. **13**: 68.
2. BAUM, J., W. SUKI & E. P. FRENKEL. Localization of erythropoietin in the kidney by immunofluorescence. In preparation.

INVESTIGATIONS ON AN IMMUNOASSAY OF ERYTHROPOIETIN

P. G. L. C. Krugers Dagneaux, R. Goudsmit and H. W. Krijnen

Central Laboratory of the Netherlands Red Cross Blood Transfusion Service, Amsterdam, Netherlands

It is presently possible to perform determinations of plasma erythropoietin, but such procedures are fraught with difficulties. The current methods bear the handicap inherent in bioassay: they are insensitive, time-consuming and expensive in that they require animals and many materials. Since the antigenicity of human urinary erythropoietin has been established by Schooley and Garcia,[1] one may hypothesize that an immunoassay is theoretically possible. This would be a vast improvement when compared to current methods, but such an immunoassay is not possible without first obtaining a specific antibody.

We were able to produce a precipitating neutralizing antibody against human erythropoietin by injecting rabbits with a human plasma-erythropoietin preparation. As the antigen used for immunization contained several other human plasma proteins besides erythropoietin, precipitating antibodies directed against these proteins were produced at the same time and several precipitation lines were obtained with the agar diffusion technique (FIGURE 1). The antiserum showed a continuous precipitation line with human, rat and rabbit erythropoietin using the same technique (FIGURE 1). By using this cross reactivity, we were able to produce an antiserum specifically directed against human erythropoietin and not against other human plasma proteins.

We immunized rabbits with a rat erythropoietin preparation. Although the produced antiserum showed several precipitation lines with rat erythropoietin preparations, only one was seen with a human erythropoietin preparation, as well as with a rabbit erythropoietin preparation (FIGURE 2). The antiserum showed only one precipitation line in the α_1 globulin range with a human and a rabbit erythropoietin preparation in the immunoelectrophoresis (FIGURE 3).

The antiserum depressed the endogenous erythropoietin activity in the normal rat (TABLE 1) and neutralized human erythropoietin in the polycythemic hypoxic mouse assay (TABLE 2). We were able to dissociate the erythropoietin activity from an immune precipitate of a human erythropoietin preparation and this antiserum at pH 2.5 followed by Sephadex G 200 gelfiltration (TABLE 3). The anti-rat erythropoietin antiserum again showed only one precipitation line in the α_1 globulin range with the aforementioned dissociation product in the immunoelectrophoresis as did an anti human erythropoietin antiserum.

To investigate the possibility of an immunoassay of erythropoietin, we carried out some preliminary experiments with different plasma samples using the agar diffusion technique. With normal plasma a precipitation line was seen up to a dilution of 1:4. With plasma of patients with aplastic anemia a precipitation line up to a dilution of 1:256 was seen. Plasma of two patients with chronic nephritis, uremia and anemia did not give any visible reaction.

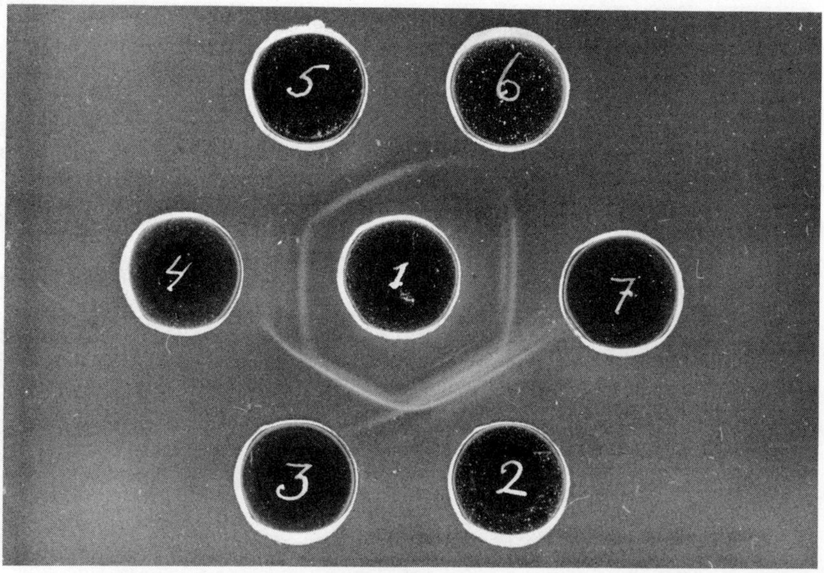

FIGURE 1. Precipitation lines obtained with agar diffusion technique.
1 = antihuman EP antiserum
2 = antigen used for immunization
3 = purified human erythropoietin
4 = rabbit erythropoietin
5 = rat erythropoietin
6 = sheep erythropoietin
7 = human urinary erythropoietin

TABLE 1
RABBITS IMMUNIZED WITH ACTIVE RAT ERYTHROPOIETIN

		% ^{59}Fe Incorporation	
	No.	Mean	Range
Normal rabbit serum	4	22.2	(25.1 – 19.2)
Rabbit 1	5	8.1	(9.8 – 5.0)
Rabbit 2	5	15.4	(21.0 – 10.7)
Rabbit 3	3	9.1	(10.3 – 7.7)

TABLE 2
POLYCYTHEMIC MICE

	Number of Animals	% ^{59}Fe Incorporation Mean	Range
Saline	4	0.6	0.4 – 0.8
Human erythropoietin	5	34	22 – 47
Human erythropoietin + anti-rat EP antiserum	4	5.9	5.3 – 6.7

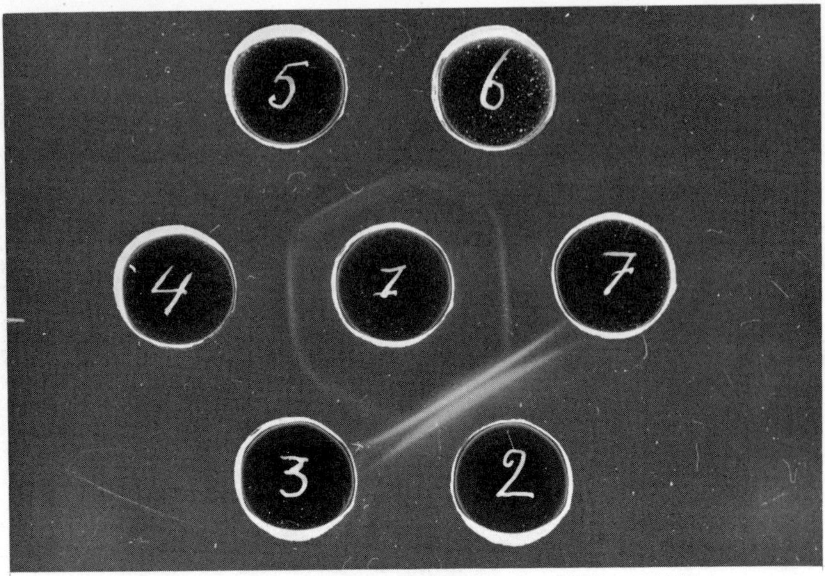

FIGURE 2. Precipitation lines obtained with agar diffusion technique.
1 = anti-rat EP antiserum
2 = antigen used for immunization
3 = purified rat erythropoietin
4 = rabbit erythropoietin
5 = human erythropoietin
6 = sheep erythropoietin
7 = human urinary erythropoietin

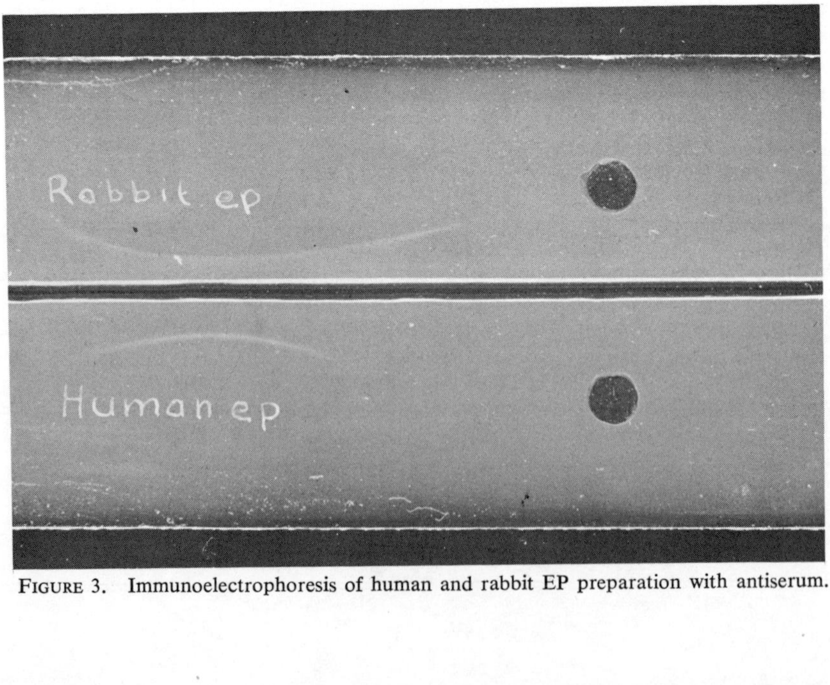

FIGURE 3. Immunoelectrophoresis of human and rabbit EP preparation with antiserum.

TABLE 3
POLYCYTHEMIC MICE

	Number of Animals	% ^{59}Fe Incorporation Mean	Range
Saline	4	0.6	0.5 – 0.7
Erythropoietin from immunoprecipitate	4	21	13 – 34

References

1. SCHOOLEY, J. C., J. F. GARCIA, L. N. CANTOR & V. W. HAVENS. 1967. A summary of some studies on erythropoiesis using antierythropoietin immune serum. This Annal.

Part VI. Endocrine and Drug Influences on Erythropoiesis

FURTHER OBSERVATIONS ON THE MECHANISM BY WHICH ANDROGENS AND GROWTH HORMONE INFLUENCE ERYTHROPOIESIS*

Howard A. Meineke and Roger C. Crafts

Department of Anatomy, University of Cincinnati College of Medicine, Cincinnati, Ohio

The process of erythropoiesis is controlled by a hormone, erythropoietin, and other hormones seem to have an influence on this process as well. The manner in which these other hormones influence erythropoiesis is problematical but, as can be seen in FIGURE 1, it may be simply (1) by increasing the general metabolic rate, thereby creating an anoxic condition; or more specifically, (2) by influencing the precursors of erythropoietin; (3) by the production of this substance; (4) by activating it in some manner; (5) by stimulating the stem cells directly; or (6) by enhancing maturation of the stem cells once they have been started toward the erythroid series by erythropoietin.

Thyroxin has already been reported[1] to influence erythropoiesis in a non-calorigenic fashion and to influence metabolism as well; and testosterone was found to increase ^{59}Fe uptake in the polycythemic mouse by Fried *et al.*[2] This was accomplished in the absence of any change in oxygen consumption.[3] Considerable attention has been given recently to the manner by which androgens increase the rate of erythropoiesis. Recent reports[3,4] have hypothesized that androgens exert their influence by increasing production of erythropoietin by the kidney, and this hypothesis has been substantiated[5–7] by the finding that the plasma of animals treated with androgens alone or in combination with anoxia[5,6] or cobalt[7] contains an increased titer of a substance which will stimulate erythropoiesis. Naets and Wittek,[8] on the other hand, have claimed that androgens act either by augmenting the action of erythropoietin on the stem cells or by influencing a later stage of erythropoiesis. In either case, the presence of erythropoietin is mandatory. Even more recently Reisner[9] has found that androgens will stimulate erythropoiesis in cultures of marrow cells, and Fried and Gurney[10] feel that androgens may alter the kidney in such a manner as to make it respond more vigorously to an anoxic stimulus.

Growth hormone has not received as much attention as the androgens in spite of the fact that the manner in which it stimulates erythropoiesis has never been elucidated. That it does affect this process has been shown by several groups.[11]

The present work was performed in an attempt to resolve the question of how androgens and growth hormone stimulate erythropoiesis.

Methods and Materials

Rats used in this experiment were two to three months of age and of the Sprague-Dawley (Holtzman) strain. All animals were fed Purina Chow ad libitum plus lettuce once a week. Completeness of hypophysectomies was checked carefully with a binocular dissecting scope and by adrenal weights. Nephrectomies were done by the usual dorsal approach.

Oxygen consumptions were calculated by the method of Holtkamp *et al.*[12] Rats were placed in the lower chamber of a 200 mm Frühling and Schultz desiccator; the upper chamber contained baskets of ascarite and dehydrite for absorption of

* This work was supported by grant AM 00476 from the National Institute of Health, Bethesda, Md.

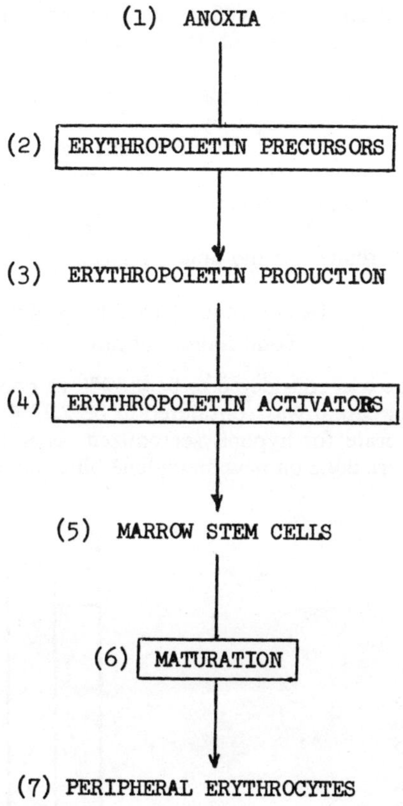

FIGURE 1. Steps by which erythrocytes are produced in response to anoxia.

Co_2 and water, respectively. This desiccator was connected with a 500 ml linear or volume recording spirometer which, in turn, was attached to the oxygen supply. Oxygen was placed in the spirometer; the amount used by the rat was recorded directly on a kymograph placed beside the spirometer. Rats were allowed a stabilizing period before measurements were started, the oxygen consumed being recorded for 10 min while the animal was at rest; the figure obtained was then corrected to standard temperature and pressure, and the final result expressed as liters consumed/m^2 of body surface/hour according to the following formula:

$$\text{l/sq. m/hr} = \frac{v}{t} \times \frac{P}{760} \times \frac{273}{T} \times \frac{10{,}000}{(\text{wt})^{2/3} \times 10} \times \frac{1}{1000}$$

where, $\frac{v}{t}$ = ml of oxygen used over time in hours, P = barometric pressure, T = temperature in the desiccator, $\frac{10{,}000}{(\text{wt})^{2/3} \times 10}$ a means of converting weight to surface area, and $\frac{1}{1000}$ simply a means of converting to liters. The temperature inside the desiccator showed very little change. As fasting hypophysectomized animals for 12 hr occasionally induced a hemoconcentration, fasting had to be avoided. These results are therefore subject to the error that the process of digestion might induce.

Rate of erythropoiesis was determined by the amount of ^{59}Fe incorporated into newly formed erythrocytes and by reticulocyte counts. Intravenous injections of 1 μc of ^{59}Fe were given at 4:00 P.M. the day before autopsy. Eighteen hours later 0.5 ml of blood was removed via heart puncture and its activity determined in a well-type scintillation counter. This figure was doubled to represent activity in 1.0 ml of blood. Red cell utilization was calculated on the basis of radioactivity recovered related to the amount given; the following formula was used:

$$\text{Percent incorporation} = \frac{\text{Counts/min} \times \text{total blood volume}}{\text{Total counts per min injected}}$$

The total blood volume was considered to be 4.87% of body weight unless given a transfusion, in which case it was considered to be 5.23%.[13] These figures have been found to be accurate for hypophysectomized, as well as for normal, rats. Reticulocyte counts were done on new methylene blue stained smears, 1,000 cells being counted.

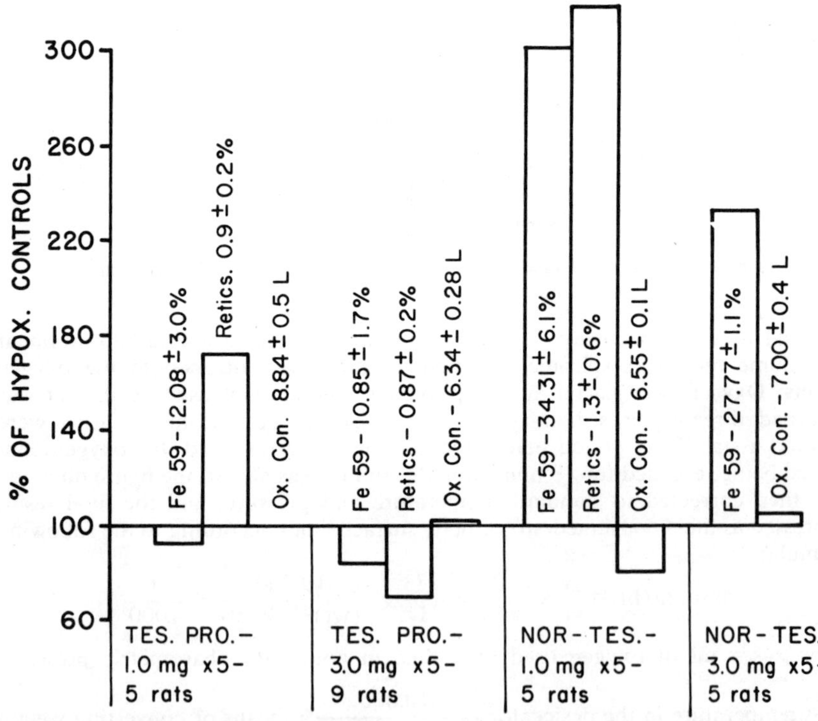

FIGURE 2. Effects of five daily injections of 1.0 or 3.0 mg of testosterone propionate or of nortestosterone on ^{59}Fe uptake, reticulocyte percentage, and on oxygen consumption in adult female rats hypophysectomized two weeks previous to injections. The data are graphed as percent of hypophysectomized controls, but the actual figures obtained are presented as well. ± = S.E.

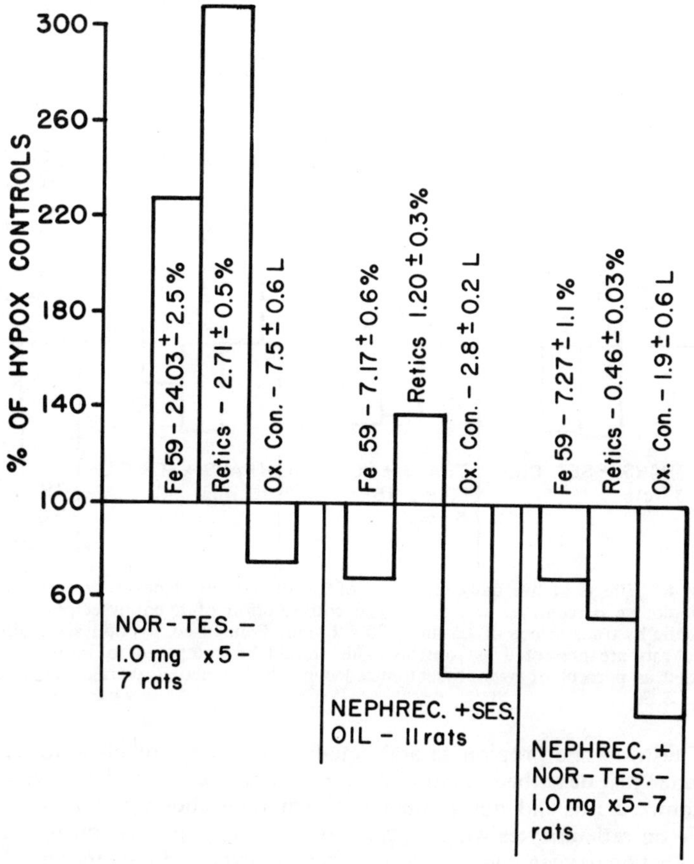

FIGURE 3. Effects of five daily injections of 1.0 mg of nortestosterone on ^{59}Fe uptake, reticulocyte percentages, and oxygen consumption of hypophysectomized rats which were nephrectomized 48 hr before autopsy. Treated hypophysectomized rats with intact kidneys are presented for comparison. The data are graphed as percent of hypophysectomized controls but the actual averages are presented as well. ± = S.E.

PROCEDURE AND RESULTS

Unless otherwise indicated, the experiments have been performed as follows. Adult two to three-month-old rats were hypophysectomized and allowed to remain untreated for two weeks at which time they were relatively plethoric with an arrested erythropoiesis; any response in such animals could be attributed to the agent injected. Furthermore, such animals are relatively free of endogenous hormone influences. The material to be tested was then injected daily at 9:00 A.M. for a period of five days, oxygen consumption determinations and autopsies occurring in the morning of the sixth day; ^{59}Fe was injected at 4:00 P.M. on the fifth day. An equal number of rats served as hypophysectomized controls.

Androgens

FIGURE 2 shows the results obtained when assaying 1.0 and 3.0 mg daily injec-

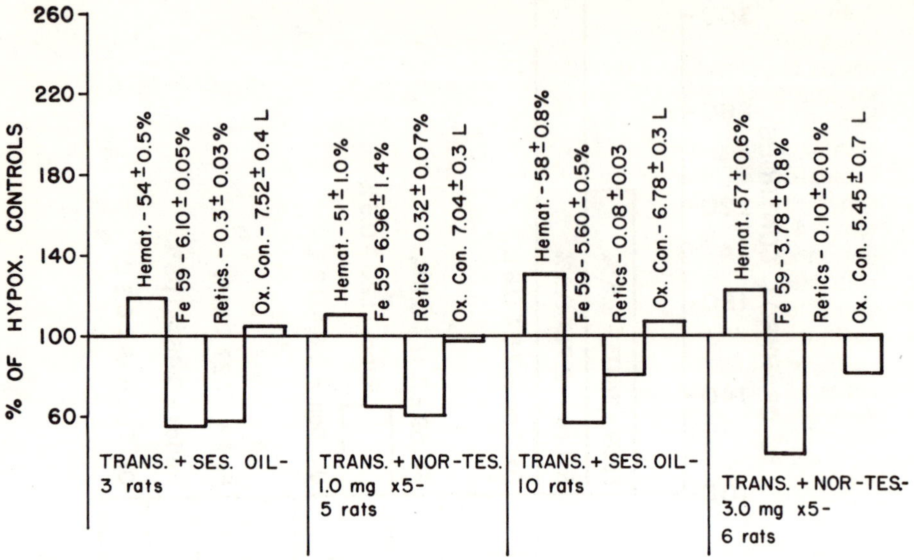

FIGURE 4. Effects of five daily injections of 1.0 or 3.0 mg of nortestosterone on ^{59}Fe uptake, reticulocyte percentage, and on oxygen consumption of hypophysectomized rats made polycythemic by transfusions of 3.5 ml of 70% blood. Transfused, hypophysectomized, sesame oil-treated rats are presented as controls. This should be compared to FIGURE 2. The data are graphed as percent of hypophysectomized controls but actual averages are presented as well. ± = S.E.

tions of testosterone propionate and equally-sized doses of nortestosterone** in the manner just described. Testosterone propionate at these dose levels in hypophysectomized rats did not stimulate ^{59}Fe uptake and was not uniform in its influence on reticulocytes when compared to the hypophysectomized controls; it has no effect on oxygen consumption. Nortestosterone, on the other hand, induced a profound rise in rate of erythropoiesis as judged by ^{59}Fe uptake and reticulocyte level; this hormone resembled testosterone propionate in having no effect on oxygen consumption. The nortestosterone influenced erythropoiesis by some other means than through increasing oxygen need.

In an attempt to determine whether this effect of nortestosterone was associated in some manner with erythropoietin, a group of hypophysectomized rats was treated with nortestosterone in the above fashion but, in addition, the kidneys were removed 48 hr before autopsy. These data are compared with those obtained in nephrectomized sesame oil-treated hypophysectomized rats and with those found in hypophysectomized rats treated with nortestosterone in the presence of intact kidneys. The results obtained are presented in FIGURE 3.

Removal of the kidneys for the last 48 hr of the treatment eliminated the response to nortestosterone found in hypophysectomized rats with intact kidneys. These findings are similar to those obtained by Gurney and Fried[14] and can be interpreted to mean that nortestosterone stimulates production of erythropoietin, as has been stated by others,[3–7] or could indicate that the presence of erythropoietin is necessary for androgen action, as has been presented by Naets and Wittek.[8]

** The nortestosterone was Nilevar® from G. D. Searle Co.

In an attempt to solve this problem, another group of hypophysectomized rats was treated with 1.0 or 3.0 mg of nortestosterone in the same manner as indicated above, but were also given a transfusion of 3.5 ml of 70% blood two days before the injections started. It was assumed that such a transfusion in already plethoric hypophysectomized rats would induce a marked decrease in erythropoietin, if not eliminate it completely. Data from transfused, noninjected rats are presented for comparison. These data are presented in FIGURE 4. The transfusion induced the expected decrease in ^{59}Fe uptake and reticulocyte levels in these hypophysectomized rats, and these results were not significantly changed by injections of nortestosterone. Therefore, an excess of erythrocytes in hypophysectomized rats with intact kidneys completely eliminated the rather marked stimulus to ^{59}Fe uptake and reticulocyte percentage found in the nontransfused hypophysectomized rats treated with nortestosterone.

These results are difficult to explain if androgens induce their effects by stimulating an increased production of erythropoietin; they favor the hypothesis that androgens in some manner interact with erythropoietin.

Growth Hormone

Growth hormone was studied in a manner similar to that utilized in the inves-

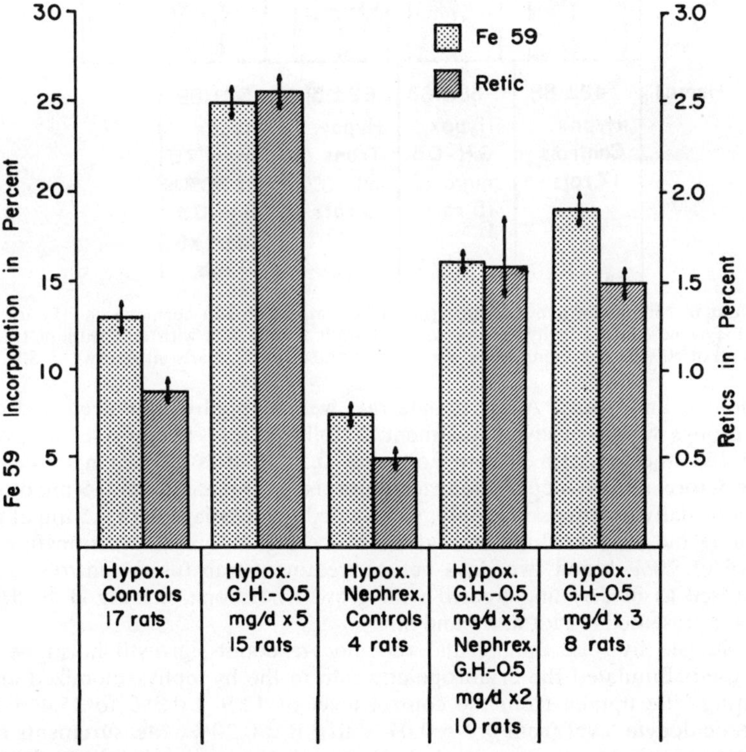

FIGURE 5. Effects of five daily injections of 0.5 mg of growth hormone on ^{59}Fe uptake and reticulocyte percentage in hypophysectomized adult female rats which were nephrectomized 48 hr before autopsy. Noninjected hypophysectomized and hypophysectomized-nephrectomized rats as well as hypophysectomized rats injected for three days are presented for comparison. Arrows = S.E.

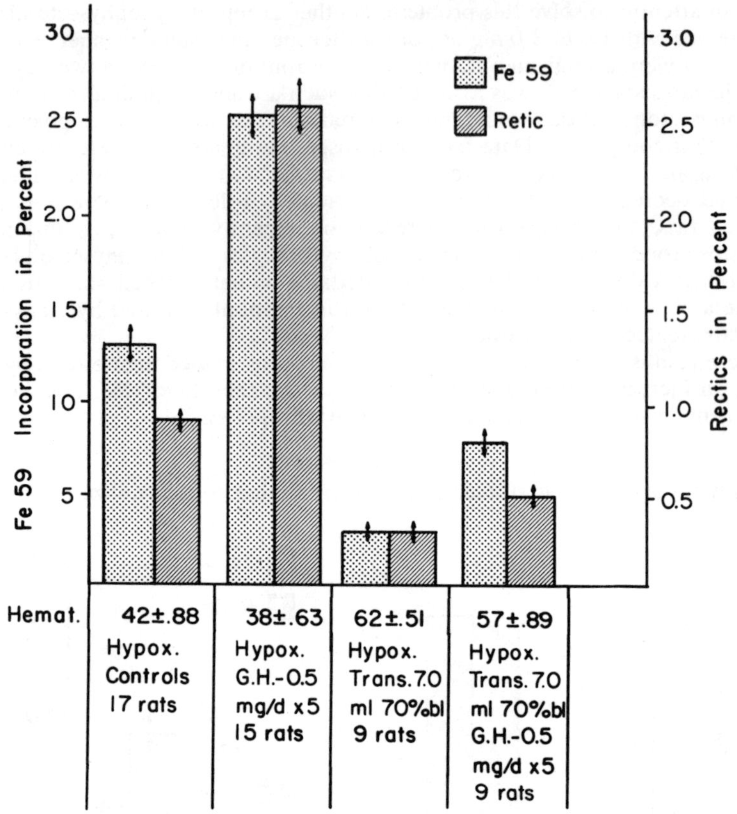

FIGURE 6. Effects of five daily injections of 0.5 mg of growth hormone on ^{59}Fe uptake and reticulocyte percentage in hypophysectomized adult female rats with and without transfusion of 7.0 ml of 70% blood. Noninjected rats are presented for comparison. Arrows = S.E.

tigation of androgens. Adult female rats were hypophysectomized and divided into groups which received treatment as follows: (1) hypophysectomized controls; (2) injected with growth hormone, 0.5 mg/d × 5; (3) nephrectomized 48 hr before autopsy-nephrectomized controls; (4) treated with 0.5 mg of growth hormone daily for three days only; (5) treated for five days with 0.5 mg of growth hormone but also nephrectomized 48 hr before autopsy; (6) transfused with 7.0 ml of 70% blood two days before treatment-transfused controls; and (7) transfused as in (6) and treated with growth hormone, 0.5 mg/d × 5. These data are presented in FIGURES 5 and 6.

As judged by ^{59}Fe uptake and reticulocyte counts, growth hormone in the dose used stimulated the erythropoietic rate in the hypophysectomized animals, elevating ^{59}Fe uptake from the control level of 12.9 ±0.9% to 25.4 ±1.2%† and reticulocyte level from 0.9 ±0.07% to 2.6 ±0.20%. Measurements of oxygen consumption in these animals indicated that this stimulus to erythropoiesis was not secondary to an increased oxygen need.

Nephrectomy 48 hr before autopsy (FIGURE 5) induced an expected decrease

† Standard error of the mean.

in rate of ^{59}Fe uptake (7.7 ±0.62%) and reticulocyte level (0.5 ±0.09%). Growth hormone treatment throughout the five-day period (three days before nephrectomy and two days after surgery) elevated these parameters in such animals to 16.4 ±1.24% for ^{59}Fe uptake and 1.6 ±0.29% for the reticulocyte level. Comparing these figures to those obtained in the growth hormone-treated nonnephrectomized group (25.4 and 2.6%) shows that the nephrectomy did influence the effectiveness of growth hormone injection; in fact it lowered it to what was found in animals treated with growth hormone for three days only (19.2 ±1.42% for ^{59}Fe uptake and 1.5 ±0.10% for the reticulocyte level). These data would indicate that growth hormone requires the presence of the kidneys to be effective, but, as with nortestosterone, these results can be interpreted either as erythropoietin production by growth hormone, or that the presence of erythropoietin is necessary for erythropoietic stimulation by this hormone.

Once again, in an attempt to determine in which manner growth hormone acts on erythropoiesis, another group of hypophysectomized rats was transfused with 7.0 ml of 70% blood two days before growth hormone injections were started. The results obtained are shown in FIGURE 6. Transfused untreated hypophysectomized rats are given for comparison.

Transfusion induced the expected decrease in ^{59}Fe uptake (3.2 ±0.43%) and in reticulocyte level (0.27 ±0.03%). In contrast to the results obtained with the nortestosterone, the growth hormone treatment in such transfused animals did elevate the ^{59}Fe uptake slightly but significantly to 8.04 ±0.67% and the reticulocyte level to 0.53 ±0.08%. Therefore, growth hormone induced its effects in a manner different from that shown by the nortestosterone, probably by inducing production of erythropoietin by the kidneys.

Discussion

Androgens are recognized as substances having a stimulating effect on erythropoiesis, and have been associated with the higher peripheral red cell counts found in males when compared to females. The present experiment with nortestosterone indicates that the action of this hormone is not related to the oxygen need of the animal, results similar to those of Gurney and Fried.[3] These data indicate further that the erythropoietic action of androgens is dependent on the presence of the kidneys, which also is in agreement with Gurney and Fried.[14]

However, at this point a divergence of opinion has developed. In the present experiment extreme plethora eliminated any response to nortestosterone, a result difficult to explain if androgens induce an increased production of erythropoietin. Our findings would indicate that the erythropoietic action of androgens is related, in some manner, to the specific action of erythropoietin rather than to its production. The exact mechanism is still problematical but we agree with Naets and Wittek[8] who feel that androgens act either by augmenting the action of erythropoietin on the stem cells or by influencing a stage of erythropoiesis after cellular differentiation; in either case "a présence d'érythropoiétine serait indispensable."[8]

Fried, *et al.*,[2] in their first paper on the role of androgens in erythropoiesis, found that testosterone propionate would stimulate ^{59}Fe uptake in the polycythemic mouse, but their results indicated a small response; they "were not able to restore erythropoiesis to anything approaching the normal rate even by repeated massive doses of testosterone."[2] These results can be explained on the basis of androgen interacting with erythropoietin. Since they used the polycythemic mouse, they undoubtedly decreased erythropoietin to minimal levels, thus decreasing the effectiveness of the androgen.

In subsequent papers 3 & 4, Gurney and Fried introduced quite convincing evidence that the response to a given dose of androgen decreased with increasing plethora of the animal. Assuming increased plethora induces a decrease in erythropoietin, we once again have obtained evidence that the effect of androgen is dependent upon the amount of erythropoietin available. These results are difficult to explain on the basis of increased production by the kidney. Furthermore, these authors point out that erythropoietin and testosterone have a synergistic action,[3] a point difficult to explain on a production basis but easily understood if androgen stimulates maturation of the stem cells pushed toward the erythroid series by erythropoietin. The same interpretation can be given to the synergisms found when cobalt and testosterone[7] are injected or when testosterone is combined with anoxia.[3]

In contrast is the work of Mirand *et al.*[5] and Fried and Gurney[6] in which the plasma of animals treated with testosterone contained an elevated amount of a substance which would stimulate erythropoiesis, and their finding that the plasma of animals treated with a combination of hypoxia and testosterone would influence ^{59}Fe uptake to a greater degree than plasma from animals treated with either stimulus alone, and more than one would expect from merely adding the responses obtained from the two stimuli. These results indicate that androgen acts by inducing an increase in the amount of erythropoietin released from the kidneys.

Thus, a dichotomy exists, one set of data indicating that the effectiveness of androgen is dependent upon the amount of available erythropoietin, a point difficult to understand if androgens stimulate an increased production of erythropoietin, and another set of data showing that androgens do induce a greater production of a substance into the plasma which will stimulate erythropoiesis.

Since others [2–8] have shown that short-term treatment with testosterone propionate will increase the rate of erythropoiesis, and it is well known that long-term treatment with this hormone will enhance erythropoiesis, our negative results with this hormone demand discussion. The explanation may be that the hypophysectomized rat two weeks after surgery is less sensitive to testosterone than at other times due to the presence of a minimum amount of erythropoietin. This point is being investigated as well as reasons for the greater effectiveness of the nortestosterone.

One other point demands discussion. It was a bit surprising to find that the androgen-treated nephrectomized rats exhibited no response whatsoever. One would have expected that the three days of injection while the animals had intact kidneys would have induced a detectable stimulus. However, it should be noted that we were measuring ^{59}Fe uptake during only the last 18 hr of life and the reticulocyte level at the point of autopsy. Possibly this adds support to the contention that androgens do not induce an increased production of erythropoietin, which would be detectable 48 hr later, but actually do interact with erythropoietin.

In conclusion, since androgens are less effective under conditions which decrease the amount of erythropoietin and are completely inactive under conditions which eliminate erythropoietin, it would seem that they act in some manner in conjunction with erythropoietin rather than induce an increase in erythropoietin production. This role of androgens is noncalorigenic and is not dependent upon the presence of the hypophysis. It might be added that in our hands, nortestosterone is more effective than testosterone propionate.

Growth hormone, on the other hand, seems to be effective in stimulating ^{59}Fe uptake and reticulocytosis in the severely plethoric hypophysectomized rat, and, at the same time, is dependent upon the kidney to be effective. This would indicate that it may indeed be involved with production of erythropoietin by the kidney. It also should be noted, in contrast to the nortestosterone, that growth hormone in the animals nephrectomized 48 hr before autopsy exhibited a respone to the first three days of injections when kidneys were intact. This may be evidence of an increased production of erythropoietin. The role of growth hormone is non-calorigenic and is not dependent on the presence of the hypophysis.

Summary

Both nortestosterone and growth hormone will stimulate erythropoiesis in hypophysectomized rats as judged by increases in ^{59}Fe uptake and reticulocyte levels. This action is abolished by nephrectomy. Transfusions in the already plethoric hypophysectomized rats completely eliminated the erythropoietic effect of the androgen but did not abolish the response to growth hormone. These results are explained on the basis that androgens are not effective in the severely plethoric animals because they are dependent upon interaction with erythropoietin, and that growth hormone acts by inducing its production by the kidney.

Acknowledgment

The technical assistance of Beverly Rouse, Andrew Luther and Susan Onken is greatly appreciated.

References

1. Meineke, H. A. & R. C. Crafts. 1964. Evidence for a noncalorigenic effect of thyroxin on erythropoiesis as judged by radioiron utilization. Proc. Soc. Exp. Biol. Med. **117:** 520.
2. Fried, W., R. DeGowin & C. W. Gurney. 1964. Erythropoietic effect of testosterone in the polycythemic mouse. Proc. Soc. Exp. Biol. Med. **117:** 839.
3. Gurney, C. W. & W. Fried. 1965. Further studies on the erythropoietic effect of androgens. J. Lab. Clin. Med. **65:** 775.
4. Fried, W. & C. W. Gurney. 1965. The use of mild plethora to demonstrate an erythropoietic effect from small amounts of androgen. Proc. Soc. Exp. Biol. Med. **120:** 519.
5. Mirand, E. A., A. S. Gordon & J. Wenig. 1965. Mechanism of testosterone action in erythropoiesis. Nature **206:** 270.
6. Fried, W. & C. W. Gurney. 1965. Erythropoietic effect of plasma from mice receiving testosterone. Nature **206:** 1160.
7. Janda, W. E., W. Fried & C. W. Gurney. 1965. Combined effect of cobalt and testosterone on erythropoiesis. Proc. Soc. Exp. Biol. Med. **120:** 443.
8. Naets, J. & M. Wittek. 1964. Étude du mécanisme d'action des androgènes sur l'érythropoïése. C. R. Acad. Sci. **259:** 3371.
9. Reisner, Jr. E. H. 1966. Tissue culture of bone marrow. II. Effect of steroid hormones on hematopoiesis in vitro. Blood **27:** 460.
10. Fried, W. & C. W. Gurney. 1966. The erythropoietic response to testosterone in male and female mice. J. Lab. Clin. Med. **67:** 420.
11. Crafts, R. C. & H. A. Meineke. 1959. The anemia of hypophysectomized animals. Ann. N. Y. Acad. Sci. **77:** 501.
12. Holtkamp, D. E., S. Ochs, C. C. Pfeiffer & A. E. Heming. 1955. Determination of oxygen consumption of groups of rats. Endocrinology **56:** 93.
13. Gallagher, N. I., D. Q. Hagen, J. M. McCarthy & R. D. Lange. 1961. Response of starved rats and polycythemic rats to graded doses of erythropoietin. Proc. Soc. Exp. Biol. Med. **106:** 127.
14. Gurney, C. W. & W. Fried. 1965. The mechanism of action of androgens on erythropoiesis. J. Clin. Invest. **44:** 1057 (abstr.)

EFFECTS OF ANGIOTENSIN, NOREPINEPHRINE AND RENAL ARTERY CONSTRICTION ON ERYTHROPOIETIN PRODUCTION*

James W. Fisher, Alan Samuels and James Langston

Department of Pharmacology, University of Tennessee Medical Units, Memphis, Tenn.

Introduction

Erythropoietin production has been found to be increased following renal artery constriction in rabbits.[1,2] An increase in radioactive iron incorporation in red cells has also been reported in hypophysectomized rats injected with angiotensin.[3] Piliego *et al.*[4] have demonstrated a rise in erythropoietin levels in plasma of normal humans following angiotensin infusions as well as increased erythropoietic activity of kidney extracts from rats treated with angiotensin. However, other workers[5,6] have been unable to demonstrate an acute effect of angiotensin in mice or rats.

Angiotensin and norepinephrine infusions into dogs are known to produce a decrease in renal blood flow.[7,8] Therefore, it is quite possible that the erythropoietic effects seen with angiotensin could be due to increased erythropoietin production as the result of a decrease in renal blood flow. Because of the inconclusive results seen with angiotensin in mice and rats we decided to study the relationship between renal artery blood flow and erythropoietin production in dogs. In the present studies erythropoietin production was compared in dogs where renal blood flow was reduced with pressor drugs or mechanical constriction of the renal artery. Plasma levels of erythropoietin, renal artery blood flow, femoral arterial blood pressure, urine production and hematocrit values were measured in dogs following infusions of angiotensin or norepinephrine as well as after constriction of the renal artery with a modified Goldblatt clamp. Erythropoietin production was also sudied in polycythemic mice and fasted rats following acute injections of angiotensin and norepinephrine.

Materials and Methods

Male and female mongrel dogs anesthetized with pentobarbital (30 mg/kg) were used in these studies. Renal artery blood flow was measured with the use of a Square Wave electromagnetic flowmeter. An electromagnetic probe was applied directly to the left renal artery through an anterior abdominal incision. Mean femoral arterial blood pressure was measured with a Statham pressure transducer and grass polygraph. Urine was collected throughout the experiment via a bladder catheter. Microhematocrits were determined at hourly intervals on carotid arterial blood using heparinized capillary tubes. Synthetic angiotensin[1] or norepinephrine[2] (L-arterenol bitartrate) in saline were infused intraarterially at a rate of 1.0 ml/min with the use of an AL-2E sigmamotor infusion pump. The infusions were made through polyethylene tubing inserted through the left femoral artery into the abdominal aorta to a level of approximately 1½″ above the renal arteries. Saline was infused into the abdominal aorta of five dogs at a rate of 1.0 ml/min and served as the controls. The left renal artery was constricted with a modified Goldblatt clamp and renal blood flow monitored with the electromagnetic flowmeter probe placed peripheral to the clamp. The 7 mm diameter probe

* Supported by USPHS Grant AH–02973–07.

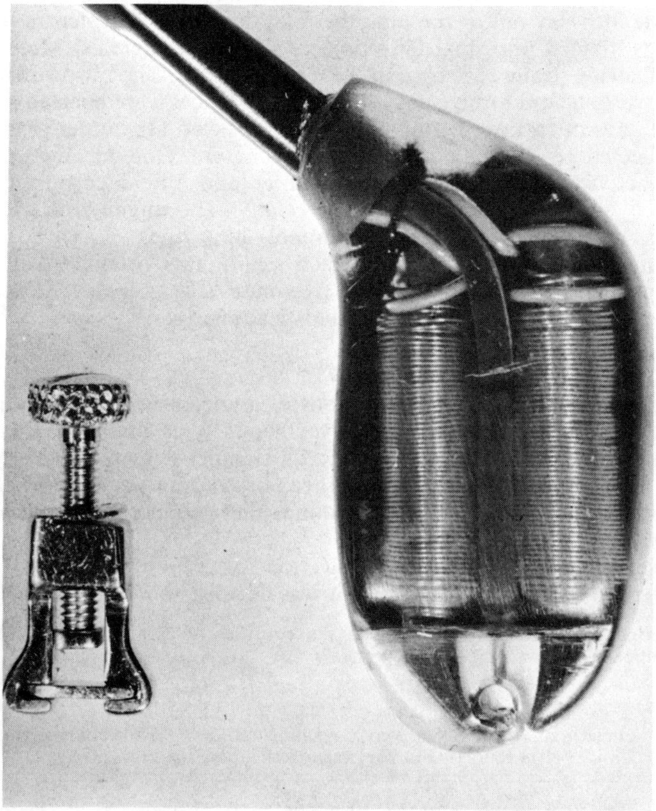

FIGURE 1. Modified Goldblatt clamp and 7 mm diameter electromagnetic flowmeter probe used in the renal artery constriction and blood flow studies in dogs.

and stainless steel clamp are shown in FIGURE 1. The kidneys were removed at the termination of all experiments, fixed in formalin, and stained with hematoxylin and eosin for histological studies. Approximately 40 ml of blood was removed from the carotid artery initially and at hourly intervals. The blood was heparinized, centrifuged, and plasma removed for erythropoietin assay. The red cells were resuspended in saline and infused into the dog within 10–15 min after the blood was withdrawn.

The plasma samples were assayed in polycythemic mice via a modification of the method of DeGowin *et al.*[9] Male Swiss-Webster strain mice were injected with 1 mg of iron dextran s.c. prior to being placed at 0.5 atm for three weeks. On the day the mice were removed from the low pressure tank each mouse was injected i.p. with 1 ml donor mouse blood at hematocrit 70. On the fifth day out of the tank each mouse was injected with 1 ml plasma three times at five-hour intervals. Each mouse was injected with 0.5 μc ^{59}Fe citrate on the seventh posthypoxia day, completely exsanguinated three days later and ^{59}Fe incorporation in RBC determined.

The polycythemic mice receiving angiotensin or norepinephrine were treated exactly the same way as that of the mice receiving dog plasma with the exception that on the fifth day out of the tank the total dosage of angiotensin or norepinephrine was divided into three injections at five-hour intervals. Male rats of the Sprague-Dawley strain were used in these experiments. The rats used in the fasted rat assay were starved for five days. The test substances were injected in the second and third days of fasting, 1.0 μc ^{59}Fe citrate injected i.v. on the fourth day, and blood collected 18–20 hr later via cardiac puncture. One ml blood was counted for radioactivity with a scintillation counter and ^{59}Fe incorporation in RBC determined via the technique of Fried *et al.*[10] The angiotensin (Hypertensin-CIBA)** or norepinephrine (L-arterenol bitartrate, Winthrop) was suspended in corn oil before being injected s.c. in rats or mice. All dosages of norepinephrine are expressed as the free base L-arterenol. The technique of analysis of variance was used in the statistical analyses.[11]

Results

TABLE 1 shows the results of injections of angiotensin and norepinephrine on ^{59}Fe incorporation in red cells of polycythemic mice and fasted rats. Neither angiotensin nor norepinephrine produced a significant increase in ^{59}Fe incorporation in RBC of polycythemic mice. Sheep erythropoietin and the 500-μg dose of norepinephrine were the only compounds that produced a significant increase in ^{59}Fe incorporation in fasted rats.

Because the data following acute injections of pressor substances in mice and rats have been inconclusive thus far, it was decided to study erythropoietin pro-

** Hypertensin-CIBA furnished through the courtesy of Dr. William E. Wagner, Ciba Pharmaceutical Co.

TABLE 1

EFFECTS OF ANGIOTENSIN AND NOREPINEPHRINE ON ^{59}Fe INCORPORATION IN RBC OF POLYCYTHEMIC MICE OR FASTED RATS

Treatment	Total Dose (Units or μg/Animal)	No. Animals	Percent ^{59}Fe Incorporation in RBC
	Polycythemic Mice		
Oil vehicle	—	11	.45 ± .35
Erythropoietin*	1.0	10	8.12 ± 1.96*
Angiotensin†	50	8	.61 ± .12
Angiotensin	100	7	.96 ± .32
Norepinephrine‡	25	4	.75 ± .76
	Fasted Rats		
Oil vehicle	—	19	3.77 ± .88
Erythropoietin§	2.0	9	6.74 ± 2.5*
Angiotensin	50	14	4.03 ± 2.0
Angiotensin	100	15	4.38 ± 2.1
Angiotensin	150	10	4.47 ± 2.2
Norepinephrine	250	8	5.29 ± 1.9
Norepinephrine	500	8	6.65 ± 1.7*

* Significantly different from oil vehicle controls at 1% level.

** Step III (Lot 147192A) erythropoietin from plasma of phenylhydrazine anemic sheep in corn oil vehicle. (dosage in units)

† Synthetic Angiotensin amide in corn oil vehicle. (dosage in μg)

‡ L-arterenol bitartrate in corn oil vehicle. (dosage in μg)

§ Standard B from National Institute of Medical Research, Mill Hill, London, England. (dosage in units)

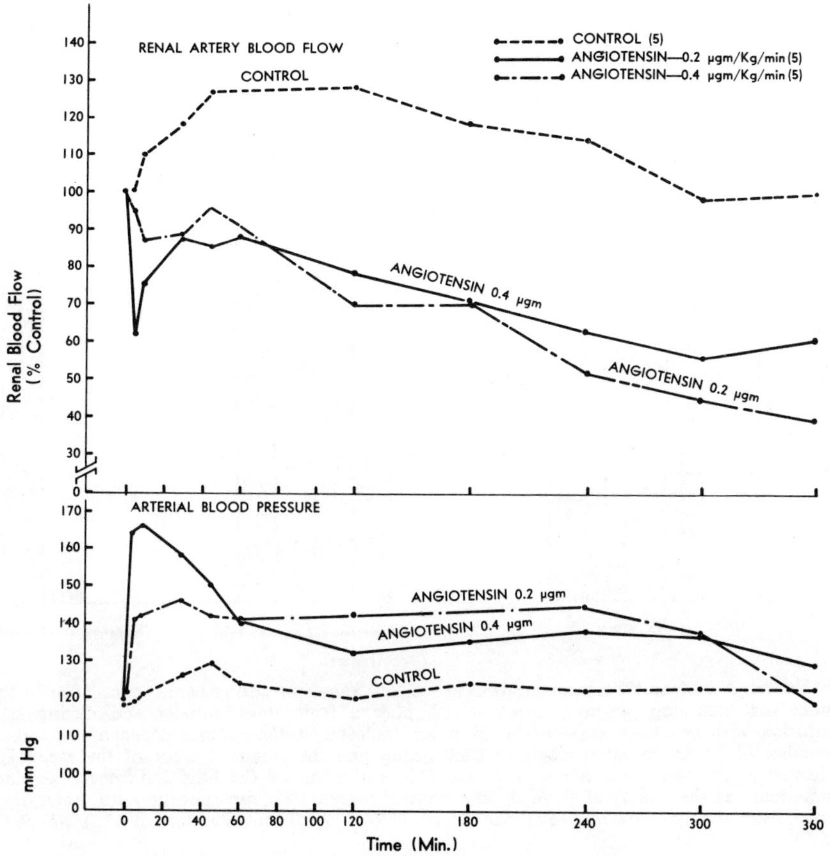

FIGURE 2. Mean renal artery blood flow and femoral arterial blood pressure during intra-arterial infusion of saline or angiotensin. The number enclosed in parenthesis following each dosage indicates the number of dogs in the groups.

duction in dogs following intraarterial infusion of angiotensin or norepinephrine.

The preinfusion levels of renal blood flow were given a value of 100%; the effects of angiotensin at several times during a six-hour infusion period were calculated from this level. The initial renal artery blood flows for all groups fell within a range of 6.5–11.0 ml/kg/min. FIGURE 2 shows the decrease in renal blood flow and rise in arterial blood pressure in dogs during six hr infusion with angiotensin or saline. A gradual increase in renal arterial blood flow was seen with intraarterial saline infusions which reached a plateau after 40 min and gradually returned to control levels after 300 min. Arterial pressure was uniformly maintained throughout the infusion of saline in the control group. Both dosages of angiotensin produced a rapid fall in renal blood flow and immediate rise in arterial pressure. The renal blood flow started to return toward normal after 5–10 min but after 45 min began a gradual decline which eventually reached levels of 40–60% of the initial flow after 360 min.

FIGURE 3 shows the graded increases seen in plasma levels of erythropoietin during infusion of dosages of 0.2 and 0.4 μg angiotensin as compared with

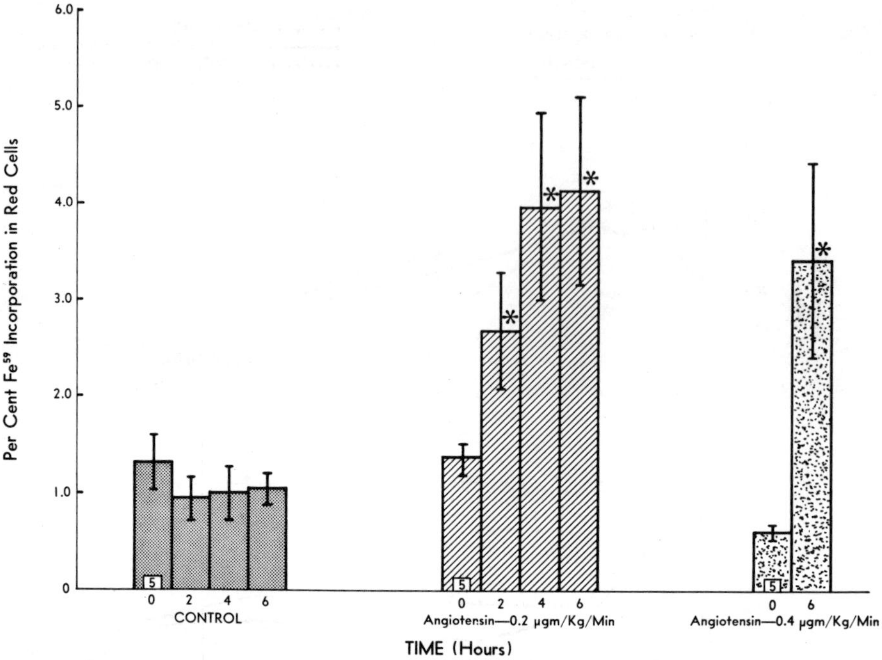

FIGURE 3. Mean ^{59}Fe incorporation in red cell values in polycythemic mice (five to seven mice for each dog plasma) injected with plasma from dogs initially and during six hr infusion with saline or angiotensin. Number enclosed at the bottom of each bar indicates number of perfusion experiments in each group and the standard error of the mean is indicated at the top of each bar. Asterisk (*) at the top of the bars indicates a significant difference at the 1% level from 0 time control. Mean ^{59}Fe incorporation for polycythemic mice used as saline controls (57) was .44 ± .05% and 1.0 unit Standard B (53) was 9.31 ± .75%.

saline controls. Significant increases in erythropoietin titers were found after two, four and six hr infusion of a dosage of 0.2 μg and after six hr with 0.4 μg angiotensin. There was no significant difference at six hr between the 0.2 and 0.4 μg dosages of angiotensin on erythropoietin production.

FIGURE 4 shows the decrease in renal blood flow produced with norepinephrine (0.4 μg/kg/min) and renal artery constriction with a modified Goldblatt clamp. There was an immediate decrease in renal blood flow at the beginning of the intraarterial infusion of norepinephrine. However, after 5–10 min there was a marked increase in renal blood flow. After 45 min the renal blood flow was still above the initial flow and comparable to the increase seen with the saline control infusion. After 60 min infusion with norepinephrine there was a gradual decline in renal blood flow which eventually reached 47% of the initial flow after six hr infusion. The decline in renal blood flow with norepinephrine was not as rapid as that seen with angiotensin. The mean arterial pressure was only moderately elevated during the first four hr infusion with norepinephrine and returned to normal at five and six hr. The blood flow was maintained between 30–40% of the initial control value with the renal artery clamp for a six-hour period. It was necessary to make frequent adjustments in the clamp to maintain the reduced renal blood flow because of the tendency of the renal blood flow to return toward normal.

FIGURE 5 shows the increases in plasma levels of erythropoietin seen with a 0.4 μg dosage of norepinephrine or renal artery constriction with the clamp. The plasma erythropoietin levels were significantly elevated two, four and six hr after renal artery constriction and after six hr infusion of norepinephrine when compared with the initial plasma levels. The histological studies did not reveal evidence of degenerative changes in any of the kidneys following angiotensin or norepinephrine infusions. However, there was slight to moderate cloudy swelling in the tubules and slight glomerular congestion seen in the histological sections from the renal artery clamp group.

The mean hematocrit values were moderately increased in the norepinephrine infusion (from 49 $\pm$ 2.9% to 53 $\pm$ 2.7%) and in the renal artery clamp (from 42 $\pm$ 2.0% to 54 $\pm$ 2.5%) experiments; however, the hematocrit values in the saline control and angiotensin infusion studies were essentially the same throughout the infusion. Urine production was less than normal in the saline controls (approx. .12 ml/min) and renal artery clamp experiments (approx. .08 ml/min) but slightly greater in the norepinephrine (approx. 0.3 ml/min) and 0.2 μg

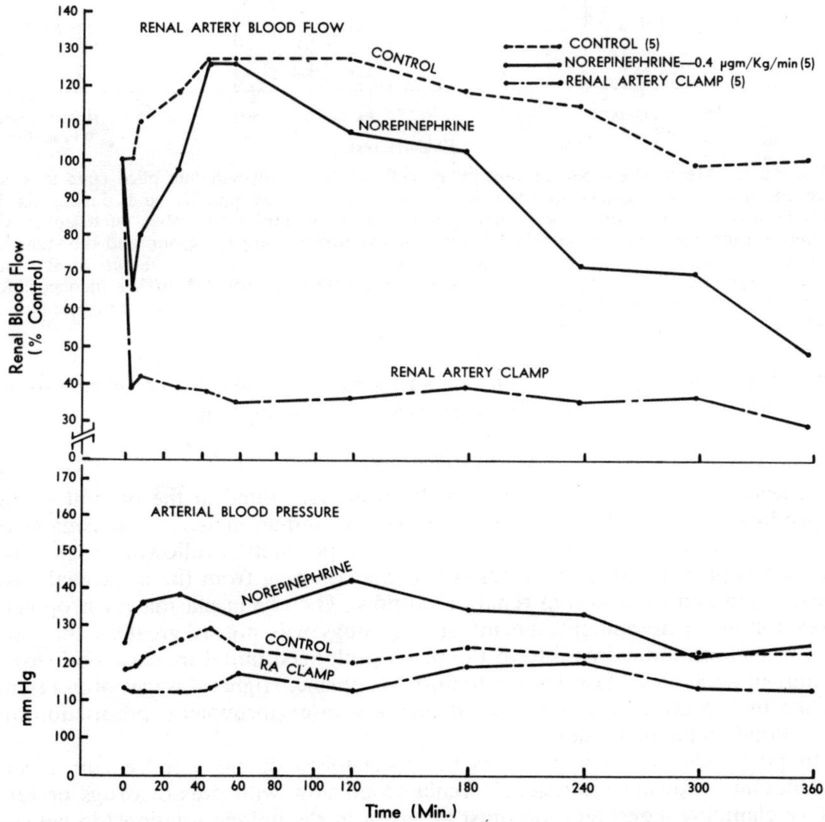

FIGURE 4. Mean renal artery blood flow and femoral arterial blood pressure during intra-arterial infusion of saline or norepinephrine or renal artery clamping. The number in parenthesis following each dosage or group indicates the number of animals in this group.

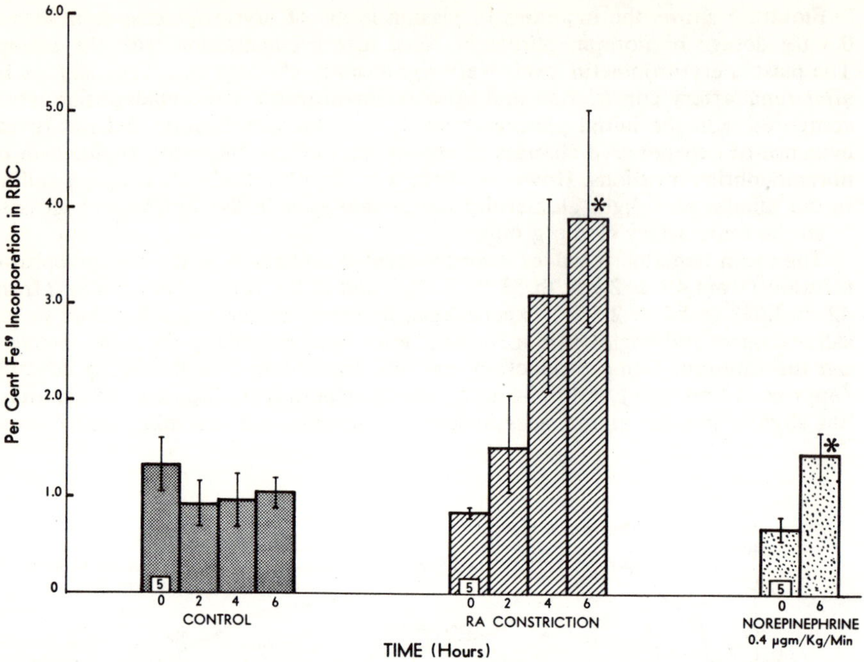

FIGURE 5. Mean ^{59}Fe incorporation in red cell values in polycythemic mice (five to seven mice for each dog plasma) injected with plasma from dogs initially and during six hr infusion with saline or norepinephrine or renal artery clamping. Number enclosed at the bottom of each bar indicates number of perfusion experiments in each group and the standard error of the mean is indicated at the top of each bar. Asterisk (*) at the top of the bars indicates significantly different at the 1% level from 0 time control. Mean ^{59}Fe incorporation for polycythemic mice used as saline controls (58) was 0.47 ± .05% and 1.0 unit Standard B (39) was 9.75 ± .96%.

dose of angiotensin (.19 ml/min) experiments. The low rate of urine production is attributed to the pentobarbital used as the anesthetic.

Discussion

Infusion of angiotensin in dogs has been demonstrated in the present studies to produce a gradual decline in renal blood flow and an increase in plasma levels of erythropoietin. The increased erythropoietin production following angiotensin infusion is probably due to the renal hypoxia resulting from the intrarenal vasoconstriction and reduction in renal blood flow. The rise in plasma erythropoietin titers following norepinephrine infusion in dogs was not as great as that seen with angiotensin, due possibly to the more prolonged initial increase and slower decline in renal blood flow seen with norepinephrine. Higher dosages of norepinephrine may produce a more marked increase in erythropoietin production and reduction in renal blood flow.

In postulating renal hypoxia as the mechanism of enhanced erythropoietin production following reduction in renal blood flow with pressor drugs or renal artery clamping, consideration must be given to the unique relationship between blood flow and oxygen extraction from arterial blood in the kidney. In contrast to other organs, a moderate reduction in renal blood flow results in a decrease in renal uptake of oxygen.[12] Only when blood flow is reduced to the limit where glomerular filtration ceases (less than 1.0 ml/g/min) and reabsorption of sodium is reduced does the kidney extract more oxygen per ml of blood in response to reduction in blood flow. When renal blood flow in the dog is reduced below a certain level, probably in the range of 35–45% of normal, there is a sharp rise in arteriovenous oxygen difference.[12] This may be the critical level of reduction in renal blood flow where sufficient renal hypoxia occurs to provide the adequate stimulus for erythropoietin production.

The tendency for reduction in renal blood flow to recover during renal artery clamping[13] or infusion of norepinephrine[8] is postulated to be due to an active autoregulatory mechanism for regulating renal blood flow which is controlled by a sensitive feedback mechanism. It is not known whether the gradual initial increase in renal blood flow seen with the saline infusions in our experiments is due to autoregulation or to an effect of the infusion fluid. Even though the renal blood flow was at a lower level for a longer period of time in the renal artery constriction experiments than with the low dose of angiotensin, plasma levels of erythropoietin were higher throughout the infusion with angiotensin. Angiotensin probably has a more selective effect on renal vessels within the kidney to modify intrarenal blood flow and may result in a more marked reduction in blood flow in critical vascular beds in the kidney near the site of erythropoietin.

The secondary increase in renal blood flow following the initial drop seen in our angiotensin infusion experiments is probably also caused by autoregulation. It has been reported that infusion of norepinephrine in dogs reduced cortical blood flow markedly while medullary flow was not significantly changed.[14] The glomerular tuft[15] and juxtaglomerular cells[16] have been suggested as sites of production or release of erythropoietin. It is quite possible that both norepinephrine and angiotensin produced a more marked decrease in cortical blood flow in our experiments than that reflected in the renal artery blood flow measurements, rendering glomeruli in the outer cortex sufficiently hypoxic to stimulate erythropoietin production.

Waldman and Bradley[17] found increased amounts of erythropoietin in the blood serum as well as saline extracts of a tumor in a patient with pheochromocytoma and associated polycythemia. This type of tumor is known to contain high amounts of norepinephrine[18] Frohlich *et al.*[19] have recently reported erythrocytosis associated with renal artery stenosis and hypertension. In addition, Piliego *et al.*[20] have reported an increase in plasma levels of erythropoietin in patients with heart failure and have suggested reduction in renal arterial blood flow as a possibility for the enhanced erythropoietin production in this condition. It is quite possible that moderately high dosages of pressor substances for a prolonged period of time, such as those reported by Piliego *et al.* in rats,[4] are sufficient to produce enough reduction in renal blood flow and renal hypoxia to stimulate erythropoietin production.

The reasons for our failure, as well as those of other workers,[5,6] to stimulate erythropoiesis in fasted rats and polycythemic mice with angiotensin may have been due to the shorter duration of treatment or route of administration. The plethoric state or short duration of treatment of the polycythemic mouse may account for its failure to respond to angiotensin and norepinephrine. Angiotensin is also known to be rapidly degraded by peptidases in serum, plasma and other tissues. This may also account for the variable effects on erythropoietin production in different species reported by other investigators.[5,6] Testosterone,[21] cobalt[22] and triiodothyronine[23] are also less effective in polycythemic mice. Marked plethora may also render the kidney or other sites more resistant to stimuli that enhance erythropoietin production. Fasted rats may have failed to respond to angiotensin and low dosages of norepinephrine because of the short duration of treatment.

Summary

Angiotensin and norepinephrine infusions in dogs produced a decrease in renal artery blood flow, an increase in mean arterial blood pressure and significant increases in plasma levels of erythropoietin. Constriction of renal arteries in dogs with a renal artery clamp sufficient to reduce renal blood flow to 30–40% of normal also resulted in a significant elevation in plasma erythropoietin titers after six hr. Angiotensin failed to produce a significant erythropoietic effect in polycythemic mice and fasted rats. Norepinephrine produced a slight erythropoietic effect in fasted rats but failed to produce a significant effect in polycythemic mice. Angiotensin and norepinephrine are postulated to stimulate erythropoietin production in dogs as the result of renal vasoconstriction and reduction in renal blood flow.

Acknowledgments

The authors gratefully acknowledge the technical assistance of Mrs. Judy Parker and Mr. Carroll Osburn in these studies and are also indebted to Dr. Y. C. Kim, Pathology Dept., Baptist Memorial Hospital, Memphis, Tenn. for his histological evaluation of the kidneys.

References

1. Takaku, F., N. Hirashima & E. Nakao. 1962. Studies on the mechanism of erythropoietin production. I. Effect of unilateral constriction of the renal artery. J. Lab. Clin. Med. **59:** 815.
2. Fisher, J. W., R. Schofield & D. D. Porteous. 1965. Effects of renal hypoxia on erythropoietin production. Brit. J. Haemat. **11:** 382.
3. Fisher, J. W. & J. J. Crook. 1962. Influence of several hormones on erythropoiesis and oxygen consumption in the hypophysectomized rat. Blood **19:** 557.
4. Piliego, N. & P. Rossini. 1963. The hemodynamic factors in the renal secretion of erythropoietin. IV. Increase of erythropoietin after infusion of synthetic angiotensin. Rass. Fisiopatol. Clin. Terap. **35:** 687.
5. Bilsel, Y. C., J. E. Wood & R. D. Lange. 1963. Angiotensin II and erythropoiesis. Proc. Soc. Exp. Biol. Med. **114:** 475.
6. Mann, D. L., R. M. Donati & N. I. Gallagher. 1966. Effect of renin, angiotensin II and aldosterone on erythropoiesis. Proc. Soc. Exp. Biol. Med. **121:** 1152.
7. Swann, H. G. & R. L. Zapalac. 1964. Threshold for pressor and renal ischemic effects of angiotensin. Proc. Soc. Exp. Biol. Med. **117:** 879.
8. Langston, J. B., A. C. Guyton, J. H. Depoipter & G. G. Armstrong, Jr. 1962. Changes in renal function resulting from norepinephrine infusion. Amer. J. Physiol. **202:** 893.
9. DeGowin, R. L., D. Hofstra & C. W. Gurney. 1962. The mouse with hypoxia-induced erythremia, an erythropoietin bioassay animal. J. Lab. Clin. Med. **60:** 846.
10. Fried, W., L. F. Plzak, L. O. Jacobson & E. Goldwasser. 1956. Erythropoiesis. II. Assay of erythropoietin in hypophysectomized rats. Proc. Soc. Exp. Biol. Med. **92:** 203.
11. Dixon, W. J. & F. J. Massey, Jr. 1957. Introduction to statistical analysis. 2nd Ed. : 139. McGraw-Hill Co., Inc. New York, N. Y.
12. Thaysen, J. H., N. A. Lassen & O. Munck. 1961. Sodium transport and oxygen consumption in the mammalian kidney. Nature **190:** 919.
13. Schmid, Jr., H. E. & P. S. Merrill. 1962. Characteristics of pressure-flow regulation by the kidney. J. Applied Physiol. **17:** 201.
14. Pilkington, L. A., R. Binder, J. C. M. DeHaas & R. F. Pitts. 1965. Intrarenal distribution of blood flow. Amer. J. Physiol. **208:** 1107.
15. Fisher, J. W., G. W. Taylor & D. D. Porteous. 1965. Localization of erythropoietin in glomeruli of sheep kidney by the use of a fluorescent antibody technique. Nature **205:** 611.
16. Osnes, S. 1960. Influence of the pituitary on the erythropoietic principle produced in the kidney. Brit. Med. J. **1:** 1153.

17. WALDMANN, T. A. & J. E. BRADLEY. 1961. Polycythemia secondary to the pheochromocytoma with production of an erythropoiesis-stimulating factor by the tumor. Proc. Soc. Exp. Biol. Med. **108:** 425.
18. PITCAIRN, D. M. & W. B. YOUMANS. 1950. The nature of pressor substances in pheochromocytomas. Circulation **2:** 505.
19. FROHLICH, E. D., R. C. TARAZI, H. P. DUSTEN, R. W. GIFFORD, JR. & I. H. PAGE. 1965. Polycythemia in hypertension: another clue to renal arterial disease. Clin. Res. **13:** 554 (Abstr.).
20. PILIEGO, N. & P. ROSSINI. 1963. Effective haemodynamic factors in renal secretion of erythropoietin. II. Increase of plasma erythropoietin in heart failure. Rass. Fisiopatol. Clin. Terap. **35:** 421.
21. GURNEY, C. W. & W. FRIED. 1965. Further studies on the erythropoietic effect of androgens. J. Lab. Clin Med. **65:** 775.
22. FISHER, J. W., D. D. PORTEOUS, K. HIRASHIMA & S. C. TSO. 1966. Effects of cobalt on the activity of sheep erythropoietin in kidney homogenates. Prox. Soc. Exp. Biol. Med. In press.

ANDROGEN ACTIONS ON ERYTHROPOIESIS*

Albert S. Gordon, Edwin A. Mirand, Jeffrey Wenig, Robert Katz
and Esmail D. Zanjani

Department of Biology, Graduate School of Arts & Science, New York University, New York, N. Y., and the Roswell Park Memorial Institute, Buffalo, N. Y.

It is now firmly established that sex steroids exert significant effects on the erythron and blood-forming organs of endocrine-deficient and intact animals.[1–5] Until recently, explanations as to the mechanisms by which these hormones influence erythropoiesis have been largely speculative. Among the suggestions offered was that hormonal action on erythropoiesis was secondary to more primary effects exerted on general body metabolism which, in turn, determined the oxygen requirements of the animal and, consequently, the need for red cells.[4,6,7] In this regard, although removal of the hypophysis,[5,8,9] testis,[5,10] thyroid[5,9] or adrenal[5,9,11] was found to result in an anemic state correctable by administration of the lacking hormones, the response of such endocrinectomized animals to sufficient intensities of hypoxia remained essentially unaltered.[5,12,13] This led us to conclude that the role of hormones in erythropoiesis was facultative rather than obligatory and that the fundamental action of the endocrine system was to reinforce rather than to exercise a primary control over red cell formation.[14]

This study in confined largely to experiments dealing with the mechanisms of androgen action on erythropoiesis. It will demonstrate that the effects are mediated, at least in part, through the production of the circulating erythropoiesis-stimulating factor (ESF or erythropoietin).

Our studies with androgen have been conducted in four species of animals, namely, rats, mice, rabbits and tamarins.[15] In this paper emphasis will be placed on experiments carried out in rats and rabbits.

Plasma Donor Rats

Two hundred and ten adult female Sprague-Dawley rats (250–300 g) received i.m. injections of 12.5 mg of long-acting testosterone cyclopentylpropionate (TCP) (Depo-testosterone, Upjohn Co.) in one ml of suspending fluid once every seven days. Another group of 210 rats were administered the same schedule of TCP injections but, in addition, were exposed to hypoxia (10% oxygen) for 30 hr before they were killed. At various intervals the rats were exsanguinated, the bloods were heparinized and the plasmas corresponding to the different groups were pooled, frozen and stored at $-20°$ C.

Assay of Plasmas

Adult female Ha/ICR Swiss mice, rendered plethoric by i.p. injections of homologous red cells, were employed to determine the erythropoiesis-stimulating activity of plasma from the androgen-treated rats.[15] Six mice were used to assay each plasma sample. Each test mouse received three daily s.c. injections of 0.5 ml of plasma. One μc of ^{59}Fe was administered i.v. on the fourth day and the percent of radioiron incorporated into the circulating red cells determined on the fifth day. Mice with hematocrits lower than 60% at the end of the experiment were eliminated.

* Supported by grants 5–R01–HE03357–09, AI–04506, CA–02728 and CA–07745 from the National Institutes of Health, U.S.P.H.S.

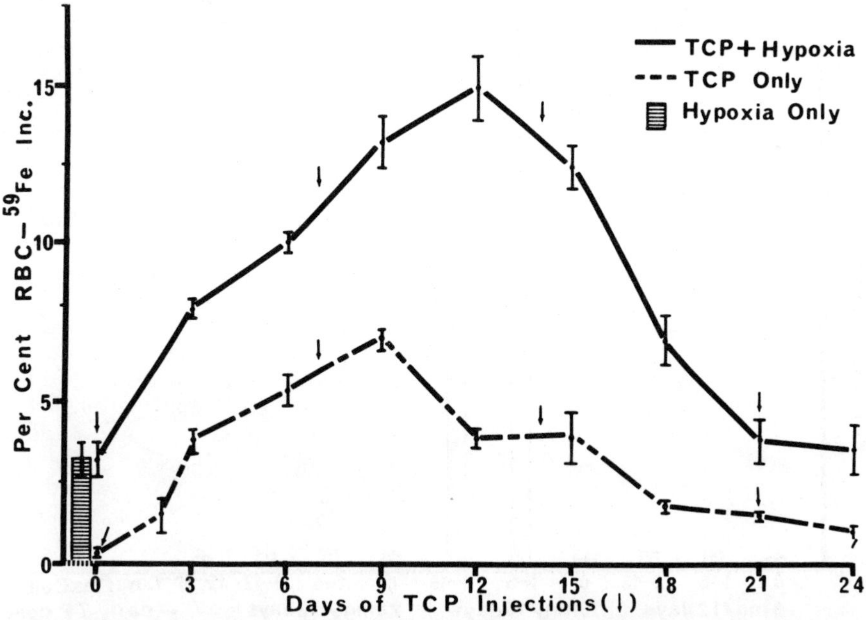

FIGURE 1. Erythropoietic effects of plasma from rats given testosterone cyclopentylpropionate and/or hypoxia. (Data reproduced from paper in Nature.[15])

It will be noted from FIGURE 1 that erythropoiesis-stimulating activity was found in the plasma of the donor rats by the third day after androgen administration. Maximal activity was detectable by the ninth day. It then tended to decrease with time with markedly lower values noted on the 24th day (three days after the third injection of TCP). It is also to be observed that the rats subjected to the same TCP regimen, but in addition, exposed to hypoxia just prior to exsanguination, exhibited significantly greater plasma activity than would be expected from the additive effects of TCP and the hypoxic stimulus applied separately. Essentially similar results have been reported by Fried and Gurney in mice.[16] Peak activity with the combined stimuli was observed at 12 days and a similar waning in the erythropoiesis-stimulating activity of the plasma was noted. At 24 days, the activity observed in the plasma of these animals was approximately equivalent to that found in the rats exposed only to the hypoxia, It would seem, therefore, that refractoriness to androgen had occurred in those animals given the combined stimuli as well as in those administered androgen alone.

It is likely that the increase in erythropoiesis-stimulating activity of the plasma of rats receiving androgen is attributable to the ESF. The plethoric mouse assay is at present the most specific for detecting the ESF.[17] Such test mice have been demonstrated to respond sensitively to the ESF and to hypoxic stimuli (hemorrhage, lowered barometric pressures, cobalt) which operate by stimulating the production of the ESF.

DOSE-DEPENDENCE OF THE ANDROGEN EFFECT

The ability of androgen to evoke production of the ESF is not only determined by the duration of treatment, as noted in FIGURE 1, but is dose-dependent as well.

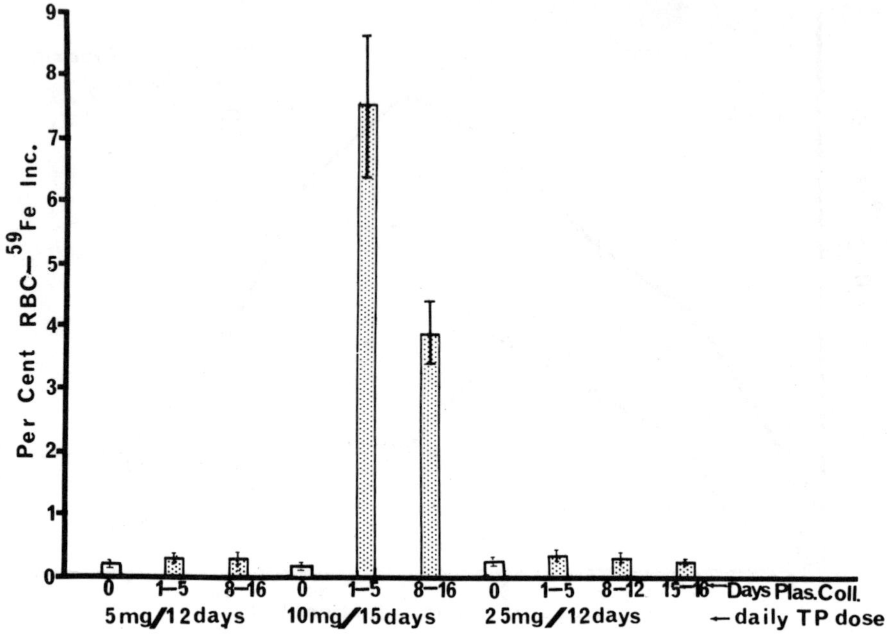

FIGURE 2. Erythropoietic effects of plasma from dogs injected daily with testosterone propionate. (Data reproduced from paper in Investigative Urology.[18])

This is seen to advantage in the dog.[18] Six adult male mongrel dogs weighing 10.0–19.1 kg were assigned to three equal groups receiving 5, 10 or 25 mg testosterone propionate (TP) i.m. daily for 12–15 days. Samples of plasmas corresponding to the first five days, the eighth through the 16th day and, in one instance, the 15th through the 16th day, were collected and separately pooled.

FIGURE 2 indicates that administration of 5 mg TP daily evoked no significant increase in the ESF titers of plasma. This was true whether the plasmas were tested at the 1–5-day or 8–16-day sampling periods. At the dose level of 10 mg TP per day, a highly significant increase in erythropoiesis-stimulating activity of plasma was noted in the samples collected and pooled during the first five days after initiation of androgen injections. Although the activity of the 8–16-day pooled samples was still significantly above normal baseline values, the effect had begun to diminish. No increase in ESF values was observed at any of the plasma sampling periods in the dogs receiving 25 mg TP per day.

A similar dose-dependency relating to androgen effects on ESF appearance has been observed in rabbits and mice.[15] It is of interest that dose-dependency also characterizes the effects of androgen on reproductive tissues. Thus the androgen influence on the testis is dependent not only on the age of the animals when treatment is begun, but also on the period over which the steroid is given, on the nature of the androgen, and on the dose administered as well.[19]

The ability of plasma obtained from androgen-injected animals to enhance erythropoiesis does not appear to be due to residual androgen in the body fluids. This is supported by several facts. Firstly, the plasma shows diminishing erythropoiesis-stimulating activity with continued injections and with increased dosages of administered androgen. In addition, quantities of plasma from androgen-treated animals, equivalent to those used for assaying their ESF content, fail to augment significantly the seminal vesicle and prostate weights in immature 8–10 g male mice (unpublished). That it also cannot be attributed to a metabolic product of androgen, which is active in much smaller quantities than the testosterone administered, is noted from recent observations[20,21] that administration of anti-ESF serum completely blocks the ability of testosterone propionate to augment erythropoiesis in mice. Indeed, this latter work provides additional strong evidence that androgens operate in erythropoiesis by stimulating production of the ESF.

Site of Androgen Action

Work by Jacobson *et al.*[22] Naets,[23] Fisher,[24] Kuratowska,[25] Mirand,[26] Reissman,[27] and others, has established that the kidneys play an important role in the production of the ESF. It seemed that it might be of interest to determine whether kidneys of rabbits that had received androgen treatment would produce ESF under conditions of perfusion.

Perfusion Apparatus

A no. 2.0 metal cannula or 15-gauge metal needle was secured to the end of a five-foot section of 25 mm internal diameter tygon tubing extending from the housing of a sigmamotor finger pump through which it passed (FIGURE 3). The other end of the tubing, emanating from the housing in the opposite direction, was connected to the sidearm of an Erlenmeyer filtering flask of 50 ml capacity. The neck of the flask was closed by a one-hole rubber stopper in which a piece of glass tubing extended from the bottom of the flask to approximately 5 cm above the stopper. Another five-foot section of tygon tubing was connected to the glass

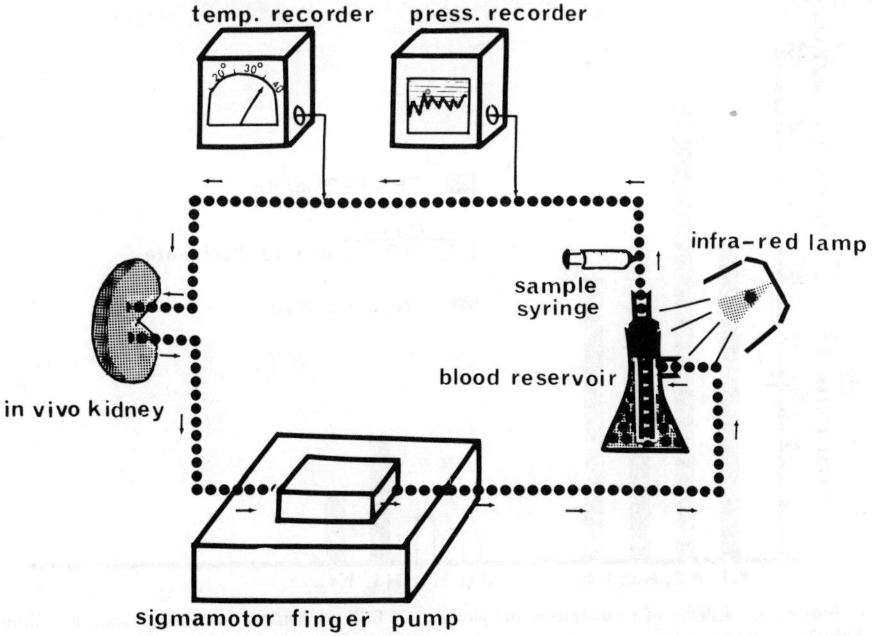

FIGURE 3. Schematic representation of system for perfusion of rabbit kidneys.

tubing extending from the flask. The open end of this section of tubing was attached to a no. 1.5 metal cannula or a 15-gauge metal needle. Three connections were interposed in this section of tubing: One was a three-way valve from which blood could be withdrawn through a syringe or materials added to the system; the second was a connection for an electronic temperature recording device; and the third, for a pressure register in the form of a precalibrated transducer connected to a polygraph recorder. An infrared lamp, positioned alongside the reservoir, was used as the source of heat to maintain the temperature of the system at 37° C.

Before all perfusion studies, 50 ml of whole blood obtained from normal rabbits was heparinized and delivered into the reservoir of the system. A small additional amount of blood was placed into a separate beaker. The two ends of tubing connected to the metal cannulas or needles were inserted into this beaker, below the blood level and the pump turned on. This procedure was used to eliminate air spaces and to prime the apparatus for operation.

Operative Procedure

The animals were anesthetized with nembutal given i.v. in a dose of 30 mg/kg and then secured to an operating board in a dorsal recumbent position. A longitudinal perimedial incision was made from approximately 5 cm below the xiphoid process to the lower abdominal region. The left kidney was located and the renal artery, vein and ureter were exposed. Four 2-0 silk strands were placed between the renal artery and vein, two drawn distal to and two proximal to the kidney. One 2-0 silk strand was placed around the ureter. One of the distal strands was looped around the renal vein, pulled tight and knotted, thereby occluding the

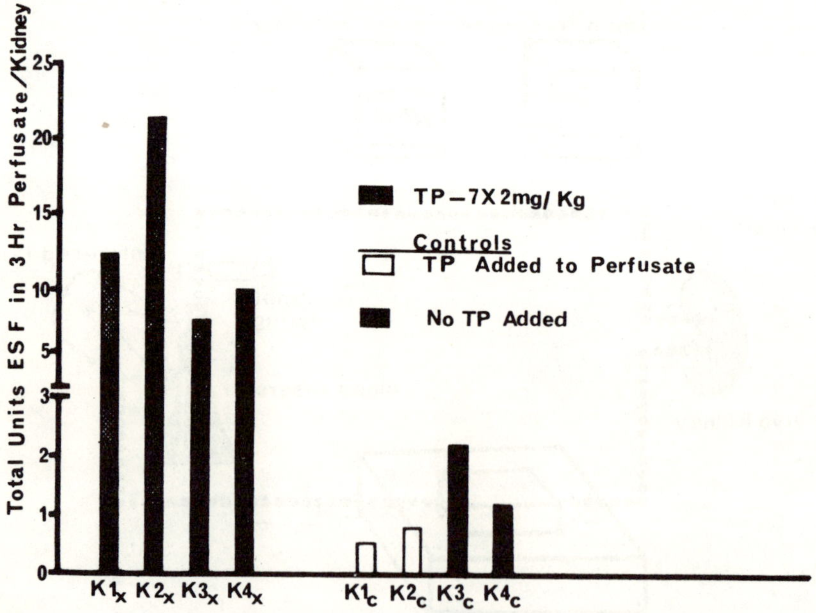

FIGURE 4. Effects of testosterone propionate on ESF formation during perfusion of rabbit kidneys.

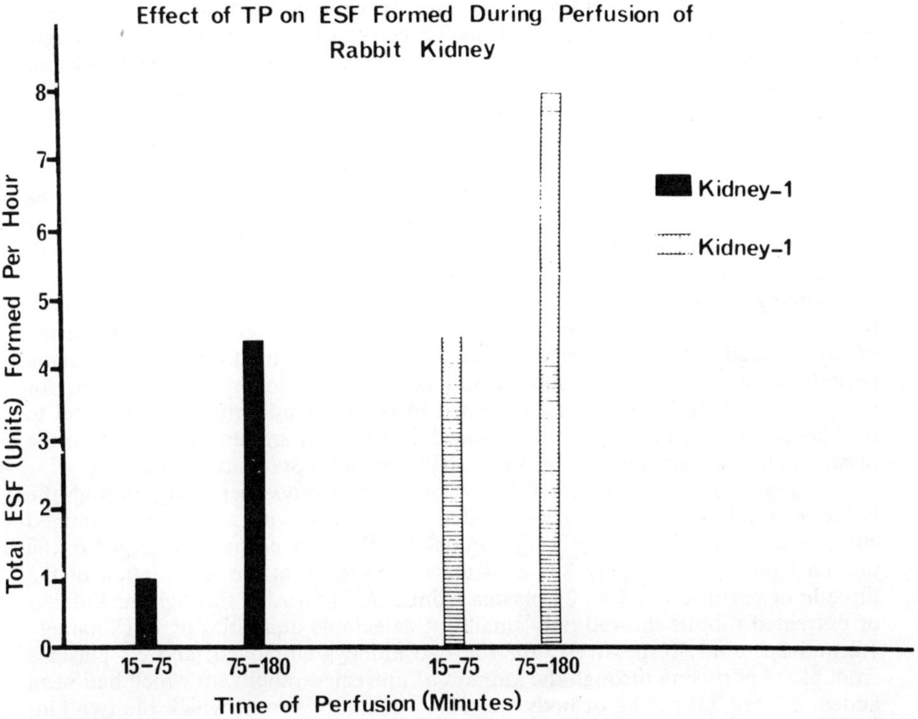

FIGURE 5. Time study of effects of testosterone propionate on ESF appearance during perfusion of rabbit kidneys.

vessel lumen. A small nick was then made in the renal vein near this ligature while tension applied to the proximal strand looped around the vein prevented blood loss. The no. 2.0 metal cannula or the 15-gauge needle from the perfusion apparatus was diverted into the slit in the vein and inserted about 3 cm towards the kidney where it was firmly tied in place by tightening the second 2-0 silk strand around it and the blood vessel. The same procedure was employed to insert the no. 1.5 metal cannula or 15-gauge needle into the renal artery. A 15-gauge metal needle was also inserted into the ureter and secured firmly by tightening the silk thread previously placed around it. With the apparatus now attached to the kidney via the renal artery and vein, the pump was turned on to a predetermined setting equivalent to 90–110 mm Hg. Temperature checks were made by inserting the electronic temperature probe into the system. A schematic representation of the perfusion system is shown in FIGURE 3.

Perfusion Procedures

Eight adult male New Zealand rabbits (2.2–4.0 kg) were employed for the kidney perfusions. A group of four rabbits received 2 mg/kg daily of TP for seven days. On the eighth day, the rabbits were exsanguinated and their kidneys were perfused in situ with 50 ml of normal homologous rabbit blood. Kidneys from two untreated normal rabbits were likewise perfused in situ with 50 ml of normal rabbit blood. In addition, kidneys from two normal rabbits were perfused with 50 ml normal blood to which 2 mg TP per kg of original rabbit body weight had been added to the blood at the commencement of perfusion. All perfusions were carried out for three hr with no extra oxygen admitted to the system. The perfusions were conducted under these relatively hypoxic conditions with the hope that the potentiating effects of androgen on ESF production might be seen to better advantage.

At the end of the perfusion period, the perfusates were heparinized and the plasmas assayed as a single 0.75 ml dose in hypoxia-induced polycythemic mice according to the method of Weintraub *et al.*[28] Six mice were employed to assay each of the plasmas.

Knowing the hematocrit of the normal rabbit blood employed as the perfusate to be 40 $\pm$ 2%, it was possible to calculate the total ESF content of the plasma of the circulating 50 ml of perfusing blood at the end of the three-hour perfusion period. Since the log dose-response of RBC-radioiron incorporation values for the plasmas of these perfusates, as tested in polycythemic mice, was parallel to that obtained for Erythropoietin Standard A, the total amount of activity in the plasma could be calculated in terms of Erythropoietin Standard A units.

It will be noted from FIGURE 4 that: 1) plasma of blood perfusing through the kidneys of rabbits that had been treated for a week with androgen contained considerable quantities of ESF. The values for the four perfusions ranged in the plasma from approximately 8.1–21.4 units per kidney at the termination of the three-hour perfusion period; 2) plasma from blood perfusing through the kidneys of untreated rabbits showed only small but detectable quantities of ESF, namely 1.2 and 2.2 units, respectively, for the two kidneys employed; and 3) plasmas from blood perfusing through the kidneys of untreated rabbits, to which had been added, 2.5 mg TP per kg of body weight of the rabbits from which the two kidneys were obtained, possessed only 0.8 and 1.2 units.

It is thus apparent that blood perfused through kidneys obtained from previously androgenized rabbits contains considerably greater quantities of ESF than does either of the two control groups. The data also indicate that the presence of these relatively large amounts of ESF cannot be attributed to any potentiative influence of free circulating androgen on whatever small amounts of ESF that might have been present in the normal blood being used as the perfusate.

A point of interest relates to the finding that increasing amounts of ESF appear to be formed as the perfusion proceeds. The results obtained for two representative kidneys, obtained from rabbits treated daily for one week with 2.5 mg TP per kg body weight, are indicated in FIGURE 5. After complete exsanguination, these kidneys were also perfused with 50 ml normal rabbit blood. Samples of perfusate were removed at 15, 75 and 180 min after initiation of perfusion and the plasmas tested for ESF content. In calculating total ESF levels in the plasmas of the perfusates, account was taken of the volumes of perfusate removed at the 15- and 75-min sampling times.

FIGURE 5 indicates that, in the case of the first kidney, a total of 0.93 units per hour were formed in the first period (15–75 min) and 4.36 units per hour in the second period (75–180 min). For the other kidney, 4.42 units were produced per hour in the first period and 7.97 units per hour during the second period. The explanation for this increase in ESF appearance with increasing time of perfusion is not clear. Since the perfusions were conducted under relatively hypoxic conditions (no extra oxygen supplied), it is possible that increasing degrees of oxygen lack, associated with the later periods of perfusion, engendered the production of greater quantities of ESF from these kidneys obtained from androgenized rabbits.

Renal Mechanisms Underlying the Erythropoiesis-Stimulating Action of Androgens

Experiments in Rabbits

Attempts were made to determine the renal mechanisms involved in the stimulatory action of androgens on erythropoiesis. We have recently demonstrated the existence in normal and hypoxic kidneys of a factor (the renal erythropoietic factor or REF) that is present in large quantities in the light mitochondrial fraction.[29,30] Although this factor is not erythropoietically active when administered alone i.p. to plethoric mice, it engenders the production of the functional ESF when it is incubated in vitro with normal serum. Evidence recently obtained indicates that the REF functions in an enzymatic capacity upon a serum substrate[31] to produce the ESF.

In the present experiments, seven adult female New Zealand rabbits were injected daily for seven days with 2 mg TP per kg body weight. On the eighth day, the rabbits were exsanguinated and their kidneys removed. The procedure for extracting the REF and the description of the incubation procedure are outlined in FIGURE 6.

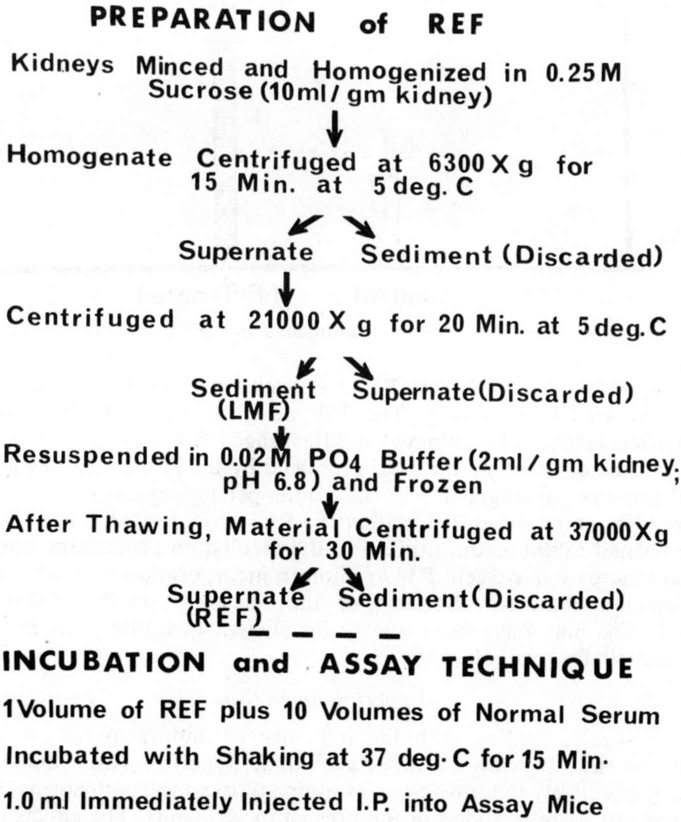

FIGURE 6. Flow diagram for preparation of the REF and method of its incubation with normal serum.

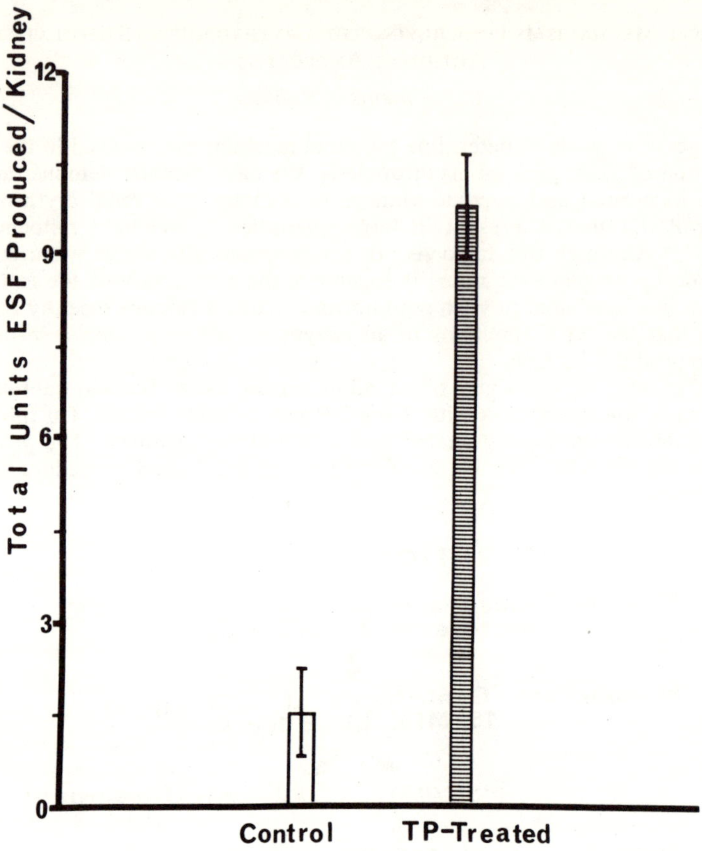

FIGURE 7. Effects of testosterone propionate on REF production in rabbits.

It will be noted from FIGURE 7 that a week's treatment with androgen significantly increased REF activity. The ESF generated by the REF from the seven androgenized rabbits (14 kidneys) used averaged 9.9 ± 0.85 (S.E.$_{m}$) units per kidney. On the other hand, the ESF produced by the REF from five normal rabbits (10 kidneys) averaged 1.5 ± 0.72 units per kidney.

It should be emphasized that neither the REF from testosterone-treated rabbits nor the normal rabbit serum utilized in the incubation procedures produced any significant increase in percent RBC-radioiron incorporation in polycythemic mice when injected alone i.p. Because of the relatively small amounts of REF employed, this may have been due to insufficient quantities entering the blood to interact with the serum factor.

Experiments in Rats

Further studies dealing with the influence of androgens on the REF were extended to rats. In view of reports[32,33] that hypertransfused animals do not respond as effectively to testosterone as nonplethoric ones, both normal and hypertransfused rats were included in the present experiments. The effects of hypoxia in both types of animals were also investigated.

Androgen Studies. In all experiments adult male rats (250–300 g) of the Long-Evans strain served as serum and REF donors. Two parameters of erythropoietic activity were employed: a) the titers of ESF in the serum and b) the quantity (or activity) of the REF. One group of five rats received a single i.m. injection of 12.5 mg long-acting testosterone cyclopentylpropionate (TCP) in 0.25 ml cottonseed oil. Another group of five constituting the controls were administered 0.25 ml of the vehicle, cottonseed oil. Ten additional rats were rendered plethoric by i.p. injections, on two successive days, of 10 ml of whole heparinized blood* obtained from normal male rats. Five of these plethoric rats were given a single i.m. injection of 12.5 mg TCP while the other five received only the cottonseed oil. All injections were made four days after the second transfusion. Hematocrits at this time ranged from 65–70%. All four groups were exsanguinated six days after the injections, the bloods allowed to clot at 5° C and the sera corresponding to the different groups pooled. The kidneys of the four groups were also separately pooled and subjected to the procedure shown in FIGURE 6 for extraction of the REF. Incubations of the REF with normal rat serum were conducted in reaction vessels left open to the atmosphere and the reactions were stopped at the end of the incubation period by submerging the reaction flasks in ice water.

Hypoxia Studies. These experiments were patterned along the lines of those conducted with androgen except that hypoxic hypoxia was used as the erythropoietic stimulus. A group of five normal adult male rats were subjected to 0.4 atm in a decompression chamber for 16 hr. A second group of five rats constituted the untreated unexposed controls. An additional 10 rats were made plethoric by two successive daily i.p. injections of 10 ml of whole homologous blood. Of

* We have found that whole blood is superior to saline suspensions of red cells in producing experimental plethora. With the former procedure there is less tendency of coating of the peritoneal lining with red cells and therefore, a more efficient induction of the plethoric state is achieved.

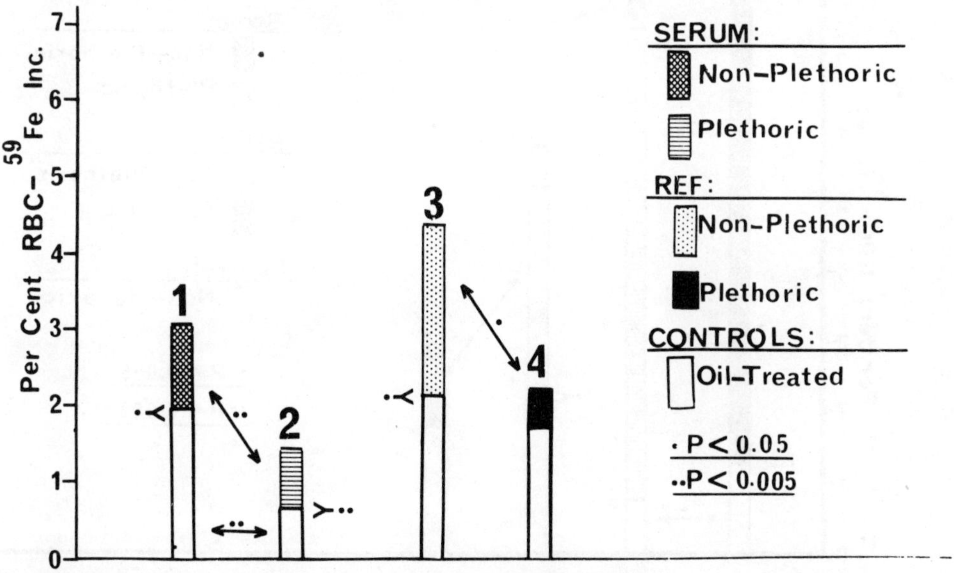

FIGURE 8. ESF content of serum and REF activity in androgen-treated rats. (Reprinted from Gordon *et al.* 1966. Proc. Soc. Exp. Biol. Med. **123:** 475–478).

these, five were subjected to 0.4 atm for 16 hr while the remaining five comprised the unexposed plethoric controls.

Directly following the period of hypoxia, the exposed and unexposed rats were exsanguinated and the sera and kidneys of each of the groups collected and separately pooled. The REF was extracted from the kidneys and incubated with normal rat serum as shown in FIGURE 6.

Methods of Assay. The sera and incubates of REF-serum were examined for erythropoietic activity in hypoxia-induced polycythemic mice. Five to six mice were used to assay each sample. Each mouse received either 1.0 ml of serum or 1.0 ml of the incubate as a single i.p. injection on the third day after interruption of the hypoxia. They were injected i.v. on the fifth day with an amount of ^{59}Fe in 0.2 ml saline recording at 150,000 cpm. All mice were killed on the sixth day and the percent RBC-radioiron incorporation estimated.[28]

Results for Androgen-Treated Group. In FIGURE 8, bar 1 indicates that sera from normal, nonplethoric rats administered a single injection of TCP exhibited greater erythropoiesis-stimulating activity than sera from the vehicle-treated animals. Sera obtained from cottonseed oil-injected controls appeared to have slightly stimulated RBC-radioiron incorporation values in assay mice. This effect, however, has not been observed in other experiments. The androgen also caused a small but statistically significant increase in the ESF content of the sera from hypertransfused rats (FIGURE 8, bar 2). It will be noted, however, that the quantity of the ESF detected in plethoric rat sera was significantly less than in nonplethoric rats administered the same dose of TCP. Bar 3 indicates that TCP also caused a considerable increase in the REF activity in nonplethoric rats. A small,

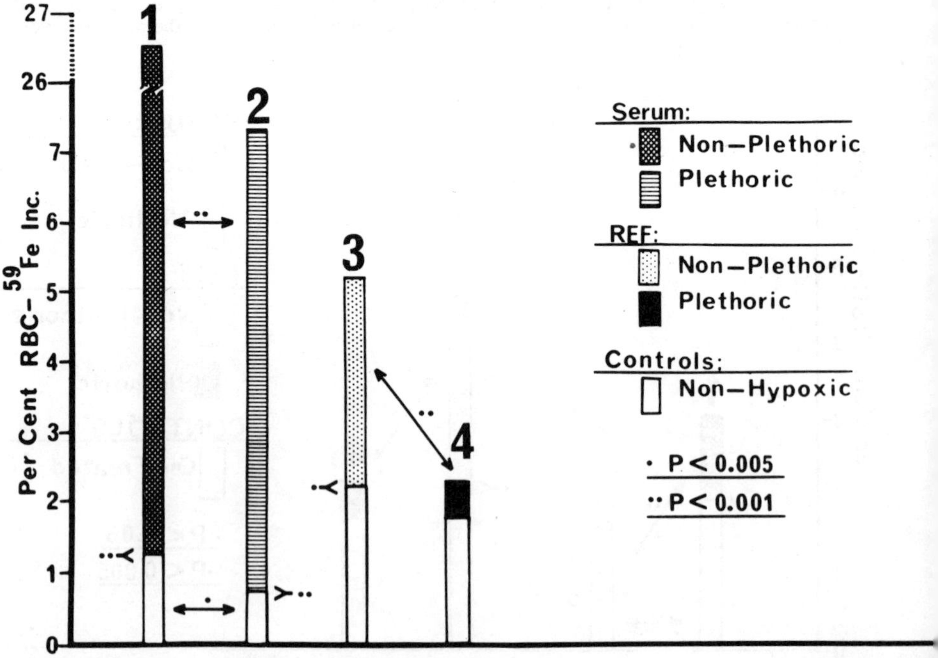

FIGURE 9. ESF content of serum and REF activity in rats exposed to hypoxia. (Reprinted from Gordon *et al.* 1966. Proc. Soc. Exp. Biol. Med. **123**: 475–478).

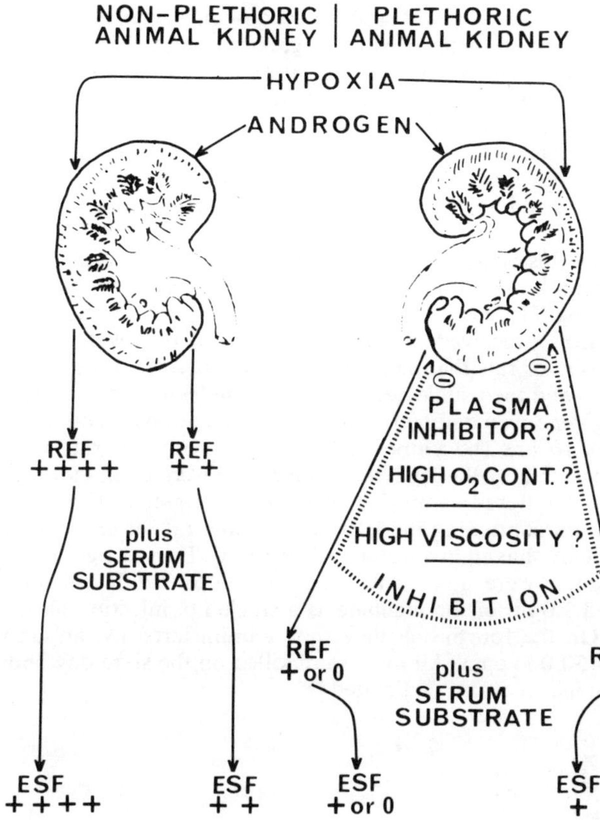

FIGURE 10. Possible renal mechanisms by which androgen, hypoxia and the plethoric state alter ESF production.

statistically insignificant elevation in REF activity resulted from treatment of hypertransfused rats (bar 4). The extent of activity in these animals was thus definitely less than that noted in the normal nonplethoric group.

Results for Hypoxia-Exposed Group. In FIGURE 9, bar 1 indicates that exposure to hypoxia resulted in a highly significant increase in ESF titers in the sera of normal rats. The rise noted in serum ESF in the hypoxia-exposed hypertransfused rats was considerably smaller than that in the nonplethoric group exposed to the same stimulus (bar 2). TCP also induced a considerable increase in REF activity in nonplethoric rats (bar 3) but was ineffective in this regard in the hypertransfused group (bar 4).

These studies show that the rise in serum ESF, induced by androgen or hypoxia, is positively correlated to the increase in REF activity evoked by these two stimuli in normal rats. Hypertransfusion appears to inhibit the appearance of the ESF in response to either androgen or hypoxia, apparently due to an inhibitory influence on elaboration of the REF in these plethoric animals. The mechanism by which plethora operates to inhibit the production or activation of the REF remains conjectural. Several possibilities are suggested in FIGURE 10. Its relation to the possible presence of an inhibitor in the blood of hypertransfused animals[34,35] should be investigated. It might also be a consequence of an increased oxygen supply to the kidneys associated with the greater numbers of circulating erythrocytes, or it might be caused by some as yet unclear action exerted by the higher blood viscosity associated with the plethoric state.[36,37]

Effects of Testosterone and/or Hypoxia on the REF. Experiments reported earlier in this paper have indicated that the influence of the combined stimuli of androgen and hypoxia on the erythropoiesis-stimulating action of plasma in rats is greater than the additive effects of each administered alone. It seemed possible that this might stem from an action on the REF.

To investigate this possibility, the following experiments were conducted. Four groups of four adult male Long-Evans rats (250–280 g) were established. Group 1 received 0.4 mg TP in 0.2 ml cottonseed oil daily for seven days. The rats of group 2 (controls) received 0.2 ml cottonseed oil on seven consecutive days. Group 3 consisted of rats that had been injected daily for seven days with 0.4 mg of the androgen and then subjected to 0.4 atm for 16 hr. The animals comprising group 4 were given seven daily injections of 0.2 ml cottonseed oil and also exposed to 0.4 atm for 16 hr. The kidneys of the four groups of rats were separately pooled and extracted for the REF in the manner described in FIGURE 6. The incubation procedure differed somewhat in these experiments. Here, equal volumes of the supernatant containing the REF and normal rat serum were incubated for 10 min while being shaken in a water bath at 37° C. Five to eight hypoxia-induced polycythemic mice were used to test each of the four different incubates. Each mouse received 1.0 ml of the incubate as a single i.p. injection on the third post-hypoxia day. On the fourth day they were administered i.v. an amount of ^{59}Fe registering at 150,000 cpm. All mice were killed on the sixth day and the percent RBC-radioiron incorporation estimated.[28]

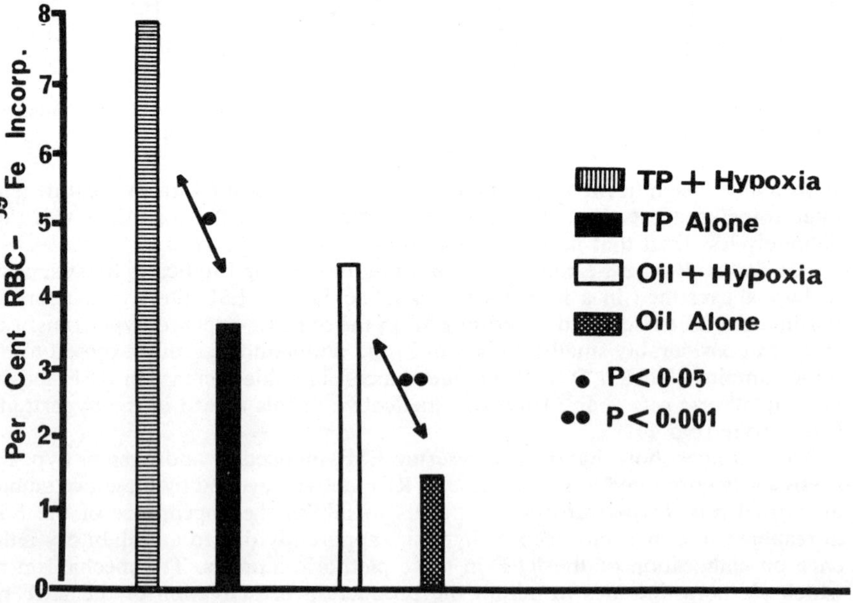

FIGURE 11. REF activity in rats treated with testosterone propionate and/or exposed to hypoxia.

It is clear from FIGURE 11 that the REF activity induced by the combined stimuli of androgen and hypoxia was considerably greater than that produced by either the androgen or hypoxia treatment applied alone. The effects on REF activity evoked by the combined stimuli appear to be additive rather than synergistic, the latter phenomenon being characteristic of the ESF response to the two stimuli administered together (see above). This does not necessarily preclude the possibility that the effects exerted on the REF in vivo by the two stimuli are of a different order than can be predicted on the basis of the arbitrarily chosen amounts of REF and serum used in the in vitro incubation system.

Discussion

Several suggestions have been made with regard to the mechanisms by which androgens influence the processes of erythropoiesis. These include: 1) a direct action on the responsive cells of the blood-forming organs;[38,39] 2) a potentiation of the effects of the ESF;[33] and 3) a stimulation of the production of the ESF.[15,16] The present results may be interpreted to provide additional evidence for the concept that the action of androgen on erythropoiesis is achieved through an enhancement of the production of the ESF. Moreover, androgen is capable of potentiating the stimulatory effects of hypoxia on ESF production, in agreement with findings by Fried and Gurney.[16]

The involvement of a renal mechanism in the stimulation of erythropoiesis by androgen is seen from the inability of testosterone to stimulate erythropoiesis in nephrectomized mice.[21] Similarly, while androgen augments the erythropoietic response to hypoxia in intact mice, it fails to produce this action in mice binephrectomized just prior to exposure to hypoxia.[40] Moreover, as shown in the present paper, perfusion of kidneys from previously androgenized rabbits with normal blood under hypoxic conditions results in continued production of the ESF over a three-hour perfusion period.

It is further shown that the rise in serum ESF caused in normal rats by androgen or hypoxia is positively correlated to the increase in REF evoked by these two stimuli. Similarly, the ability of androgen to enhance the effects of hypoxia on ESF production appears to stem from the greater REF activity evoked by the combined stimuli than by either one applied alone.

The experiments reported here lend further support to the participation of a dual component mechanism in the evocation of the ESF: one, present in the kidney (REF), probably functioning in an enzymatic capacity and the second, a serum component serving as the substrate. In this regard, estrogens administered in large doses have been demonstrated to depress erythropoiesis by inhibiting production of the ESF.[40] Unlike the situation for the stimulatory effects of androgen, the depressing action of estrogen on erythropoiesis may not require the presence of the kidney.[40] It has been proposed that estrogens operate here by inhibiting the generation of an ESF precursor substrate through a suppressing action on protein synthesis in the liver which has been recently shown to participate in the production of the ESF.[31] In this sense, the mechanism of ESF elaboration can be analogized to the production of the blood pressure-elevating factor, angiotensin.

Hammond[41,42] has recently demonstrated that administration of normal human plasma to some patients with chronic hypoplastic anemia, refractory to other forms of treatment, caused an increase in red cell production. These results are of considerable interest and importance because they support the concept that the basic lesion in these particular subjects may relate to an abnormality in the serum component. It is also possible that those of Hammond's patients who exhibited refractoriness to the normal human plasma, apart from an abnormal marrow, possess a defective REF which could result from inhibited synthesis or reduced activity of this factor. In this regard, although the plasma ESF appears to mount to high levels in patients with severe hypoplastic anemia, it should be remembered that these plasmas are tested in relatively normal assay animals in which an incomplete or defective ESF or REF could undergo activation. In this connection, the fall in plasma ESF noted in those aplastic anemia patients exhibiting a response to testosterone[43] may be the result of an ability of the androgen to convert an incomplete or faulty REF or ESF in these subjects into a more normally operating one effective in smaller quantities. Another possibility is that the quantities of ESF required to stimulate erythropoiesis in such aplastic anemia subjects may exceed the elevated amounts already present in their body fluids. In this situation, the benefit that derives from androgen could relate to the ability of this steroid to enhance production or potentiate the action of the ESF.

That relative refractoriness to the ESF may actually exist in some situations is seen from recent experiments in mice with hereditary anemias[44] in which much larger than usual quantities of ESF are required for at least some stimulation of erythropoiesis.[45] Although the basic lesion here is a refractoriness of the hematopoietic cells to ESF, the possibility cannot be completely precluded that an abnormal ESF[46,47] may be generated in such mice. In this connection the observation[21] that androgen can apparently stimulate erythropoiesis and ESF production in WW^v mice is of interest since hereditary anemias of this type may represent, to a degree, an animal counterpart of the relatively refractory hypoplastic anemias in man.

With regard to other possible modes of androgen action, doubt has been cast on a direct action of this steroid on erythropoiesis in view of recent experiments indicating that addition of water-soluble testosterone to rabbit bone marrow cells, in a wide range of dosage, actually inhibited or exerted no influence on ^{59}Fe uptake by the marrow cells.[48] This was true whether the suspending medium contained normal or anemic rabbit serum. Others[33,49] have proposed that testosterone potentiates the action of ESF on responsive marrow cells. However, it has been demonstrated[50,51] that consecutive small doses of ESF evoke a greater effect on erythropoiesis than would be expected from the additive effects of the individual doses administered alone. Thus it is still possible here that androgen is operating by increasing the production of the ESF which adds to the effect of exogenously-administered ESF or that produced endogenously by hypoxia.

It is our present opinion that the major pathway by which androgen stimulates erythropoiesis in rodents and the lower primate (tamarin) is through its capacity to cause an increase in the amount or activity of the REF. Moreover, it appears that androgen potentiates the erythropoietic response to hypoxia on a similar basis. The mechanism by which androgen accomplishes this may represent yet another manifestation of its ability to stimulate enzyme systems involved in nucleic acid and protein anabolism not only in reproductive organs but in a number of nonreproductive tissues as well.[52] Since both androgen and hypoxia stimulate the production of the REF, and as a consequence, the ESF, it remains to be determined why the erythropoietic response occurs considerably more rapidly to the latter stimulus than to the former. Perhaps hypoxia activates a later step than does androgen in the series of interlocking synthetic reactions[53] leading to the formation of the REF. It is also possible that androgen is concerned largely with the synthesis of REF while hypoxia triggers its release.

Finally, it is suggested that the members of the endocrine system, especially the adenohypophysis, gonads, adrenal and thyroid, exert their well-documented influences on erythropoiesis, at least in part, by regulating the production and/or action of the ESF. However, the possibility that other pathways are also involved cannot at present be completely excluded.

Summary and Conclusions

Evidence is presented in support of the concept that androgens enhance erythropoiesis in mice, rats and dogs by increasing production of the erythropoiesis-stimulating factor (ESF or erythropoietin). The ability of hypoxia to stimulate elaboration of the ESF is potentiated by prior treatment with androgen. Maximal plasma ESF levels, in response to injections of a long-acting androgen, testosterone cyclopentylpropionate, occur in rats within approximately a week; thereafter the titers fall, attaining normal values by about three to four weeks after start of treatment.

Considerable amounts of ESF are formed during perfusion of kidneys of rabbits that had been treated daily for a week with androgen. This effect is not reproduced by direct addition of androgen to blood being perfused through kidneys of untreated rabbits. Androgen administration to rabbits causes a marked rise in the quantity (or activity) of the renal erythropoietic factor (REF). This principle, itself only weakly active or totally inactive when injected alone, engenders the production of the ESF when incubated in vitro with normal serum.

The appearance of increased amounts of the ESF in the sera of rats following treatment with androgen or exposure to hypoxia is accompanied by augmented production (or activity) of the REF. Greater amounts of the REF are generated by the combination of androgen and hypoxia treatment rather than by either stimulus alone. The conclusion is reached that androgen and hypoxia stimulate erythropoiesis in rodents by increasing the production of the active REF.

Plethora, induced in rats by hypertransfusion, results in a marked decrease in REF activity in response to androgen or hypoxia. This probably constitutes the mechanism by which plethora inhibits production of the ESF.

It is proposed that the endocrine system plays a significant role in erythropoiesis by influencing the production of the ESF as a result of alterations in the formation of the REF and/or the serum factor with which the REF interacts.

References

1. Vollmer, E. P. & A. S. Gordon. 1941. The effect of sex and gonadotropic hormones upon the blood picture of the rat. Endocrinology **29:** 828–837.
2. Crafts, R. C. 1946. Effects of hypophysectomy, castration and testosterone propionate on hemopoiesis in the adult male rat. Endocrinology **39:** 401–413.
3. Gordon, A. S. & H. A. Charipper. 1947. The endocrine system and hemopoiesis. Ann. N. Y. Acad. Sci. **48:** 615–637.
4. Gordon, A. S. 1954. Endocrine influences upon the formed elements of blood and blood-forming organs. Rec. Prog. Horm. Res. **10:** 339–394.
5. Van Dyke, D. C., A. N. Contopoulos, B. S. Williams, M. E. Simpson, J. H. Lawrence & H. M. Evans. 1954. Hormonal factors influencing erythropoiesis. Acta Haemat. **11:** 203–222.
6. Crafts, R. C. & H. A. Meineke. 1959. The anemia of hypophysectomized animals. Ann. N. Y. Acad. Sci. **77:** 501–517.
7. Jacobson, L. O., E. Goldwasser & C. W. Gurney. 1959. Control of red cell formation. *In* The Kinetics of Cellular Proliferation. F. Stohlman, Jr., Ed. : 344–356. Grune and Stratton. New York, N. Y.
8. Vollmer, E. P., A. S. Gordon, I. Levenstein & H. A. Charipper. 1939. Effects of hypophysectomized on the blood picture of the rat. Endocrinology **25:** 970–977.

9. Crafts, R. C. 1941. The effects of endocrines on the formed elements of the blood. I. The effects of hypophysectomy, thyroidectomy and adrenalectomy on the blood of the female rat. Endocrinology **29**: 596–605.
10. Steinglass, P., A. S. Gordon & H. A. Charipper. 1941. Effect of castration and sex hormones on blood of the rat. Proc. Soc. Exp. Biol. Med. **48**: 169–177.
11. Gordon, A. S., S. J. Piliero & D. Landau. 1951. The relation of the adrenal to blood formation in the rat. Endocrinology **49**: 497–511.
12. Feigin, W. M. & A. S. Gordon. 1950. Influence of hypophysectomy on the hemopoietic response of rats to lowered barometric pressures. Endocrinology **47**: 364–369.
13. Piliero, S. J. 1959. Influence of hypoxic stimuli upon blood formation in endocrine-deficient animals. Ann. N. Y. Acad. Sci. **77**: 518–542.
14. Gordon, A. S. 1957. Influence of humoral factors on erythropoiesis. Am. J. Clin. Nut. **5**: 461–472.
15. Mirand, E. A., A. S. Gordon & J. Wenig. 1965. Mechanism of testosterone action in erythropoiesis. Nature **206**: 270–272.
16. Fried, W. & C. W. Gurney. 1965. Erythropoietic effect of plasma from mice receiving testosterone. Nature **206**: 1160–1161.
17. Camiscoli, J. F., A. H. Weintraub & A. S. Gordon. 1967. Comparative assay of erythropoietin standards. Ann. N. Y. Acad. Sci. This Annal.
18. Mirand, E. A., G. S. Johnston, G. P. Murphy & A. S. Gordon. 1966. Effects of testosterone on renal hemodynamics and erythropoietin release in dogs. Investig. Urol. **4**: 203–207.
19. Albert, A. 1961. The mammalian testis. *In* Sex and Internal Secretions. W. C. Young, Ed. : 305–365. Williams and Wilkins. Baltimore, Md.
20. Schooley, J. C. 1966. Inhibition of erythropoietic stimulation by testosterone in polycythemic mice receiving antierythropoietin. Proc. Soc. Exp. Biol. Med. **122**: 402–403.
21. Fried, W. & C. W. Gurney. 1967. The erythropoietic stimulating effects of androgens. Ann. N. Y. Acad. Sci. This Annal.
22. Jacobson, L. O., E. Goldwasser, C. W. Gurney, W. Fried & L. Plzak. 1959. Studies of erythropoietin: the hormone regulating red cell production. Ann. N. Y. Acad. Sci. **77**: 551–573.
23. Naets, J. P. 1963. The role of the kidney in erythropoiesis in the dog. *In* Hormones and the Kidney. P. C. Williams, Ed. : 175–186. Academic Press. New York, N. Y.
24. Fisher, J. W. & B. J. Birdwell. 1961. The production of an erythropoietic factor by the in situ perfused kidney. Acta Haematol. **26**: 224–232.
25. Kuratowska, Z., B. Lewartowski & E. Michalak. 1961. Studies on the production of erythropoietin, by isolated perfused organs. Blood **18**: 527–534.
26. Mirand, E. A., T. C. Prentice & W. R. Slaunwhite. 1959. Current studies on the role of erythropoietin on erythropoiesis. Ann. N. Y. Acad. Sci. **77**: 677–702.
27. Reissmann, K. R. 1963. Erythropoietin formation in the kidney. *In* Hormones and the Kidney. P. C. Williams, Ed. : 195–200. Academic Press. New York, N. Y.
28. Weintraub, A. H., A. S. Gordon & J. F. Camiscoli. 1963. Use of the hypoxia-induced polycythemic mouse in the assay and standardization of erythropoietin. J. Lab. Clin. Med. **62**: 743–752.
29. Contrera, J. F. & A. S. Gordon. 1966. Erythropoietin: production by a particulate fraction of rat kidney. Science **152**: 653–654.
30. Contrera, J. F. & A. S. Gordon. 1967. Role of the kidney in erythropoietin production. Ann. N. Y. Acad. Sci. This Annal.
31. Katz, R., G. W. Cooper, A. S. Gordon & E. D. Zanjani. 1967. Studies on the site of production of erythropoietin. Ann. N. Y. Acad. Sci. This Annal.
32. Gurney, C. W. & W. Fried. 1965. Further studies on the erythropoietic effect of androgen. J. Lab. Clin. Med. **65**: 775–782.
33. Naets, J. P. & M. Wittek. 1966. Mechanism of action of androgens on erythropoiesis. Amer. J. Physiol. **210**: 315–320.
34. Krzymowski, T. & H. Krzymowska. 1962. Studies on the erythropoiesis-inhibiting factor in the plasma of animals with transfusion polycythemia. Blood **19**: 38–44.
35. Whitcomb, W. H. & M. Z. Moore. 1965. The inhibitory effect of plasma from hypertransfused animals on erythrocyte iron incorporation in mice. J. Lab. Clin. Med. **66**: 641–651.
36. Erslev, A. J. 1966. The erythropoietic effect of hematocrit variations in normovolemic rabbits. Blood **27**: 629–636.
37. Erslev, A. J. & E. B. Thorling. 1967. Erythropoietin in erythropoiesis. Ann. N. Y. Acad. Sci. This Annal.

38. ERSLEV, A. J. 1962. Erythropoietin and testosterone in vitro. Proc. IX Cong. Int. Soc. Hematol. **3:** 143–148.
39. REISNER, JR. E. H. 1966. Tissue culture of bone marrow. II. Effect of steroid hormones on hematopoiesis in vitro. Blood **27:** 460–469.
40. MIRAND, E. A. & A. S. GORDON. 1966. Mechanism of estrogen action in erythropoiesis. Endocrinology **78:** 325–332.
41. HAMMOND, G. D. 1962. Discussion on physiology of erythropoietin. *In* Erythropoiesis. L. O. Jacobson and M. Doyle, Eds. : 270–273. Grune and Stratton. New York, N. Y.
42. HAMMOND, G. D. 1967. Studies on the production and utilization of erythropoietin in chronic anemias and in aplastic crisis. Ann. N. Y. Acad. Sci. This Annal.
43. GARDNER, F. H. & D. G. NATHAN. 1966. Androgens and erythropoiesis. III. Further evaluation of testosterone treatment of myelofibrosis. New Eng. J. Med. **274:** 420–426.
44. KEIGHLEY, G., E. S. RUSSELL & P. H. LOWY. 1962. Response of normal and genetically anemic mice to erythropoietin stimulation. Brit. J. Haemat. **8:** 429–441.
45. KALES, A., W. FRIED & C. W. GURNEY. 1964. The erythropoietic defect in a congenitally anemic mouse. Clin. Res. **12:** 347.
46. MIRAND, E. A. & T. C. PRENTICE. 1964. The ability of genetically anemic mice (WW^v) to respond only to erythropoietin from WW^v mice. Amer. Zool. **4:** 422.
47. MIRAND, E. A. & G. GUTMAN. 1963. The inability of genetically anemic mice to respond to various erythropoietin preparations. Amer. Zool. **3:** 551.
48. MCDONALD, T. P. 1967. Effects of testosterone on bone marrow cells. Ann. N. Y. Acad. Sci. This Annal.
49. MEINEKE, H. A. & R. C. CRAFTS. 1967. Further observations on the mechanism by which androgens and growth hormone influence erythropoiesis. Ann. N. Y. Acad. Sci. This Annal.
50. GURNEY, C. W., N. WACKMAN & E. FILMANOWICZ. 1961. Studies on erythropoiesis. XVII. Some quantitative aspects of the erythropoietic response to erythropoietin. Blood **17:** 531–546.
51. FOGH, J. 1966. A sensitive erythropoietin assay on mice exposed to CO-hypoxia. Scand. J. Clin. Lab. Invest. **18:** 33–44.
52. FRIEDEN, E. H. 1964. Sex hormones and the metabolism of amino acids and proteins. *In* Actions of Hormones on Molecular Processes. G. Litwack and D. Kritchevsky, Eds. 509–559. J. Wiley and Sons. New York, N. Y.
53. TATA, J. R. 1964. Biological action of thyroid hormones at the cellular and molecular levels. *In* Actions of Hormones on Molecular Processes. G. Litwack and D. Kritchevsky, Eds. : 58–131. J. Wiley and Sons. New York, N. Y.

THE INTERRELATIONSHIPS OF THE ENDOCRINE AND ERYTHROPOIETIC SYSTEMS IN THE RAT WITH SPECIAL REFERENCE TO THE MECHANISM OF ACTION OF ESTRADIOL AND TESTOSTERONE*

Sam J. Piliero, Paul T. Medici and Clara Haber**

Department of Pharmacology, Geigy Research, Division of Geigy Chemical Corporation, Ardsley, N. Y.

and the Department of Biology, St. John's University, Graduate School of Arts & Science, Jamaica, N. Y.

The immense concentration of attention to the problems surrounding the control of erythrocyte production has culminated in firmly establishing erythropoietin as a major governing factor of red cell production or release.[1] In assessing the overall phenomenon of erythrocytopoiesis, however, it is clearly evident that uncertainties still prevail as to: 1) the specific nature of the erythrocytogenic stimulus attributed to erythropoietin, and 2) the precise character of the stimuli capable of augmenting its production and release.

That certain classically well-defined hormones influence red cell production has been amply documented. Changes in metabolic patterns have been suggested as the primary manifestation of hormonal administration. Needless to say, therefore, it is extremely difficult to relate the nature of the response of erythropoietic tissues to any specific hormonal effect.

A relationship has been known to exist between the gonadal hormones and the status of erythrocyte levels in the rat, male hormones maintaining the dominant erythrocytogenic activity as reflected by higher red cell levels in males and castrated females. Furthermore, estrogens have been highly effective in depressing red cell production in rats[2–6] whereas exogenously administered androgens evoked accelerated erythropoiesis.[2–4, 6–10]

Recent studies have sought to elucidate the nature of the gonadal steroid effect on erythropoietic tissues per se or via an indirect mechanism involving another organ.[11–15] While this question remains unresolved, the evidence does point to a fundamentally indirect action of these steroids.

In an attempt to resolve certain questions concerning the primary role of gonadal hormones in erythropoiesis, a comprehensive study was made of the blood and tissues of rats subjected to large doses of estrogenic and androgenic hormones.

Materials and Methods

Two hundred and seventy-six young adult female rats of the Long Evans strain, weighing 160 to 165 g were employed. All animals were fed a standard laboratory ration and kept at temperatures of 70 to 80° F.

Peripheral blood from the tail was employed for all procedures. Red cell counts were made in duplicate and were required to agree to within $\pm$ 4%. Reticulocyte counts were made from dry smears of peripheral blood stained with new methylene blue.[16] One thousand erythrocytes were counted and the reticulocytes expressed as a percentage of these. Hemoglobin concentrations were determined by the acid hematin and cyanmethemoglobin methods with a photoelectric colorimeter. Duplicate hematocrit determinations from heparinized blood, spun at

* Supported in part by Public Health Service research grant HE 03374–08 from the National Heart Institute and a research grant from the Intercounty Blood Banks, Inc., Jamaica, N. Y.

** Taken in part from a thesis submitted in partial fulfillment of the requirements for a Ph.D. at St. John's University.

12,000 rpm for seven min, were made by a capillary micromethod and were required to agree to within ± 1 mm. Icterus indices were determined by comparing the plasma columns of the hematocrit tubes with a set of standard solutions of potassium dichromate.[17] Serum bilirubin determinations were made by the method of Malloy and Evelyn as modified by Ducci and Watson.[18] The percentage of radioiron incorporation into the circulating red cells (RBC-^{59}Fe) was determined at 48 hr after injection by the method of Gordon *et al.*[19] The percentage ^{59}Fe uptake by the bone marrow was determined on a suspension of marrow in saline six hr after the i.v. injection of ^{59}Fe. Control hematologic determinations were carried out in all animals before experimental treatment was begun. The experimental groups were established as follows:

Experiment 1: Effects of Estradiol Treatment for Four Weeks. Forty-two rats were given daily s.c. injections of 2.0 mg estradiol valerate (Delestrogen, E. R. Squibb & Sons) for varying periods of time up to four weeks. Nine were sacrificed on the tenth day, nine on the 20th day, and the remainder (24) on the 30th day following treatment. Also included were 42 sesame oil-injected control animals.

Experiment 2: Effects of Combined Estradiol-Erythropoietin Treatment for Four Weeks. Twenty-seven animals were given s.c. injections of 2.0 mg estradiol valerate daily plus 3 cobalt units of sheep plasma erythropoietin (Armour) given every other day for the duration of the experiment. Appropriate controls consisted of 27 animals in each of the following three groups which included rats treated with 2.0 mg estradiol, animals injected every other day with 3 cobalt units of erythropoietin, and a sesame oil-injected group.

Experiment 3: Effects of Testosterone Treatment for Four Weeks. Forty-two rats were given daily s.c. injections of testosterone propionate (Oreton, Schering Corp.) for varying periods of time up to four weeks, nine of which were sacrificed on the tenth day, nine on the 20th day, and 24 on the 30th day following treatment. An equal number of sesame oil-injected control animals were included.

At the termination of the observation periods all rats were anesthetized lightly with ether and exsanguinated by cardiac puncture. Bone marrow differentials were made on smears stained with May-Grunwald or treated by the peroxidase method of Ralph.[20] Other bone marrow smears were prepared for the demonstration of Perl's reaction for nonhemoglobin iron.[21] In some cases, marrow weight and nucleated cell numbers were determined by the method of Lo Bue *et al.*[22] A portion of the marrow suspension was treated with new methylene blue stain and smears were made for enumeration of the percentage of reticulocytes present. Similarly, spleen preparations were made, stained and examined for nucleated erythroid cells and reticulocyte percentages.

Besides gross observations and weight changes at the time of autopsy, bone marrow, liver, spleen, and kidney tissues were removed and fixed for routine and special histological and histochemical analyses. Special procedures included Perl's reaction for nonhemoglobin iron, Wilson's stain for hyalin droplet degeneration, and Bowie's stain for examination of the juxtaglomerular cells of the kidney.

RESULTS†

Experiment 1

The effects of daily injections of estradiol upon the blood elements for a period of four weeks are shown in FIGURES 1 and 2. It will be noted (FIGURE 1) that

† All statements made in this section regarding differences among the means of the different groups of animals compared are based on statistical analyses for probability values derived from the distribution of Fisher's t. P values of <0.05 have been considered significant.

after four weeks of treatment with massive doses of this agent, the red blood cells, hemoglobin and hematocrit values are significantly lowered. Mean corpuscular volume is decreased (58.0 ± 0.31 to 54.8 ± 0.70), while the mean corpuscular hemoglobin concentration remains unchanged. Regarding icterus index and bilirubin determinations, no significant changes are found to accompany the anemia.

Peripheral blood reticulocyte percentages (FIGURE 2) are observed to be lowered at five and ten days after treatment but subsequent elevations are seen throughout the remaining period of treatment. Bone marrow reticulocyte values of animals sacrificed at 10 days after estrogen treatment indicate that significant increases occur which persist throughout the injection period. However, this increase in most cases is due to the presence of old forms rather than increased numbers of young reticulocytes.

From a quantitative standpoint (FIGURE 2), the most significant alteration seen in estradiol-treated rats is the decrease in total marrow nucleated cellular elements and even more significant is the decrease in actual numbers of nucleated erythrocytes.

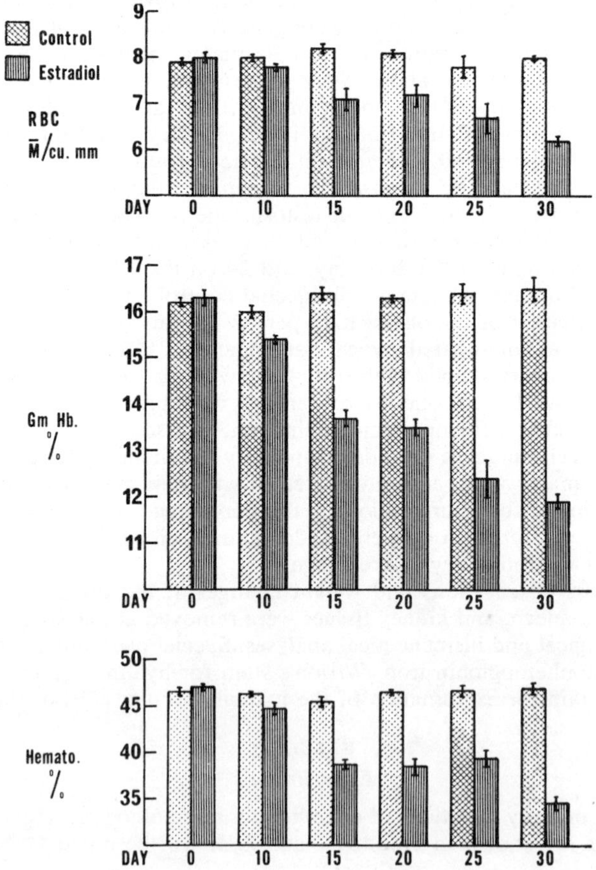

FIGURE 1. Effects of estradiol upon erythocytic values. Vertical lines through the bars represent ± 1 standard error of the mean.

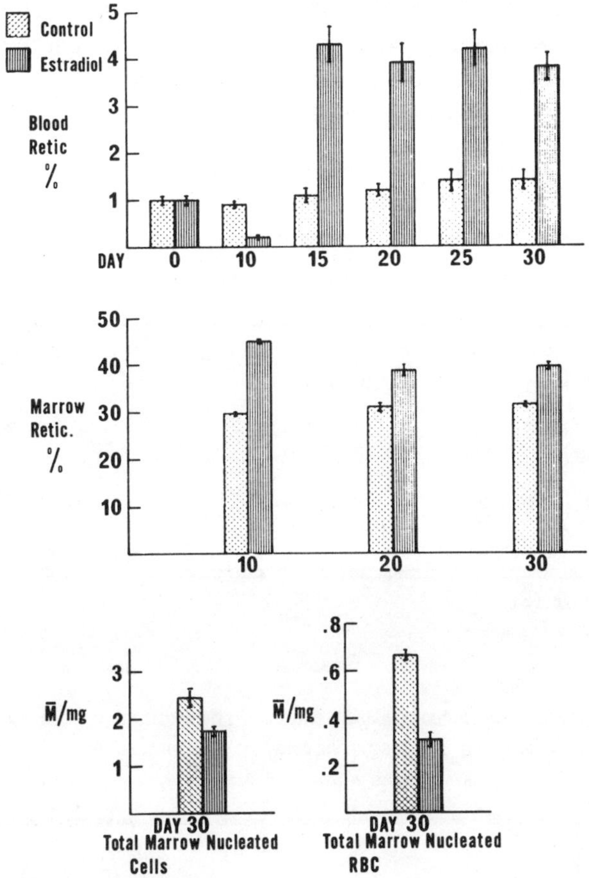

FIGURE 2. Effects of estradiol upon peripheral blood and bone marrow reticulocytes. Also shown are quantitative estimates of bone marrow cellularity. Vertical lines through the bars represent ± 1 standard error of the mean.

TABLE 1 indicates that 10 days of estradiol treatment significantly reduces the ability of both peripheral blood and bone marrow erythrocytes to utilize iron. By 30 days, in the estradiol group, an increase in peripheral blood iron utilization is seen in comparison to controls.

The effects of estradiol on organ weights is shown in TABLE 2. Significant gains in liver weight are noted during the entire experimental period while spleen and kidney weights remained unaltered.

The architecture of the spleen of estradiol-treated rats appears somewhat disrupted and reveals a marked increase in hemosiderin deposition (FIGURE 3, A & B). Perl's reaction for nonhemoglobin iron (FIGURE 3, C & D) also indicates an increase in iron deposition in the red pulp of the spleen of estrogenized animals in comparison to controls. That an increase in the nonhemoglobin iron content also occurs in kidney sections of treated animals is revealed in the comparative sections shown in FIGURE 4, A–C. Iron deposition in bone marrow smears is found to be

TABLE 1

EFFECTS OF ESTRADIOL AND TESTOSTERONE UPON ^{59}Fe UPTAKE BY PERIPHERAL BLOOD AND BONE MARROW ERYTHROCYTES

(Means ± Standard Errors)

Treatment	Days	% Radioiron incorp. Peripheral RBC (48 hr. uptake)	% Radioiron incorp. Bone Marrow RBC (6 hr. uptake)
Controls	10	6.2 ± 0.31 (12)*	2.1 ± 0.17 (3)
(Sesame Oil)	30	10.8 ± 0.19 (12)	
Estradiol	10	3.7 ± 0.10 (6)	1.5 ± 0.14 (3)
(2.0 mg daily)	30	13.9 ± 0.81 (6)	
Testosterone	10	12.5 ± 0.30 (6)	3.1 ± 0.14 (3)
(5.0 mg daily)	30	10.7 ± 0.37 (6)	

( )* Number of rats.

TABLE 2

EFFECTS OF ESTRADIOL, COMBINED ESTRADIOL-ERYTHROPOIETIN AND TESTOSTERONE TREATMENTS UPON ORGAN WEIGHTS/100 GM. BODY WEIGHT

(Means ± Standard Errors)

	Days	Liver (g)	Spleen (g)	Kidney (g)
Controls	10 (25)*	3.7 ± 0.11	0.18 ± 0.03	0.32 ± 0.07
(Sesame oil)	20 (12)	4.0 ± 0.17	0.16 ± 0.02	0.27 ± 0.02
	30 (19)	3.8 ± 0.07	0.18 ± 0.02	0.33 ± 0.02
Estradiol	10 (15)	4.3 ± 0.14	0.17 ± 0.01	0.30 ± 0.06
(2.0 mg daily)	20 (9)	5.0 ± 0.07	0.15 ± 0.02	0.25 ± 0.04
	30 (15)	4.8 ± 0.08	0.13 ± 0.01	0.31 ± 0.01
Erythropoietin	10 (6)	3.4 ± 0.12	0.27 ± 0.02	0.34 ± 0.05
(3 Cobalt units	20 (6)	3.3 ± 0.09	0.29 ± 0.03	0.35 ± 0.03
every other day)	30 (6)	3.6 ± 0.07	0.27 ± 0.01	0.37 ± 0.03
Estradiol + Erythropoietin	10 (6)	3.5 ± 0.08	0.21 ± 0.03	0.38 ± 0.03
(2.0 mg (3 Cobalt units	20 (6)	4.1 ± 0.10	0.25 ± 0.01	0.32 ± 0.06
daily) every other day)	30 (6)	3.5 ± 0.11	0.28 ± 0.02	0.34 ± 0.04
Testosterone	10 (15)	3.4 ± 0.06	0.25 ± 0.03	0.36 ± 0.02
(5.0 mg daily)	20 (9)	3.7 ± 0.10	0.19 ± 0.01	0.40 ± 0.01
	30 (15)	3.6 ± 0.08	0.23 ± 0.02	0.47 ± 0.03

( )* Number of rats

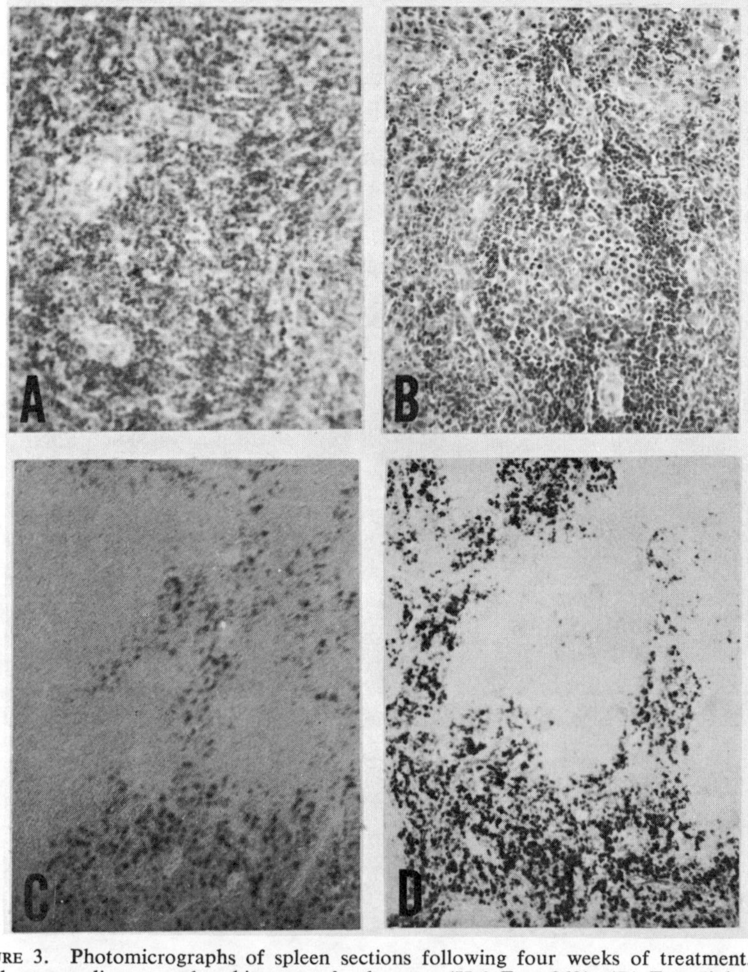

FIGURE 3. Photomicrographs of spleen sections following four weeks of treatment. (A) Control rat revealing normal architecture of pulp areas (H & E × 269). (B) Estradiol-treated rat revealing a somewhat disrupted architecture. A marked increase in hemosiderin deposition is evident (H & E × 269). (C) Control rat revealing the appearance of Perl's reaction for non-hemoglobin iron. Dark granules representing iron deposits are seen almost exclusively in the red pulp areas (× 196). (D) Estradiol-treated rat revealing Perl's reaction. Note the increase in iron deposition in comparison to the control section (× 196).

too variable, with iron occurring in macrophages and in addition freely distributed over the smears and not confined to cells. Thus, the observed slight increase seen especially in macrophages of only a few of the bone marrow smears of animals treated with estradiol do not permit a positive judgment. Regarding liver sections stained for Perl's reaction, sections from estradiol animals appear no different from control sections and reveal a normal distribution of iron granules in the parenchymal cells. However, if one takes into account that the size of the liver of the estradiol-treated group is enlarged, then perhaps it can be assumed that an increase in iron deposition does occur.

Observation of kidney sections examined for the presence of hyalin droplets (tiny, dark, rounded granules smaller than renal nuclei in size) reveals hyalin droplet degeneration of the tubular cells of estradiol-treated animals (FIGURE 5, B & D) accompanied by a moderate vacuolization of the cytoplasm in comparison to control sections (FIGURE 5, A & C). Kidney sections stained and studied for the extent of juxtaglomerular cell granulation reveal that the extent of granulation in both groups is of a similar magnitude.

FIGURE 6, B illustrates the somewhat disrupted architecture of the liver with cells revealing a loss of cytoplasmic detail, vacuolization and blurred cellular outlines in a section of liver from an estradiol-treated rat. In contrast, note the normal cellular pattern and distinct cell outlines of a liver section taken from a control rat (FIGURE 6, A).

The observations of bone marrow sections parallel those made on the smears.

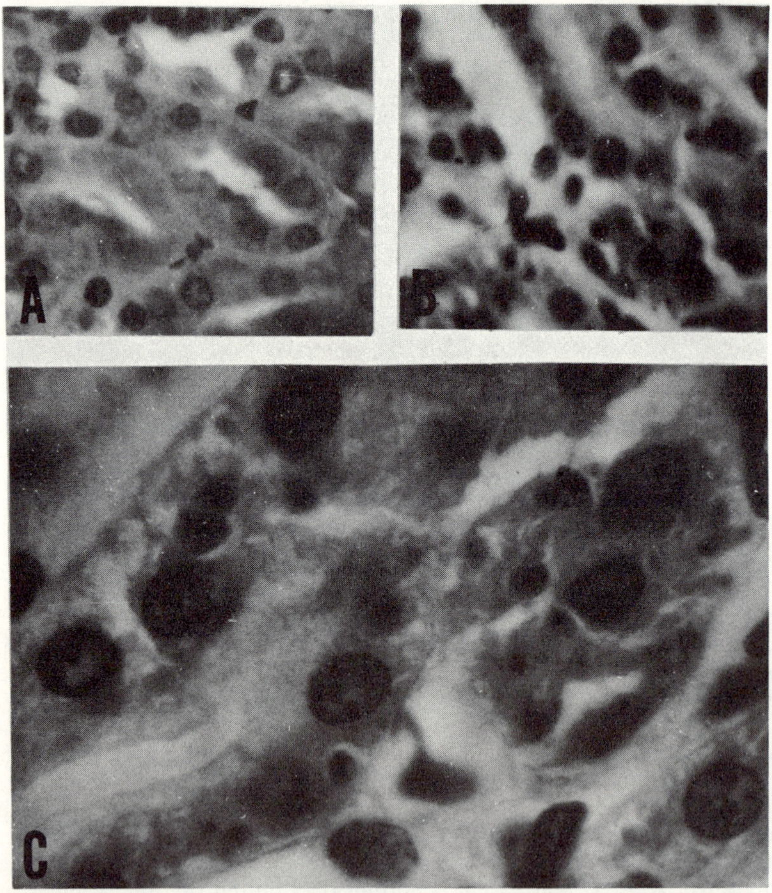

FIGURE 4. Photomicrographs of kidney sections following four weeks of treatment. (A) Control rat for Perl's reaction. Few granules are present (× 1120). (B) Estradiol-treated rat revealing Perl's reaction. Note the increase in iron deposits which are visible as small dark granules in sacs (× 1120). (C) Estradiol-treated rat for Perl's reaction taken at a higher magnification. The granules appearing in sacs are obvious (× 2453).

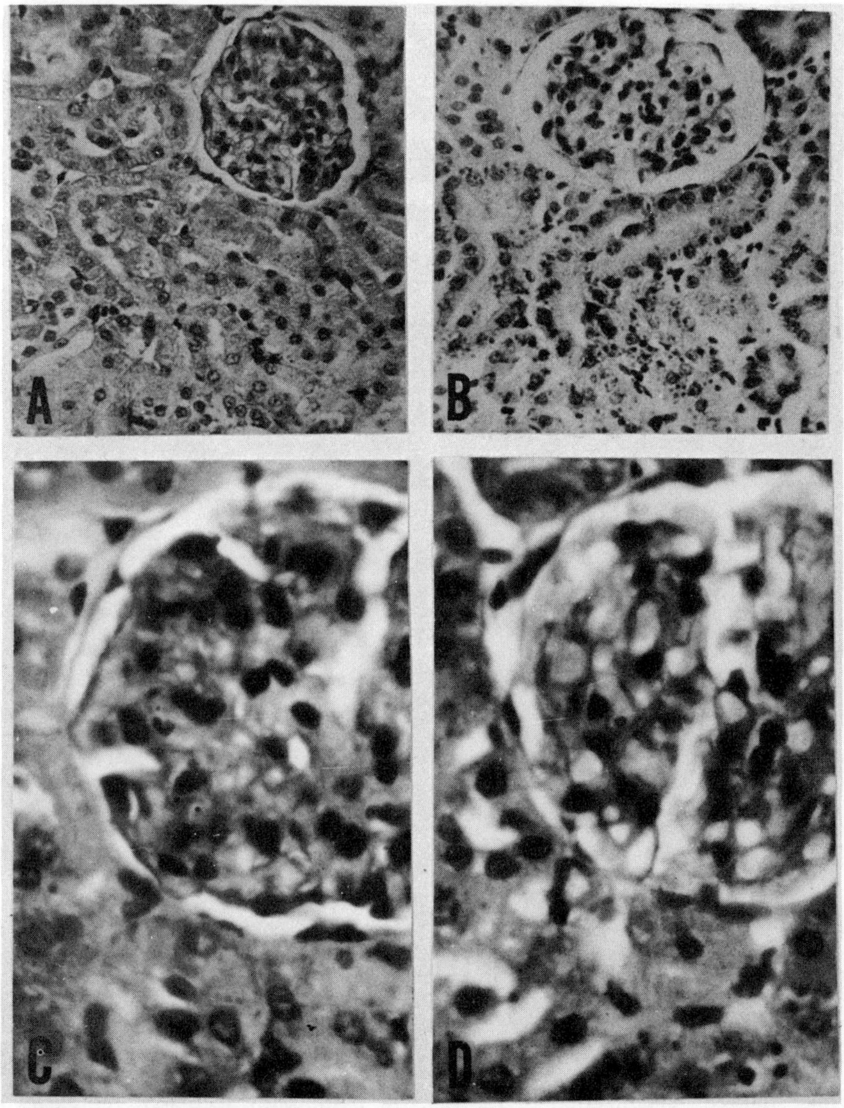

FIGURE 5. Photomicrographs of kidney sections following four weeks of treatment. (A) Control rat for the presence of hyalin droplet degeneration which would appear as tiny dark granules smaller than the nuclear elements. Note that these granules are virtually absent (Wilson stain $\times$ 568). (B) Estradiol-treated rat. Numerous hyalin droplets are evident in the tubules (Wilson stain $\times$ 568). (C) Control rat at a higher magnification. Note the absence of hyalin droplets (Wilson stain $\times$ 1120). (D) Estradiol-treated rat. At this magnification, hyalin droplets are obvious. Moderate vacuolization of the cytoplasm also appears to be present (Wilson stain $\times$ 1120).

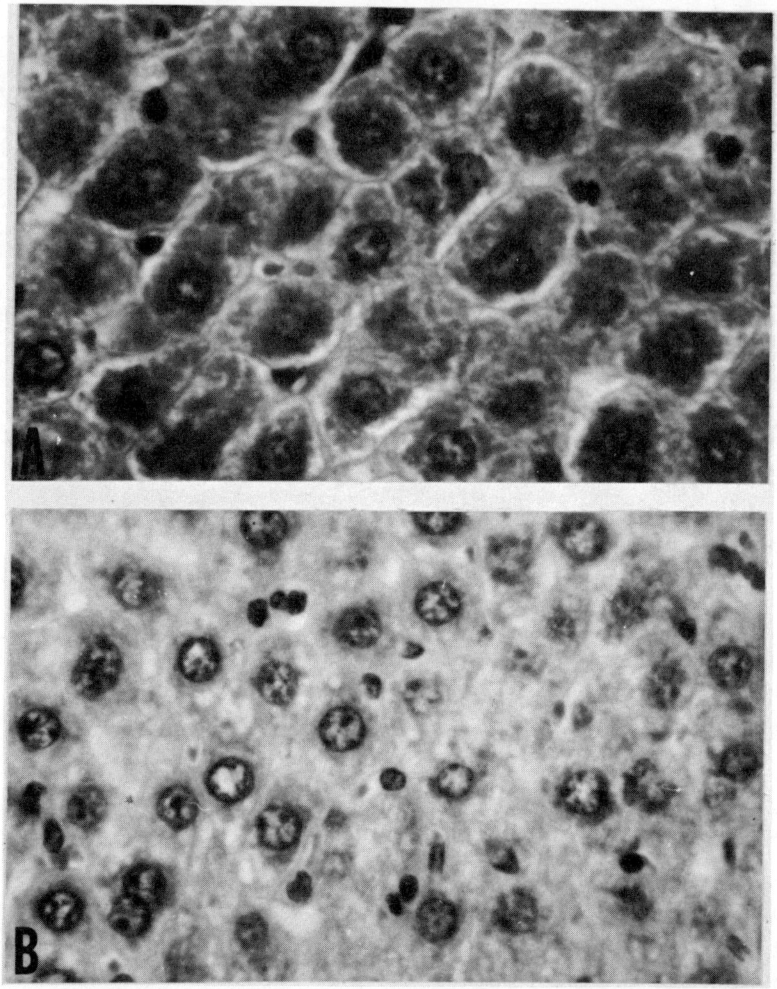

FIGURE 6. Photomicrographs of liver sections following four weeks of treatment. (A) Control rat. This section reveals a normal architecture with cells having distinct outlines. Testosterone treated animals were similar and revealed no changes in comparison to controls (H & E × 1120). (B) Estradiol-treated rat. Especially note the blurred cell outlines (H & E × 1120).

Thus, marked vacuolization of the marrow tissue with decreased cellularity is observed in the estradiol-treated rat compared to controls (FIGURE 7, A–D).

Experiment 2

FIGURE 8 shows the results of peripheral blood studies of combined estradiol-erythropoietin-treated animals in comparison to the various control groups employed. Combined estradiol-erythropoietin treatment for four weeks offsets the depressing action of massive doses of estradiol on hemoglobin and hematocrit values. Also noted is that erythropoietin prevented estradiol from exerting its usual early depressing effect on peripheral blood reticulocytes at the 10-day period of treatment. The subsequent elevations seen in reticulocyte percentages appear to be of a similar magnitude in the combined-treated animals, estradiol and erythropoietin groups. A comparison of peripheral blood and bone marrow reticulocyte percentages of the various groups is shown in FIGURE 9. At the 30-day period of treatment, increases in these values are still evident in the combined-treated group and estradiol-treated animals.

At the 10-day period, peripheral blood iron uptake percentages reveal significant increases in the combined-injected group (7.4 ± 0.35) in comparison to the estradiol-treated group (3.7 ± 0.10). Animals treated solely with erythro-

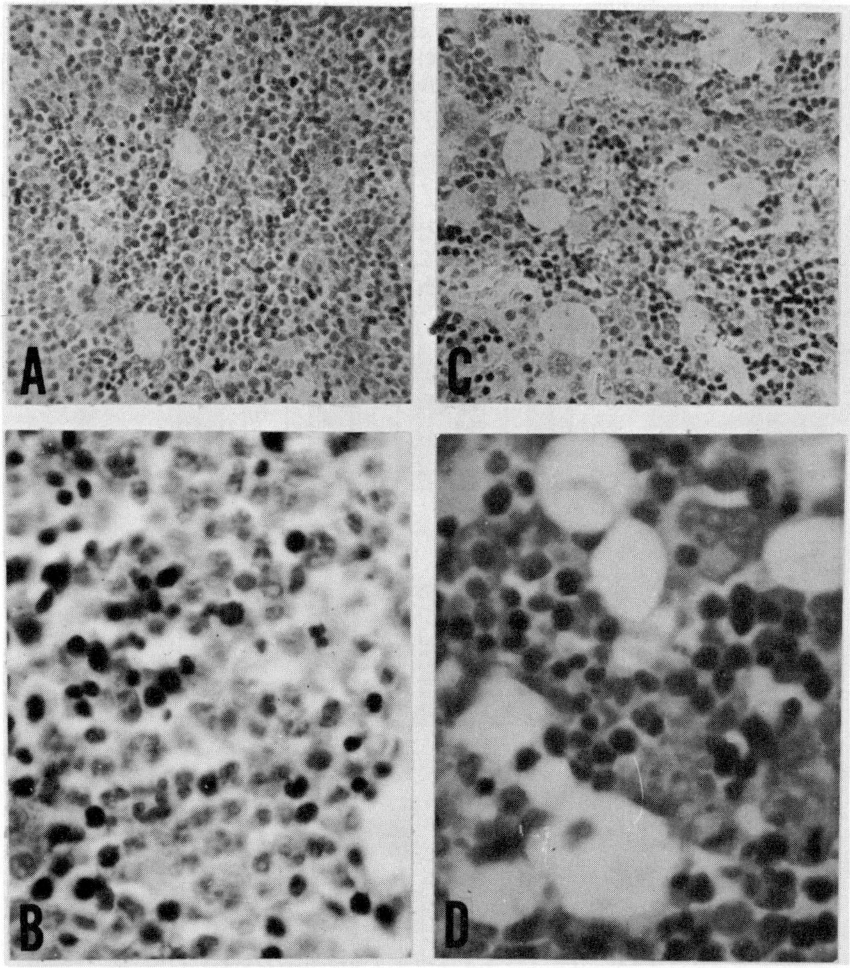

FIGURE 7. Photomicrographs of bone marrow sections. (A) Control rat. Note the normal architecture and erythroid/myeloid distribution (H & E × 568). (B) Control rat taken at a higher magnification (H & E × 1120). (C) Estradiol-treated rat. Note the decrease in cellularity and the increase in vacuolization (H & E × 568). (D) Estradiol-treated rat at a higher magnification (H & E × 1120).

poietin are found to have elevated iron uptake percentages to 14.8 ± 0.15.

The depression in marrow nucleated erythrocyte percentages seen in estradiol-treated rats (FIGURE 9) is overcome by the simultaneous administration of erythropoietin. The effectiveness of the amount of erythropoietin employed to increase the marrow nucleated erythrocytic percentages in intact animals is also demonstrated. FIGURE 9 also shows that estrogen brings about a rise in splenic nucleated erythrocytes. However, the amount of erythropoietin used in this study seems to exert very little effect on the numbers of these elements. The splenic nucleated erythrocyte percentages of combined estradiol-erythropoietin-treated animals reveal no differences from the estradiol-injected group.

Examination of the organ weights (TABLE 2) shows increases in the splenic weights in the combined estradiol-erythropoietin and erythropoietin groups as compared to estradiol- and sesame oil-injected controls. Moreover, the striking increase in liver weight of the estradiol-treated animals is no longer present in the combined estradiol-erythropoietin rats. Kidney weights reveal no changes in

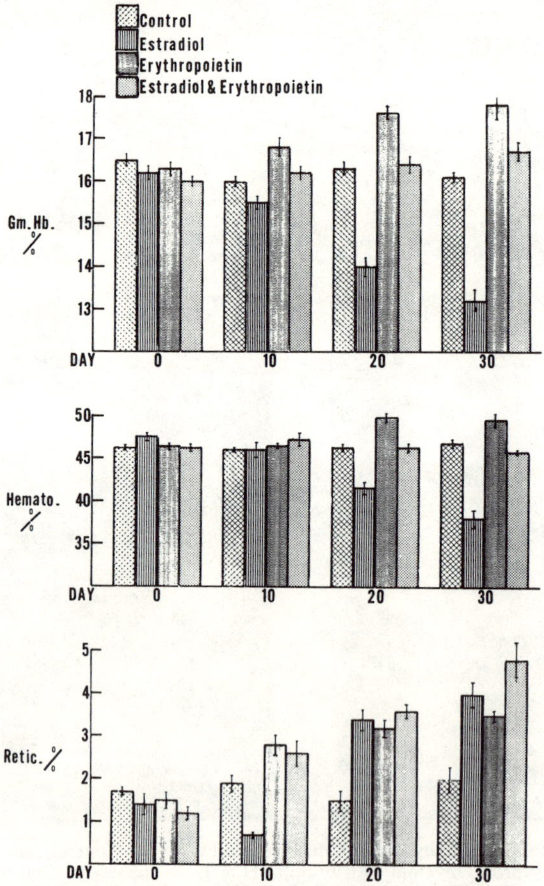

FIGURE 8. Effects of combined estradiol-erythropoietin treatment upon erythrocytic values. Vertical lines through the bars represent ± standard error of the mean.

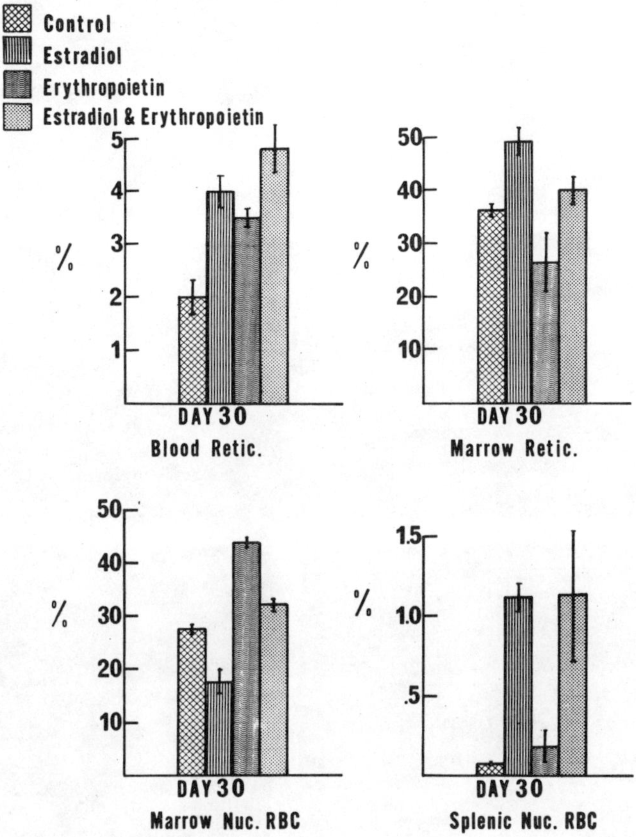

FIGURE 9. Effects of combined estradiol-erythropoietin treatment upon peripheral blood and bone marrow reticulocytes. Also shown are the nucleated erythrocyte percentages of bone marrow and splenic preparations. Vertical lines through the bars represent ± 1 standard error of the mean.

the four groups of this series. Except for bone marrow sections, histologic examinations of the other organs cited have not been completed. Bone marrow sections from combined estradiol-erythropoietin-treated animals (FIGURE 10, A) reveal the increased marrow cellularity and diminished vacuolization in contrast to the marrows of estradiol-treated rats depicted in FIGURE 7, C and D.

Experiment 3

The effects of testosterone treatment for a period of four weeks upon the blood elements are shown in FIGURES 11 and 12. Significant increases in hemoglobin and hematocrit values are quite evident while the increases in numbers of circulating erythrocytes are not as striking (FIGURE 11). Mean corpuscular volume calculations reveal that following protracted testosterone treatment (30 days), there is a significant increase in cell size (59.4 ± 0.19 to 61.4 ± 0.63). Accompanying this change is a slight decrease in mean corpuscular hemoglobin concentration of these animals (35.5 ± 0.30 to 33.6 ± 0.16).

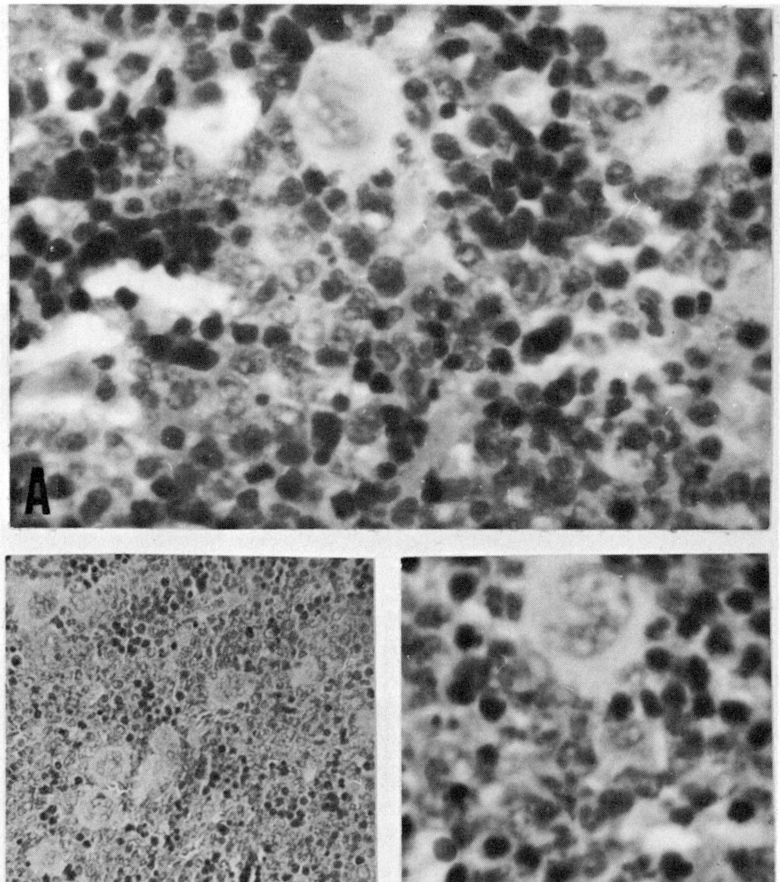

FIGURE 10. Photomicrographs of bone marrow sections. (A) Combined estradiol-erythropoietin-treated rat. Note the increased marrow cellularity and lack of vacuolization in comparison to FIGURE 7, D (H & E × 1120). (B) Testosterone-treated rat. Note the hypercellularity of the marrow in comparison to FIGURE 7, A (H & E × 568). (C) Testosterone-treated rat at a higher magnification. A definite increase in nucleated erythroid elements is evident in comparison to FIGURE 7, B (H & E × 1120).

FIGURE 12 reveals increases in the number of peripheral blood reticulocytes approximating those values observed in the erythropoietin-injected animals (FIGURE 8). At 10 days after testosterone treatment the percentage of marrow reticulocytes is significantly lower than control levels but subsequently, no changes can be detected. The myelograms of testosterone-treated rats reveal significant increases in the percentages of nucleated erythroid elements at the 30-day period (23.9 ± 2.5 to 32.2 ± 1.3). However, the increase does not approach that seen in erythropoietin-injected animals (FIGURE 9). Splenic nucleated erythrocyte percentages are not significantly different in the treated (0.86 ± 0.14) and control groups (0.74 ± 0.20).

The pattern of radioactive iron uptake in androgen-stimulated animals is shown in TABLE 1. Analysis of the data discloses that exposure to treatment produces significant increases in iron utilization by 10 days in both peripheral blood and bone marrow samples. However, by 30 days, the peripheral blood iron uptake values have returned to within control limits.

TABLE 2 shows the effects of testosterone on organ weights. The only significant change noted is the increase in kidney weight especially evident by 20 and 30 days following treatment.

Histologically, the splenic architecture appears normal and sections treated for Perl's reaction reveal similar or slightly decreased iron deposits in the testosterone-treated groups as compared to controls. Similarly, liver sections were no different from controls (FIGURE 6, A). Kidney iron deposition was minimal and was comparable to that seen in control animals. Regarding observations for the presence

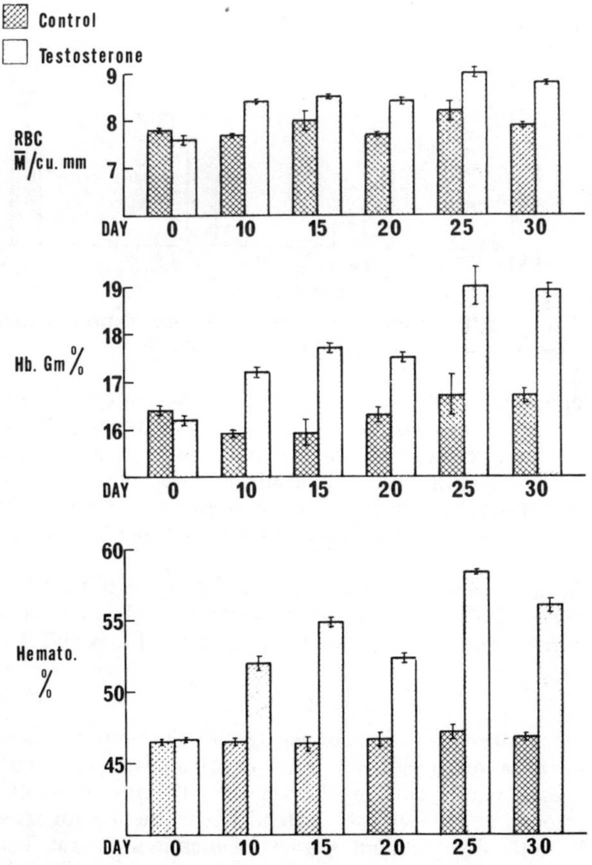

FIGURE 11. Effects of testosterone upon erythrocytic values. Vertical lines through the bars represent ± 1 standard error of the mean.

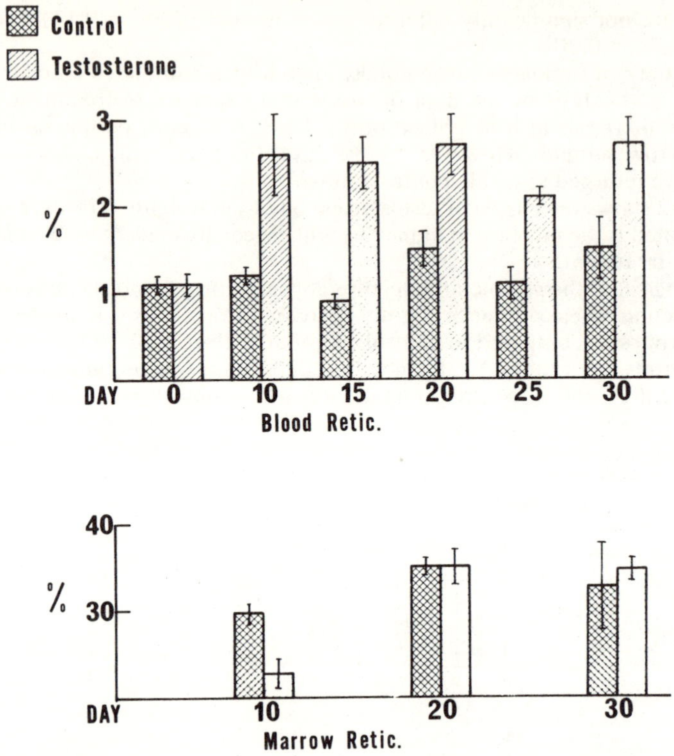

FIGURE 12. Effects of testosterone upon blood and bone marrow reticulocytes. Vertical lines through the bars represent ± 1 standard error of the mean.

of hyalin degeneration, none was apparent. However, suggestions of increases in kidney glomerular and tubular sizes were seen. The kidneys of a small group of animals treated with testosterone for 10 days and specifically stained for the appearance of the juxtaglomerular apparatus revealed marked increases in juxtaglomerular cell granulation in comparison to controls but this change was not apparent in a large number of animals examined at the 30-day period following treatment.

Examination of bone marrow sections in testosterone-treated rats (FIGURE 10, B & C) revealed hypercellularity of the marrow with an evident increase in nucleated erythroid elements as compared to controls (7, A and B.).

Discussion

Although the suppressive actions of estrogens[3,5,23,24] and the contrasting stimulatory activities of androgens[2,9,10,25–29] on erythropoiesis have been well documented, the present study further characterizes the responses of rats to these agents. As demonstrated previously, extended treatment with massive doses of estradiol results in the development of a severe anemia in the rat. That this anemia is not due to cellular destruction is shown by the failure to note elevated icterus indices and bilirubin levels in these animals. This type of evaluation was especially important since increased iron deposition, which is often a sign of hemolysis, was noted in various tissues studied.

Since increases in the percent of radioactive iron uptake has been a valid criterion for enhanced erythropoiesis by the bone marrow, this parameter was also included. Our data show that at 10 days following estradiol treatment, the uptake of iron by peripheral erythrocytes is significantly less than that of control values. However, at the 30-day period, despite the noted severe anemia, the erythrocyte uptake of iron at this time is higher than those of control animals and consonant with the observed increases in peripheral blood reticulocytes. The accompanying decrease in marrow iron uptake in the estradiol animal seems to indicate that the production rate or turnover was not increased to compensate for the decrease in erythroid elements which may be the result of depressed erythropoietin activity. The importance of turnover, in addition to actual numbers of erythroid cells, has been suggested by other investigators[29–31] and may provide a possible explanation for the anemia-producing effects of estradiol. In addition, the increased phagocytosis of iron by large outstretched reticuloendothlial cells noted in the spleens of estradiol-treated rats presents the possibility that these cells have been stimulated to engulf iron which has not been utilized in hemoglobin production by the early erythrocytic forms. It therefore appears that estradiol is, in some way, altering the ability of marrow erythroid elements to utilize iron.

The depressing effects on peripheral blood reticulocytes reported by Dukes and Goldwasser[5] vary somewhat with the observations made in this investigation. That is, while at 10 days highly significant decreases in circulating reticulocytes were observed, marrow reticulocyte levels were elevated, which indicates a possible defect in the release of these elements into the circulation. However, while at the 15-day period and for the duration of the experiment, peripheral blood reticulocytes remained higher than control levels, marrow percentages, although maintained at higher levels than the controls but not as great as those seen at the 10-day period, reveal that these reticulocytes were mainly of the older type. This fact would indicate an inhibition of marrow erythroid maturation or a delayed release of relatively mature reticulocytes into the circulation. It is of interest to note that female castrated rats treated with estrogens similarly reveal decreases in marrow cellularity and increases in peripheral blood reticulocytes.[2,7,32] In the present study, the increase in peripheral blood reticulocytes may possibly be accounted for by a number of these cells coming from the marrow (in view of the fewer numbers of cells present in comparison to the number noted at the 10-day period) and possibly from the spleen as their source. It is conceivable that the spleen regains some of its early erythropoietic activity during the marrow depression stage in an attempt to compensate for the anemic state. In view of the suggestion by Fruhman and Fisher[33] and Gordon *et al.*[34] that the release of reticulocytes might be a major activity of erythropoietin, our results imply a decrease in erythropoietin production.

Moreover, Dukes and Goldwasser[5] have reported that estrogens exert a negative control over red cell formation by interfering with stem-cell differentiation, considered by many investigators to be the prime mode by which erythropoietin exerts its effect. While our study does not offer direct evidence for inhibition of stem-cell differentiation, other than the decrease in numbers of marrow cells, it is possible that this mechanism also induces the anemia of estradiol treatment.

Relative to studies on cellular size, Winkert *et al.*[40] and Stohlman[41] have reported macrocytic changes in peripheral erythrocytes following treatment with erythropoietin. In this study, the decrease in mean corpuscular volume could be a reflection of lowered titers of erythropoietin. In addition, injections of erythropoietin into estrogenized rats for a prolonged period of time, prevented the changes seen in animals receiving estradiol alone.

The observed increases in iron-laden hyalin droplets within the renal tubular cells as well as the tubular vacuolization noted in the estradiol-treated group are manifestations of kidney damage. It appears that some of the features of the anemia secondary to renal disease are also characteristic of that which results from estradiol treatment, namely, depressed marrow activity, possible prolonged reticulocyte maturation time, and preferential storage of iron in tissues. Since erythropoietin has been shown to be elaborated chiefly, though not exclusively, by the kidney,[35–39] the kidney damage noted in the estradiol-treated animals of this study could result in depressed erythropoietin production which, as previously stated, may account for the anemia.

Mirand and Gordon[15] have recently demonstrated that the erythropoiesis-inhibiting effects of estrogen are evident in nephrectomized as well as in intact mice. Furthermore, they have presented evidence suggesting that estrogens inhibit erythropoiesis by suppressing the production of an extrarenal precursor of erythropoietin from the liver that requires activation by a kidney mechanism for elaboration of functional circulating erythropoietin. The observed liver changes seen in our study seem to be in accord with their proposal that estrogens act by inhibiting the production of a liver precursor substance.

Recently, the clinical effectiveness of testosterone in various refractory anemias,[26,42,43] which may possibly be mediated by stimulating erythropoietin production, has created further interest in the mechanism of action of this steroid. Furthermore, the work of Vollmer *et al.*[3,44] has demonstrated that long-term administration of testosterone exerts an erythropoietic-stimulating effect in rodents that is especially striking in the castrated or hypophysectomized animal. Pursuing the problem further, Fried *et al.*[45,46] presented evidence that combinations of cobalt and testosterone act synergistically to increase erythropoietin levels in the plasma of normal mice. Similarly, our data suggest that extended treatment with massive doses of testosterone accelerates the rate of red cell maturation to functionally effective erythrocytes. Moreover, the observed increase in mean corpuscular volume may be indicative of increased erythropoietic activity. In addition, the observed hypercellularity of the bone marrow with increased marrow nucleated cell numbers is another sign of enhanced erythropoiesis.

The fact that peripheral blood reticulocytes are elevated and of the young variety, concomitant with increased uptake of iron at 10 days after testosterone treatment, indicates an increase in turnover. The importance of turnover rate in erythropoiesis has been previously considered.[27,29,31,47,48] Our findings of a slight decrease in iron deposition in the tissues under the influence of testosterone may be the result of an accelerated use of iron in hemoglobin synthesis. Therefore, along with the observed marrow hypercellularity, these findings are suggestive of increased erythropoietin production.

Analysis of the 30-day iron uptake levels indicate normal percentages and can possibly be explained on the basis of the studies by Kochakian[49] and Brande[50] in that androgens apparently do not continue to elicit their stimulatory effects indefinitely.

The general anabolic effects must also be considered as a possibility in increasing erythropoietin production.[43] Testosterone may act by elevating the metabolic rate, thus increasing the demand for oxygen beyond the immediate supply of oxygen to tissues. Recently, Nathan and Gardner[51] have demonstrated that androgen-treated female rats exhibited an accelerated rate of erythropoiesis producing a gain in total red cell volume out of proportion to the accretion of lean tissue. Therefore, in the female rat, this erythropoietic response appears to be independent of the effects of testosterone on body composition.

Of particular interest is the work of Mirand and Gordon[15] which presents evidence that plasma from testosterone-treated animals augmented the iron uptake response to hypoxia in intact mice but did not produce this effect in bilaterally nephrectomized mice. Therefore, it appears that the stimulatory action of testosterone requires the presence of the kidneys. Our studies offer collateral evidence of kidney involvement. In accord with the findings of Selye[52] a significant increase in kidney size was noted in this experiment. Although evidence for the production of erythropoietin by renal juxtaglomerular cells is indirect, in this investigation an increase in renal juxtaglomerular cell granularity was observed at 10 days following testosterone administration. The lack of similar increases at 30 days appears to agree with observations indicative of a maximal early stimulatory erythropoietic effect following testosterone administration.

Summary and Conclusions

Prolonged administration of massive doses of estradiol in young adult female rats results in a severe anemia. In estradiol-treated rats it appears that the anemia is not due to cellular destruction but attributable to depressed erythropoietin production as well as to impaired iron utilization. Histologic examination of the kidneys from such animals shows increases in iron-laden droplets within the tubular cells, indicating degenerative changes of this organ. That depressed erythropoietin production may be the case is further substantiated by our findings that injections of sheep plasma erythropoietin administered over a prolonged period prevent the changes seen in rats receiving estradiol alone. The observed liver changes appear to be in accord with the proposal by Mirand and Gordon[15] that estrogens act by inhibiting the production of liver precursor substance.

Our studies utilizing large doses of testosterone indicate that the erythroid stimulatory effects of this hormone may be the result of an increase in erythropoietin production. In contrast to the findings in estrogen-treated rats, the paucity of iron in tissues under the influence of testosterone seems to indicate an accelerated use of iron for hemoglobin synthesis. Consistent with signs of enhanced erythropoiesis is the noted increase in kidney weight and the observed increase in renal juxtaglomerular cell granulation at 10 days following testosterone administration. Thus, it appears that the erythroid stimulatory action is mediated via the renal tissue.

References

1. Gordon, A. S. 1959. Hemopoietine. Physiol. Rev. **39:** 1.
2. Steinglass, P., A. S. Gordon & H. A. Charipper. 1941. Effect of castration and sex hormones on blood of the rat. Proc. Soc. Exp. Biol. Med. **48:** 169.
3. Vollmer, E. P. & A. S. Gordon. 1941. Effect of sex and gonadotropic hormones upon the blood picture of the rat. Endocrinology. **29:** 828.
4. Van Dyke, D. C., A. N. Contopoulos, B. S. Williams, M. S. Simpson, J. H. Lawrence & H. M. Evans. 1954. Hormonal factors influencing erythropoiesis. Acta Haemat. **11:** 203.
5. Dukes, P. P. & E. Goldwasser. 1961. Inhibition of erythropoiesis by estrogens. Endocrinology **60:** 21.
6. Medici, P. T., C. Haber & S. J. Piliero. 1964. Effects of estradiol and testosterone on erythropoiesis. Am. Zool. **4:** 343.
7. Finkelstein, G., A. S. Gordon & H. A. Charipper. 1944. The effect of sex hormones on the anemia induced by hemorrhage in the rat. Endocrinology **35:** 267.

8. CRAFTS, R. C. 1954. The value of a high protein diet in the prevention of anemia in hypophysectomized adult female rats by means of thyroxine and androgen therapy. Endocrinology **54**: 542.
9. SAHA, J. 1962. The effect of testosterone propionate on haemopoiesis in experimental haemolytic anemia in rats. Ann. Biochem. Exp. Med. **22**: 249.
10. ASCHKENASY, A. Effets de la thyroxine, de la cortisone et des androgènes sur la réticulocytose sanguine et sur l'incorporation du Fe-59 dans les érythrocytes et dans certains organes chez des rats carences en protéines. Compt. Rend. Soc. Biol. **157**: 91.
11. FRIED, W., R. DE GOWIN & C. W. GURNEY. 1964. Erythropoietic effect of testosterone in the polycythemic mouse. Proc. Soc. Exp. Biol. Med. **117**: 839.
12. NAETS, J. P. & M. WITTEK. 1964. Etude de mécanisme d'action des androgènes sur l'érythropoïèse. Compt. Rend. Acad. Sci. **259**: 3371.
13. GURNEY, C. W. & W. FRIED. 1965. Further studies on the erythropoietic effect of androgens. J. Lab. Clin. Med. **65**: 775.
14. MIRAND, E. A., A. H. WEINTRAUB, A. S. GORDON, T. C. PRENTICE & J. T. GRACE, JR. 1965. Erythropoietic activity of untreated and deproteinized normal human plasma. Proc. Soc. Exp. Biol. Med. **118**: 823.
15. MIRAND, E. A. & A. S. GORDON. 1966. Mechanism of estrogen action in erythropoiesis. Endocrinology **78**: 325.
16. BRECHER, G. 1949. New methylene blue as a reticulocyte stain. Am. J. Clin. Pathol. **19**: 895.
17. CASELLA, R. L. & S. J. PILIERO. 1964. A simple, rapid microicterus test for estimating the degree of jaundice. Conn. Med. **28**: 103.
18. DUCCI, H. & C. J. WATSON. 1945. The quantitative determination of serum bilirubin with special reference to the prompt-reacting and the chloroform-soluble types. J. Lab. Clin. Med. **30**: 293.
19. GORDON, A. S., J. WINKERT, B. DORNFEST & C. SIEGEL. 1959. Studies on the actions and properties of the circulating erythropoietic stimulating factor. Ann. N. Y. Acad. Sci. **77**: 650.
20. RALPH, P. H. 1941. The histochemical demonstration of hemoglobin in blood cells and tissue smears. Stain Technol. **16**: 105.
21. LILLIE, R. 1954. Histopathologic technic and practical histochemistry. : 243–244, Blakiston Co. New York.
22. LO BUE, J., B. DORNFEST, A. S. GORDON, J. HURST & H. QUASTLER. 1963. Distribution in rat femurs determined by cell enumeration and iron-59 labeling. Proc. Soc. Exp. Biol. Med. **112**: 1058.
23. GORDON, A. S. & H. A. CHARIPPER. 1947. The endocrine system and hemopoiesis. Ann. N. Y. Acad. Sci. **48**: 615.
24. CRAFTS, R. C. 1941. The effects of endocrines on the formed elements of the blood. Endocrinology **29**: 606.
25. MCCULLOUGH, E. & R. JONES. 1942. Effect of androgens on the blood count of man. J. Clin. Endocr. **2**: 243.
26. GARDNER, F. & J. PRINGLE. 1961. Androgens and erythropoiesis. Arch. Int. Med. **107**: 846.
27. KENNEDY, J. 1962. Stimulation of erythropoiesis by androgenic hormones. Ann. Int. Med. **57**: 917.
28. SHAHIDI, N. 1963. Morphologic and biochemical characteristics of erythrocytes in testosterone induced remission in patients with acquired and constitutional aplastic anemia. J. Lab. Clin. Med. **62**: 294.
29. SILVER, R., D. JENKENS & R. ENGLE. 1964. Use of testosterone and busulfan in the treatment of myelofibrosis with myeloid metaplasia. Blood **23**: 341.
30. MEINEKE, H. A. & R. C. CRAFTS. 1957. Further observations on the effect of cortisone and thyroxine on the blood picture of hypophysectomized rats. Blood **12**: 11.
31. VAN DYKE, D. C., H. ANGER & M. POLLYCOVE. 1964. The effect of erythropoietic stimulation of marrow distribution in man, rabbit and rat as shown by iron-59 and iron-52. Blood **24**: 356.
32. CRAFTS, R. C. 1948. The effects of estrogens on the bone marrow of the adult female dog. Blood **3**: 276.
33. FRUHMAN, G. J. & S. FISHER. 1962. The short-term effects of a single dose of erythropoietin upon reticulocytes in starved rats. Experientia. **18**: 1.
34. GORDON, A. S., J. LO BUE, B. DORNFEST & G. COOPER. 1962. Reticulocyte and leukocyte release from isolated perfused rat legs and femurs. *In* Erythropoiesis. L. O. Jacobson & M. Doyle, eds. : 321. Grune & Stratton. N. Y.

35. JACOBSON, L. O., E. GOLDWASSER, W. FRIED & L. PLZAK. 1957. Rose of kidney in erythropoiesis. Nature **179:** 633.
36. ERSLEV, A. J. 1962. Erythropoietin in vitro. *In* Erythropoiesis. L. O. Jacobson & M. Doyle, eds. : 275. Grune & Stratton. N. Y.
37. KORST, D. R., E. P. FRENKEL, L. COUSINEAU & E. E. MUIRHEAD. 1962. Erythropoietin studies in human renal abnormalities: Correlative renal explant attempts in rat and dog. *In* Erythropoiesis. L. O. Jacobson & M. Doyle, eds. : 374. Grune & Stratton. N. Y.
38. NAETS, J. P. & A. HEUSE. 1962. Measurement of erythropoietic stimulating factor in anemic patients with or without renal disease. J. Lab. Clin. Med. **60:** 365.
39. TAKAKU, P., K. HIROSHIMA & K. NAKAO. 1962. Studies on the mechanism of erythropoietin production. I. Effect of unilateral constriction of the renal artery. J. Lab. Clin. Med. **59:** 815.
40. WINKERT, J., A. S. GORDON, P. T. MEDICI, S. J. PILIERO, A. L. LUHBY & M. TANNENBAUM. 1958. Erythropoietic stimulatory activity of urine from anemic human subjects. Proc. Soc. Biol. Med. **97:** 191.
41. STOHLMAN, F. 1961. Humoral regulation of erythropoiesis. IV. Mechanism of action of erythropoietin in the irradiated animal. Proc. Soc. Exptl. Biol. Med. **107:** 751.
42. KENNEDY, B. J. & A. S. GILBERTSON. 1957. Increased erythropoiesis induced by androgenic hormone therapy. New Eng. J. Med. **256:** 719.
43. SHAHIDI, N. T. & L. K. DIAMOND. 1961. Testosterone induced remission in aplastic anemia of both acquired and congenital types: Further observations in twenty-four cases. New Eng. J. Med. **264:** 953.
44. VOLLMER, E. P., A. S. GORDON & H. A. CHARIPPER. 1942. Effect of hormones on erythropoiesis in the hypophysectomized rat. Endocrinology **31:** 619.
45. FRIED, W. & C. W. GURNEY. 1965. Erythropoietic effect of plasma from mice receiving testosterone. Nature **206:** 1160.
46. JANDA, W. E., W. FRIED & C. W. GURNEY. 1965. Combined effect of cobalt and testosterone on erythropoiesis. Proc. Soc. Exp. Biol. Med. **120:** 443.
47. CRAFTS, R. C. & H. A. MEINEKE. 1957. Influence of the pituitary on hemopoiesis. Am. J. Clin. Nut. **5:** 542.
48. ERSLEV, A. J. & J. HUGHES. 1960. The influence of environment on iron incorporation and mitotic division in a suspension of normal bone marrow. Brit. J. Haem. **6:** 414.
49. KOCHAKIAN, C. D. & J. A. WEBSTER. 1958. Effect of testosterone propionate on the appetite, body weight and composition of the normal rat. Endocrinology **63:** 737.
50. BRANDE, P. F. 1960. The Influence of Androgen on Protein Metabolism of Normal and Tumor-Bearing Rats. Thesis submitted to the Graduate School of Rutgers, The State University, New Brunswick, N. J.
51. NATHAN, D. G. & F. H. GARDNER. 1965. Effect of large doses of androgen on rodent erythropoiesis and body composition. Blood **26:** 411.
52. SELYE, H. 1939. The effect of testosterone on the kidney. J. Urol. **42:** 637.

THE ERYTHROPOIETIC-STIMULATING EFFECTS OF ANDROGENS

W. Fried and C. W. Gurney

Veterans Administration West Side Hospital and the Department of Medicine, University of Chicago, Chicago, Ill.

Introduction

Several authors have reported that testosterone is capable of stimulating erythropoiesis in some patients with various types of anemias.[1–3] More knowledge of the mechanism by which testosterone affects erythropoiesis might improve our understanding of the pathogenesis of these anemias and thereby lead to a more rational basis for their therapy with androgens. Blacher first suggested that the sex hormones influence erythropoiesis after he described differences in the red blood counts of male and female fowl.[4] Shortly thereafter Juhn and Domm showed that these differences were dependent on the presence of intact gonads in the male.[5] Vollmer *et al.*[6,7] showed that testosterone propionate stimulated erythropoiesis in female rats, in castrated male rats and in hypophysectomized rats.

In this paper we shall report the results of studies on the mechanism by which androgens and other anabolic steroids stimulate erythropoiesis in mice. We will also discuss the effect of testosterone on mice with anemia resulting from mutation at the W locus. Finally we shall speculate on the relationship between these findings and the way that testosterone stimulates erythropoiesis in anemic patients.

The Effect of Testosterone on Male and Female CBA & DBA Polycythemic Mice

Mice made polycythemic by transfusion are sensitive indicators of erythropoietic-stimulating substances.[8] We therefore measured the ability of testosterone to stimulate erythropoiesis in polycythemic mice. Male and female CBA and DBA mice were used. The mice were made plethoric by transfusion with 0.5 cc of packed RBC's on each of two consecutive days. On the same two days, they were injected s.c. with either 2.5 mg of testosterone in 0.1 cc of sesame oil, or with 0.1 cc of sesame oil. ^{59}Fe was administered i.v. four days after the second injection, and the 72-hour incorporation into the red blood cells was determined and expressed as a percentage of the injected dose of iron. The results are shown in FIGURE 1.

While testosterone caused the iron incorporation into RBC's of female DBA mice to rise from about 0.5% to over 15%, male DBA mice were not significantly stimulated by the same dose. The response of female CBA mice to testosterone was similar to that of female DBA mice. Testosterone, however, increased the rate of iron incorporation into RBC's of CBA male mice from 1.4% to only 3.6%.

In both species tested here, testosterone greatly stimulated erythropoiesis in female mice, but stimulated that of males to a lesser degree if at all. It is also noteworthy that ^{59}Fe incorporation of male CBA mice was less completely inhibited by plethora than was that of female CBA mice.

Since female polycythemic mice are sensitive to the erythropoietic effects of androgens, we used them to compare the ability of testosterone and that of a primarily anabolic steroid to stimulate erythropoiesis.

Comparison of the Effect of Testosterone and of Nandralone Phenylpropionate on Erythropoiesis

Testosterone propionate or nandralone phenylpropionate (2.5 mg/0.1 cc

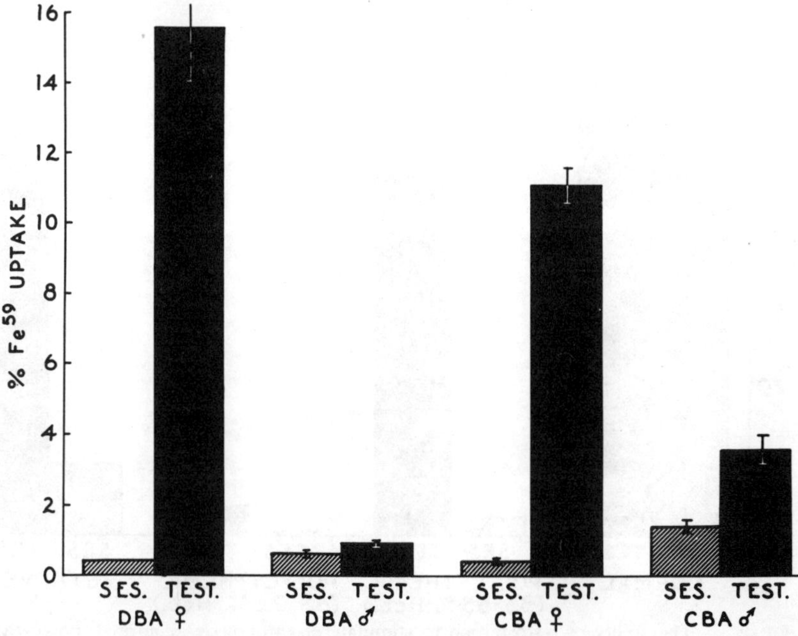

FIGURE 1. The effect of testosterone on male and female CBA & DBA polycythemic mice.

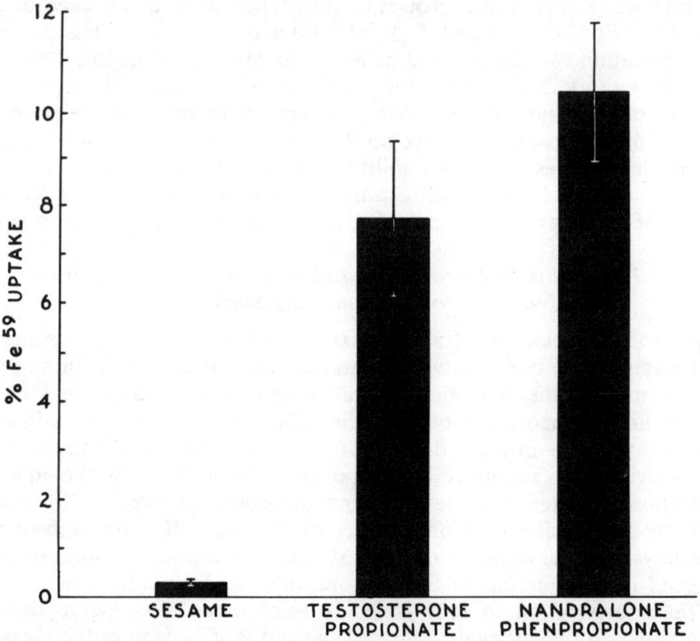

FIGURE 2. Comparison of the effect of testosterone and of nandralone phenylpropionate on erythropoiesis.

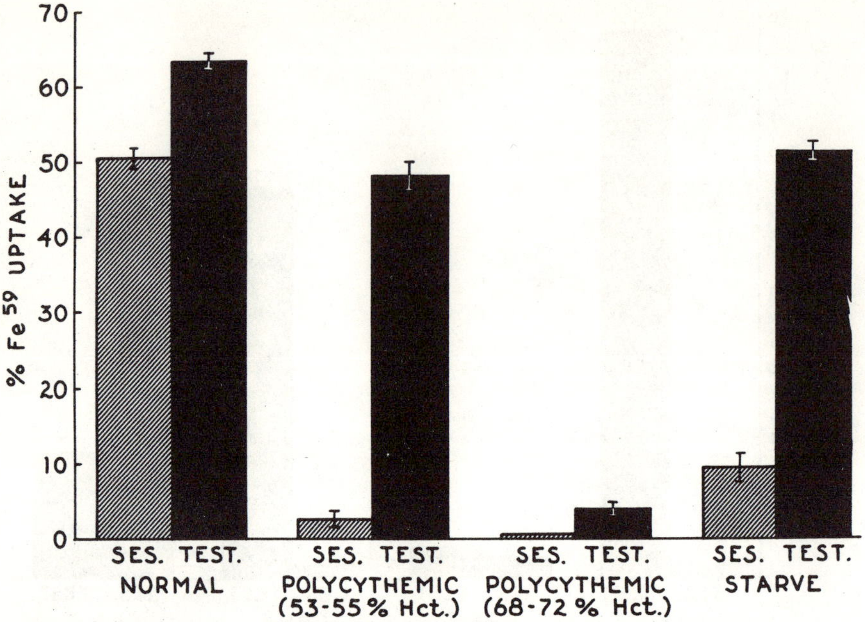

FIGURE 3. The ability of testosterone to stimulate erythropoiesis in normal, polycythemic and starved mice.

sesame oil) was injected into groups of polycythemic mice on each of two consecutive days. Four days later 0.5 μc of ^{59}Fe was injected i.v. The percentage of iron incorporation was determined as in the previous experiment. The results are recorded in FIGURE 2. Controls that received only sesame oil incorporated less than 0.5% of the injected iron. Mice injected with testosterone propionate or nandralone phenylpropionate took up 7.6 and 10.5%, respectively. This experiment indicates that testosterone's ability to stimulate erythropoiesis is not a function of its androgenic properties. Studies are currently in progress to determine the ability of other primarily anabolic steroids to stimulate erythropoiesis.

The Ability of Testosterone to Stimulate Erythropoiesis in Normal, Polycythemic and Starved Mice

Testosterone propionate (2.5 mg in 0.1 cc of sesame oil) or sesame oil was given on each of two consecutive days to normal, polycythemic, or starved mice. Ninety-six hr after the last injection, all mice received 0.5 μc of ^{59}Fe and the 72-hour radioiron incorporation into the RBC's was determined and expressed as a percentage of the injected dose. FIGURE 3 illustrates the results. Normal mice which received only sesame oil incorporated about 50% of the injected iron whereas those injected with testosterone incorporated over 62%. Mice made plethoric by transfusion with only 0.2 cc of packed RBC's on each of two consecutive days had hematocrits of 53–55% and incorporated only about 2% of the injected iron. Injection of testosterone into mildly plethoric mice increased their ^{59}Fe incorporation to over 45%. In mice made more polycythemic (Hct 68–72%) by two injections of 0.8 cc of packed RBC's, iron uptake was reduced to 0.2%. Testosterone increased this to only 3.5%. Mice, starved by removing all food for four days prior to receiving iron, incorporated only 9% of the injected iron. Injection of testosterone increased this to over 50%.

This experiment indicates that testosterone can stimulate erythropoiesis, as measured by ^{59}Fe incorporation in normal mice. When erythropoiesis is reduced, either by mild plethora or by starvation, the effect of testosterone becomes more apparent. Testosterone stimulates erythropoiesis in very plethoric mice to a lesser degree than it does in less plethoric mice. This contrasts with the effect of erythropoietin which stimulates erythropoiesis in polycythemic mice independently of their degree of plethora.[9] This difference in the way that testosterone and erythropoietin stimulate erythropoiesis in polycythemic mice can best be explained by postulating that testosterone's effect is mediated by erythropoietin. Accordingly, as the degree of plethora increases, endogenous erythropoietin production decreases and testosterone's ability to stimulate erythropoiesis decreases. Testosterone may stimulate erythropoiesis either by increasing the production of erythropoietin or by increasing the erythropoietic response to erythropoietin. The first of these possibilities was tested in the next experiment.

The Effect of Testosterone on ^{59}Fe Incorporation and on ESF Titers

Female CBA mice were made polycythemic by transfusion as in the previous experiments. All mice received ^{59}Fe four days after the second transfusion of packed RBC's. At various times prior to receiving ^{59}Fe, groups containing eight mice each were injected s.c. with 5 mg of testosterone propionate. The 72-hour ^{59}Fe incorporations of these groups of mice was determined and recorded in the solid line of FIGURE 4.

Normal CBA female mice were divided into groups containing 20 mice each. All received 5.0 g of testosterone on day zero. At various times afterward, as shown in the abscissa of FIGURE 4, mice were exsanguinated and the plasma was collected and assayed for erythropoietic stimulating factor (ESF). ESF titers were determined on 0.5 cc of plasma, using the polycythemic mouse assay of DeGowin.[10] The ESF titers are plotted on the dotted line in FIGURE 4 as the percentage ^{59}Fe incorporation of the assay mice.

^{59}Fe incorporation was greatest five days after receiving testosterone. On the

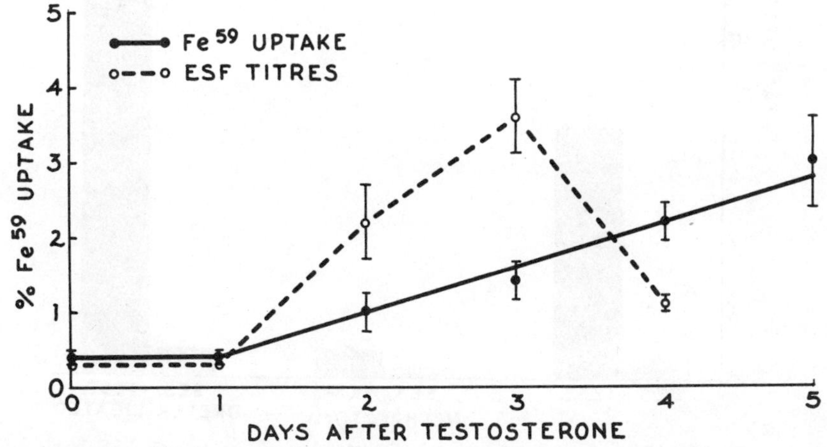

FIGURE 4. The effect of testosterone on ^{59}Fe incorporation and on ESF titers.

other hand, others have shown that iron uptake was maximal only two days after receiving erythropoietin.[11] The plasma ESF levels were highest three days after testosterone injection.

The data support one of the conclusions drawn from the previous results, i.e., that testosterone increases erythropoietin production. Since plasma ESF titers were highest 48 hr prior to the largest ^{59}Fe uptakes, it is likely that the increase in iron uptake was the result of the increase in plasma ESF titers.

Erythropoietin titers of mice and rats produced in response to hypoxia, anemia and cobalt have been shown to be dependent on the presence of the kidneys.[12,13] The following experiment was performed to determine the role of the kidneys in producing the elevated ESF titers observed following injection with testosterone.

The Effect of Nephrectomy and of Ureter Ligation on Plasma ESF Levels after Testosterone

This experiment investigates the effect of nephrectomy and of ureter ligation on ESF levels after testosterone. Mice were given 2.5 mg of testosterone propionate on each of two consecutive days. Forty hr after the last injection, bilateral nephrectomies were performed on some, bilateral ureter ligations on others, and still others were unoperated. Eight hr postoperatively, or 48 hr after the last injection of testosterone, mice were exsanguinated and plasma was collected and assayed for ESF activity. FIGURE 5 shows the results. Plasma of unoperated mice treated with testosterone resulted in over 7% iron incorporation into assay mice whereas plasma of control mice resulted in less than 0.5%. Eight hr after bilateral

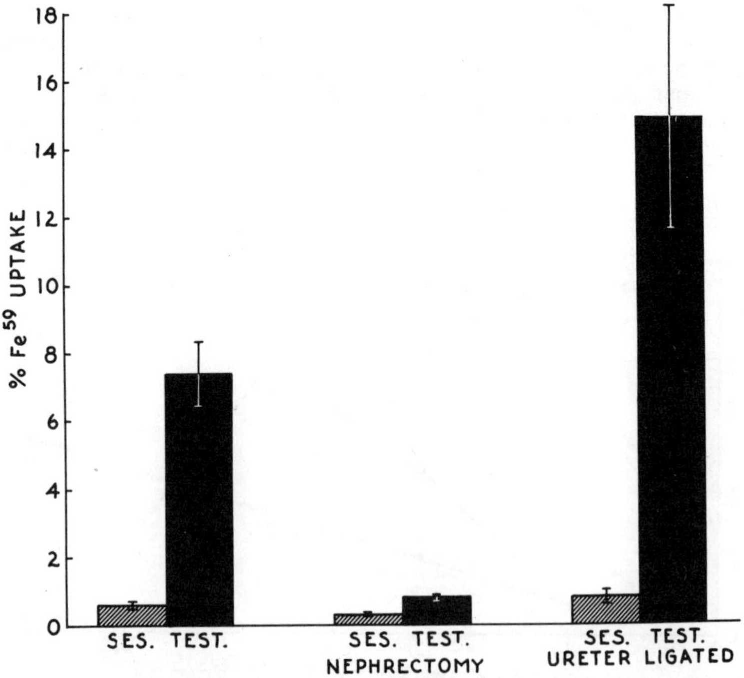

FIGURE 5. The effect of nephrectomy and of ureter ligation on plasma ESF levels, after testosterone.

nephrectomy no ESF activity was detectable. Mice injected with testosterone and whose ureters were ligated for eight hr had ESF titers over two times greater than those of unoperated, testosterone-treated mice. The increase in plasma ESF after testosterone, like that after hypoxia, is dependent on the kidneys. The increase in plasma ESF observed after ureter ligation is even greater than that in unoperated mice. Mitus reported that erythrocytosis occurs in some mice following ureter ligation. They suggested that increased renal medullary pressure stimulates erythropoiesis.[14] Such a mechanism may also account for our findings. However, it is also possible that the decreased rate of ESF excretion in an animal whose ureters have been ligated may result in higher plasma titers.

The Effect of Anti-Erythropoietin Plasma on ESF Activity of Plasma from Testosterone-Treated Mice

The above experiments suggest that the erythropoietic effect of testosterone is partially or wholly mediated by a plasma ESF which is dependent on the kidney for its production. We next investigated whether or not this ESF is immunologically related to an erythropoietin produced in response to hypoxia. Plasma was obtained from mice injected with 2.5 mg of testosterone propionate two and three days prior to harvest. Six cc of this plasma (test-plasma) was then incubated with either 0.6 cc of plasma containing antierythropoietin activity (anti-E*) or 0.6 cc of plasma from a normal rabbit (NRP). After one hour of incubation, the mixtures were placed overnight in the refrigerator at 4° C after which the precipitate was removed. One cc of the supernatant was then assayed for erythropoietin activity. To test the potency of the anti-E, 0.7 units of erythropoietin was added to 7 cc of NRP.

One cc of the respective mixture prepared as described above was then assayed. The results are shown in FIGURE 6. The Anti-E completely abolished the ESF activity in the plasma of testosterone-treated mice, suggesting that this ESF activity results from an erythropoietin which is identical to that mediating the erythropoietic response to hypoxia. We may therefore conclude that testosterone, at least partially, increases erythropoiesis by stimulating the kidneys to produce more erythropoietin. The following experiment was performed to determine whether or not testosterone stimulates erythropoietin production by potentiating the effect of hypoxia, or whether it can act independent of the degree of hypoxia.

The Effect of Hypoxia and of Polycythemia on the ESF Levels after Testosterone

All mice received 2.5 mg of testosterone on each of two consecutive days. Polycythemic mice were transfused with 0.5 cc of packed RBC's on the same two days. Hypoxic mice were exposed to 0.5 atm for six hr beginning 42 hr after the final injection of testosterone. All mice were exsanguinated and their plasma collected 48 hr after the last injection of testosterone. The plasma was then assayed for erythropoietin activity. The results are illustrated in FIGURE 7.

Plasma from normal mice injected with testosterone caused an iron uptake of over 3.5% in assay mice whereas that of polycythemic mice injected with testosterone resulted in less than 0.5% uptake. Plasma from mice exposed to six hr of hypoxia resulted in about 2.5% incorporation and plasma from mice injected with testosterone prior to being made hypoxic resulted in an uptake which

* Antierythropoietin plasma was prepared and provided by Dr. Robert D. Lange according to a technique which has been described elsewhere.[15]

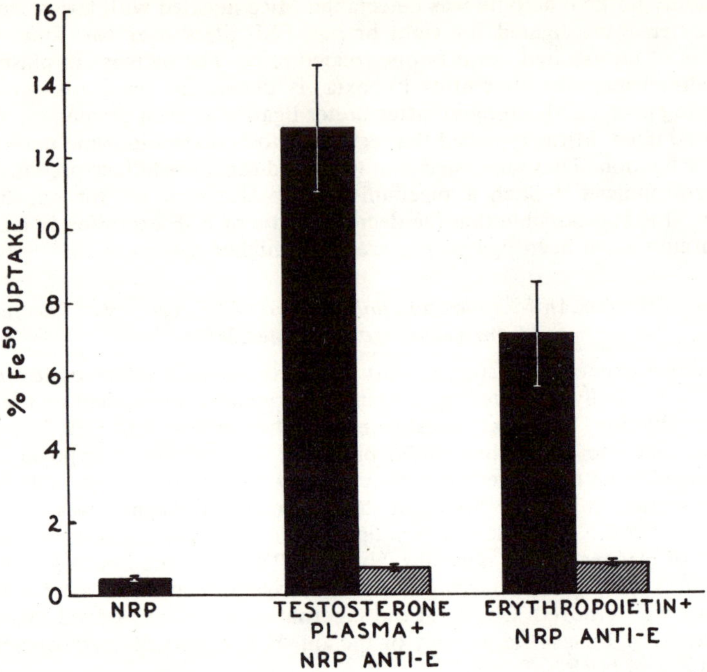

FIGURE 6. The effect of antierythropoietin plasma on ESF activity of plasma from testosterone-treated mice. Black bars represent plasmas without addition of Anti-E NRP. Striped bars represent plasmas after incubation + Anti-E NRP.

was over five times this high. This experiment suggests that testosterone potentiates the effect of hypoxia on erythropoietin production so that for any given level of hypoxia a greater than expected amount of erythropoietin is produced. Some of the morphologic and metabolic changes induced by testosterone in the kidneys of female and castrated male rodents are well documented.[16–18] We suggest the possibility that testosterone stimulates erythropoiesis by so altering the kidney that it produces more erythropoietin than usual in response to any given stimulus.

Although these experiments clarify the mechanism by which testosterone stimulates erythropoiesis in lower mammals, it is by no means clear to what extent such a mechansm acts in humans. Since patients with anemias responsive to testosterone often have elevated plasma erythropoietin levels, prior to androgen therapy it has been considered unlikely that testosterone could increase erythropoiesis by further increasing the erythropoietin titers.

Several varieties of hereditary anemias occur in mice. One such has been described in mice bearing the genotype WW_v. Plasma of such mice contains high titers of erythropoietin. When WW_v mice are made plethoric by transfusion, they do not respond to erythropoietin unless it is given in repeated large doses.[19] We performed the following experiments to determine whether and how testosterone affects the anemia of WW_v mice.

The Effect of Testosterone and of Hypoxia on the Hematocrits of WW_v Mice

Adult WW_v mice were divided into three groups containing 10 mice each. Hematocrits were measured by the capillary tube method using blood from the retroorbital venous sinus. One group was then injected with 2.5 mg of testosterone every other day for two weeks and one group was made hypoxic by exposure to 0.5 atm for two weeks. The third group remained untreated. After two weeks hematocrits were repeated. The results are recorded in FIGURE 8.

There was no change in the hematocrits of untreated mice. Those of mice injected with testosterone rose from 39.5% to over 46%. The hematocrits of hypoxic mice rose from 40% to 52%. Both testosterone and hypoxia significantly reduced the degree of anemia of mice with genotype WW_v. This suggests that although the erythropoietin titers of these mice were already elevated, further elevations were necessary to overcome the refractoriness of their bone marrow. The following experiment measures the effect of hypoxia and of testosterone on the erythropoietin titers.

Effect of Hypoxia and of Testosterone on Erythropoietin Titers of WW_v Mice

WW_v mice were divided into three groups containing 12 mice each. One group received 2.5 mg of testosterone on each of two consecutive days. Their plasma was collected 48 hr later for erythropoietin assay. The second group was made hypoxic for 12 hr by exposure to 0.5 atm and their plasma was collected and assayed immediately afterwards. The third group remained untreated prior to collection of its plasma for assay. Erythropoietin assays were performed using 0.4 cc of plasma. The results are shown in FIGURE 9. Plasma from CF_1 mice produced no significant increase in the ^{59}Fe uptake of the assay mice whereas that of WW_v mice resulted in over 13% incorporation. Plasma of WW_v mice

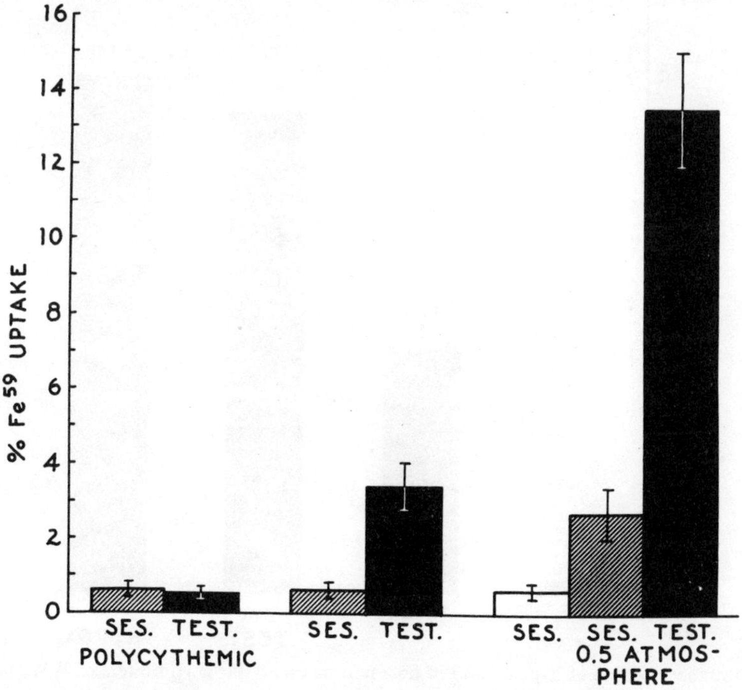

FIGURE 7. The effect of hypoxia and of polycythemia on the ESF levels after testosterone.

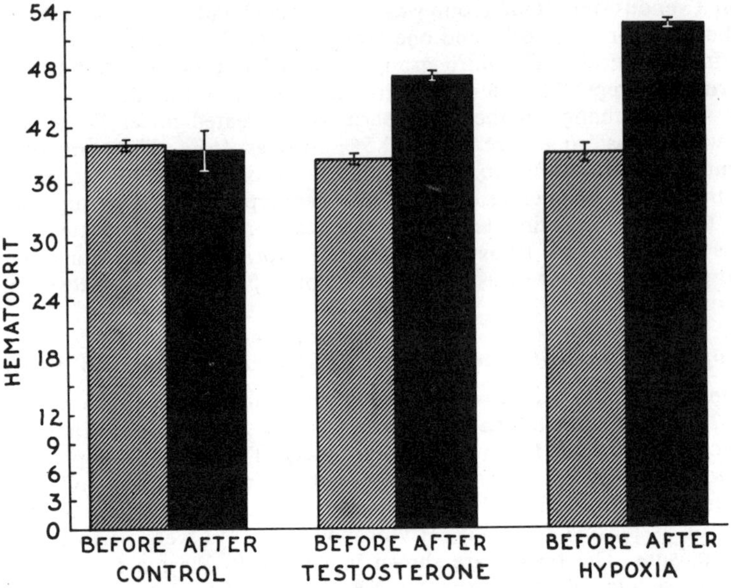

FIGURE 8. The effect of testosterone and of hypoxia on hematocrits of WW_v mice.

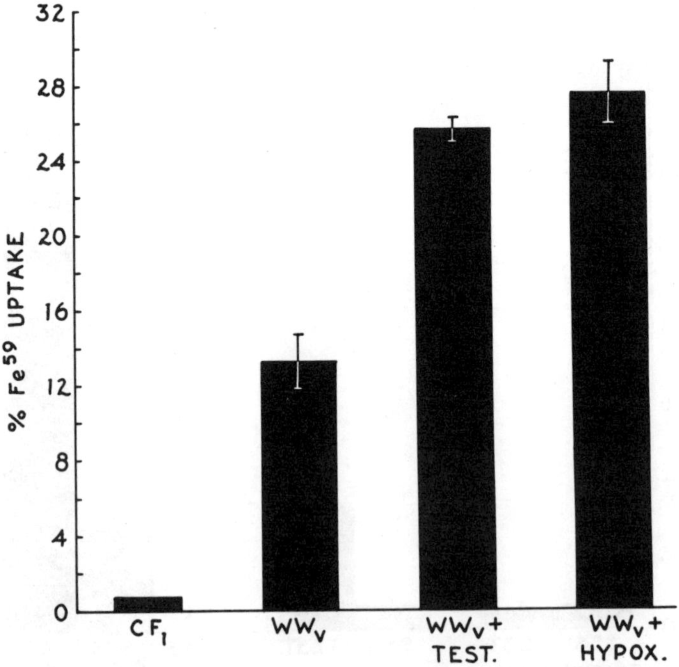

FIGURE 9. Effect of hypoxia and of testosterone on erythropoietin titers of WW_v mice.

which received testosterone increased the iron uptake to about 25% and that of hypoxic mice to almost 28%.

Since WW_v mice have been shown to be relatively refractory to erythropoietin, it is not unreasonable to presume that their rate of erythropoiesis might be increased by further elevation of the erythropoietin titers even if their plasma erythropoietin titers are elevated prior to therapy. Accordingly, both testosterone and hypoxia increase erythropoiesis of these mice and may do so by further increasing their erythropoietin levels.

It is conceivable that some testosterone-responsive anemias in humans have been caused by bone marrow damage resulting in a relative refractoriness to erythropoietin. Testosterone may then increase the erythropoietin titers to a level sufficient to elicit a response by the damaged marrow.

Summary

1) Testosterone stimulates erythropoiesis of female normal, polycythemic and starved mice. Erythropoiesis of males is affected to a much lesser degree.

2) The anabolic steroid, nandralone phenylpropionate, stimulates erythropoiesis to the same extent as does testosterone.

3) Evidence is presented supporting the concept that testosterone stimulates erythropoiesis in mice by altering the kidney so that more erythropoietin is produced for any given stimulus.

4) We suggest that some anemias in humans may result from a relative refractoriness to erythropoietin, and that testosterone may act here by increasing the erythropoietin titers to a point where the bone marrow can respond.

5) In support of this possibility, we described the response of WW_v mice to testosterone. WW_v mice are relatively refractory to erythropoietin and have high circulating titers. Testosterone increases these titers even higher and their anemia is ameliorated.

References

1. Kennedy, B. J. & A. S. Gilbertson. 1957. New Eng. J. Med. **256**: 719.
2. Gardner, F. H. & J. C. Pringle, Jr. 1961. New Eng. J. Med. **264**: 103.
3. Shahidi, U. T. & L. K. Diamond. 1961. New Eng. J. Med. **264**: 953.
4. Blacher, L. J. 1926. Trans. Lab. Exp. Biol. Moscow. **1**: 9.
5. Juhn, M. & L. V. Domm. 1930. Am. J. Physiol. **34**: 656.
6. Vollmer, E. P. & A. S. Gordon. 1941. Endocrinology **29**: 828.
7. Vollmer, E. P., A. S. Gordon & H. A. Charipper. 1942. Endocrinology **31**: 619.
8. Jacobson, L. O., E. Goldwasser & C. W. Gurney. 1960. Ciba Symposium on Haemopoiesis. : 423. London. J. E. Churchill Ltd.
9. Gurney, C. W. & W. Fried. 1965. J. Lab. Clin. Med. **65**: 775.
10. DeGowin, R. L., D. Hofstra & C. W. Gurney. 1962. Proc. Soc. Exper. Biol. Med. **110**: 48.
11. Gurney, C. W., R. L. DeGowin, D. Hofstra & J. Byron. 1962. *In* Erythropoiesis. : 151. Grune and Stratton. New York & London.
12. Jacobson, L. O., E. Goldwasser, W. Fried & L. Plzak. 1957. Trans. Assn. Amer. Phys. **70**: 305.
13. Naets, J. P. 1958. Nature **181**: 1134.
14. Mitus, W. J., P. Galbraith, M. Gollerken & K. Toyama. 1964. Blood **24**: 343.
15. Pavlovic-Kentera, V., R. D. Lange, J. P. Lewis & E. Gardner, Jr. 1965. Jugoslav. Physiol. Pharmacol. Acta. **1**: 15.
16. Selye, H. 1939. Urology **42**: 637.
17. Frieden, E. H. 1964. *In* Actions of Hormones on Molecular Processes. : 509.
18. Korenchevsky, V., M. Dennison & A. Kohn-Speyer. 1933. Biochem. J. **27**: 557.
19. Thompson, M. W., E. C. McFarland & E. S. Russel. 1963. Proc. XIth Int. Genet. Cong.

THE MECHANISM OF ACTION OF ANDROGENS ON ERYTHROPOIESIS*

J. P. Naets and M. Wittek

Laboratoire de Médecine Expérimentale et Laboratoire de Biologie Clinique de l'Hôpital Brugmann, Université Libre de Bruxelles et Fondation Médicale Reine Elisabeth, Belgique

Introduction

The beneficial effect of androgens on erythropoiesis in patients with several hematological disorders has been well established.[1–4] Experimentally it has been shown that orchiectomy reduces the erythropoietic activity, whereas androgen administration stimulates the erythropoiesis of castrated or hypophysectomized animals.[5–8] However, the mechanism of action of these substances was, till recently, unexplained. From the observation that androgens amplify the response to hypoxia as well as to exogenous erythropoietin, it was inferred that androgens act by potentiation of erythropoietin.[9] Recent investigations suggest that these steroids act mainly by enhancing the production of this hormone.[10,11]

This paper presents the results of our studies concerning the effect of androgens on erythropoiesis in rodents.

Materials and Methods

Normal or polycythemic female and normal male TO mice, weighing 20–25 g were used in randomized groups of six animals. Polycythemia was achieved either by transfusion (transfused polycythemic mice = TP mice) or by hypoxia (hypoxic polycythemic mice = HP mice). Transfusion consisted of i.p. injection of 1 ml homologous blood (hematocrit 75%) for two consecutive days, and hypoxia was produced in mice previously injected i.p. with 1 mg iron as iron dextran (Imferon) by exposure to simulated altitude (340 mm Hg for three weeks), following the methods described by Degowin *et al.*[12,13]

Erythropoiesis was measured by ^{59}Fe incorporation into red cells, or determination of red cell mass. Radioiron incorporation was determined by injecting 0.5 μc ^{59}Fe Cl_3 in a vein of the tail. In polycythemic mice, the injection was performed eight days after the second transfusion or removal from the altitude chamber (two days after the last injection of androgens). Blood samples for radioactivity counts were taken by heart puncture, 72 hr after the injection of ^{59}Fe in polycythemic mice, and after 20 hr in the case of normal mice.

Testosterone propionate§, (0.2–6 mg, dissolved in 0.2 ml peanut oil) was injected two, four and six days before ^{59}Fe administration. Experiences with two anabolic steroids, nandrolone phenylpropionate (Durabolin)† and methylandrostenolone enanthate (Primobolan)‡ followed the same schedule. In chronic experiments, animals received on the first day 1 mg iron i.p. as iron dextran, and testosterone propionate was injected two or three times a week during a period of seven to 60 days. Control groups in all experiments were injected with the vehicle only. Red cell mass was determined by the ^{51}Cr dilution method.[14] Hemoglobin concentration was measured by oxyhemoglobin method, and hematocrits by a micromethod. Iron determinations were performed by the method of Peters

* This work was performed under Contract Euratom U.L.B. – Pise no. 063–4 BIAC.

§ Kindly provided by Roussel, Paris, France.

† Durabolin – Organon, Oss. Holland.

‡ Primobolan – Shering, Berlin, Germany.

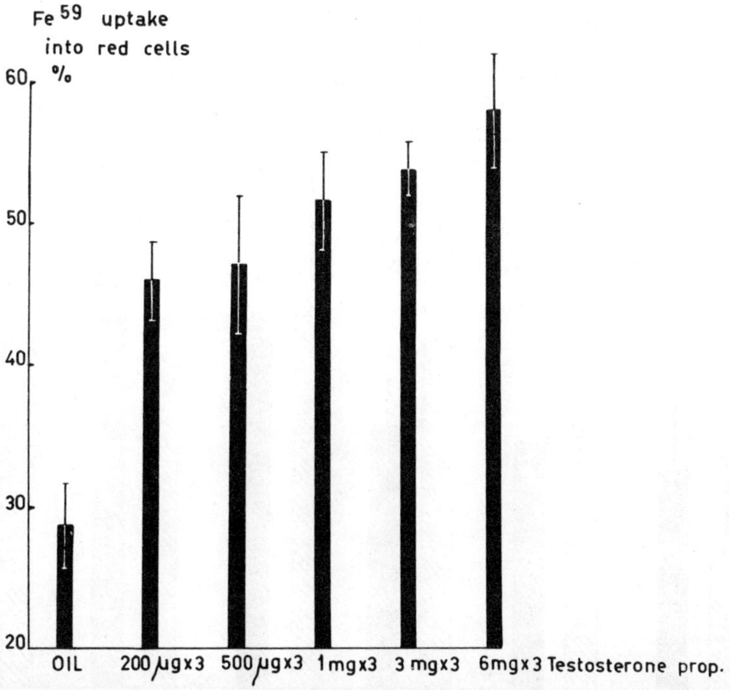

FIGURE 1. Erythropoietic response of normal TO female mice to increasing doses of testosterone propionate. Uptake measured 20 hr after ^{59}Fe injection. Vertical lines represent standard error of the mean.

et al.[15] in almost all of the experiments. Pooled plasma from groups of 18 normal or polycythemic mice was utilized. No difference in plasma iron level was observed between the testosterone-treated groups and the oil-injected controls, or between hypoxic and transfused polycythemic mice.[16]

Determinations of erythropoietin plasma level were performed on pooled plasma of TO mice (15 mice/group) or Wistar rats (180–230 g), (five rats/group) of both sexes, following the methods of Degowin *et al.*[12,13] Blood was collected two days after the last injection of testosterone by puncture of the heart in mice or the abdominal aorta in rats; the pooled plasma was stored until assay at $-10°$ and injected into TP or HP mice six days after the second transfusion or after removal from the altitude chamber. Erythropoietin plasma titer is expressed in ^{59}Fe percent incorporation into red cells of recipient polycythemic mice, or in standard B units* by reference to a dilution curve.

RESULTS

Effect of Androgens on Erythropoiesis in Mice

Effect of Short-Term Administration of Testosterone Propionate, Nandrolone Phenylpropionate and Methylandrostenolone Enanthate on the Incorporation of ^{59}Fe into Red Cells of Normal and Polycythemic Mice

Testosterone propionate, administered in increasing doses (0.2–6 mg) three times a week, enhances the incorporation of ^{59}Fe into red cells of normal female

* Provided by The Department of Biological Standards, Medical Research Council of Great Britain, London.

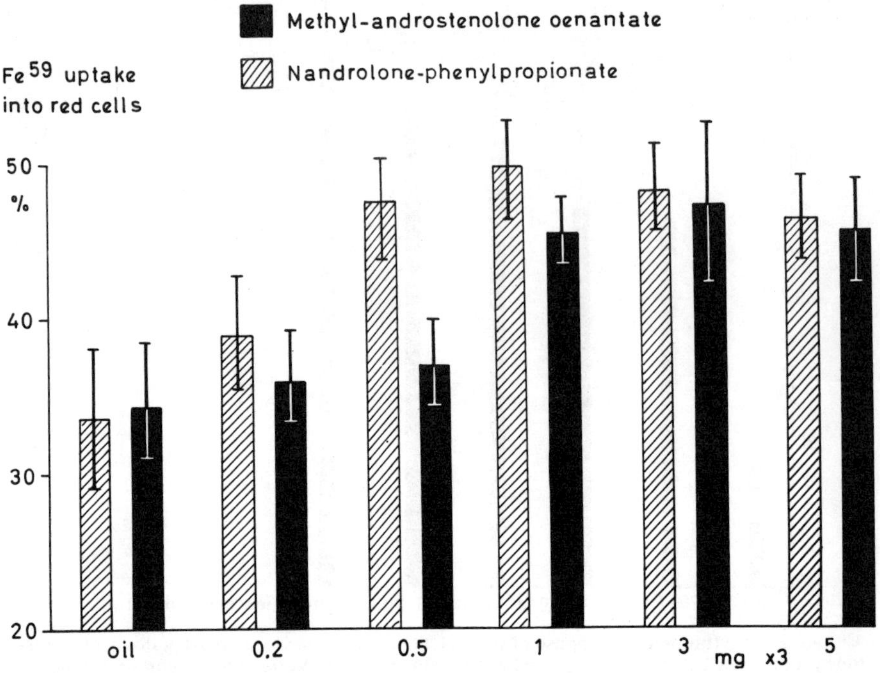

FIGURE 2. Effect of anabolic steroids (methylandrostenolone enanthate and nandrolone phenylpropionate) on erythropoiesis of normal male mice. Erythropoiesis is measured by the ^{59}Fe incorporation into red cells as a function of the administered dose. Vertical bars represent standard error of the mean.

mice from 28.5 to 58% (FIGURE 1). A similar effect is observed with both anabolic steroids, nandrolone phenylpropionate and methylandrostenolone enanthate (FIGURE 2). Within the range of utilized doses the erythropoietic response is not proportional. The stimulating effect of a single dose of testosterone propionate (6 mg), requires a delay of four days between administration and injection of radioiron to manifest itself (FIGURE 3).

In hypoxic polycythemic mice, the response to androgens (0.5–6 mg, three times a week) is proportional to the injected dose (FIGURE 4). ^{59}Fe incorporation into red cells increase with a threshold and a log-dose response, followed by a plateau averaging 7.5%. In HP as in normal mice, a single dose of testosterone propionate (6 mg) is effective only after four days. No increase of erythropoiesis is detectable 50 hr after androgen administration, which is contrary to the effect observed after this delay with erythropoietin or with cobalt. In TP mice, in contrast to the effect observed in HP mice, there is only a slight elevation of ^{59}Fe incorporation.

Effect of Chronic Administration of Testosterone Propionate on Red Cell Mass and ^{59}Fe Uptake into Red Cells

Chronic administration of testosterone propionate (3 × 3 mg a week for seven to 60 days) to male and female normal mice results in a moderate but constant rise of the red cell mass which is statistically significant and a function of the

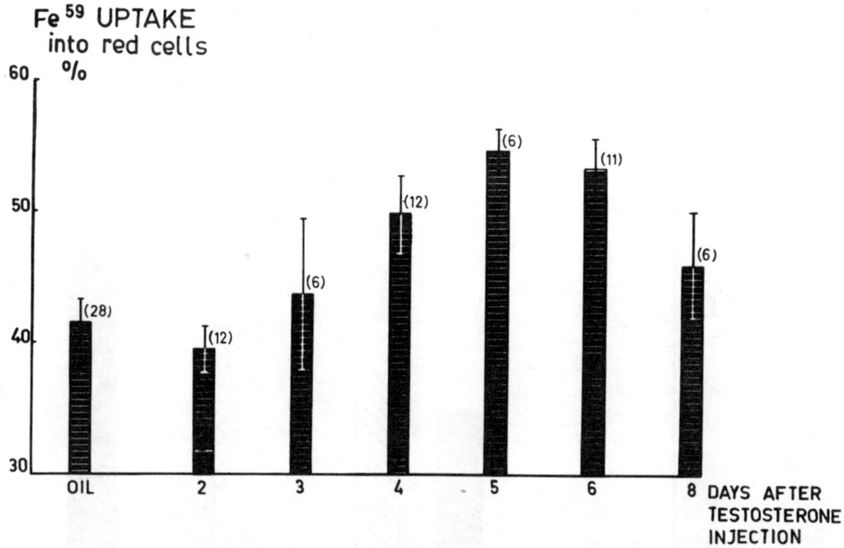

FIGURE 3. Erythropoietic response of normal mice to a single dose of testosterone propionate (6 mg) as a function of time between administration and injection of radioiron. Vertical bars indicate SE of mean. Number of mice are in parentheses.

(Reproduced by courtesy of the Amer. J. Physiol. **210:** 315, 1966).

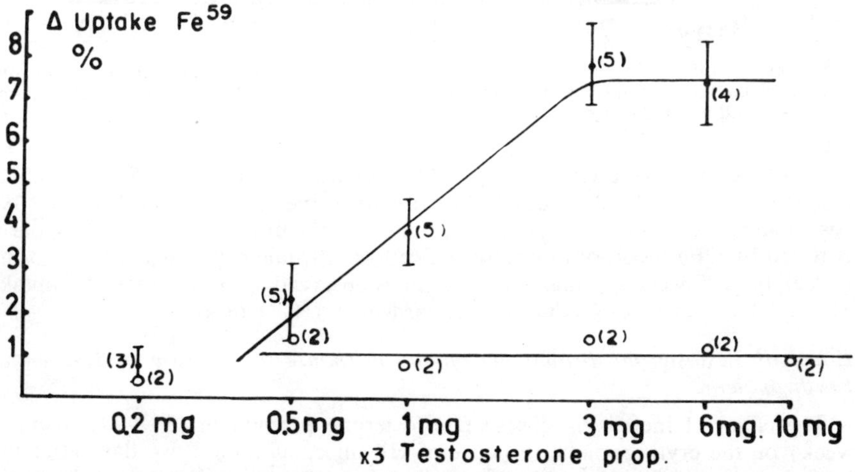

FIGURE 4. Comparative effect of increasing doses of testosterone on the erythropoiesis of hypoxic (●) and transfused (○) polycythemic mice. Number of experiments performed are in parentheses. Vertical bars indicate SE of the mean.

(Reproduced by courtesy of the Amer. J. Physiol. **210:** 315, 1966).

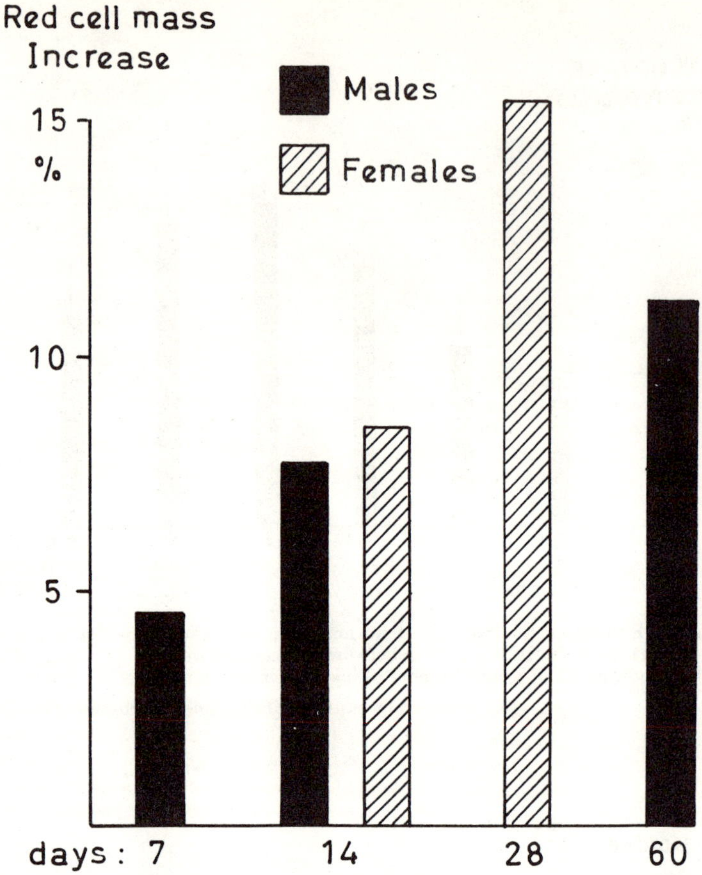

FIGURE 5. Effect of testosterone propionate on red cell mass in male and female normal mice as a function of duration of treatment. Results are expressed in percent increase of red cell mass of oil-injected controls.

duration of treatment (FIGURE 5). This increase amounts to 8.5 and 15.5%, respectively, for 14 and 28 days of treatment in the females, and 7.8 and 13% for 14 and 60 days of treatment in the males. On the other hand, if erythropoiesis is tested by ^{59}Fe incorporation into red cells in chronic experiments (3×3 mg a week for 1–5 weeks) a maximal increase is observed after one week ($\triangle$ uptake 15.8%) that decreases gradually afterwards to 1.7% (FIGURE 6).

Effect of Testosterone Propionate on the Response to Hypoxia or Exogenous Erythropoietin

The effect of increasing doses of testosterone propionate (3×0.5–6 mg a week) on the erythropoietic response of HP mice, submitted two days after the last injection to a short hypoxic stimulation (four hours at 340 mm Hg), is shown in TABLE 1. ^{59}Fe was injected i.v. two days after hypoxic stimulation, and incorporation was measured 72 hr afterwards. Incorporation into red cells in response to hypoxia is amplified by previous androgen treatment. The observed increase is

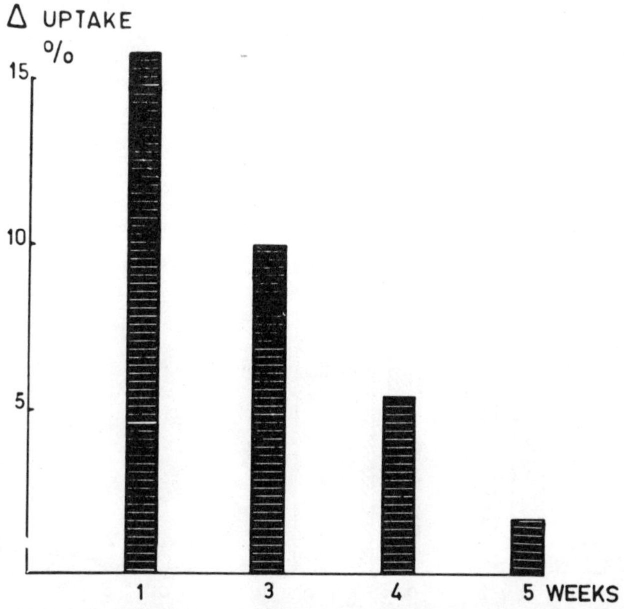

FIGURE 6. Erythropoietic response of normal mice to testosterone propionate (3 mg × 3/week) as a function of the duration of administration. △ Uptake represents the difference between ^{59}Fe incorporation of testosterone and corresponding oil-injected controls.

(Reproduced by courtesy of the Amer. J. Physiol. **210:** 315, 1966).

TABLE 1

ERYTHROPOIETIC RESPONSE OF HP MICE TO HYPOXIA OR EXOGENOUS ERYTHROPOIETIN ALONE OR AFTER TREATMENT WITH ANDROGENS

Testosterone Propionate Doses Administered mg × 3	Testosterone Propionate Alone St. B units	Hypoxia 340 mm Hg/4 hr St. B units	Erythropoietin 1.25 St. B units
0		0.47	1.25
0.5	0.08	1.11	0.75
1	0.07	2.80	3.15
3	0.23	5.40	3.17
6	0.19	4.20	>6.00

proportional to the injected dose, and exceeds the predictable additive effect of both individual stimulations. Oil-injected controls responded to hypoxia alone by increase in ^{59}Fe incorporation corresponding to the effect of 0.47 Standard B units whereas testosterone-treated animals exposed to the same hypoxic stimulation gave a response amounting to 5 Standard B units. The same amplification occurs if HP mice treated with androgens are injected with exogenous sheep erythropoietin.** The administration of 1.25 Standard B units in androgen-treated HP mice elicited an increase in ^{59}Fe incorporation higher than the response to 6 Standard B units. Amplification of the effect of exogenous erythropoietin is proportional to the doses of androgens administered.

** Prepared by Armour & Co. (Chicago), Research Division, and distributed by the Hematology Study Section of the Division of Research Grants, National Institutes of Health, Bethesda, Md.

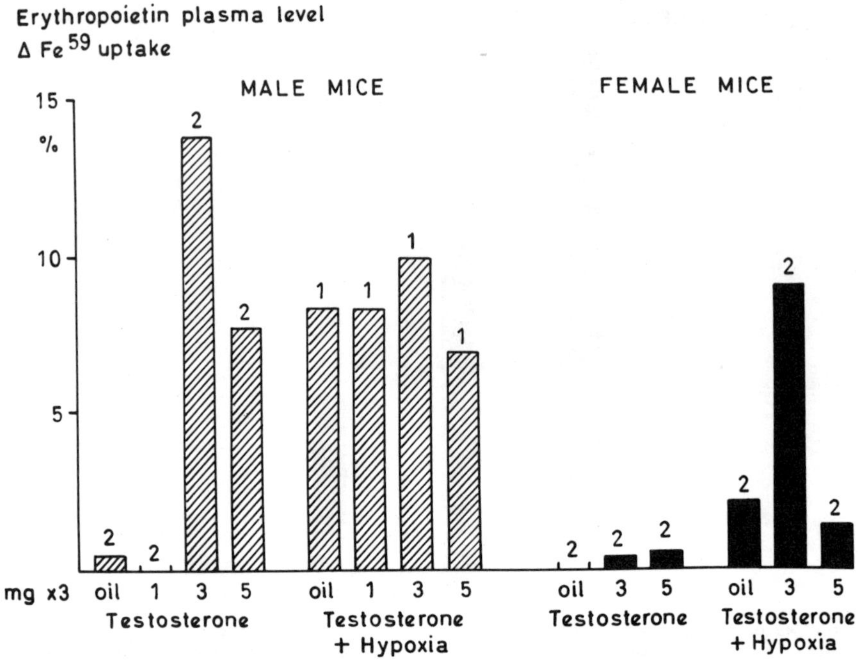

FIGURE 7. Effect of testosterone propionate alone, or combined to hypoxia (2 hr 30 min at 340 mm Hg), on erythropoietin plasma titer in male and female normal mice. Erythropoietin plasma titer is expressed as ^{59}Fe incorporation into red cells of recipient polycythemic mice. Figures on the top indicate the number of experiments.

Effects of Androgens on Erythropoietin Plasma Titer

After androgen treatment erythropoietin plasma titer increases in males but is not measurable in females. A 13.8% increase of ^{59}Fe incorporation into red cells is induced in TP mice injected with the plasma of male mice given testosterone propionate (3 × 3 mg a week) whereas no increase is elicited with the plasma of female mice under the same conditions (0.37%).

If androgen-treated mice are submitted to a short exposure to hypoxia (2 hr 30 min at 340 mm Hg), the erythropoietin response to this stimulation is again different in both sexes. Erythropoietin plasma titer in males is not significantly increased by androgens (9.88%) as compared to oil-injected controls (8.27%) whereas an evident elevation is observed in females: 8.95% in androgen-treated animals against 2.6% in the controls (FIGURE 7). This fact could possibly be related to a maximal response to hypoxia in males.

Direct measurements of erythropoiesis with ^{59}Fe incorporation also show the influence of sex on the response to the combined effect of androgens and hypoxia. FIGURE 8 shows that while both sexes respond identically to androgens alone, amplification of hypoxia by androgens occurs only in females.

Effect of Androgens on Erythropoietin Plasma Level in Rats

Wistar rats of both sexes were injected with testosterone propionate (10, 30 and 50 mg, dissolved in 0.5 ml peanut oil) three times a week. Erythropoietin

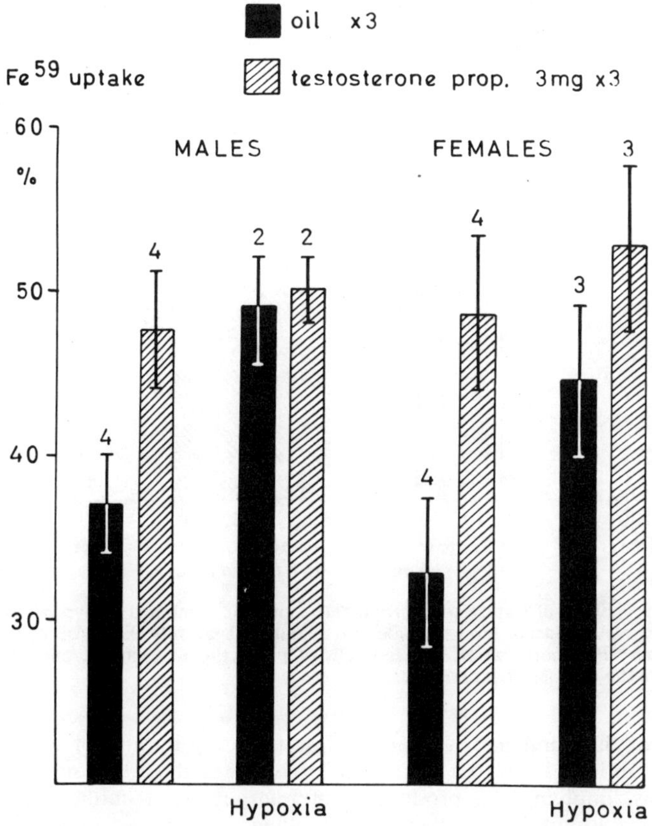

FIGURE 8. Effect of testosterone propionate (3 × 3 mg) alone, or combined to hypoxia (2 hr 30 min at 340 mm Hg), on the ^{59}Fe uptake of male and female normal mice. Figures on the top indicate the number of experiments. Vertical bars indicate standard error of the mean.

plasma titer was measured after androgens alone or combined with hypoxia. No erythropoietin response was elicited by androgens alone, either in male or in female rats. A moderate but statistically significant amplification of the effect of hypoxia was observed in androgen-treated males (12 or 20 hr at 340 mm Hg). In females the response was not significant in spite of a more severe hypoxic stimulus: 21 hr at 320 mm Hg (FIGURE 9).

DISCUSSION

The stimulating effect of androgens on erythropoiesis is confirmed in this study. Testosterone propionate, as well as anabolic steroids, significantly increases ^{59}Fe incorporation into red cells in male and female mice. Furthermore, testosterone propionate induces a moderate but significant increase in red cell mass, amounting to 15% after four weeks of treatment. Similar increases have been observed by Van Dyke *et al.*[8] in the rat and Jepson *et al.*[17] in mice. To explain this effect on red cell mass, there are two possible hypotheses: there is either an

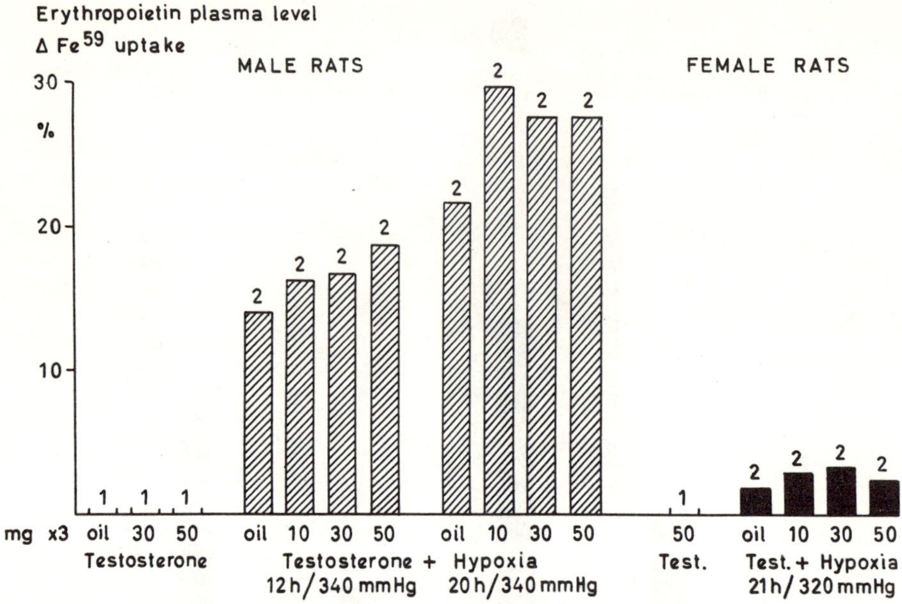

FIGURE 9. Effect of testosterone propionate alone, or combined to hypoxic stimulation, on the erythropoietin plasma level of male and female Wistar rats. Erythropoietin plasma level expressed as ^{59}Fe incorporation into red cells of polycythemic recipient mice. Figures on the top indicate the number of experiments.

increase of the number of stem cells differentiating by unit of time into normoblasts, or an increase in the number of divisions of the erythroid cells. The latter hypothesis, implying the production of microcytes, is unlikely as we did not observe any modification of m.c.v. following chronic androgen administration. The theoretical mechanisms involved in the stimulation of stem cell differentiation could be the following:

1. Effect on stem cell differentiation (erythropoietin-like effect).
2. Increased production of erythropoietin.
3. Potentiation of erythropoietin (a greater number of stem cells being differentiated for a given amount of erythropoietin).

If the effect of testosterone propionate is tested on polycythemic mice, results are different whether plethora has been achieved by hypoxia or by transfusion. An evident increase of ^{59}Fe incorporation occurs in HP mice whereas in TP mice only a slight elevation is observed. It is inferred that testosterone, contrary to erythropoietin, does not have a direct action on stem cell differentiation. Accordingly, 50 hr after a single injection of testosterone, this delay corresponding to a maximal effect on stem cell differentiation following erythropoietin,[18] there was no detectable effect on ^{59}Fe incorporation, even in HP mice. This discrepancy between HP and TP mice with regard to their responsiveness to androgens is not clearly understood. Iron plasma levels are similar in HP and TP mice,[16] the red cell mass is no lower in HP than in TP mice. Furthermore, both types of assay animals are equally sensitive to exogenous erythropoietin: ^{59}Fe incorporation after 0.3 units of sheep erythropoietin averages 6.5% in HP and 5.8% in TP mice. It could be that HP mice are more susceptible to produce erythropoietin than TP mice, a hypothesis consistent with the observation that the erythropoietic response to hypoxia or cobalt is higher in HP than in TP mice.[19] As residual erythropoiesis is higher in HP than in TP mice, at least with our strain and our experimental schedule, it could be suggested that androgens require the persistence of some erythropoietic activity to exert their effect on erythropoiesis. The erythropoietic response of mild plethoric TP mice to androgens, reported by others, is in agreement with both these hypotheses.[20]

The erythropoietic response of HP mice to a short stimulation is amplified by previous androgen administration to an extent that exceeds the additive effects of androgens and hypoxia alone. This amplification could be due either to an increased production of erythropoietin in response to hypoxia or to an effect of potentiation of endogenous erythropoietin by androgens. The observation of higher erythropoietin titers following hypoxia in female mice previously treated with androgens is an argument in favor of the former hypothesis. However, the effect of exogenous erythropoietin on erythropoiesis is also amplified by androgens. This observation, confirmed by others,[21] could again be explained by increased production of erythropoietin or potentiation. Potentiation could be due to a direct effect of testosterone on the stem cell by increasing its sensitivity to erythropoietin. However, as androgens increase the production of endogenous erythropoietin, the observed amplification could be explained, as has been suggested by Gurney *et al.*[21] by the synergic effect of two consecutive doses of endogenous and exogenous erythropoietin.[22] The fact that after androgen treatment alone the erythropoietin plasma titer of the normal TO mice is not measurable and the erythropoiesis of HP mice is only slightly increased does not favor the latter hypothesis.

Potentiation confirms the observation of only moderate effects of androgens on red cell mass in chronic experiments. Homeostatic regulation must probably intervene in response to the effect of potentiation to reduce the production of endogenous erythropoietin. This view is supported by the progressive reduction of the erythropoietic response after five weeks of treatment measured by ^{59}Fe incorporation. The $\triangle$ uptake averages 15.8% after one week and decreases gradually to 1.7% after five weeks of treatment.

Effect of androgens on erythropoietin plasma titer is different from one sex to another. Furthermore, strain and interspecific differences seem to exist. For instance, our TO female mice do not respond to androgens by a measurable elevation of the erythropoietin plasma titer, contrary to CBA female mice.[23] Conversely, TO male mice respond whereas CBA males do not. Androgens do not increase erythropoietin plasma titer of Wistar rats to measurable levels either in males or in females, and amplify the erythropoietin response to hypoxia in males only. The erythropoietic response to androgens, measured in mice by ^{59}Fe incorporation or by the red cell mass, is similarly increased in both sexes, in spite of the differences in erythropoietin plasma level. These results indicate that the erythropoietic action of androgens is not clearly related to an effect on the production of erythropoietin. Consequently, it seems difficult to adopt a definite position with regard to the mode of action of androgens on erythropoiesis, and moreover to extrapolate experimental data on rodents to man. That androgens do increase erythropoietin production under certain experimental conditions seems an established fact. However, this mode of action could not explain all the experimental data or the beneficial action of testosterone in certain cases of medullary hypoplasia with a high erythropoietin plasma level.

Summary

The effect of androgens has been studied in normal and hypoxic (HP) or transfused (TP) polycythemic mice and in normal rats. Stimulating effects of androgens and anabolic steroids have been demonstrated by increase of red cell mass and ^{59}Fe incorporation into red cells. Furthermore, a similar amplification of the response to a short hypoxic stimulus or a single dose of erythropoietin has been observed after androgen treatment.

Administration of testosterone increases the erythropoietin plasma titer in normal male but not in female mice. Conversely, androgens amplify the erythropoietin plasma titer in response to hypoxia only in females. In rats, plasma titer is not increased by androgens and an amplified effect of hypoxia is only observed in males. It is concluded that the effect of androgens on erythropoiesis is due to an increased production of erythropoietin and/or potentiation of the action of erythropoietin on stem cells.

References

1. Shahidi, N. T. & L. K. Diamond. 1959. Testosterone-induced remission in aplastic anemia. Amer. J. Dis. Child. **98:** 293.
2. Shahidi, N. T. & L. K. Diamond. 1961. Testosterone-induced remission in aplastic anemia of both acquired and congenital types. New Eng. J. Med. **264:** 953.
3. Gardner, F. H. & J. C. Pringle. 1961. Androgens and erythropoiesis. I. Preliminary clinical observations. Arch. Intern. Med. **107:** 846.
4. Kennedy, B. J. 1962. Stimulation of erythropoiesis by androgens hormones. Ann. Intern. Med. **57:** 917.
5. Steinglass, P., A. S. Gordon & H. A. Charipper. 1941. Effect of castration and sex hormones on blood of rat. Proc. Soc. Exp. Biol. Med. **48:** 169.
6. Arvy, L. 1943. Le retentissement de la castration sur l'hématopoïèse du coq domestique. Sang. **15:** 334.
7. Crafts, R. C. 1946. The effects of hypophysectomy, castration, and testosterone propionate on hemopoiesis in the adult male rat. Endocrinology **39:** 401.
8. Van Dyke, D. C., A. M. Contopoulos, B. S. Williams, M. E. Simpson, J. H. Lawrence & H. M. Evans. 1954. Hormonal factors influencing erythropoiesis. Acta Haematol. **11:** 203.
9. Naets, J. P. & M. Wittek. 1964. Etude du mécanisme d'action des androgènes sur l'érythropoièse. Compt. Rend. Acad. Sci. (Paris) **259:** 3371.
10. Mirand, E. A., A. S. Gordon & J. Wenig. 1965. Mechanism of testosterone action in erythropoiesis. Nature **206:** 270.
11. Fried, W. & C. W. Gurney. 1965. Erythropoietic effect of plasma from mice receiving testosterone. Nature **206:** 1160.
12. Degowin, R. L., D. Hofstra & C. W. Gurney. 1962. A comparison of erythropoietin bioassays. Proc. Soc. Exp. Biol. Med. **110:** 48.
13. Degowin, R. L., D. Hofstra & C. W. Gurney. 1962. The mouse with hypoxia-induced erythremia, an erythropoietin bioassay animal. J. Lab. Clin. Med. **60:** 846.
14. Read, R. C. 1954. Studies of red-cell volume and turnover using radiochromium. New Eng. J. Med. **250:** 1021.
15. Peters, T., J. Giovanniello, L. Apt & J. F. Ross. 1956. A simple improved method for the determination of serum iron. J. Lab. Clin. Med. **48:** 280.
16. Naets, J. P. & M. Wittek. 1966. Mechanism of action of androgens on erythropoiesis. Amer. J. Physiol. **210:** 315.
17. Jepson, J. H. & L. Lowenstein. 1964. Effect of prolactin on erythropoiesis in the mouse. Blood **24:** 726.
18. Filmanowicz, E. & C. W. Gurney. 1961. Studies on erythropoiesis. XVI. Response to a single dose of erythropoietin in polycythemic mouse. J. Lab. Clin. Med. **57:** 65.
19. Naets, J. P. & M. Wittek. To be published.
20. Fried, W., R. Degowin & C. W. Gurney. 1964. The erythropoietic effect of testosterone in polycythemic mice. Proc. Soc. Exper. Biol. Med. **117:** 839.
21. Gurney, C. W. & W. Fried. 1965. Further studies on the erythropoietic effect of androgens. J. Lab. Clin. Med. **65:** 775.
22. Gurney, C. W., N. Wackman & E. Filmanowicz. 1961. Studies on erythropoiesis. XVII. Some quantitative aspects of the erythropoietic response to erythropoietin. Blood **17:** 531.
23. Fried, W. & C. W. Gurney. 1966. The erythropoietic response to testosterone in male and female mice. J. Lab. Clin. Med. **67:** 420.

HEMOLYSIS AND ERYTHROPOIESIS

III. THE EFFECT OF HEMOLYSIS AND HEMOLYSATES ON ERYTHROPOIESIS*

L. Sánchez-Medal and Juan Labardini

Department of Hematology, Instituto Nacional de la Nutrición, México

The prevailing concept that erythropoiesis is under the control of a single substance, erythropoietin, whose production depends exclusively on the balance between supply and demand of oxygen at tissue level,[1,2] is not consistent with data obtained in hemolytic processes and in experimental conditions resembling them. These data will be the subject of the present report.

In compensated hemolytic disease increased erythrocytic production occurs in the absence of the hypoxic effect of anemia. Pertinent data from two personal cases and from cases reported in the literature[3–8] in that situation are given in TABLE 1.

Polycythemia may be observed in patients with mild hemolytic disorders. This situation has been reported in hereditary spherocytic and ovalocytic hemolytic disease,[9,9a] and data on two personal cases with autoimmune idiopathic hemolytic disease are shown in TABLE 2. Pertinent to this point is the observation by Stohlman[10] that compensated hemolysis after plastic ball valve prosthesis in dogs may produce a mild rise in hematocrit; in one of the animals it increased from 48 to 50–56 percent.

In hemolytic anemia erythrocytic production is greater than in other anemias with similar hemoglobin deficit. This was generally accepted several decades ago[11] but, to our knowledge, had not been proven. Our own observations[12,13] have shown that in hemolytic anemia, whether hereditary or autoimmune, erythrocytic production is greater than in iron, folate or vitamin B_{12} deficiency anemias of similar degree under adequate therapy, as estimated by:

1) Maximal absolute reticulocyte counts observed in 132 cases of the three types of anemia. The average value in hemolytic anemia was 2–2.5 times that of the deficiency anemias (TABLE 3). In hemolytic anemia, as many as four million reticulocytes per cubic millimeter of blood have been observed.[14]

2) The rate of hemoglobin rise per day obtained in 245 cases. This rate was about the same in both iron deficiency and megaloblastic anemias and about 50 percent greater in the autoimmune hemolytic cases responding to corticosteroids (TABLE 4).

3) Estimations of the red cell production in patients with severe anemia by means of balance studies showed an average production of 8.4 times normal in the hemolytic anemias, whereas they were much lower in the megaloblastic and ferropenic anemias (4.2 and 2.9 times normal, respectively). As shown in FIGURE 1, five out of six cases of hemolytic anemia had production rates from 5.1 to 14.8, whereas only one out of 13 cases of the other two groups had a rate slightly above five. These balance studies were made by considering the red cell volume measured with ^{51}Cr, at the beginning and end of the study and the red cells destroyed during that period.[13]

Experimental work performed in our laboratory in the past seven years. The main findings have been obtained by the intraperitoneal injection, once or twice

* The experimental studies reviewed in this paper were supported by a grant from Laboratorios Carnot, Mexico.

TABLE 1

CASES WITH COMPENSATED HEMOLYTIC DISEASE AND INCREASED ERYTHROCYTIC PRODUCTION

Reference	Diagnosis*	Sex and Age	Hb.	EV‡ ml/kg	Ashby T	^{51}Cr T½	E.P.**
Letman[3]	H. Sph.	M–11	11.9	—	16	—	6.7
Erlandson[4]	H. Sph.	M– 3	12.1	24.3	—	25	2.1
Erlandson[4]	H. Sph.	F– 4	12.2	20.1	—	8	5.8
Motulsky[5]	H. Nonshp.	M–23	12.4	28.2	13	—	7.9
Crosby[6]	H. Sph.	M–"young"	13	21.5	—	11	7.1
Erlandson[4]	H. Sph.	F– 7	13.7	19.1	—	12	3.7
Jandl[7]	H. Sph.	M–18	13.9	†	—	11.9	5.14
Boiron[8]	H. Sph.	M–20	(47)§	—	—	21	2.5
Personal	H. Sph.	F–47	14	24	—	11.8	3.41
Personal	Id. Autoimm.	F–30	15.7	21.5	—	17	2.16

* H. Sph. = hereditary spherocytosis; H. Nonsph. = hereditary nonspherocytic hemolytic disease; Id. Autoimm. = idiopathic autoimmune hemolytic disease.
** E.P. = erythrocytic production in times normal.
† Calculated as above average on data presented by the AA.
‡ EV. = volume of circulating erythrocytes.
§ Represents hematocrit, as hemoglobin was not given.

TABLE 2

POLYCYTHEMIA IN TWO FEMALES WITH AUTOIMMUNE HEMOLYTIC ANEMIA*

Case Reg.	Hb, g/100 ml	Ht. Percent	EV ^{51}Cr** ml/kg
HEN 35073	16.9 17.	49.2 48.8	28.44 26.38
HEN 23059	18.1 18.2	52.7 54.2	27.72 26.88
Normal values	15.2 ± 0.97	45.4 ± 2.1	20.2 – 26.0

* The clinical history of these cases is given in the *Appendix*.
** EV ^{51}Cr = volume of circulating erythrocytes estimated with ^{51}Cr-labeled cells.

TABLE 3

MAXIMAL RETICULOCYTE VALUES (IN UNITS)* IN ANEMIC PATIENTS RESPONDING TO ADEQUATE THERAPY

Degree of Anemia (Hb. g/100 ml)	Iron Deficiency No. Cases	Iron Deficiency Rets.	Megaloblastic No. Cases	Megaloblastic Rets.	Hemolytic** No. Cases	Hemolytic** Rets.
6 or less	28	409	16	601	15	1177
6.05 – 8	19	403	13	496	7	1039
8.05 – 10	14	303	7	429	13	646
Ratios:	1		1.37		2.57	

* The units were obtained by multiplying the percent reticulocyte figure by the hematocrit.
** Includes cases of autoimmune hemolytic anemia treated with corticosteroids, and hereditary disease with no therapy.

TABLE 4

RATE OF HEMOGLOBIN RISE (IN MG/100 ML OF BLOOD/DAY) IN ANEMIC PATIENTS RESPONDING TO ADEQUATE THERAPY

Degree of Anemia (Hb. g/100 ml)	Iron Deficiency No. Cases	Hb.	Megaloblastic No. Cases	Hb.	Hemolytic No. Cases	Hb.
6.0 or less	31	345	18	341	18	558
6.05 – 8.0	38	282	16	272	6	394
8.05 – 10.0	46	216	19	198	12	325
10.05 – 12.0	15	202	16	199	10	242
Ratios:	1.03		1.0		1.5	

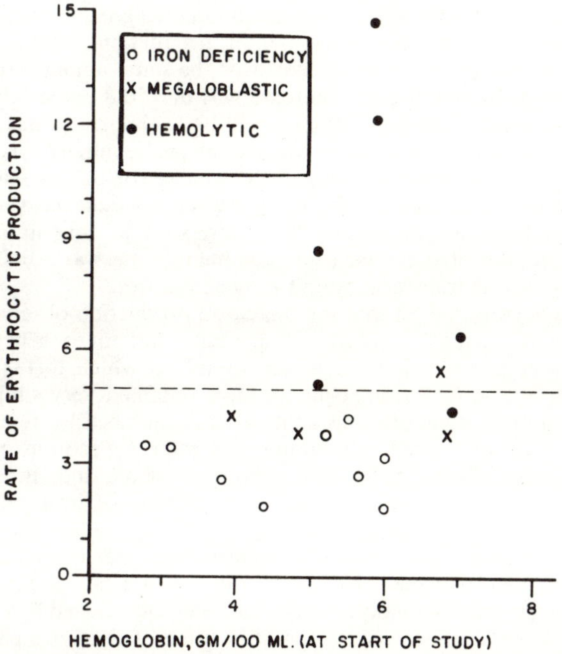

FIGURE 1. Erythrocytic rates in hemolytic, megaloblastic and iron deficiency anemias.

daily, of autohemolysates into dogs (1.5 ml/kg/day) and isohemolysates into Wistar rats (10 ml/kg/injection) previous to the evaluation of erythropoiesis by different parameters. These studies have shown that the hemolysates produce:

1) An increase in the ^{59}Fe incorporation into hemoglobin from 26.98 $\pm$ 1.81 (S.E.) percent to 43.43 $\pm$ 2.33 (p less than 0.001) in normal rats receiving four daily injections.[15]

2) An increase in the ^{59}Fe incorporation from 1.92 $\pm$ 0.42 to 24.98 $\pm$ 3.64 (p less than 0.001) and in reticulocytes from 0.004 $\pm$ 0.003 to 1.17 $\pm$ 0.2 (p less than 0.001) in hypertransfused polycythemic rats receiving injections twice daily for four days.

3) Increases in ^{59}Fe incorporation from 6.6 $\pm$ 0.45 to 31.35 $\pm$ 2.11 (p less than 0.001), in reticulocytes (0.35 vs. 2.03 percent) and in the relative number

of normoblasts in bone marrow (12 vs. 26.3 percent) and spleen 0.20 vs. 0.79 percent) in rats starved for four days and injected daily for four days. These effects in the fasting rat do not seem to depend on the amount of protein given as hemolysate since the daily administration of 1 ml/100 g of animal weight of a balanced mixture of the essential amino acids** and of a normal rat liver homogenate containing 0.32 g of liver/ml did not significantly increase the ^{59}Fe incorporation into the hemoglobin (8.96 ± 1.27 and 7.0 ± 0.43, respectively, vs. 5.6 ± 0.45).

4) A moderate but significant polycythemia in normal rats when injected twice daily for 21 days. The red cell volume increased from 2.60 ± 0.07 to 3.15 ± 0.03 ml/100 g (p less than 0.001). Similar effects, though less marked, have been induced with smaller amounts of hemolysate for shorter periods.

5) An increase in erythrocytic production in bled anemic dogs. Daily injection of an autohemolysate increased hemoglobin production in 60.7 percent and red cell volume production in 56.8 percent over the same animal production during a control period. In one dog this increase was of 150.8 percent.[16]

Although some of our observations could be explained, as has been suggested, on the basis that heme iron is more available or preferentially used in hemoglobin synthesis,[17] this latter explanation does not suffice for others. Thus, preferential utilization of the heme iron by the normal animal would have decreased rather than increased the incorporation of ^{59}Fe, more so if, as done in our experimental models, the amount of heme iron gives as hemolysate was 5,000 times or more the amount given as transferin-bound radioactive iron.

It has also been proposed that the increased production observed in hemolytic anemias is related to the chronicity of the process and not to its hemolytic nature.[2] To our knowledge, there is no adequate study on which this statement can be based. In opposition to this concept we have obtained very similar productions in a normal human male after an acute anemia induced by removing, in a few hours, 52 percent of his red cell volume and after 2.5 months of anemia maintained by repeated phlebotomies. Throughout the whole study the subject received 100 mg of iron-IM (as iron-dextran†) and 150 mg of iron per os (as ferrous fumarate) daily.

Studies on the effect of hemolysis on erythropoiesis performed by other authors, most of them done between 1908 and 1935,[18–21] are consistent with those presented, although with methodology that has been questioned.[22] Very few investigations have been done in recent years, but three of them are particularly interesting. Brown *et al.*,[23] following a methodology similar to some in our studies, observed the same effect of hemolysates and heme compounds on the ^{59}Fe incorporation into the hemoglobin. Erslev[24] found in vitro differences in the effect of erythropoietin on rabbit bone marrow cells obtained from normal, acutely bled anemic and nonanemic hemolysing animals. The differences observed led him to believe in an enlarged stem cell pool in the hemolytic states. Finally, García and Schooley[25] have reported that antierythropoietin was incapable of completely neutralizing the stimulatory effect of serum obtained from sheep and rabbit with phenylhydrazine anemia in spite of accomplishing complete neutralization of sera belonging to hypoxic rats, sheep and rabbit and to an anemic human being.

** This mixture was kindly supplied by Labs. Farmacobiológicos, Mexico, and had the following composition per 50 ml: lysine 1.32 g, leucine 1.29 g, valine 1.02 g, isoleucine 0.93 g, phenylalanine 0.75 g, threonine 0.57 g, arginine 0.48 g, methionine 0.45 g, histidine 0.33 g and tryptophane 0.30 g.

† We are indebted to Farm. Lakeside de Mexico for the Imferon provided for this study.

It seems to us that the only explanation for the clinical and experimental observations reviewed in this presentation is that the red cell components released by hemolysis exert a stimulatory effect on erythropoiesis, as we suggested in 1962.[26] It seems very likely that such an action plays a role in the regulation of erythropoiesis at least in some pathological conditions.

Summary

Data has been presented showing that: 1) in compensated hemolytic disease increased erythrocytic production occurs in the absence of the hypoxic effect of anemia; 2) in occasional cases of mild hemolysis, polycythemia may be observed; 3) erythrocytic production is greater in hemolytic anemia than in other anemias with similar hemoglobin deficit; and 4) administration of hemolysate increases the speed of recovery from bled anemia in dogs and increases the number of reticulocytes and the ^{59}Fe incorporation into the hemoglobin in rats with either normal or depressed erythropoiesis secondary to hypertransfusion polycythemia or starvation. In rats it also produced an increase in the number of erythroblasts in bone marrow and spleen and polycythemia, as estimated by total erythrocyte volume determinations with ^{59}Fe-labeled RBC.

These data are considered to indicate that RBC constituents have an erythropoietic stimulatory effect and that it is very probable that they play a role in the control of erythropoiesis.

Appendix

Clinical Histories of Patients with Polycythemia and Hemolytic Anemia

HEN 35073. A 22-year-old female came to the hospital with a two-year history of relapsing anemia, jaundice and fever. A diagnosis of autoimmune hemolytic anemia was made and she was treated with corticosteroids. One year later the spleen was removed with improvement, although during the following two years she continued having a positive direct Coombs and a 2–3% reticulocytosis. Shortly after splenectomy hematocrit rose to 48–52% and has remained stable at that level. Six months after splenectomy ^{51}Cr red cell volume determinations were made twice two weeks apart and in both, results were above normal limits (28.44 and 26.38 ml/kg).

HEN 23059. A female was seen first in 1955, when she was 29 years old, with acute hemolytic anemia that responded to corticosteroid therapy. In the following four years she continued having microspherocytosis, positive direct Coombs and moderate reticulocytes with a high hematocrit (50–54%). In 1960, a second hemolytic crisis supervened that was easily controlled with prednisone. After that, hematocrit rose again and has remained about 50–57%. Two years after the last corticosteroid treatment, the erythrocyte volume was determined with ^{51}Cr on two separate occasions, 24 days apart. Results were 27.72 and 26.88 ml/kg. At that time the spleen was not palpable, reticulocytes were 2–2.8% and direct Coombs and bromelin reactions were positive.

References

1. Jacobson, L. O., E. Goldwasser, C. W. Gurney, W. Fried & L. Plzak. 1959. Studies of erythropoietin: the hormone regulating red cell production. Ann. N. Y. Acad. Sci. **77:** 551.
2. Simon, E. R. & C. A. Finch. 1966. Red cell manual : 9. Univ. Press. Seattle, Wash.
3. Letman, H. 1959. Red cell destruction in the anaemias. A. Stiftsbogtrykkerie, Copenhagen. (Case 52).
4. Erlandson, M. E., I. Schulman & C. H. Smith. 1959. Studies on congenital hemolytic syndromes. II. Rates of destruction and production of erythrocytes in hereditary spherocytosis. Pediatrics **23:** 462. (Cases 6, 9, 10).

5. MOTULSKY, A. G., W. H. CROSBY & H. RAPPAPORT. 1954. Hereditary nonspherocytic hemolytic anemia. Blood **9**: 749. (Case 3).
6. CROSBY, W. H. & J. H. ACKEROYD. 1952. The limit of hemoglobin synthesis. Amer. J. Med. **13**: 273. (Case 1).
7. JANDL, J. H., M. S. GREENBERG, R. H. YONEMOTO & W. B. CASTLE. 1956. Clinical determination of the sites of red cell sequestration in hemolytic anemias. J. Clin. Invest. **35**: 842. (Case 2).
8. BOIRON, M., L. MEEUS-BITH, C. PAOLETTI, M. TUBIANA, J. BOUSSER & J. BERNARD. 1958. La mesure de la production érythrocytaire chez l'homme à l'aide du chrome radioactif. Rev. Hémat. **13**: 171. (Case C).
9. HEILMEYER, L. 1946. Enfermedades de la sangre. Ed. Labor, Barcelona, : 264 and 281.
9a. GANSSLEN, M. 1922. Über hämolytischen Ikterus. Nach 25 eigenen Beobachtungen und 10 Milzexstirpationen. Dtsch. Arch. Klin. Med. **140**: 210.
10. STOHLMAN, JR., F. 1959. Observations on the physiology of erythropoietin and its role in the regulation of red cell production. Ann. N. Y. Acad. Sci. **77**: 551.
11. MCMASTER, P. D. & H. HAESSLER. 1921. The factor determining the spread of red marrow during anemia. J. Exp. Med. **34**: 579.
12. SANCHEZ-MEDAL, L., H. M. RODRIGUEZ & E. QUINTANAR. 1958. Medición de la actividad eritropoyética en diferentes tipos de anemia. Proc. VII Reunión Asociación Investigación Pediátrica. México, 1958, : 205.
13. SANCHEZ-MEDAL, L., J. PIZZUTO, H. M. RODRIGUEZ & L. ESPOSITO. Hemolysis and erythropoiesis. II. Reticulocytosis and rate of hemoglobin rise in hemolytic and deficiency anemias. To be published.
14. BATY, J. M. 1930. Congenital hemolytic jaundice with a high reticulocyte count. Amer. J. Med. Sci. **179**: 546.
15. SALAS, M., J. F. SMYTH, L. SANCHEZ-MEDAL, E. RODRIGUEZ & J. LABARDINI. 1963. The effect of hemolysates in increasing the ^{59}Fe hemoglobin incorporation in rats. Med. Exper. **8**: 159.
16. SANCHEZ-MEDAL, L., J. LABARDINI & A. LORIA. 1963. Hemolysis and erythropoiesis. I. Influence of intraperitoneal administration of whole hemolysates on the recovery of bled dogs, as measured by changes in the total erythrocytic volume. Blood **21**: 586.
17. KEENE, W. R. & J. H. JANDL. 1964. Uptake of hemoglobin and blood cells by bone marrow. Clin. Res. **12**: 226.
18. ITAMI, S. 1908. Ein experimentellen Beitrag-zur-Lehre von der extramedullaren Blutbildung bei Anämien. Arch. Experim. Path. Pharm. **60**: 76.
19. RITZ, H. 1909. Studies über Bluttregeneration bei experimentellen Anämien. Folia Haemat. Zentr., **8**: 186.
20. OKA, A. 1932. Influence of the red cell constituents of erythrocytes and various organs on recovery from experimental anemia. Japan. J. Exp. Med. **10**: 203.
21. MILLER, D. K. & C. P. RHOADS. 1934. The effect of hemoglobin injections on erythropoiesis and erythrocyte size in rabbits rendered anemic by bleeding. J. Exp. Med. **59**: 333.
22. GRANT, W. C. & W. S. ROOT. 1952. Fundamental stimulus for erythropoiesis. Physiol. Rev. **32**: 499.
23. BROWN, J. R., N. ALTSCHULER & J. A. D. COOPER. 1963. Erythropoietic effect of red blood cell components and heme-related compounds. Proc. Soc. Exp. Biol. Med. **112**: 840.
24. ERSLEV, A. J. 1964. The role of erythropoietin in the control of red cell production. Medicine **43**: 661.
25. GARCIA, J. F. & J. C. SCHOOLEY. 1963. Immunological neutralization of various erythropoietins. Proc. Soc. Exp. Biol. Med. **112**: 712.
26. SANCHEZ-MEDAL, L. 1962. Hemolisis y actividad eritropoyética. Rev. Invest. Clin. (México) **14**: 199.

OBSERVATIONS ON THE EFFECT OF TESTOSTERONE AND HYDROCORTISONE ON ERYTHROPOIESIS*

Bertil E. Glader, Walter A. Rambach and Howard L. Alt

Department of Medicine, Northwestern University Medical School, Chicago, Ill.

The erythropoietic-stimulating effect of testosterone has been recognized for many years. The utilization of this androgen, or synthetic analogues, has become commonplace in the treatment of specific human anemias. Over the past few years the mechanism of this effect has come under extensive scrutiny in laboratory animals. However, the effect of large doses of corticosteroids on erythropoiesis in normal animals has received relatively little attention although the use of testosterone and hydrocortisone in humans has been directed toward a concept of their being erythropoietic stimuli. Little is known about the relationship of the activity between these two steroids and erythropoiesis; yet they have been used jointly in the treatment of refractory anemia.

Current concepts have been developed by a number of investigators relating testosterone and erythropoietin. Extensive work has not clearly related corticosteroids and erythropoietin in normal animals. In our work we have attempted to study the interaction of testosterone and hydrocortisone with erythropoietin in the normal rat, utilizing iron, tritiated glycine and tritiated thymidine kinetics, and morphological studies.

Female albino rats of Sprague-Dawley strain, weighing 180–220 g were utilized. Iron-59 incorporation into bone marrow, spleen and erythrocytes was determined by standard techniques.[1] Hemoglobin was isolated from a hemolysate by acetone precipitation followed by washes with water, acetone, acetone-ether and ether. The appearance of ^{59}Fe in hemoglobin was used as an index of iron uptake into heme. Globin was isolated by the method of Fanelli and Antonini[2] following 72-hr labeling with tritiated glycine. Recovery of radioactivity was accomplished by standard oxygen combustion techniques.[3] Tritiated thymidine incorporation into splenic tissue, representing DNA utilization, was studied with methods previously reported.[3]

Effect of Testosterone on Erythropoiesis

Four days after a single injection of testosterone propionate there is a significant increase in ^{59}Fe incorporation into peripheral erythrocytes (TABLE 1). Splenic incorporation and clearance of ^{59}Fe are also increased while no significant differences are noted in the bone marrow. These results are similar to those we have previously reported for erythropoietin,[1] and they again show the sensitive ability of splenic measurements to reflect erythropoiesis. Supplementing these data are the results presented in TABLE 2. Here, tritiated thymidine uptake is seen to be increased after testosterone administration although not to the same extent as that induced by erythropoietin. No change is noted in the thymus and intestine, which were used as control lymphoid tissues. Splenic imprints in both groups of animals reveal normoblastic proliferation which is quite similar to that noted in our prior studies with erythropoietin.[3] In the current experiments the smaller response to testosterone as compared to that with erythropoietin is probably related to dose since ^{59}Fe uptake into peripheral erythrocytes is lower in androgen- than in erythropoietin-treated animals.

* This work was supported in part by grant no. AH05289–05 from the National Institute of Health.

TABLE 1
EFFECT OF TESTOSTERONE ON ERYTHROPOIESIS

	^{59}Fe Incorporation (Percent Injected Dose)	
	6 hr	24 hr
Blood		
Control	10.8 ± 4.0 (5)	26.0 ± 2.9 (5)
Testosterone (10 mg × 1)	21.4 ± 3.4 (5)*	43.9 ± 4.7 (5)*
Spleen		
Control	2.6 ± 2.0 (5)	2.0 ± 0.3 (5)
Testosterone (10 mg × 1)	6.8 ± 1.4 (5)*	2.3 ± 0.3 (5)
Bone Marrow		
Control	28.0 ± 6.0 (5)	15.6 ± 1.8 (5)
Testosterone (10 mg × 1)	28.3 ± 3.7 (5)	14.5 ± 1.6 (5)

* p value less than 0.01.
( ) = number of experimental animals.

TABLE 2
EFFECT OF TESTOSTERONE ON THYMIDINE KINETICS

	Thymidine-^{3}H Incorporation (Percent Injected Dose per Gram Dry Tissue Weight)		
	Control	Testosterone (10 mg × 1)	Erythropoietin (5 Units Standard B×2)
Spleen	5.7 ± 1.8 (25)	7.2 ± 2.3 (22)*	11.3 ± 2.1 (5)**
Thymus	2.6 ± 0.5 (6)	2.8 ± 0.5 (6)	—
Intestine	9.0 ± 1.7 (6)	7.5 ± 0.7 (6)	—
72 hr RBC ^{59}Fe incorporation	42.4 ± 5.5 (21)	58.5 ± 6.0 (24)**	71.2 ± 2.8 (5)**

* p value less than 0.05.
** p value less than 0.01.
( ) = number of experimental animals.

From the above results it is apparent that testosterone is capable of stimulating erythropoiesis. Since it has been noted that the free erythrocyte protoporphyrin increases in cases of human anemia treated with testosterone,[4] it is possible that the stimulus to erythropoiesis might reside in a differential effect on heme and globin synthesis. In TABLE 3 the response of heme and globin synthesis to testosterone and erythropoietin is recorded. The factorial increase in isotope incorporation above control levels is seen to be the same for heme and globin. There does not appear to be a specific differential effect of testosterone on heme and globin synthesis, and no difference between the action of testosterone and erythropoietin is apparent.

In the dehydrated, relatively polycythemic rat, ^{59}Fe incorporation into the red blood cells of control and testosterone-treated animals is inversely related to the hematocrit (TABLE 4). However, as the degree of polycythemia is increased, the relative effect of testosterone in responding animals remains constant. Similar results have been reported in hypertransfused mice.[5] It is significant, however, that our animals, which are polycythemic to an extent that no effect of testostrone can be observed, remain capable of an increased ^{59}Fe incorporation into erythrocytes following erythropoietin administration (TABLE 5). Consequently, it is unlikely that testosterone, in contrast to erythropoietin, exerts its primary action at the stem cell level.

The current experiments suggest that testosterone in some manner augments erythropoietin production or activation. Such an interpretation is consistent with the previously suggested hypotheses of other workers.[6,7] In addition, there does not appear to be a specific effect of the hormone on erythrocyte maturation, which is different from that of erythropoietin. However, the possibility that testosterone exerts more than one action on erythropoiesis can not be ruled out, and further studies at the biochemical level are necessary before the role of androgens in erythropoiesis will be completely understood.

Effect of Hydrocortisone on Erythropoiesis

In contrast to testosterone, hydrocortisone seems to depress erythropoiesis. After four days' treatment with relatively large doses of hydrocortisone acetate, a reduction in erythropoiesis is manifested by a decreased ^{59}Fe incorporation into

TABLE 3

EFFECT OF TESTOSTERONE ON HEMOGLOBIN SYNTHESIS

	72-Hr Isotope Incorporation into Globin and Hemoglobin (Percent Injected Dose per Gram Protein)	
	Globin (glycine-^{3}H)	Hemoglobin (^{59}Fe)
Control	0.18 ± 0.02 (6)	16.9 ± 2.7 (6)
Testosterone (10 mg × 1)	0.27 ± 0.03 (6)	28.7 ± 1.1 (6)
Erythropoietin (5 units Standard B × 2)	0.37 ± 0.08 (6)	33.8 ± 3.3 (6)

( ) = number of experimental animals.

TABLE 4

EFFECT OF HEMATOCRIT ON THE ERYTHROPOIETIC ACTION OF TESTOSTERONE

	24-Hr ^{59}Fe Incorporation (Percent Injected Dose)		
Average Hematocrit	Control	Testosterone (10 mg × 1)	Percent Increase
39.0	31.6 ± 6.3 (6)	47.0 ± 6.6 (6)	48.7
49.4	12.8 ± 2.5 (6)	18.0 ± 5.7 (6)	40.6
51.5	6.7 ± 1.2 (5)	9.4 ± 0.9 (6)	40.3
54.9	3.2 ± 0.7 (6)	2.8 ± 0.5 (6)	—

( ) = number of experimental animals.

TABLE 5

COMPARISON OF THE RESPONSES TO TESTOSTERONE AND ERYTHROPOIETIN IN THE DEHYDRATED POLYCYTHEMIC RAT

	24-Hr ^{59}Fe Incorporation (Percent Injected Dose)
Control	2.8 ± 0.3 (6)
Testosterone (10 mg × 1)	2.4 ± 0.6 (6)
Erythropoietin (0.5 units Standard B × 4)	19.1 ± 4.5 (6)
Testosterone (10 mg × 1) + Erythropoietin (0.5 units Standard B × 4)	17.2 ± 3.4 (6)

( ) = number of experimental animals.

TABLE 6
EFFECT OF HYDROCORTISONE ON ERYTHROPOIESIS

	^{59}Fe Incorporation (Percent injected dose)		
	Bone Marrow (6 hr)	Bone Marrow (24 hr)	Red Blood Cells (24 hr)
Control	25.6 ± 4.3 (15)	13.0 ± 2.2 (15)	29.6 ± 7.0 (10)
Hydrocortisone (10 mg/day × 4)	30.8 ± 7.0 (16)**	29.3 ± 7.4 (15)*	14.4 ± 5.2 (10)*
Control	29.7 ± 3.9 (6)	16.0 ± 3.3 (11)	32.8 ± 6.5 (21)
Hydrocortisone (1 mg/day × 4)	28.3 ± 0.5 (6)	21.8 ± 3.1 (11)*	25.8 ± 3.7 (20)*
Control	—	17.2 ± 1.8 (6)	35.8 ± 5.9 (6)
Hydrocortisone (1 mg/day × 21)	—	23.3 ± 3.1 (6)*	20.1 ± 5.1 (6)*
Control	28.7 ± 3.0 (6)	16.0 ± 3.1 (6)	32.9 ± 4.8 (6)
Dehydrated rats	14.4 ± 2.4 (6)*	14.5 ± 3.0 (6)	4.2 ± 0.7 (6)*

* p value less than 0.01.
** p value less than 0.02.
( ) = number of experimental animals.

red blood cells and a slower clearance of the label from the marrow (TABLE 6). Similar results are seen after three weeks of hydrocortisone injections. It is noteworthy that this effect of hydrocortisone is seen only with pharmacological doses of the drug. In our hands the administration of physiological amounts of the corticosteroid (0.5 mg/kg body weight) has no apparent effect on erythropoiesis in normal rats.

These results are unlike those seen in the hypophysectomized rat[8,9] or the adrenalectomized rat[10] where small quantities of the adrenal cortical hormones have been reported to augment erythropoiesis. This discrepancy in the erythropoietic effect of corticosteroids is most probably related to whether the hormone is administered in replacement doses to a deficient animal or given in larger than physiological amount to normal animals. A similar phenomenon is seen in biochemical processes where the rate of reaction is inhibited in the presence of excess substrate.

In the acute experiments, the animals lose weight and this is associated with some reduction of plasma volume. This could decrease erythropoietin formation as is the case in the deliberately dehydrated rat, which we have used as an erythropoietin assay animal. However, in the hydrocortisone-treated animals there is no reduction in ^{59}Fe incorporation in the bone marrow, as noted in the dehydrated rat (TABLE 6). This suggests that the hydrocortisone suppression is due to an action other than a reduction in erythropoietin production. Cohen and Gardner[11] have arrived at a similar conclusion while studying the effect of triamcinalone on the erythropoietic response to phenylhydrazine hemolysis in rabbits.

Effect of Hydrocortisone on Erythropoietin-Stimulated Erythropoiesis

When hydrocortisone-treated rats are given erythropoietin simultaneously, the resultant ^{59}Fe incorporation into peripheral erythrocytes is essentially the same as that seen when erythropoietin is administered alone (TABLE 7). This result is seen in both normal and dehydrated, relatively polycythemic rats. On the basis of these findings, it would not appear that hydrocortisone influences the action of erythropoietin on the bone marrow. However, it remains possible that erythropoietin is capable of overcoming, and thus masking, the inhibitory effect of hydrocortisone on the bone marrow.

Effect of Hydrocortisone on Testosterone-Stimulated Erythropoiesis

When hydrocortisone-treated animals are given testosterone simultaneously, there is a significant increase in the ^{59}Fe clearance from the bone marrow and an increased incorporation into red blood cells (TABLE 8). It is interesting to note, however, that the ^{59}Fe uptake in peripheral erythrocytes of animals treated with both hydrocortisone and testosterone is not greater than when testosterone is given alone. In fact, the response with both drugs together is less than that seen when only the androgen is given. This is unlike the response seen in hydrocortisone-treated animals given erythropoietin. The difference in response between

TABLE 7

EFFECT OF HYDROCORTISONE ON ERYTHROPOIETIN-STIMULATED ERYTHROPOIESIS

	24-Hr RBC ^{59}Fe Incorporation (Percent injected dose)
Control	38.5 ± 4.1 (5)
Hydrocortisone (1 mg/day × 4)	23.2 ± 4.1 (5)
Erythropoietin (5 units Standard B × 2)	48.7 ± 3.2 (5)
Hydrocortisone (1 mg/day × 4) + Erythropoietin (5 units Standard B × 2)	50.8 ± 6.3 (5)
Control	29.1 ± 7.4 (6)
Hydrocortisone (10 mg/day × 4)	17.6 ± 5.1 (6)
Erythropoietin (5 units Standard B × 2)	49.3 ± 2.0 (6)
Hydrocortisone (10 mg/day × 4) + Erythropoietin (5 units Standard B × 2)	44.5 ± 4.3 (6)
Polycythemic rats:	
Control	4.5 ± 1.6 (12)
Hydrocortisone (1 mg/day × 4)	2.8 ± 0.5 (12)
Erythropoietin (0.5 units Standard B × 4)	19.2 ± 4.4 (12)
Hydrocortisone (1 mg/day × 4) + Erythropoietin (0.5 units Standard B × 4)	15.9 ± 4.8 (12)

( ) = number of experimental animals.

TABLE 8

EFFECT OF HYDROCORTISONE ON TESTOSTERONE-STIMULATED ERYTHROPOIESIS

	24-Hr ^{59}Fe Incorporation (Percent injected dose)	
	Red Blood Cells	Bone Marrow
Control	37.0 ± 3.9 (10)	
Hydrocortisone (1 mg/day × 4)	23.3 ± 3.3 (10)	
Testosterone (10 mg × 1)	44.0 ± 6.2 (10)	
Hydrocortisone (1 mg/day × 4) + Testosterone (10 mg × 1)	37.3 ± 3.7 (10)	
Control	35.8 ± 5.9 (6)	17.2 ± 1.8 (6)
Hydrocortisone (1 mg/day × 21)	20.1 ± 5.1 (6)	23.3 ± 3.1 (6)
Testosterone (10 mg/day × 21)	40.5 ± 5.6 (6)	12.0 ± 2.3 (6)
Hydrocortisone (1 mg/day × 21) + Testosterone (10 mg/day × 21)	34.3 ± 10.2 (6)	16.4 ± 3.4 (6)

( ) = number of experimental animals.

testosterone- and erythropoietin-treated hydrocortisone animals may reflect the dosages employed. However, the possibility that hydrocortisone in some manner limits the maximal response of testosterone can not be ruled out. If the mechanism of action for testosterone, as suggested by others, is to increase the production of erythropoietin, then hydrocortisone given in large doses may act by depressing the formation of erythropoietin.

Summary

(1) General observations are reported on the erythropoietic effects of testosterone and hydrocortisone when given in pharmacological doses to normal rats.

(2) There are no specific effects of testosterone that are different from those of erythropoietin.

(3) Large doses of hydrocortisone appear to depress erythropoiesis as revealed by iron-59 kinetic studies. Whether this effect is due to some action on maturation and release of cells from the bone marrow or is possibly related to a decrease in erythropoietin production has not been established.

(4) It has been noted that the erythropoietic effect of testosterone, in both long- and short-term studies, is reduced by the administration of hydrocortisone.

(5) Hydrocortisone has little effect on erythropoiesis stimulated by exogenous erythropoietin.

Acknowledgments

We are indebted to Mrs. Gerlinde Louis and Miss Rosemary Ashworth for their excellent technical assistance.

References

1. Rambach, W. A., H. L. Alt & J. A. D. Cooper. 1957. Blood **12:** 1101.
2. Fanelli, A. Rossi & E. Antonini. 1958. Biochim. Biophys. Acta **30:** 608.
3. Kurtides, E. S., W. A. Rambach, H. L. Alt & J. C. Wurster. 1963. J. Lab. Clin. Med. **61:** 23.
4. Shahidi, N. T. 1963. J. Lab. Clin. Med. **62:** 294.
5. Gurney, C. W. & W. Fried. 1965. J. Lab. Clin. Med. **65:** 775.
6. Mirand, E. A., A. S. Gordon & J. Wenig. 1965. Nature **208:** 270.
7. Fried, W. & C. W. Gurney. 1965. Nature **206:** 1160.
8. Crafts, R. C. & H. A. Meineke. 1959. Ann. N. Y. Acad. Sci. **77:** 501.
9. Evans, E. S., D. C. Van Dyke & L. L. Rosenberg. 1964. Endocrinology **75:** 758.
10. Fruhman, G. J. & A. S. Gordon. 1955. Endocrinology **57:** 711.
11. Cohen, P. & F. H. Gardner. 1965. J. Lab. Clin. Med. **65:** 88.

THE EFFECT OF TESTOSTERONE ON THE UPTAKE OF TRITIATED THYMIDINE BY THE BONE MARROW OF CHILDREN*

W. Jacobson,** R. L. Sidman† and L. K. Diamond‡

*Strangeways Research Laboratory, Cambridge, England,***
Departments of Pediatrics and Neuropathology, Harvard Medical School, Boston, Mass.†
and
Research Hematology Division of the Medical Department of Children's Hospital Medical Center, Boston, Mass.‡

Introduction

Twenty-five years ago McCullagh and Jones (1941 & 1942) administered testosterone to patients with hypogonadism and observed that this hormone had a stimulating effect on the human bone marrow and especially on erythropoiesis.

These findings have been confirmed in numerous reports on patients who were given testosterone in an attempt to counteract the progression of malignancy, e.g. mammary carcinoma (Talbot *et al.*, 1949; Adair *et al.*, 1949; Kennedy and Gilbertsen, 1957; and Kennedy, 1962), or myelofibrosis (Rosenthal *et al.*, 1943, and Erf *et al.*, 1944). Shahidi and Diamond (1959, 1961) used testosterone and corticosteroids successfully in the treatment of children with aplastic anemia. Gardner and Pringle (1961a & b) showed the value of testosterone in adult patients whose bone marrows were in a depressed state secondary to a variety of malignancies including reticuloses and multiple myeloma. Recently West (1965) noted that the anemia associated with chronic lymphatic leukemia, myelofibrosis, or hypoplastic marrow activity, responded favorably to testosterone in about one-third of the patients. Gardner and Pringle (1961a) and Rørdam (1965) reported a beneficial effect of testosterone in multiple myelomatosis, and Hartmann *et al.*, (1965) observed a similar action of an androgen (fluoxymesterone) in patients with paroxysmal nocturnal hemoglobinuria. Kennedy (1964) also found that this compound stimulates erythropoiesis in chronic lymphatic leukemia.

In the clinical trials by Shahidi and Diamond the addition of prednisone (up to 15 mg daily) to the treatment with testosterone (in dosages from 20 to 40 mg per day) gave a better response in the marrow than testosterone alone. Of 40 children treated by this regimen 16 (eight boys and eight girls) showed a definite and sustained increase in the activity of the bone marrow.

Two closely connected questions presented themselves: 1) What is the mechanism through which testosterone operates on an aplastic marrow; and 2) why did over half of the children fail to respond?

The hypothesis that testosterone may act as a metabolic regulator exerting its effect through an initiating reaction in nucleic acid synthesis has been helpful in an attempt to answer these questions. When testosterone is given systemically, the first observable response in an aplastic marrow is proliferation of the few remaining erythroblasts, some of which are found in mitotic division (W. Jacobson, unpublished observations). Such cells must have synthesized a tetraploid complement of deoxyribonucleic acid and their intense cytoplasmic basophilia indicates that ribonucleic acid also is relatively abundant.

In order to determine whether testosterone directly stimulates nucleic acid synthesis, suspensions of bone marrows from 12 children with various disorders (not all hematological) were incubated with tritiated thymidine in the presence and absence of testosterone. In the following sections autoradiographic data are

* This study was supported in part by research grants from the John A. Hartford Foundation and the National Institutes of Health (H2405).

presented which show that five of the 12 marrows incorporated considerably more tritiated thymidine into DNA in the presence of testosterone, two responded only moderately, and five failed to respond.

Material and Methods

Material. The 12 bone marrows studied in this investigation were obtained from children at the Children's Hospital Medical Center, Boston. Two were apparently normal bone marrows, one from a patient with an extradural spinal tumor, and the other from a child who had recovered from an infection. The other patients had been hospitalized with neutropenia (2), aplastic anemia (2, one of the Fanconi type), hypoplastic anemia (during successful treatment with prednisone), idiopathic thrombocytopenia, hemolytic anemia (of unknown type), microcytic anemia, acute leukemia (untreated), and paroxysmal nocturnal hemoglobinuria. This last patient, now 14 years old, had aplastic anemia years ago and was one of two original cases that showed a remarkable spontaneous recovery during puberty.

Brief clinical notes concerning the 12 patients whose bone marrow samples form the basis of this work are given below. They will be referred to by their numbers and are presented here in the sequence in which the bone marrow aspirations were performed.

No.	Name.	Age.	Length of incubation.	Diagnosis
1.	Michelle D.	11 years	18 hr	Acute infection. Normal marrow, after recovery.
2.	Peter F.	6 years	18 hr	Idiopathic thrombocytopenia, untreated.
3.	Charles S.	9 years	18 hr	Acute leukemia, untreated. (95% "blasts" in marrow).
4.	Kendra S.	2 years	4 hr	Neutropenia, untreated.
5.	Susan S.	12 years	20 hr	Hemolytic anemia, unknown cause.
6.	William T.	3 years	5 hr	Aplastic anemia, on prednisone only and not responding. Subsequently failed to respond to testosterone.
7.	James O'L.	8/12 years	6 hr	Hypoplastic anemia, while responding to prednisone.
8.	Thomas M.	9 years	6 hr	Aplastic anemia (Fanconi's) Poor response to medication.
9.	Michael S.	10 years	4 hr	Neutropenia with hemolytic anemia. On corticosteroid therapy.
10.	Kathleen H.	15 years	20 hr	Normal marrow; extradural spinal tumor.
11.	Bruce U.	14 years	4 hr	Recovered aplastic anemia, not on treatment; recently paroxysmal nocturnal hemoglobinuria.
12.	Michael B.	6/12 years	5 hr	Microcytic anemia, due to iron deficiency

Incubation of Marrows and Preparation of Smears. As soon as the marrows were obtained, they were placed in 1.5–3.0 ml of sterile cold Tyrode's salt solution containing 0.1% glucose in a small precooled tube. The tubes were gently shaken, then rested in crushed ice. Within a few minutes the content was aseptically distributed into four sterile tubes: the first was kept as control, to the second 2.88 μg. testosterone had been added, the third contained 2 μc of tritiated thymidine (^{3}H-thymidine, specific activity 2.0 c/mM) in 0.002 ml of sterile water, and the fourth contained both 2.88 μg testosterone and 2 μc of the ^{3}H-thymidine. The testosterone was introduced to tubes two and four as follows: a stock solution was prepared by dissolving 2.88 mg testosterone in 0.1 ml ethanol; this was added slowly to 9.9 ml ice-cold sterile Tyrode's salt solution containing 0.1 ml of normal adult male serum. Then 0.01 ml of this stock suspension, containing 2.88 μg testosterone, was placed in a tube to which the aliquot of marrow suspension was added. All four tubes were sealed and incubated for 2 to 20 hr at 37° C. The volumes in tubes three and four were kept approximately equal, while the amount of marrow suspension used ranged between 0.4 and 1.0 ml, according to the size of the bone marrow sample. At the end of the incubation period the supernatant was pipetted off and smears were prepared from the sediment. All smears were fixed in absolute methanol for 10 min and were dried in air. Autoradiographs were made by dipping the slides in Kodak NTB_2 liquid emulsion (Kopriwa & Leblond, 1962). They were then drained and placed in light-tight boxes in a dry-ice chest at −70° C for 42 hours. The slides were returned to the darkroom and were developed in Kodak Dektol developer for three min at 68° F, placed in Kodak acid fixer for five min and then washed in running tap water for one hour. The preparations were either transferred to methanol and stained immediately or air-dried and stained later. A modified May-Grunwald and Giesma procedure was used: the slides were stained for one to two hr in a saturated solution of May-Grunwald's dye which had been diluted with an equal volume of methanol; they were then transferred without washing to a dilute Giesma solution (1:20) for 6 to 18 hr, washed in glass-distilled water, and air-dried.

Extraction Procedure. In order to determine whether the radioactivity was in the DNA and/or in the RNA fraction of the cells, some methanol-fixed and air-dried smears of marrows incubated with ^{3}H-thymidine or ^{3}H-thymidine and testosterone, were extracted with 5% trichloracetic acid in water at 90° C for 15 min to remove most of the DNA and RNA; or they were extracted with 10% perchloric acid in water at 37°C for 15 min to remove most of the RNA only. The slides were rinsed in water, air-dried and autoradiographs were then prepared as described above.

Classification of Cells. Immature white and red cells were classified as follows: immature white cells included myeloblasts, myelocytes, metamyelocytes and any lymphoblasts that might be present, e.g. in the marrow of the patient with acute leukemia; small lymphocytes and mature granulocytes were excluded. The group of immature red cells included all nucleated red cells. To avoid irregular distribution of cell types on the slides, counts were made in blocks of 250–350 cells. Within each block the slide was scanned systematically by means of a mechanical stage. A total of 1000 immature cells (in five bone marrows) or 2000 immature cells (in seven bone marrows) was considered satisfactory for obtaining percentage figures of immature red or white cells with grains. Deviations from these figures are mentioned specifically in the text.

Grain Counts. These were made with an oil immersion objective (NA 1.3; 2 mm, apochromat) and a × 15 eye piece. They were recorded for the individual cells, but cells with approximately 100 grains or more were recorded as having 110 grains as it was found impossible to obtain accurate figures for such high counts. After the grain counts of the individual cells had been completed, two values were determined for both immature white cells and erythroblasts respectively: 1) the percentages of labeled immature white and red cells, and 2) the average grain count for labeled white and red cells. This latter figure was obtained by dividing the total number of grains in immature white cells and erythroblasts respectively by the number of labeled cells of each type. In addition, immature white cells and erythroblasts with grains were then grouped according to whether they had 1–10, 11–20 grains, etc., up to 91–100 and over 100 grains/cell; those in the last class were recorded to have 110 grains. The one or two grains occasionally found over mature red and white cells were disregarded.

In the two types of control slides from marrows incubated in the salt solution and without ^{3}H-thymidine and either with or without testosterone, no immature white or red cells with more than two grains were found; the total number of grains over immature cells were invariably less than 40 among 1000 immature cells. Thus the results from the marrows exposed to ^{3}H-thymidine were not affected by such low 'background' values.

Results

General Principles of Assessing the Results Obtained by Grain Counts

Two distinct parameters serve to evaluate a positive effect of testosterone on bone marrow cells: the hormone may either cause more cells to take up labeled thymidine and/or induce those cells that are in the synthetic period of the intermitotic phase to incorporate more ^{3}H-thymidine. These two parameters are readily expressed by histograms, where the ordinate represents the percentage of cells containing tritium and the abscissa the average grain count of those labeled

Table 1

Results Obtained from Five Out of Twelve Bone Marrows Responding to Testosterone with Increased Uptake of Tritiated Thymidine*

No., Patient and Diagnosis	Incubation		Immature Whites	Erythroblasts	No. of Immature Cells Counted
1. Michelle D., 11 yr, normal marrow after infection	18 hr	C	9.5% (73)	13% (38)	1000
		T	25% (92)	29% (32)	1000
5. Susan S., 12 yr, hemolytic anemia	20 hr	C	9.7% (88)	22.0% (32)	2000
		T	9.0% (87)	34.6% (55)	2000
9. Michael S., 10 yr, neutropenia hemolyt. anemia	4 hr	C	3.6% (35)	2.4% (14)	2000
		T	11.7% (91)	14.2% (58)	2000
10. Kathleen H., 15 yr, normal marrow extra-dural tum.	20 hr	C	5.2% (86)	6.7% (58)	2000
		T	7.8% (90)	21.5% (89)	2000
12. Michael B., 6/12 microcyt. anemia	5 hr	C	5.4% (77)	7.5% (39)	1000
		T	9.8% (72)	10.3% (60)	1000

* Percent of immature white and red cells with grains are given, and average grain counts for these in parenthesis.

C = controls (incubated without testosterone); T = incubated with testosterone.

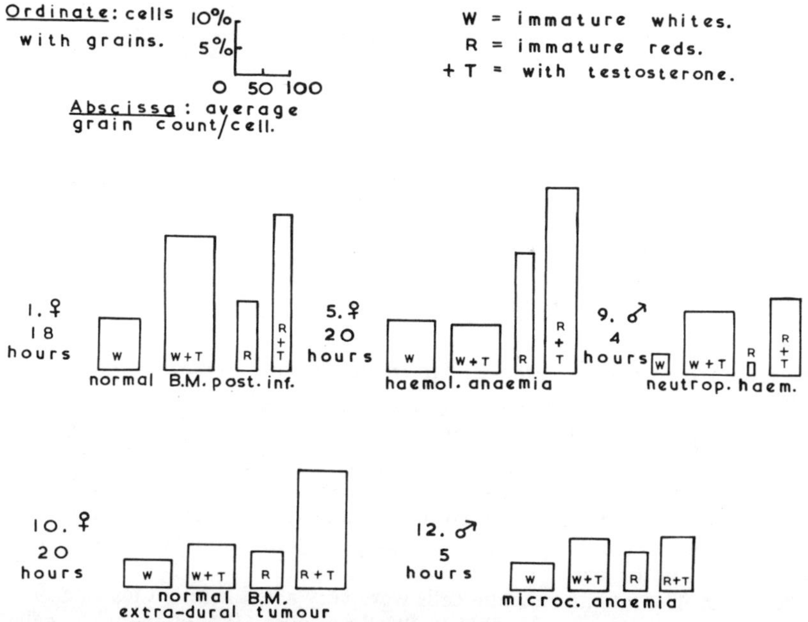

FIGURE 1. Histograms showing the results obtained from autoradiographs of five marrows (out of a total of 12) that responded to testosterone with an increased uptake of tritiated thymidine. Ordinate: percentage of immature white or red cells with grains; abscissa: average grain count per cell with grains. Area = 'product of activity'.

cells; thus the area of each rectangle represents the 'product of activity':

Percent of cells with grains × average grain count per labeled cell

Within each marrow sample these two parameters and their 'product of activity' were used to compare the results obtained in the absence and presence of testosterone. Allowance was also made for the fact that if the average grain count per cell had been close to 100 grains, it would have been impossible to determine any further stimulation of thymidine uptake.

The bone marrows examined can be conveniently arranged in three groups according to their response to incubation with testosterone:

1. Bone marrows that responded with an increase in thymidine uptake; this group comprised the five marrows of patients 1, 5, 9, 10 and 12 (TABLE 1 and FIGURE 1).
2. Bone marrows that showed only a slight increase in thymidine uptake; these were the two marrows of patients 2 and 8 (TABLE 2 and FIGURE 2).
3. Bone marrows that failed to respond to testosterone during the incubation period; this group consisted of the five bone marrows of the patients 3, 4, 6, 7, and 11 (TABLE 3 and FIGURE 3).

Comments on the Bone Marrows

The following brief comments are intended to clarify particular points among the findings. The full details are given in TABLES 1–3 and FIGURES 1–3.

TABLE 2

RESULTS OBTAINED FROM TWO OUT OF TWELVE BONE MARROWS THAT RESPONDED TO TESTOSTERONE WITH ONLY SLIGHTLY INCREASED UPTAKE OF TRITIATED THYMIDINE*

No., Patient and Diagnosis	Incubation		Immature Whites	Erythroblasts	No. of Immature Cells Counted
2. Peter F., 6 yr, idiopath. thrombocytopen.	18 hr	C	9.3% (43)	13.0% (19)	1000
		T	11.0% (67)	16.6% (30)	1000
8. Thomas M., 9 yr, aplastic anemia (Fanconi's)	6 hr	C	4.9% (103)	5.1% (88)	2000
		T	4.8% (99)	10.3% (67)	1670

* For details see footnote to TABLE 1.

The Five Marrows that Responded to Incubation with Testosterone

Patient 1: Under the influence of testosterone the percentage of labeled erythroblasts increased from 13% to 29%, but the average grain count per labeled erythroblast did not rise. This was because more erythroblasts with grain counts below 40 grains per cell were found in the incubate with testosterone than in that without it. Thus testosterone caused more than twice the number of erythroblasts to take up thymidine, but the resultant average grain count was slightly lowered from 38 to 32 grains per cell.

Patient 5: The immature white cells were very active without testosterone, and the average grain count per cells was 88. Since over 60% of the white cells had more than 100 grains per cell, it would have been impossible to detect any but a very conspicuous increase of grains per cell. The number of labeled erythroblasts and the average grain count increased.

Patient 9: This patient's marrow showed a striking response to testosterone both in the number of immature white and red cells taking up labeled thymidine, as well as in the average number of grains per cell. The incubation time of four hr was one of the shortest in the series.

Patient 10: The average grain count among the immature white cells was already high without testosterone. The comment made on the bone marrow of patient 5 applies equally to this specimen. The erythroblast response to testosterone was striking.

Patient 12: Testosterone induced more immature white and red cells to take up thymidine, but the average grain count among the immature white cells did

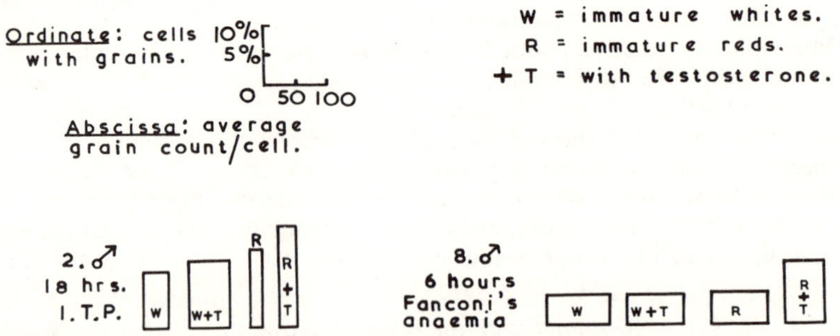

FIGURE 2. Histograms of the results obtained from autoradiographs of two marrows (out of a total of 12) that showed only a slightly increased uptake of tritiated thymidine when incubated with testosterone. For details of symbols see legend to FIGURE 1.

TABLE 3

RESULTS OBTAINED FROM FIVE OUT OF TWELVE BONE MARROWS THAT FAILED TO RESPOND TO TESTOSTERONE DURING INCUBATION WITH TRITIATED THYMIDINE*

No., Patient and Diagnosis	Incubation		Immature Whites	Erythroblasts	No. of Immature Cells Counted
3. Charles S., 9 yr, acute leukemia	18 hr	C	10.8% (77)	20.5% (70)	1000
		T	11.0% (94)	22.3% (48)	1000
4. Kendra S., 2 yr, neutropenia	4 hr	C	8.1% (75)	14.9% (65)	2000
		T	7.7% (64)	13.6% (46)	2000
6. William T., 3 yr, aplastic anemia	5 hr	C	7.4% (65)	8.3% (48)	2000
		T	7.8% (72)	7.8% (44)	2000
7. James O'L., 8/12, hypoplastic anemia	6 hr	C	12.9% (104)	17.2% (40)	1000
		T	9.4% (56)	15.1% (21)	1000
11. Bruce U., 14 yr, parox. noct. hemoglobinuria	2 hr	C	6.1% (64)	12.1% (71)	2000
		T	6.1% (93)	11.2% (77)	1500

* For details see footnote to TABLE 1.

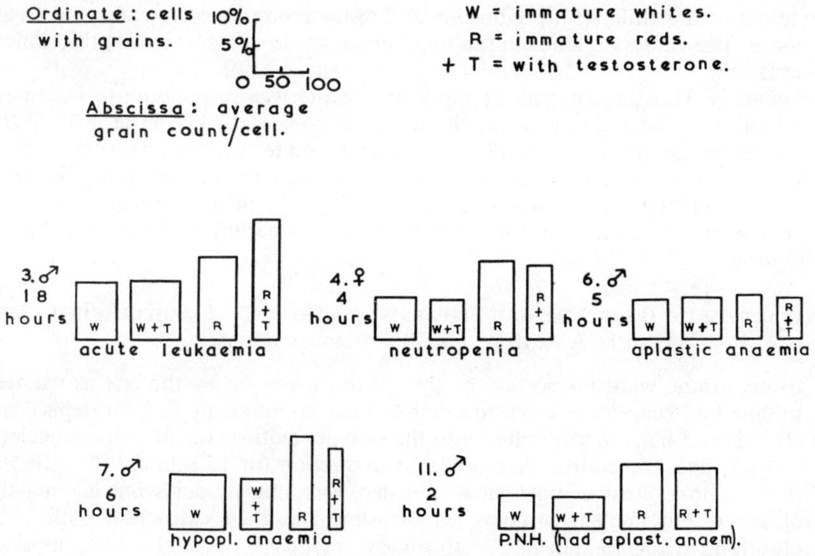

FIGURE 3. Histograms of the results obtained from autoradiographs of five marrows (out of a total of 12) that failed to respond with an increase in uptake of tritiated thymidine when incubated with testosterone. For details of symbols see legend to FIGURE 1.

not increase. This was mainly due to a three-fold increase of cells with less than 50 grains. The 'product of activity' of both cell lines is much increased.

The Two Marrows with a Slight Response to Testosterone

The only comment on this group concern *Patient 8*. In this bone marrow two thousand immature cells from the incubate without testosterone were counted, but only 1670 immature cells were available from the incubate with testosterone. Percentage figures for immature white cells were the same, with and without testosterone; the corresponding average grain counts were 103 and 99. Among the erythroblasts incubated with testosterone the average grain count dropped from 88 to 67. This was mainly due to an increase in the number of erythroblasts with a grain count below 70 grains per cell. The 'product of activity' of the immature red cells is slightly increased.

The Five Marrows That Did Not Respond to Testosterone

Patient 3: The drop in the average grain count among erythroblasts incubated with testosterone was caused mainly by an increase of cells with less than 50 grains per cell.

Patient 4: A possible explanation for the drop in average grain count of the erythroblasts in the incubates from 65 in the controls to 46 with testosterone may be the small number of immature red cells found in the smears prepared from the testosterone incubate; there were only 286 among 2000 cells, in contrast to 449 erythroblasts among 2000 immature cells in the film prepared from the controls, and therefore, the difference may not be significant.

Patient 6: At the time the bone marrow was taken, this patient with aplastic anemia had been on prednisone alone, without benefit. Subsequent prolonged treatment of the child with prednisone and testosterone failed to cause a marrow response. The values obtained in this experiment are in agreement with the clinical observation.

Patient 7: This patient with hypoplastic anemia was responding to treatment with prednisone at the time when the bone marrow was taken. The drop in the thymidine uptake of the erythroblasts incubated with testosterone from an average of 40 grains per cell in the controls to 21 was not observed in any other marrow.

Patient 11: This patient was in remission from the aplastic anemia which he had had several years ago. At the present time he has paroxysmal nocturnal hemoglobinuria.

Extraction of Bone Marrow Smears with Hot 5% Trichloracetic Acid (TCA) and Warm 10% Perchloric Acid

To determine what proportion of the tritium taken up by the cell as tritiated thymidine had been transferred to other cellular components (e.g. proteins) and whether it had been incorporated into the polynucleotides of the cells, especially into DNA, two procedures were used: 1) extraction for 15 min at 90° with 5% TCA to remove most of both ribo- and deoxyribonucleic acids but leaving the cytoplasmic and nuclear proteins on the slides; and 2) extraction with 10% perchloric acid for 15 min at 37° to remove mainly RNA and leaving most of the DNA and proteins in the cells. Sufficient material was available to perform the first extraction of slides of the marrows of four patients (4, 5, 9, and 10) and the second extraction on the slides of the marrows of three patients (4, 5, and 10). In most of these extraction procedures, 1000 immature cells from the incubates

TABLE 4

RESULTS OBTAINED AFTER EXTRACTION WITH 5% TRICHLORACETIC ACID AT 90° C FOR 15 MINUTES TO REMOVE MOST OF THE DNA AND RNA FROM MARROWS*

Case No. and Incubation Time		Immature Whites	Immature Reds	No. of Cells Counted
4. 4 hr	C	8.1% (75) → 3.6% (11)	14.9% (65) → 4% (7)	1000
	T	7.7% (64) → 2.1% (8)	13.6% (46) → 5% (8)	1000
5. 20 hr	C	9.7% (88) → 3.3% (19)	22.0% (32) → 11% (11)	1000
	T	9.0% (87) → 3.7% (20)	34.6% (55) → 16.3% (14)	1000
9. 4 hr	C	3.6% (35) → 2.8% (9)	2.4% (14) → 2.2% (6)	1000
	T	11.7% (91) → 4.7% (9)	14.2% (58) → 3.5% (5)	1000
10. 20 hr	C	5.2% (86) → 2.4% (30)	6.7% (58) → 4.1% (11)	1000
	T	7.8% (90) → 3.4% (13)	21.5% (89) → 11.7% (10)	1000

* The grain counts are much reduced in immature white and immature red cells. The changes are indicated by the first % figures representing % of cells with grains in unextracted smears; the second % figures represent % of cells with grains on extracted smears; in brackets are given the average grain counts/cell.

C = controls (incubated with tritiated thymidine without testosterone).

T = incubated with tritiated thymidine and testosterone.

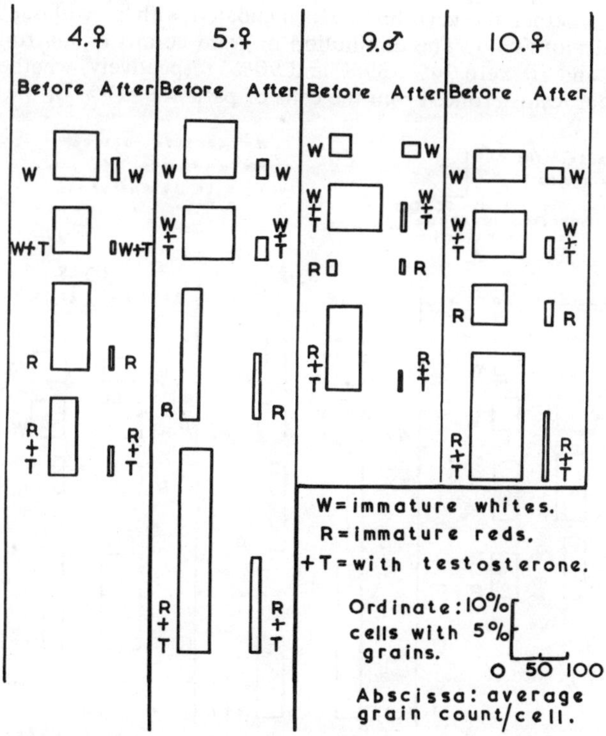

FIGURE 4. Histograms showing the effect of extraction of bone marrow smears with 5% trichloracetic acid at 90° C for 15 minutes to remove most of the DNA and RNA. Autoradiographs were made on one slide before extraction and on another slide from the same marrow incubate after extraction. For details of symbols see legend to FIGURE 1.

TABLE 5

RESULTS OBTAINED AFTER EXTRACTION WITH 10% PERCHLORIC ACID AT 37° C FOR 15 MINUTES TO REMOVE MAINLY RNA*

Case No. and Incubation Time		Immature Whites	Immature Reds	No. of Cells Counted
4. 4 hr	C	8.1% (75) → 7.6% (53)	14.9% (65) → 13.3% (54)	1000
	T	7.7% (64) → 7.1% (56)	13.6% (46) → 10.1% (57)	1000
5. 20 hr	C	9.7% (88) → 10.0% (45)	22.0% (32) → 19.6% (32)	1000
	T	9.0% (87) → 7.9% (62)	34.6% (55) → 18.3% (56)	870
10. 20 hr	C	5.2% (86) → 6.6% (74)	6.7% (58) → 8.0% (25)	1000
	T	7.8% (90) → 8.4% (76)	21.5% (89) → ** (44)	600

* The grain counts are only slightly reduced. For details see footnote to TABLE 4.

** 13 cells only.

with and without testosterone, respectively, were counted and immature white cells and erythroblasts were again recorded separately.

EFFECT OF THE EXTRACTION WITH HOT 5% TCA ON GRAIN COUNTS OF AUTORADIOGRAPHS (TO REMOVE MOST OF THE RNA AND DNA)

This procedure greatly reduced the grain counts of immature white cells and erythroblasts whether the cells had been incubated with or without testosterone (TABLE 4 and FIGURE 4). The diminution in grain counts of marrow cells from patients 4, 5, and 10 were 96%, 89% and 90%, respectively, whether incubated with or without testosterone. From the cells of patient 9, 97% of the grains were

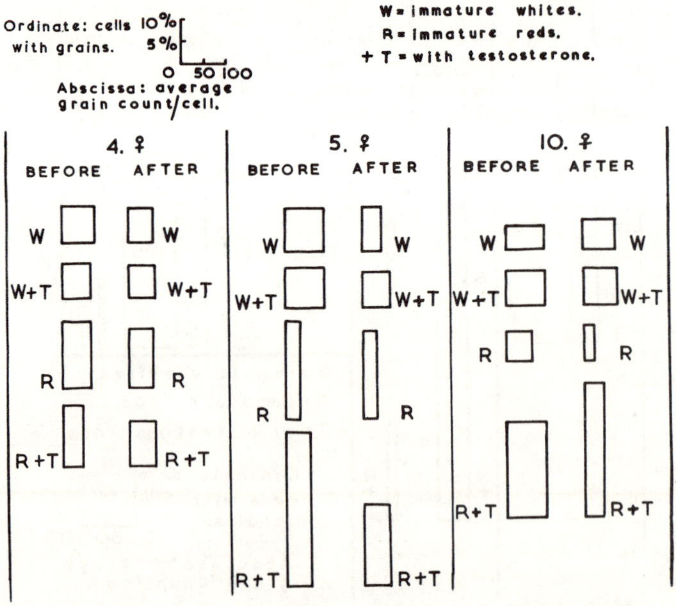

FIGURE 5. Histograms showing the effect of extraction of bone marrow smears with 10% perchloric acid at 37° C for 15 minutes to remove mainly RNA. Autoradiographs were made on one slide before extraction and on another slide from the same marrow incubate after extraction. For details of symbols see legend to FIGURE 1.

extracted from the incubate with testosterone, though from the preparation of the incubate without testosterone only 71% of the grains were lost; this unusually small reduction is unexplained. The average percentage of grains lost by extraction with hot trichloracetic acid was 90% for these four patients. Thus it can be assumed that the bulk of the tritium had not been transferred to other cellular components, e.g. cytoplasmic or nuclear proteins, which were not extracted by this procedure.

Effect of the Extraction with Warm 10% Perchloric Acid on Grain Counts (To Remove Mainly RNA)

This extraction procedure removes that fraction of thymidine that is either not incorporated into DNA or, after demethylation, has been incorporated into RNA. After the extraction the cells of the marrow of patient 4 retained 77% of their grains, those of patient 5 retained 65%, and those of patient 10 kept 78%. The average percentage of grains retained was 75%. From these results (TABLE 5 and FIGURE 5) it may be concluded that a very substantial fraction of the tritiated thymidine taken up by the cells during incubation had been incorporated into DNA.

Discussion

The autoradiograms record radioactivity (tritium) but do not indicate what species of molecules are radioactive. Several lines of evidence indicate that the silver grains represent DNA newly synthesized from ^{3}H-thymidine. Marrow cells incubated without thymidine, with or without testosterone, gave autoradiograms with negligible numbers of silver grains; nonradioactive cell constituents and the testosterone itself did not reduce silver grains. Autoradiograms of cells that had been incubated with ^{3}H-thymidine, smeared on slides and immersed in methanol and then in aqueous emulsion, contained silver grains distributed almost exclusively over cell nuclei; the radioactive label was in a relatively insoluble nuclear polymer. Most of the radioactivity was removed by hot trichloracetic and not by warm perchloric acid, properties characteristic of labeled DNA. Thus, immature red and white cells of normal and assorted diseased human marrows, like most (though not all) other cell types, incorporate thymidine almost exclusively into DNA.

Only large effects of testosterone were considered valid in this study for many reasons. The patients varied markedly in age and no three of them had the same disease. Other variables were poorly controlled, including severity of illness and therapeutic history preceding bone marrow biopsy. Examination of the Tables shows that more consistent data were obtained on the percentages of cells labeled than on the average grain counts. The grain counts are no more than semiquantitative for they are modified by many factors such as ^{3}H-thymidine dose per cell in the marrow suspensions, variations in the intracellular nucleic acid precursor pool, and local variations in cell and emulsion thickness on the slides. Another variable is the duration of marrow incubation which ranged from 2 to 20 hours. In this small series of marrows, it appears that a four-hour incubation may be as effective as longer ones; ^{3}H-thymidine incorporation (DNA synthesis) may have been limited to the first few hours. No attempt was made to determine either the latency of the response of immature blood cells to testosterone or the duration of the response.

During these relatively short incubation periods no effect of testosterone on maturation processes in the white or red cell lineage was observed, and the distribution pattern of the various stages of maturation remained very similar in the marrows whether they had been incubated with or without testosterone. The stimulation of nucleic acid synthesis in immature white and red cells is only one of the many effects of this hormone in children; some metabolic processes are stimulated, while others may be inhibited (as will be mentioned later). When confronted with such heterogeneous side effects on different components of the organism, it seems relevant to put the observations in this report into proper perspective among the multiplicity of the effects of testosterone.

Not only are there many facets to the mode of action of this steroid on different tissues, but the same tissue may respond differently during different stages of its development, an important consideration when attempting to extrapolate from the results obtained in investigations on children to related phenomena in adult patients. These problems will now be discussed.

Some Actions of Testosterone on Nonproliferating and Proliferating Tissues

In nonproliferating tissues the hormone may affect certain metabolic processes that are probably not connected with DNA synthesis, e.g. in the hypertrophy induced in individual skeletal muscle fibres which increase in diameter without mitosis.

In proliferating tissues, such as bone marrow, hair follicles, seminiferous tubules or the developing prostate and seminal vesicle, the hormone can induce mitosis by either direct or indirect action; in either case, the stimulation of mitosis must be preceded by increased synthesis of DNA.

Mitosis may be followed by cellular differentiation and synthesis of specific proteins may be induced, resulting in maturation of blood cells, keratinization of the cells of the hair follicles, spermatogenesis in the testes or secretion in such glands as the prostate and seminal vesicle. It is of interest that after puberty, once these gland cells have attained the adult size, secretion continues under the influence of the hormone while replication of DNA and mitosis are much reduced. Conversely, in other proliferating tissues such as mammary glands, endometrium and the granulosa cells of the ovarian follicles, the action of testosterone may retard the synthesis of DNA and RNA. Furthermore, the hormone may simultaneously stimulate the synthesis of DNA and inhibit other metabolic processes in the same cell line, as will be discussed later in connection with production of erythroblasts and the synthesis of hemoglobin.

Biochemical Effect of Testosterone on Bone Marrow Cells

In a previous investigation (Jacobson, 1965) it was shown that the addition of low doses of testosterone (from about 0.12 to 0.004 μmole/ml) to bone marrow lysates accelerated the activity of glucose-6-phosphate dehydrogenase (G-6-P-D). These bone marrows were from children without hematological disorders and also from those with aplastic anemia and a range of other hematological diseases. None of them had a deficiency of the enzyme. In these experiments when sufficiently low concentrations of the enzyme (contained in the bone marrow lysate) were added to the reaction mixture to be the rate-limiting factor, testosterone increased the rate of reaction by 5–15%. Neither cholesterol nor estradiol has this effect. That the enhancing effect of testosterone on the activity of G-6-P-D was dependent on the enzyme being the rate-limiting factor in the reaction was shown in experiments in which the concentration of enzyme was increased without altering the concentration of coenzyme (TPN 0.3 μmole/ml) and substrate (glucose-6-phosphate, 3.3 μmole/ml); the reaction proceeded rapidly and no effect of testosterone was demonstrable.

It is conceivable that the direct action of testosterone on the activity of this enzyme may influence the rate of nucleic acid synthesis in marrow cells in the following way. The first step in nucleic acid synthesis (whether of the DNA or RNA type) depends on the availability of ribose-5-phosphate which is derived from glucose-6-phosphate by the enzymes of the pentose-phosphate path. The first three enzymes of this path convert glucose-6-phosphate via 6-phosphogluconolactone, (which spontaneously changes into 6-phosphogluconate) and ribulose-5-phosphate to ribose-5-phosphate. Glucose-6-phosphate is a metabolite that can enter into several metabolic paths, among which are glycolysis via fructose-6-phosphate for 'energy' supply, or polymerization via glucose-1-phosphate for 'storage' as glycogen, or the pentose-phosphate shunt for 'synthesis' as mentioned above. Glucose-6-phosphate dehydrogenase is the first enzyme on the pentose-phosphate path. Testosterone may operate in aplastic bone marrows as well as in other tissues by enhancing the first reaction of the pentose-phosphate path, thus shunting glucose-6-phosphate from the crossroads of intermediate metabolism at a slightly increased rate into the channel that leads to ribose-5-phosphate. Thus more ribose-5-phosphate might be available to erythroblasts and granulocyte precursors in a bone marrow under the influence of testosterone.

Whether there is a direct connection between the increased incorporation of thymidine and the stimulating effect of testosterone on an enzyme that holds a key position in the metabolism of normally growing bone marrows, via glucose-6-phosphate dehydrogenase, cannot be stated at present. Both observed phenomena would seem to operate in the same direction.

In this connection an observation by Shahidi (1963) is of interest. He found that children with aplastic anemia under the standard treatment with testosterone and corticosteroids formed hypochromic red cells. The lowered mean concentration of corpuscular hemoglobin (excluding a concomitant iron deficiency) was caused by testosterone, since children with a pure red cell anemia with hypoplastic bone marrow under the standard treatment with corticosteroids alone did not form hypochromic red cells. Thus it appears that testosterone does not stimulate hemoglobin synthesis and in fact, may delay it, as indicated by the presence of increased free porphyrin in the erythrocytes. We have then a situation where a hormone stimulates some synthetic metabolic paths, but may delay others within the same cell.

Possible Primary Sites of Action of Testosterone on Bone Marrow and Other Tissues

Recently there have been several investigations of the effect of testosterone on the synthesizing activity of isolated cellular components. Liao and Williams-Ashman (1962) studied the rate of incorporation of amino acids into protein in ribosomal preparations from prostates of castrated rats. Testosterone added directly to this in vitro system had no effect on protein synthesis, but a day or two after the injection of hormone into a castrated animal the incorporation of amino acids in this ribosomal system was increased to the level obtained in preparations from noncastrated rats. In other words, the transfer of the labeled amino acids from s-RNA via ribosomes to protein did not respond to testosterone added directly in vitro. This interesting observation indicates that testosterone may operate, in the chain of events leading to increased protein synthesis, at a point preceding ribosomal activity. Liao (1965) observed on the ventral prostate of the castrated rat that testosterone enhances the levels of nuclear template (messenger) RNA which is complementary to DNA. Thus ribosomal activity of this gland is stimulated to synthesize more protein. Wicks and Kenney (1964) were able to show, by pulse labeling RNA in vivo, that seminal vesicles of adult rats castrated 15 hr previously synthesized 50% more RNA when the castrated animal had been injected with testosterone 20 min previously. Within 50 min after the injection of the hormone RNA synthesis had reached a plateau of two to three times that of the noninjected castrates; there was no effect at ten min after the injection. These interesting findings mean that the synthesis of a messenger-like RNA, among others, is stimulated by the injection of testosterone at a very early stage in the response of the seminal vesicle of the adult castrated rat.

The question arises as to whether these observations provide a clue to the primary action of testosterone on the bone marrow. The adult seminal vesicle of the rat, 15 hr after castration, showed only a decrease in individual cell size and responded to testosterone by resuming secretory function. It would be unlikely however for the seminal vesicle of the adult rat to undergo a proliferative (mitotic) response, as the whole organ and its cells were of mature adult size.

Thus we find that both of the investigations discussed above deal with adult glands, in which testosterone evokes increased synthesis first of RNA and, subsequently of proteins, but in contrast to its effect on immature glands, does not induce cellular multiplication. Of the three parameters of testosterone effects—increased mitosis, synthesis of RNA, and specific protein synthesis (e.g. for secretion)—the first is not a prominent feature in the accessory sex glands of the adult male rat.

By contrast, a positive response to testosterone in an aplastic marrow requires two types of cellular processes to be set in motion: 1) cellular multiplication, i.e., reduplication of all nuclear and cytoplasmic components including DNA, and 2) differentiation, i.e., the de novo synthesis of specific cell components, e.g. enzymes or hemoglobin. These latter syntheses must be preceded by the synthesis of specific ribosomal RNA, which can occur only if DNA-dependent messenger RNA has been made available. Whether some special RNA or protein induces resumption of DNA synthesis is not known. Whatever the first trigger mechanism for cell multiplication and differentiation in bone marrow may be, the de novo syntheses of purines and pyrimidines are likely to be very early stages in the response. In this connection it is of interest that one of the first steps preceding the synthesis of nucleotides is directly affected by testosterone, namely, the rate of activity of glucose-6-phosphate dehydrogenase.

The resumption of DNA synthesis in an aplastic marrow or its stimulation in a functioning marrow may precede the synthesis of specific cellular components, e.g. that of the lysosomal enzymes contained in the cytoplasmic granules of the immature granulocytes, or of hemoglobin in the erythroblasts. The formation of both these cellular constituents requires an increase in ribosomal material (RNA and protein) in the proliferating cells after completion of mitosis. The increased synthesis of DNA within a few hours of incubation with testosterone in some of the bone marrows, found in the present experiment, must be only one of the links, presumably an early one, in the chain of events expressed as a clinical response to testosterone. The observations by Wilson *et al.* (1965) on the duck's preen gland are of special interest. They found 60–100% of the testosterone-1,2-^{3}H bound to the histone of the euchromatin fraction within the cell nuclei of the gland. This indicates that testosterone operates by affecting the activity of this specific fraction of DNA.

Mirand *et al.* (1965) found that testosterone increases the level of the plasma erythropoiesis-stimulating factor (ESF, erythropoietin) in normal mice, rats, rabbits and tamarins (a primate). Similar observations were made on mice by Guerney *et al.* (1965). However, it is unlikely that the testosterone-induced remissions in children with aplastic anemia, as reportd by Shahidi and Diamond (1959 and 1961), were brought about by increased production of this factor. Measurements of erythropoietin in children with aplastic anemia have been made in our clinic and in several others, and the level was found to be markedly elevated before the testosterone treatment was begun in these patients, (unpublished data). Moreover, the lower the red cell count, the higher the erythropoietin level. Patients with aplastic anemia were unable to respond to erythropoietin administered in low or high dosages. As testosterone therapy became effective and the patient formed new red cells, the erythropoietin level fell.

Response and Failure to Respond to Testosterone

It is perplexing that while some bone marrows respond to testosterone, others do not. This applies to the clinical result, to the incorporation of thymidine by suspension of bone marrow cells, and to the activation of glucose-6-phosphate dehydrogenase (G-6-P-D) in lysates. Approximately 40% of the marrows responded to testosterone in these different systems, whether from aplastic or other patients. It is interesting that West (1965) observed similar percentages of positive responses to testosterone in a large series of patients with chronic lymphatic leukemia, myelofibrosis and 'hypoplastic' (aplastic?) anemia. In this connection attention may be drawn to the study of G-6-P-D in peripheral blood cells by Boyer *et al.* (1962) and Kirkman *et al.* (1963). These authors found that there are at least two general types of G-6-P-D (A and B) in both red and white cells; the two types could be distinguished by their electrophoretic mobility. Furthermore, in the blood cells of any given patient, each type (A and B) can be resolved into several variants, up to six isoenzymes. The protein moieties of G-6-P-D (the apoenzyme) have different charges and therefore different spatial configurations. A planar molecule like testosterone might fit better on one variant of the enzyme molecule than on another, and thus cause either activation or even steric hindrance (see below).

At present nothing is known about the isoenzymes of glucose-6-phosphate dehydrogenase in the bone marrow cells of normal children, or in those with aplastic anemia. Enlightening studies like those of Boyer and Kirkman and their colleagues have not yet been made in relation to the bone marrow in aplastic anemia. The problem need not be confined to the activation of marrow cells in children with aplastic anemia, as the hormone has been used for its stimulating effect on erythropoiesis in the treatment of adults with a variety of malignancies, and as an adjuvant in the treatment of carcinoma of the breast, where it causes a 'hindrance' of proliferation of the malignant tissue in some patients. In each of these diseases we are confronted by the same question: why do some patients respond to testosterone while others fail to? A study of the isoenzymes of glucose-6-phosphate dehydrogenase may possibly shed some light on this problem.

A comprehensive and most stimulating review of the action of steroid hormones has just been published by Williams-Ashman (1965).

Summary

Twelve bone marrows of children with a variety of diseases (not all hematological disorders) were incubated with tritiated thymidine in the absence and presence of testosterone. Five marrows responded to the hormone with greatly increased uptake of labeled thymidine. Extraction with 5% trichloracetic acid to remove most of the DNA and RNA of the cells reduced the grain counts by 90% in subsequent autoradiographs. Extraction with 10% perchloric acid to remove mainly RNA reduced the grain counts by 25%. It is concluded that under the influence of testosterone DNA synthesis in some bone marows is stimulated within a few hours.

One of the mechanisms through which testosterone may stimulate cellular proliferation in some bone marrows could be to increase the rate of activity of the enzyme, glucose-6-phosphate dehydrogenase (G-6-P-D). The idea is put forward that the failure of testosterone to stimulate other marrows may possibly be associated with the configuration of the isoenzymes of G-6-P-D.

Acknowledgment

The authors wish to acknowledge the skillful help given to them in this work and in the preparation of the manuscript by: Miss Jennifer Ambrose (Strangeways Research Laboratory, Cambridge), and Miss Sheila Sadlon (Children's Hospital, Boston, Massachusetts): Professor Dame Honor Fell, F.R.S., Director of the Strangeways Research Laboratory, and Dr. T. Fainstat (Strangeways Research Laboratory and Boston Lying-in Hospital) contributed by their continued interest and many stimulating discussions.

References

Adair, F. E., R. C. Mellors, J. H. Farrow, H. G. Woodward, G. C. Escher & J. A. Urban. 1949. The use of estrogens and androgens in advanced mammary cancer. J. Amer. Med. Assoc. **140:** 1193–1200.

Boyer, S. H., J. H. Porter & R. G. Weilbacher. 1962. Electrophoretic heterogeneity of glucose-6-phosphate dehydrogenase and its relationship to enzyme deficiency in man. Proc. Nat. Acad. Sci. **48:** 1868–1876.

Diamond, L. K., W. Jacobson & R. Sidman. 1966. Biochemical analysis of the stimulating effect of testosterone on the bone marrow of children with aplastic anemia. Proc. 10th Congr. Europ. Soc. Haematol. : 212. S. Karger. Basle and New York. In press.

Erf, L. A. & P. A. Herbut. 1944. Primary and secondary myelofibrosis, clinical and pathological study of 13 cases of fibrosis of the bone marrow. Ann. Int. Med. **21:** 863–889.

Gardner, F. H. & J. C. Pringle, Jr. 1961. Androgens and erythropoiesis. I. Preliminary clinical observations. Arch. Int. Med. **107:** 846–862.

Gardner, F. H. & J. C. Pringle, Jr. 1961. Androgens and erythropoiesis. II. Treatment of myeloid metaplasia. New Eng. J. Med. **264:** 103–111.

Gurney, C. W. & W. Fried. 1965. The mechanism of action of androgens on erythropoiesis. J. Clin. Invest. **44:** 1057.

Hartmann, R. C., D. E. Jenkins, Jr., L. C. McKee & R. M. Heyssel. 1966. Studies on P.N.H.: Iron metabolism and therapy with androgens and iron. Proc. 10th Congr. Europ. Soc. Haematology : 273–274. S. Karger. Basle and New York. In press.

Jacobson, W. 1965. The basis of treatment with steroids in some malignancies and in aplastic anemia of children. *In* The Treatment of Cancer. : 222–240. Cambridge University Press. Cambridge, England.

Kennedy, B. J. 1962. Stimulation of erythropoiesis by androgenic hormones. Ann. Int. Med. **57:** 917–936.

Kennedy, B. J. 1964. Androgenic hormone therapy in lymphatic leukemia. J. Amer. Med. Assoc. **190:** 1130–1133.

Kennedy, B. J. & A. S. Gilbertsen. 1957. Increased erythropoiesis induced by androgenic hormone therapy. New Eng. J. Med. **256:** 720–726.

Kirkman, H. N. & E. M. Hendrickson. 1963. Sex-linked electrophoretic difference in glucose-6-phosphate dehydrogenase. Amer. J. Hum. Genet. **15:** 241–258.

Kopriwa, B. M. & C. P. Leblond. 1962. Improvements in the coating technique of radioautography. J. Histochem. Cytochem. **10:** 269–284.

LIAO, S. 1965. Influence of testosterone on template activity of prostatic ribonucleic acids. J. Biol. Chem. **240**: 1236–1243.

LIAO, S. & H. G. WILLIAMS-ASHMAN. 1962. An effect of testosterone on amino acid incorporation by prostatic ribonucleoprotein particles. Proc. Nat. Acad. Sci. **48**: 1956–1964.

MCCULLAGH, E. P. & T. R. JONES. 1941. A note on the effect of certain androgens upon the red blood cell count and upon glucose tolerance. Cleveland Clinic Quart. **8**: 79–84.

MCCULLAGH, E. P. & T. R. JONES. 1942. Effect of androgens on blood counts of men. J. Clin. Endrocrinol. **2**: 243–251.

MIRAND, E. A., A. S. GORDON & J. WENIG. 1965. Mechanism of testosterone action in erythropoiesis. Nature **206**: 270–272.

RØRDAM, P. 1966. Combined treatment with melphalan and testosterone propionate of myelomatosis. Proc. 10th Congr. Europ. Soc. Haematology : 405. S. Karger. Basle and New York. In press.

ROSENTHAL, N. & L. A. ERF. 1943. Clinical observations on osteoporosis and myelofibrosis. Arch. Int. Med. **71**: 793–812.

SHAHIDI, N. T. 1963. Morphologic and biochemical characteristics of erythrocytes in testosterone-induced remission in patients with acquired and constitutional aplastic anemia. J. Lab. Clin. Med. **62**: 294–305.

SHAHIDI, N. T. & L. K. DIAMOND. 1959. Testosterone-induced remission in aplastic anemia. A. M. A. J. Dis. Child. **98**: 293–302.

SHAHIDI, N. T. & L. K. DIAMOND. 1961. Testosterone-induced remission in aplastic anemia of both acquired and congenital types. New Eng. J. Med. **264**: 953–967.

TALBOT, T. R., JR. & G. C. ESCHER. 1949. The effect of testosterone propionate on the peripheral blood and bone marrow of women with advanced inoperable carcinoma of the breast. Preliminary report. J. Clin. Endocr. **9**: 666.

WEST, W. O. 1965. The treatment of bone marrow failure with massive androgen therapy. Ohio State Med. J. **61**: 347–355.

WICKS, W. D. & F. T. KENNEY. 1964. RNA synthesis in rat seminal vesicles: stimulation by testosterone. Science **144**: 1346–1357.

WILLIAMS-ASHMAN, H. G. 1965. New facets of the biochemistry of steroid hormone action. Cancer Res. **25**: 1096–1120.

WILSON, J. D. & P. M. LOEB. 1965. Localization of testosterone-1,2-^{3}H in the preen gland of the duck. J. Clin. Invest. **44**: 1111.

EFFECTS OF ACETYLCHOLINESTERASE ON ERYTHROPOIESIS IN POLYCYTHEMIC AND MILDLY PLETHORIC MICE*

Alan I. Samuels, Lotte Moller and James W. Fisher

Department of Pharmacology, University of Tennessee Medical Units, Memphis, Tenn.

Acetylcholinesterase has been reported to produce a reticulocytosis in intact rats.[1] We were prompted to study the erythropoietic effects of acetylcholinesterase by the recent findings of Allen *et al.*[2,3] concerning a fraction of anemic mouse plasma separated by acrylamide gel electrophoresis. This esterase-positive band contained most of the erythropoietic activity in the plasma and was eserine-sensitive, suggesting the presence of cholinesterase. This erythropoietically active plasma band was also found to be testosterone-dependent.[2] The present study is a comparison of the effects of various dosages of acetylcholinesterase in polycythemic and mildly plethoric mice.

Materials and Methods

Female Swiss-Webster strain mice (20–25 g) were made polycythemic or mildly plethoric by a technique previously reported by Fried and Gurney.[4] Mice were made polycythemic by injecting 0.4 ml hematocrit 80 blood i.p. on days 1 and 2 (total 0.8 ml) of the study. The mildly plethoric mice were injected i.p. with 0.2 ml hematocrit 80 blood (total 0.4 ml) on the first two days of the study. Acetylcholinesterase** in saline was injected s.c. on days 1, 2, 3 and 4 at dosages of 25 or 200 units per day. When sheep erythropoietin† was injected, the total dose in saline was given on the fourth day in two divided doses at five-hour intervals. The mice were injected with 0.5 μc ^{59}Fe citrate i.p. on the sixth day, exsanguinated on the ninth day and ^{59}Fe incorporation in red cells determined. Microhematocrits were determined with heparinized capillary tubes. The technique of Dunnett[5,6] for comparing several treatments with a single control was used for the statistical analyses.

Results and Discussion

As seen in TABLE 1, daily dosages of 25 and 200 units of acetylcholinesterase failed to produce a significant erythropoietic effect in polycythemic mice, whereas 1.0 unit of sheep erythropoietin produced a significant increase in ^{59}Fe incorporation in red cells of polycythemic animals. A dosage of 1.0 unit sheep erythropoietin injected concurrently with 25 units acetylcholinesterase was less effective in polycythemic animals than 1.0 unit erythropoietin alone.

A dosage of 200 units acetylcholinesterase (TABLE 2) produced a significant increase in ^{59}Fe incorporation in red cells of mildly plethoric mice when compared with saline controls. A combination of 1.0 unit erythropoietin and 200 units acetylcholinesterase was less effective on ^{59}Fe incorporation in mildly plethoric mice than 1.0 unit erythropoietin alone. This may represent an antagonistic action of acetylcholinesterase on sheep erythropoietin. A slight erythropoietic effect was seen in mildly plethoric mice with the 25-unit dosage of acetylcholinesterase.

* This work was supported by USPHS grant AM–02973–07 HEM.

** Acetylcholinesterase from bovine erythrocytes containing 20,000 Ammon units per 150 mg of material was obtained from Nutritional Biochemical Corp., Cleveland, Ohio.

† Step III sheep erythropoietin was supplied by the USPHS Hematology Study Section of the National Heart Institute.

TABLE 1

EFFECTS OF ACETYLCHOLINESTERASE AND SHEEP ERYTHROPOIETIN IN POLYCYTHEMIC MICE

Group	No. Mice	Hematocrit (Percent)	Percent ^{59}Fe Incorporation in RBC
Saline control	6	56 ± 2.0	0.48 ± .17
Sheep erythropoietin 1.0 unit	7	59 ± 2.2	9.61 ± 2.49*
Acetylcholinesterase 25 units × four days	6	52 ± 2.3	0.59 ± .31
Acetylcholinesterase 200 units × four days	4	47 ± 2.5	0.36 ± .01
Acetylcholinesterase 25 units × four days plus Sheep erythropoietin 1.0 unit	7	56 ± 3.1	5.56 ± 1.58*

* Indicates significantly different from saline controls at the 1% level.
± = Standard error of the mean.

These findings are similar to those reported by Fried *et al.*[4] for testosterone. It is not known why acetylcholinesterase, as well as testosterone, is more effective in mildly plethoric than in polycythemic mice. Testosterone probably acts primarily to increase production of erythropoietin through an action on the kidney. It is quite possible that acetylcholinesterase acts through a similar mechanism, or is involved in an intermediate step in the action of testosterone on the kidney. The kidneys of mildly plethoric mice may be more responsive than those of polycythemic animals to stimuli such as testosterone and acetylcholinesterase, which appear to stimulate erythropoiesis by enhancing endogenous erythropoietin production. It is also possible that these stimuli depend upon a

TABLE 2

EFFECTS OF ACETYLCHOLINESTERASE AND SHEEP ERYTHROPOIETIN IN MILDLY PLETHORIC MICE

Group	No. Mice	Hematocrit (Percent)	Percent ^{59}Fe Incorporation in RBC
Saline control	14	48.4 ± .34	2.15 ± .61
Sheep erythropoietin 1.0 unit	14	46.9 ± 1.71	17.55 ± 3.01*
Acetylcholinesterase 25 units × four days	15	44.4 ± 1.31	3.20 ± 1.03
Acetylcholinesterase 200 units × four days	13	41.3 ± 1.11	10.40 ± 1.04*
Acetylcholinesterase 25 units × four days plus Sheep erythropoietin 1.0 unit	12	45.6 ± 1.34	17.08 ± 1.60*
Acetylcholinesterase 200 units × four days plus Sheep erythropoietin 1.0 unit	8	49.1 ± 2.48	9.39 ± 1.30*

* Indicates significantly different from saline controls at the 1% level.
± = Standard error of the mean.

certain plasma level of an erythropoietin precursor substance which is acted upon by cholinesterase to produce biologically active erythropoietin. This plasma substrate may be present in mildly plethoric animals but diminished or absent in polycythemic mice. Acetylcholinesterase may act in a manner similar to that of the renal erythropoietic factor which has been postulated to form a complex with a plasma protein to generate erythropoietin.[7]

Summary

Acetylcholinesterase has been found to exert a significant erythropoietic effect in mildly plethoric mice but did not produce an observable effect in polycythemic mice. The significance of these findings is discussed.

Acknowledgments

The authors acknowledge the technical assistance of Mrs. Judy Parker and Mr. Carroll Osburn in these studies.

References

1. Davis, J. E. 1960. Erythropoietic stimulating action of acetylcholinesterase. Proc. Soc. Exp. Biol. Med. **107:** 698.
2. Allen, R. C. & D. J. Moore. 1966. Sex-associated quantitative differences in the plasma esterases of inbred mice. Endocrinology **78:** 655.
3. Allen, R. C. & R. Hunter. To be published.
4. Fried, W. & C. W. Gurney. 1963. Use of mild plethora to demonstrate an erythropoietic effect from small amounts of androgens. Proc. Soc. Exp. Biol. Med. **120:** 519.
5. Dunnett, C. W. 1955. Multiple comparison procedure for comparing several treatments with a control. J. Amer. Stat. Assoc. **50:** 1096.
6. Dunnett, C. W. 1964. New tables for multiple comparisons with a control. Biometrics **20:** 482.
7. Kuratowska, Z., B. Lewartowski & B. Lipinski. 1964. Chemical and biologic properties of an erythropoietin-generating substance obtained from perfusates of isolated anoxic kidneys. J. Lab. Clin. Med. **64:** 226.

DISCUSSION

T. P. McDonald

University of Tennessee Memorial Research Center and Hospital, Knoxville, Tenn.

It has been repeatedly demonstrated that testosterone stimulates erythropoiesis in female mice[1–8] and rats[9] to a greater degree than in their male counterparts.[2,9,10] A number of mechanisms have been postulated to account for this effect. According to one concept, testosterone alters the kidney in some way so that it produces a greater than normal amount of erythropoietin.[2,5,11] Other workers[1,4,12] have suggested that testosterone may act directly or that the hormones may act synergistically. If the latter is true, part of the effect of testosterone on erythropoiesis could be a direct action on bone marrow cells similar to current theories of erythropoietin action.

To test this hypothesis, we have added water-soluble testosterone (testosterone hydrogen succinate sodium salt) to rabbit bone marrow cells in the presence of anemic rabbit serum as a source of erythropoietin. Young female New Zealand rabbits, weighing approximately 2.5 kg, were used. The animals were killed by exsanguination, the femurs, tibiae and humeri opened and the bone marrow spooned out into 37° C Hanks' solution. The cells were dispersed by forcing the marrow through various-sized needles and resuspended in Eagle's minimum essential medium so that each culture contained $10–15 \times 10^6$ cells. Serum and 0.03 μc of ^{59}Fe were added and the cells incubated at 37° C for 21½ hours. The cells were then washed and ^{59}Fe incorporation determined.

The results of two bone marrow cultures are shown in FIGURE 1. This graph shows that 1 mg of testosterone significantly reduced the percent ^{59}Fe uptake when compared to the saline-controls ($P < 0.01$). In addition, the tubes containing 0.5 mg of testosterone in experiment no. 92 had significantly ($P < 0.01$) lower ^{59}Fe incorporation than tubes containing 0.25 mg of testosterone or the saline-treated controls.

In FIGURE 2, data from experiment no. 95 show almost identical results with or without anemic rabbit serum as a source of erythropoietin. Again, 1 mg of testosterone significantly ($P < 0.01$) reduced the ^{59}Fe uptake. In experiment no. 96 there was a significant ($P < 0.01$) increase in ^{59}Fe incorporation due to erythropoietin, but the reduction in ^{59}Fe uptake with increased levels of testosterone was again present.

FIGURE 3 depicts the only experiment out of six in which there was a significant ($P < 0.01$) increase in uptake of ^{59}Fe by bone marrow cells due to treatment with 0.125 mg of testosterone. Also, in this experiment anemic rabbit serum failed to cause increased ^{59}Fe uptake compared to normal rabbit serum. From this experiment the possibility existed that lower doses of testosterone might be effective in producing increased ^{59}Fe uptake. Testosterone was added to tubes at doses of 7.8–31 μg and it was found that the ^{59}Fe uptakes were not different from saline-treated suspensions.

These results point to the fact that when 1 mg of testosterone is added to bone marrow cultures, ^{59}Fe incorporation is decreased. On the basis of these in vitro experiments, therefore, we cannot confirm the in vivo synergistic effect postulated between testosterone and erythropoietin. Our results also disagree with those of other investigators,[13,14] who found that testosterone accelerated erythropoiesis in vitro.

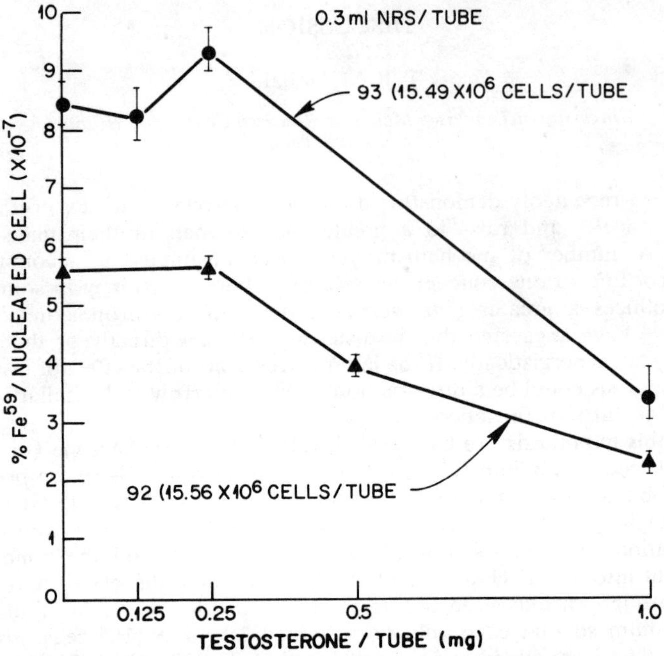

FIGURE 1. The effects of different doses of testosterone on ^{59}Fe incorporation of fresh rabbit bone marrow cells cultured in 0.3 ml/tube of autologous serum in Eagle's medium. Vertical bars indicate standard error of mean.

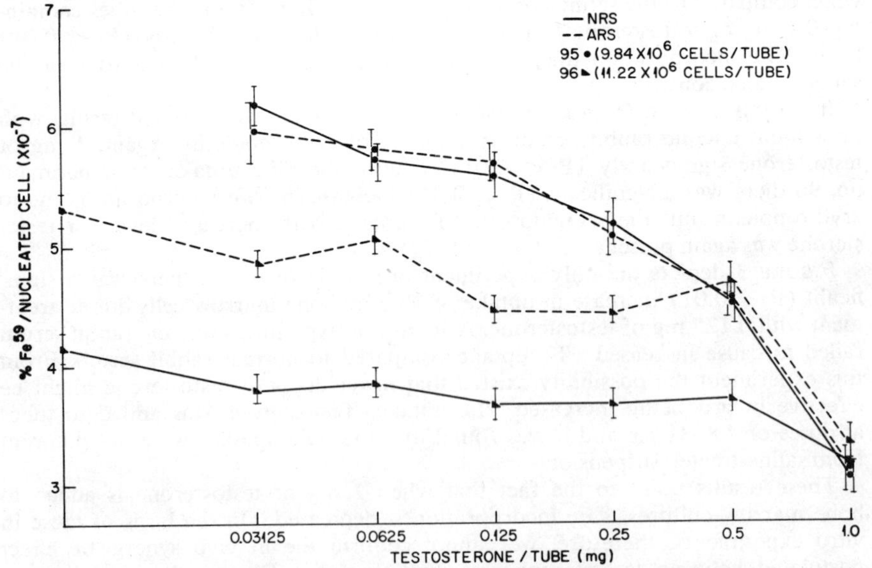

FIGURE 2. The comparison of ^{59}Fe uptake in fresh rabbit bone marrow with 0.6 ml/tube of autologous serum and 0.3 ml autologous serum plus 0.3 ml anemic rabbit serum/tube with different levels of testosterone. Vertical bars indicate standard error of mean.

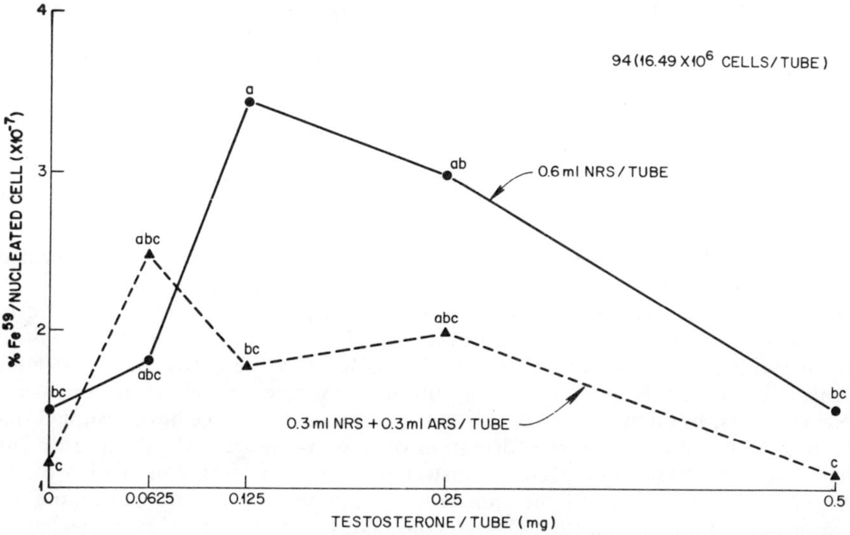

FIGURE 3. The comparison of ^{59}Fe uptake in fresh rabbit bone marrow with 0.6 ml/tube of autologous serum and 0.3 ml autologous serum plus 0.3 ml anemic rabbit serum/tube with different levels of testosterone. ABC treatment means having different superscript letters are significantly ($P < 0.01$) different using Duncan's multiple range test.

References

1. GURNEY, C. W. & W. FRIED. 1965. Further studies on the erythropoietic effect of androgens. J. Lab. Clin. Med. **65**: 775–782.
2. FRIED, W. & C. W. GURNEY. 1966. The erythropoietic response to testosterone in male and female mice. J. Lab. Clin. Med. **67**: 420–426.
3. FRIED, W. & C. W. GURNEY. 1965. Use of mild plethora to demonstrate an erythropoietic effect from small amounts of androgens. Proc. Soc. Exp. Biol. Med. **120**: 519–521.
4. JANDA, W. E., W. FRIED & C. W. GURNEY. 1965. Combined effect of cobalt and testosterone on erythropoiesis. Proc. Soc. Exp. Biol. Med. **120**: 443–446.
5. MIRAND, E. A., A. S. GORDON & J. WENIG. 1965. Mechanism of testosterone action in erythropoiesis. Nature **206**: 270–272.
6. MANN, D. L., R. M. DONATI & N. I. GALLAGHER. 1966. Relationship between erythropoietic activity of testosterone and renal mass. Clin. Res. **14**: 54 (Abstr.).
7. FRIED, W., R. DEGOWIN & C. W. GURNEY. 1964. Erythropoietic effect of testosterone in the polycythemic mouse. Proc. Soc. Exp. Biol. Med. **117**: 839–842.
8. FRIED, W. & C. W. GURNEY. 1965. Erythropoietic effect of plasma from mice receiving testosterone. Nature **206**: 1160–1161.
9. NATHAN, D. G. & F. H. GARDNER. 1965. Effects of large doses of androgen on rodent erythropoiesis and body composition. Blood **26**: 411–420.
10. MCKEE, L. C., A. B. BRILL & R. M. HEYSSEL. 1966. The mechanism of action of testosterone on erythropoiesis. Clin. Res. **14**: 91 (Abstr.).
11. GURNEY, C. W. & W. FRIED. 1965. The mechanism of action of androgens on erythropoiesis. Am. Soc. Clin. Invest. 57th Annual Meeting. : 41.
12. GURNEY, C. W. & W. FRIED. 1964. The erythropoietic effect of testosterone in the plethoric mouse. Abstracts from the 7th Annual Meeting of Am. Soc. Hemat. : 32.
13. ERSLEV, A. J. 1962. Erythropoietin and testosterone in vitro. Proc. IX Cong. Intern. Soc. Hemat. Vol. III.
14. REISNER, JR., E. H. 1966. Tissue culture of bone marrow. II Effect of steroid hormones on hematopoiesis in vitro. Blood **27**: 460–469.

Part VII. In Vitro Studies on Erythropoietin

STUDIES ON THE CONTROL OF HEMOGLOBIN FORMATION IN MARROW CELLS

Michael E. Hrinda* and Eugene Goldwasser

*Argonne Cancer Research Hospital*** and the Department of Biochemistry, University of Chicago, Chicago, Ill.*

For some time we have been engaged in testing the hypothesis that erythropoietin acts to induce erythroid differentiation by a mechanism analogous to the de-repression of gene transcription.[1] Our evidence indicates that very shortly after erythropoietin is added to rat marrow cells in vitro, there is an increase in RNA synthesis.[2] The newly-formed RNA has some of the characteristics of messenger RNA, but its identification is still not complete enough to be conclusive. Nevertheless, in the work described in this communication we have assumed that erythropoietin does cause the formation of new messenger RNA's, and on this basis we have been attempting to answer the following question: which of the newly-arising functions in the induced cell are responsible for regulating the major activity of the developing erythroid cell, i.e., hemoglobin synthesis?

In the cellular model[3] under study, we divided the process of erythroid differentiation into three distinct phases as schematized in FIGURE 1. These are sensitization, induction and specialization.

Sensitization: That phase of the cell cycle in which stem cells become competent to be induced by erythropoietin toward erythroid differentiation. We have assumed that sensitization lasts for only a short time and is reversible.

Induction: This phase includes only the primary action of erythropoietin upon sensitized cells. The result of erythropoietin action is to form a cell in the first stage of the sequence of erythroid development. Some action of the hormone has occurred but the cell is not yet at a stage that is recognizably erythroid by morphological criteria.

Specialization: In this phase all the events subsequent to primary induction take place and new cellular components, characteristic of the differentiated cell, appear. During this process some of the functions of the more primitive cells disappear. The end-product is the mature erythrocyte.

The particular emphasis in the experiments described in this paper is on the possibility that induction by erythropoietin is concerned with the regulation of hemoglobin synthesis. We have attempted to test the hypothesis that the initiation of hemoglobin synthesis resulting from erythropoietin action is the consequence of an increase in δ-aminolevulinic acid synthetase (ALA-S), and that the latter may be the enzyme that is primarily de-repressed during induction. It is known that the rate-limiting action in several heme synthesizing systems is that catalyzed by ALA-S.[4–6] If, as has been suggested,[6–9] globin synthesis is controlled by the availability of heme, then the whole sequence of reactions leading to hemoglobin formation may be regulated by the first step in the sequence. There are data showing that porphyrin synthesis by liver cells in experimental drug-induced porphyria[4] and by chick embryo cells in culture[10] is regulated by the level of ALA-S.

We attempted to determine the levels of ALA-S in short-term cultures of rat marrow cells with the results shown in TABLE 1. It is apparent that although there

* United States Public Health Service predoctoral trainee in biochemistry.

** Operated by the University of Chicago for the United States Atomic Energy Commission.

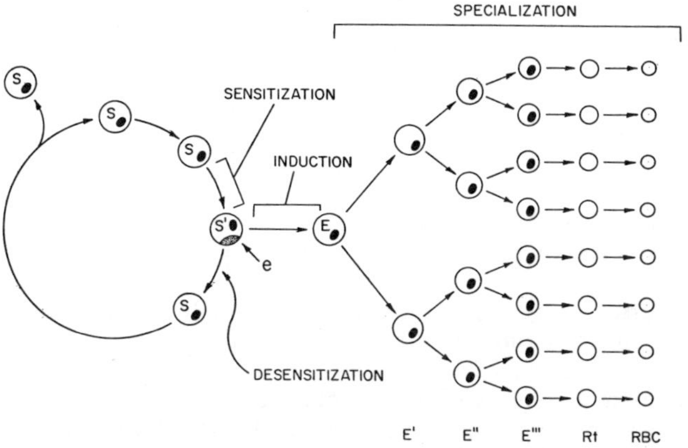

FIGURE 1. Proposed model of stem cell differentiation. S represents stem cells; S′ = sensitized stem cell; e = erythropoietin; E = first stage of erythroid differentiation; Rt = reticulocyte; and RBC = erythrocyte. The dotted area on S represents the postulated attachment site for erythropoietin.

is a measurable amount of enzyme in the cells freshly taken from the animals, there is essentially no detectable amount in the same cell population after 24 hr of culture, either with or without erythropoietin. We have no adequate explanation for the loss of enzyme activity under these conditions. Other experiments have shown that incorporation of glycine into heme by rat marrow cells proceeds linearly for at least 24 hr and is only slightly, if at all, reduced in the next three hr (TABLE 2). These data make it clear that formation of ALA from glycine does occur during the time when no ALA-S activity can be detected. Whatever the explanation may be, we are not as optimistic as we were about the possibility of directly determining the role of erythropoietin in inducing ALA-S synthesis.

We have also found that lysates of rat marrow cells can show increased heme synthesis when either ALA or protoporphyrin IX is added to the medium (TABLE 3). These data indicate that the rate-limiting reaction in porphyrin or heme synthesis in this tissue may be the formation of ALA or some earlier step leading to the sequence.

On the other hand, attempts to stimulate heme synthesis in whole cells by addition of ALA have been generally unsuccessful in our hands, indicating that exogenous ALA may not penetrate into marrow cells, in contrast to the situation with chick embryo cells.[10] When labeled ALA was added to the medium, it was incorporated into heme to an extent of about one-half percent of the amount of glycine incorporated by similar cell suspensions. Of the small amount of ALA radioactivity found in the cells, about ten times as much was present in the acid

TABLE 1

ASSAY OF ALA-S IN MARROW CELL LYSATES*

Fresh cells	1.41 mμmole ALA formed
After 24 hr in vitro	0.17 mμmole ALA formed
After 24 hr in vitro with 0.20 units of erythropoietin	0.20 mμmole ALA formed

* Each aliquot represented 10^8 nucleated cells; substrates were succinyl CoA and glycine; incubation time was 15 minutes.

TABLE 2

RATE OF INCORPORATION OF 2-^{14}C-GLYCINE IN HEME BY MARROW CELLS IN VITRO

Period	CPM Incorporated per Hour
0–24 hr	39.4
24–27 hr	33.1

insoluble fraction (nonheme-containing) as in the heme fraction. At present we interpret these findings to indicate that intracellular ALA may exist in a compartmentalized form which, in whole cells, is not freely exchangeable with added ALA.

As an alternative hypothesis for the control of hemoglobin synthesis we may consider globin formation as the step regulating the process. It is known that although there is some free protoporphyrin in mature red cells, there is no heme. In addition there is some evidence that mature red cells contain a small amount of free globin.[11] If heme synthesis were the regulatory process, the existence of free globin would not be expected.

In a test of whether globin synthesis proceeds at a fixed rate that determines the rate of heme synthesis, we have studied the inhibition of protein synthesis in marrow cell cultures by cyclohexamide. We found a surprisingly rapid inhibition of both glycine and iron incorporation into heme after addition of cyclohexamide, indicating a half-life of about 80 min for the protein components of the system. In one report the half-life of liver ALA-S in experimental porphyria was shown to be about 70 minutes.[12] This would suggest that the action of the inhibitor had been on ALA-S formation.

The half-life of the system forming heme from glycine in reticulocytes, however, is distinctly longer. From the data of Karibian and London[13] we could estimate a half-life of 3.5 hours. Our own experiments on the inhibition of reticulocyte heme synthesis by cyclohexamide (measured by ^{59}Fe incorporation) also indicates a half-life of about 3.5 hours. These data agree fairly well with one recent estimate of Granick.[10] Under conditions where whole cell protein synthesis is inhibited, cyclohexamide has no effect on the activity of the heme synthesis system in cell lysates. Since the enzyme system forming heme in reticulocytes must be very similar to, if not identical with, the system in marrow cells, the half-life of ALA-S in the marrow cell system must be considerably longer than the 80 min we found. Our interpretation of this paradox is that inhibition of the synthesis of some cellular proteins may cause the cessation of heme synthesis. Among these proteins globin may be of major importance. Although the data are not yet complete, we are tempted to formulate a control mechanism as follows (see FIGURE 2).

TABLE 3

EFFECT OF ALA AND PROTOPORPHYRIN IX ON INCORPORATION OF ^{59}FE INTO HEME BY A CELL-FREE PREPARATION OF MARROW

Substrate	Concentration	CPM/Hour
None	—	120
ALA	5×10^{-5} M	246
ALA	2×10^{-4}	397
No enzyme	—	0
None	—	133
Protoporphyrin IX	10^{-5} M	526
Protoporphyrin IX	4×10^{-5} M	2,081
No enzyme	—	16

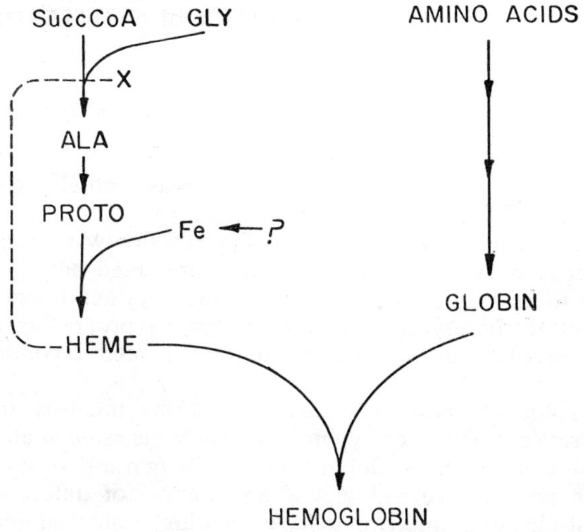

FIGURE 2. Proposed scheme for the regulation of hemoglobin synthesis. The broken line represents the direction of feedback inhibition in the heme synthetic pathway; additional control on the pathway may occur at the step of iron insertion into protoporphyrin IX.

The pathway leading to heme synthesis may be controlled at more than one step, e.g. at ALA-S, and at the step converting protoporphyrin IX to heme (heme synthetase). The system is also characterized by end-product inhibition of ALA-S by heme.[13] Granick and Levere[14] have pointed out that unless globin were present, in effect, to scavenge heme, heme synthesis would be restrained by the presence of excess heme. Initiation of globin synthesis would then be followed by increased heme synthesis, or conversely, inhibition of globin synthesis would stop heme synthesis. The action of erythropoietin, if it acts directly on this system, may be to de-repress globin synthesis and thus lead to a sharp increase in hemoglobin formation. Experiments testing these concepts are being carried out.

REFERENCES

1. JACOB, F. & J. MONOD. 1961. Cold Spring Harbor Symp. Quant. Biol. **26:** 193.
2. KRANTZ, S. B. & E. GOLDWASSER. 1965. Biochim. Biophys. Acta **103:** 325.
3. GOLDWASSER, E. 1966. Biochemical control of erythroid cell development. *In* current Topics in Developmental Biology. A. Monroy & A. A. Moscona, Eds. In press.
4. GRANICK, S. & G. URATA. 1963. J. Biol. Chem. **238:** 821.
5. LASCELLES, J. 1964. Tetrapyrrole Biosynthesis and Its Regulation. : 98–101. W. A. Benjamin. New York.
6. LEVERE, R. D. & S. GRANICK. 1965. Proc. Nat. Acad. Sci. U.S. **54:** 134.
7. BRUNS, G. P. & I. M. LONDON. 1965. Biochem. Biophys. Res. Commun. **18:** 236.
8. WAXMAN, H. S. & M. RABINOVITZ. 1965. Biochem. Biophys. Res. Commun. **19:** 538.
9. GRAYZEL, A. I., P. HÖRCHNER & I. M. LONDON. 1966. Proc. Nat. Acad. Sci. U.S. **55:** 650.
10. GRANICK, S. 1966. J. Biol. Chem. **241:** 1359.
11. WINTERHALTER, K. H. & E. R. HEUHNS. 1963. J. Clin. Invest. **42:** 995.
12. TSCHUDY, D. P., H. S. MARVER & A. COLLINS. 1965. Biochm. Biophys. Res. Commun. **21:** 480.
13. KARIBIAN, D. & I. M. LONDON. 1965. Biochem. Biophys. Res. Commun. **18:** 243.
14. GRANICK, S. & R. D. LEVERE. 1964. Heme synthesis in erythroid cells. *In* Progress in Hematology. Vol. IV. : 1. C. V. Moore & E. B. Brown, Eds. Grune and Stratton, Inc. New York, N. Y.

THE CHANGE OF HEMOGLOBIN SYNTHESIS FROM MINOR TO MAJOR IN THE COURSE OF ERYTHROBLAST MATURATION*

Henry Borsook

Kerckhoff Biological Laboratories, California Institute of Technology, Pasadena, Calif.

The point of departure of the present study was Thorell's conclusion[1] that hemoglobin synthesis does not begin in adult marrow until about the polychromatic stage of erythroblast maturation. The first reaction was disagreement based on the interpretation that ^{59}Fe incorporation represented only hemoglobin synthesis, whereas in immature erythroblasts it is incorporated mainly into ferritin: the more immature the erythroblast, the greater the proportion into ferritin.[2,3] Later work in other laboratories[4] and in Thorell's[3] tended to confirm the original conclusion.

Autoradiographic observations indicated that the intensity of protein synthesis, i.e., the rate per unit of cell volume, is nearly the same in all active erythroblasts.[5] The induction of hemoglobin synthesis is then a diversion from that of nonhemoglobin protein. Ostensibly it is an example of differentiation. Hemoglobin synthesis in adult marrow cells is inviting biological material for the study of differentiation because hemoglobin is easily measured, even in low concentration, and marrow cells are readily available.

To facilitate such a study and others, e.g., the action of erythropoietin on erythroblasts in vitro, a method was devised for segregating erythroblasts according to maturation stage in viable active state. The marrow of adult rabbits is used. The method consists of centrifugation and recentrifugation in a density gradient of bovine serum albumin for the pronormoblast fraction. The more mature erythroblast fractions are obtained from cuts in the gradient after the first centrifugation followed by absorption and differential elution from Dowex-2 spheres and recentrifugation in the BSA density gradient.**

The first observations here compare hemoglobin formation in reticulocytes from a severely anemic rabbit† with the pronormoblast fractions of normal and severely anemic rabbits. TABLE 1 gives representative composition of the pronormoblast fraction after one and two recentrifugations. Although they contained some mature erythroblasts and reticulocytes, the preponderance of pronormoblasts was sufficient to show the characteristic difference between hemoglobin synthesis in them and that which ensues later in erythropoiesis.

The cells were incubated for four hr at 37° under 95 percent oxygen and 5 percent CO_2. They were then washed by resuspension and recentrifugation several times to remove most of the free gly-2-^{14}C, homogenized in an extract of normal rabbit erythrocytes (prepared by the method of Drabkin[6]), which contains all the hemoglobin and the small amount of soluble nonhemoglobin protein in the erythrocytes. It served as a carrier in the fractionation of the proteins in the incubated cells. The hemoglobin was converted to the cyanmet derivative by the method of Drabkin and Austin,[7] dialyzed exhaustively and then chromatographed by the method of Allen *et al.*[8] for the human hemoglobins with their developer no. 1, first at 4°, then at 25°, and finally by developer no. 1 containing 4 N NaCl.

* Supported by grants from the U.S. Public Health Service (H–1624) and the U.S. Atomic Energy Commission [AT(04–3)51].

** A detailed description of all the procedures is being prepared.

† Six daily phenylhydrazine injections. The reticulocytes were 85 percent or more of the blood red cell count.

TABLE 1

REPRESENTATIVE COMPOSITION OF PRONORMOBLAST FRACTION FROM MARROW OF NORMAL AND ANEMIC RABBITS

Class of Cells	Normal*	Anemic**
	Percent	Percent
Pronormoblasts	72	84
Other erythroblasts	9	9
Nonerythroid nucleated cells	14	7
Reticulocytes	5	0

* Recentrifuged once.
** Recentrifuged twice.

FIGURE 1 shows the six chromatographic fractions obtained based on absorption at 418 mμ. None of the fractions was homogeneous. Fraction IV, which contained the major hemoglobin, and fraction V were those most nearly so. Notwithstanding their inhomogeneity the six fractions showed metabolic as well as chromatographic differences (see below).

TABLE 2 shows that when the relative cell volume (obtained by Coulter counter measurements) is taken into account, both pronormoblast fractions and the most active reticulocytes give similar values for the incorporation of gly-2-^{14}C into their proteins. The most active reticulocytes (obtained from the top of a BSA gradient) have nearly the same activity per cell as the polychromatic erythroblasts, which are the immediate antecedents of most of them. Reticulocytes lower in the gradient (designated here as of intermediate activity) were, as Marks *et al.*[9] and Glowacki and Millette[10] had noted, considerably less active. Among the fully active cells there was about a 60-fold range in the number of cells and about two-fold range in relative cell volume. Yet the values for gly-2-^{14}C incorporation per unit of cell volume were nearly the same. They confirm the previous autoradiographic observations made with labeled leucine. Evidently the protein synthesizing apparatus is fully active in all erythroblasts whatever proteins they are synthesizing and whatever their maturation state.

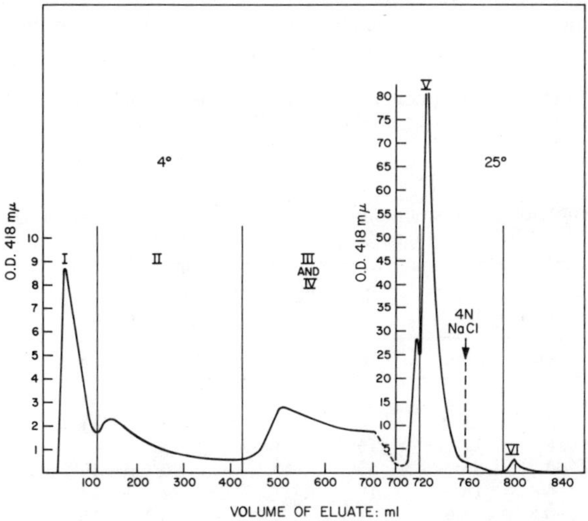

FIGURE 1. Chromatography of hemoglobins in normal rabbit blood.

TABLE 2

INCORPORATION OF GLY-2-^{14}C INTO PROTEINS AND PORPHYRINS BY RETICULOCYTES AND PRONORMOBLASTS

Cell Type	Number of Cells	Relative Volume per Cell	Incorporation by 10^6 Cells: Not Adjusted for Relative Volume per Cell	Incorporation by 10^6 Cells: Adjusted for Relative Volume per Cell
Reticulocytes most active from blood of severely anemic animals	1.62×10^9	1.06	1850	1750
Reticulocytes' intermediate activity from blood of severely anemic animal	1.38×10^9	1.00	515	515
Pronormoblast fraction from marrow of normal animals	0.278×10^9	1.44	2515	1750
Pronormoblast fraction from marrow of severely anemic animals	0.0259×10^9	1.85	4370	2350

TABLE 3 shows that the distribution of incorporated gly-2-^{14}C among the six chromatographic fractions was not the same as that of the hemoglobin (absorption at 418 mμ) or of the total protein (TABLE 4).†† Fraction V had relatively the greatest incorporation in reticulocytes; in the pronormoblast fractions, both normal and anemic, fraction I had the greatest absolute incorporation, fraction VI, the greatest relative incorporation, and fractions III and IV, the least relative incorporation.

The greatest incorporation, absolute or relative, in the pronormoblast fractions I and VI was because both their hemoglobin and nonhemoglobin protein had higher specific activities than the others (TABLES 5 & 6). Each pair of globin α and β chains had nearly the same specific activities. The porphyrins of each pair of chains also had similar specific activities but the differences relative to those

†† Estimated from the absorption at 280 mμ and the coefficient for heme absorption at 280 mμ of 0.19 $\times$ absorption of hemoglobin at 418 mμ.

TABLE 3

DISTRIBUTION OF HEMOGLOBIN (418 Mμ ABSORPTION) AND INCORPORATION OF GLY-2-^{14}C: PERCENT OF TOTAL

Fraction	Reticulocytes: Most Active		Reticulocytes: Intermediate Activity		Pronormoblasts: Normal		Pronormoblasts: Anemic	
	Hb	cpm	Hb	cpm	Hb	cpm	Hb	cpm
I	9	9	10	18	7	43	11	54
II	5	3	4	1.7	4	11	12	9
III	18	11	16	11	15	5	21	3
IV	60	55	53	41	50	12	50	8
V	6	18	16	27	24	13	5.5	6
VI	0.8	2.6	1.1	1.4	0.3	16	0.5	19

TABLE 4

DISTRIBUTION OF PROTEIN* AND INCORPORATION OF GLY-2-^{14}C: PERCENT OF TOTAL

Fraction	Reticulocytes: Most Active		Reticulocytes: Intermediate Activity		Pronormoblasts: Normal		Pronormoblasts: Anemic	
	Prot.	cpm	Prot.	cpm	Prot.	cpm	Prot.	cpm
I	18.8	9	19.1	18	32.1	43	21.6	54
II	7.6	3	5.1	1.7	7.4	11	11.5	9
III	16.7	11	13.6	11	11.0	5	17.5	3
IV	48.6	55	44.2	41	30.9	12	42.2	8
V	4.6	18	13.4	27	17.7	13	4.6	6
VI	3.7	2.6	4.5	1.4	0.7	16	2.5	19

* Absorption at 280 mμ: Total − (0.19 × 418 mμ absorption: heme).

TABLE 5

COMPARISON OF SPECIFIC ACTIVITY OF GLOBIN IN RETICULOCYTE AND PRONORMOBLAST FRACTIONS: CPM/280 NORMALIZED FOR CELL COUNT, RELATIVE CELL VOLUME AND AMOUNT OF CARRIER

Frn	Reticulocytes: Intermediate Activity*		Pronormoblasts (Normal) Hb$_1$**		Hb$_2$**	
	α	β	α	β	α	β
I	1900	2000	13250	19600	1750	1950
II	780*		920	920	—	—
III	1450	1500	300	270	180	135
IV	2150	1700	1700	1500	925	750
V	3050	3400	830	830	—	—
VI	1300*		45700*			

* Heme and globin separated by acetone-HCl and the globin fractionated by the method of Dintzis.[11]

** Intact α and β chains separated by the method of Bucci and Fronticelli[12] followed by separation of their heme and globin by acetone-HCl.

TABLE 6

COMPARISON OF SPECIFIC ACTIVITY OF PORPHYRIN (HEME) IN RETICULOCYTE AND PRONORMOBLAST FRACTIONS: CPM/395 NORMALIZED FOR CELL COUNT, RELATIVE CELL VOLUME AND AMOUNT OF CARRIER*

Frn	Reticulocytes: Intermediate Activity**	Pronormoblasts (Normal) Hb$_1$		Hb$_2$	
		α	β	α	β
I	205	428	600	80	80
II	100	46	24	—	—
III	145	32	27	34	54
IV	225	75	61	82	71
V	450	175	175	—	—
VI	235	2200*			

* See footnote to TABLE 5.

** The porphyrins extracted by acetone-HCl were fractionated into heme, proto- and copro-porphyrins. Practically all the counts were in the heme. The pronormoblast porphyrins were not fractionated.

TABLE 7

COUNTS AS HEMOGLOBIN IN THE FRACTIONS FROM RETICULOCYTES AND THE PRONORMOBLAST FRACTION: PER 10^6 CELLS

Fraction	Reticulocytes: Intermediate Activity		Pronormoblast Fraction: Normal Animal	
	Counts	Percent	Counts	Percent
I	39	9	261	47
II	19	4	24	4
III	49	11	6	1
IV	200	47	178	32
V	121	28	90	16
Total hemoglobin	428		559	
Total counts	515		2515	

in the reticulocytes were less in the heme than in the globin. This may indicate the presence of a larger pool of free heme in the pronormoblasts. In the fractionation of the pronormoblast proteins the α and β chains were separated intact; hence the porphyrins subsequently obtained from them may be considered as heme. The specific activities of hemes in fractions I and VI were higher than that of any other. It is unlikely then that the high specific activity of their globins was due to admixture of nonhemoglobin protein of very high specific activity. The specific activity of the nonhemoglobin protein in fraction I of the pronormoblasts could be estimated. It was lower than that of its Hb_1.

The data in TABLES 5 and 6 indicate that pronormoblasts form some minor hemoglobins faster than the major and the minors in other fractions. Obviously the reverse relation must ensue later in the more mature erythroblasts so that the hemoglobin of fraction IV (the major) is eventually preponderant.

TABLES 5 and 6 also show hemoglobin fractions designated Hb_2. Their specific activities are lower than those of the respective Hb_1 and of some of the reticulocyte globin fractions. Further investigation is needed in order to interpret the Hb_2 fractions.

TABLE 7 summarizes the absolute number of counts in the hemoglobin of the reticulocyte and pronormoblast fractions. In reticulocytes most was in fraction IV (the major) and in pronormoblasts, in fraction I. Some of the hemoglobin in the pronormoblast fractions IV and V was synthesized in the more mature erythroblasts and reticulocytes present.

TABLE 7 shows that 83 percent of the total counts in the reticulocytes was in hemoglobin while in the pronormoblasts it was only 22 percent, i.e., the nonhemoglobin protein had 17 and 78 percent of the total counts of the reticulocyte and pronormoblast proteins, respectively. This difference expresses the diversion of protein synthesis from nonhemoglobin protein to hemoglobin as the erythroblasts mature.

The most immature pronormoblast fractions we have obtained thus far exhibited hemoglobin synthesis. The amount was far in excess of what could be accounted for by the relatively few more mature erythroblasts present. It appears that Thorell's original conclusion needs to be modified somewhat (at least for the rabbit) as follows. Hemoglobin synthesis begins in the most immature of the recognizable erythroblasts. It consists of one or more minors and the amount is less than the nohemoglobin protein synthesized. As the erythroblast matures, synthesis of nonhemoglobin protein and of some of the minors gives way to that of the major.

Thorell's main original conclusion is confirmed by the present findings: the main synthesis of hemoglobin sets in after the pronormoblast stage. The synthesis of nonhemoglobin protein is predominant in pronormoblasts. These proteins turn over rapidly; synthesis and breakdown balance each other, with the result that the concentration of protein remains constant.[5] When their synthesis declines, breakdown continues, their concentration declines, and eventually they constitute a small fraction of the total protein. Hemoglobin does not turn over—it remains until the cell is destroyed. Because the intensity of total protein synthesis remains constant throughout the maturation of erythroblasts, when synthesis is diverted from nonhemoglobin to hemoglobin, the combined effect of decline in the former and accumulation of the latter is a steep increase in hemoglobin. This occurs sometime after the pronormoblast stage, as Thorell had seen. In studies now in progress we hope it will be possible to determine whether the steep increase in hemoglobin sets in at the basophilic or polychromatic stage, and what the effect of a high concentration of erythropoietin is.

At the San Francisco Erythropoietin Conference, evidence was presented that the main target cells of erythropoietin are antecedent to the pronormoblasts.[13–21] This conclusion may now be considered confirmed by observations on the effects of actinomycin[22–24] and erythropoietin antibodies.[25] Although it has not yet been directly demonstrated, it is to be inferred that the morphological changes in pronormoblast maturation through to the erythrocyte are not affected by actinomycin and therefore, are not to be considered as differentiation (which by definition is set in train by a newly-formed, new kind of m-RNA whose synthesis actinomycin inhibits). They appear to be analogous to the first divisions of the fertilized egg which are not affected by actinomycin.[26] The question now arises regarding the nature of the change in hemoglobin synthesis from the minors to the major in the course of maturation of the pronormoblast. Provided the appropriate m-RNA has already been formed, hemoglobin synthesis, as with all protein, is not inhibited by actinomycin. Is the change from minor to major in maturing erythroblasts also unaffected?

Some of the consequences of a high concentration of erythropoietin are analogous to those of differentiation. The resulting erythroblasts in their maturation skip the last nucleated stage; they are much shorter-lived. When sheep with hemoglobin A and B are bled, a new hemoglobin, C, appears and A diminishes. When bleeding is stopped, C disappears and A regains its former proportion.[27] It is a reasonable inference that this replacement of one hemoglobin by another is an effect of a high concentration of erythropoietin generated by the bleeding. It may be analogous to the burst of protein synthesis soon after fertilization of the egg, which is not affected by actinomycin,[1] and for which some unmasking of preformed m-RNA needs to be postulated.

References

1. Thorell, B. 1947. Acta Med. Scandinav. **129** (Suppl. 200): 1.
2. Bessis, M. 1955. Blood **10:** 272.
3. Sondhaus, C. A. & B. Thorell. 1960. Blood **16:** 1285.
4. Ackerman, G. A. 1962. Anat. Rec. **144:** 239.
5. Borsook, H. 1964. Ann. N. Y. Acad. Sci. **119:** 523.
6. Drabkin, D. 1946. J. Biol. Chem. **164:** 703.
7. Drabkin, D. & J. H. Austin. 1935–36. J. Biol. Chem. **112:** 67.

8. Allen, D. W., W. A. Schroeder & J. Balog. 1958. J. Amer. Chem. Soc. **80:** 1628.
9. Marks, P. A., R. A. Rifkind & D. Danon. 1963. Proc. Nat. Acad. Sci. **50:** 336.
10. Glowacki, E. R. & R. L. Millette. 1965. J. Molec. Biol. **11:** 116.
11. Dintzis, H. M. 1961. Proc. Nat. Acad. Sci. **47:** 247.
12. Bucci, E. & C. Fronticelli. 1965. J. Biol. Chem. **240:** PC551.
13. Jacobson, L. O., E. Goldwasser, L. F. Plzak & W. Fried. 1957. Proc. Soc. Exp. Biol. Med. **94:** 243.
14. Erslev, A. J. 1959. Blood **14:** 386.
15. Erslev, A. J. 1964. Blood **24:** 331.
16. Alpen, E. L. & D. Cranmore. 1959. *In* The Kinetics of Cellular Proliferation. F. Stohlman, Jr., Ed. : 290. New York and London.
17. Stohlman, Jr., F. 1959. Ann. N. Y. Acad. Sci. **77:** 710.
18. Stohlman, Jr., F. 1959. *In* The Kinetics of Cellular Proliferation. : 325: New York and London.
19. Matoth, Y. & E. Ben-Porath. 1959. J. Lab. Clin. Med. **54:** 722.
20. Lajtha, L. G., R. Oliver & C. W. Gurney. 1962. Brit. J. Haematol. **8:** 442.
21. Kurtides, E. S., W. A. Rambach, H. L. Alt & J. C. Wurster. 1963. J. Lab. Clin. Med. **61:** 23.
22. Philips, F. S., H. S. Schwartz, S. S. Sternberg & C. T. C. Tan. 1960. Ann. N. Y. Acad. Sci. **89:** 348.
23. Keighley, G. & P. H. Lowy. 1966. Blood **27:** 637.
24. Reissmann, K. R. & K. Ito. 1966. This Annal.
25. Schooley, J. C. 1966. This Annal.
26. Borsook, H. 1966. Biol. Rev. **41:** 1.
27. Beale, D., H. Lehmann, A. Drury & E. M. Tucker. 1966. Nature **209:** 1099.

EFFECT OF ERYTHROPOIETIN UPON HEMOGLOBIN BIOSYNTHESIS*

Lorraine M. Kraus, Iwao Iuchi and Brother Thomas Kraus, F. S. C.

Department of Biochemistry, University of Tennessee Medical Units, Memphis, Tenn.

Erythropoietin is involved in the differentiation of a multipotential cell into a cell whose major biosynthetic activity is the production of hemoglobin. Could there also be an erythropoietin effect upon hemoglobin biosynthesis?

In order to establish this erythropoietin effect, it is necessary to examine a cell population which normally synthesizes more than one hemoglobin, to separate these hemoglobins, and to establish that the separated hemoglobins are different proteins. Thereafter any change in the biosynthesis of these hemoglobins in the presence of erythropoietin might yield information as to the role of erythropoietin in hemoglobin biosynthesis. This study demonstrates that erythropoietin does affect hemoglobin biosynthesis, causing a change in the biosynthesis of the different hemoglobins present.

MATERIALS AND METHODS

Adult mice from an inbred strain of Swiss mice with a diffuse hemoglobin which separated into four bands on starch gel electrophoresis were used in this study. The cell hemolysates were prepared by the method of Drabkin[1] except that cyanmethemoglobin reagent[2] was used in place of water to lake the cells.

The hemoglobins were separated by vertical starch gel electrophoresis[3] using tris-EDTA-boric acid buffer, pH 8.6.[4] The heme was removed[5] from hemoglobin obtained from pooled blood of normal unmanipulated mice, or the hemoglobin isolated from starch gel electrophoresis. The globin was subjected to tryptic digestion and fingerprints were prepared according to the methods of Ingram[6] and Baglioni.[7] The total unfractionated globin was separated into α and β chains using countercurrent distribution by the method of Hill and Craig.[8] The isolated α and β polypeptide chains were hydrolyzed in 6 N HCl for 24 or 72 hr under N_2 and amino acid analysis of the hydrolysate was performed using a Technicon amino acid analyzer. The isolated α and β chains were subjected to tryptic digestion and fingerprints were processed as described above.

In Vitro Experiments. Normal unmanipulated mice were bled and the heparinized plasma pooled and used as normal plasma. The hemoglobin was prepared as 2 percent cyanmethemoglobin and used as unlabeled carrier hemoglobin in the electrophoretic fractionation. Bone marrow was extruded from the bones of the hind limbs of the mice with Tyrode's solution. The bone marrow was pooled, centrifuged and the supernatant was removed. The incubation mixture was prepared by adding the components in the following order:

1. pooled bone marrow cells in one ml of Tyrode's solution, approximately 300,000 nucleated cells per mm^3.
2. a) 5 ml of normal pooled plasma: control study.
   b) 5 ml of pooled plasma from mice subjected to one-half atmosphere for 12 hr: mouse erythropoietin effect.

* This investigation was supported in part by USPHS grants HE06627 and AM08592.

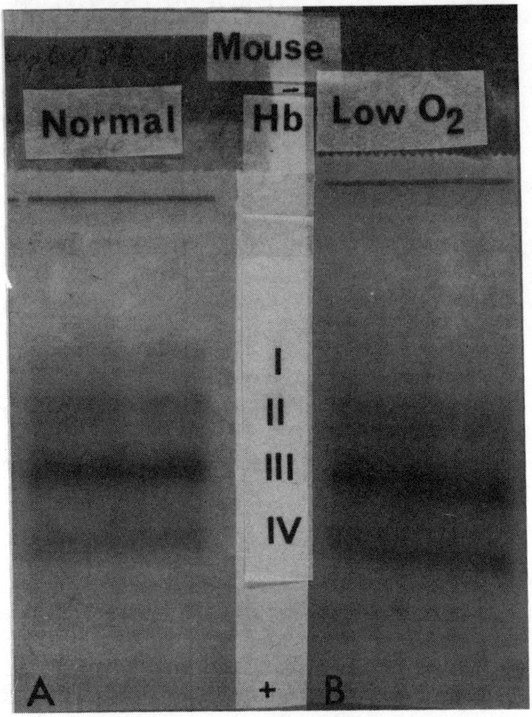

FIGURE 1. A typical starch gel electrophoretic fractionation of diffuse hemoglobin from the adult Swiss mouse at pH 8.6, 250 v for 18 hr showing the separation of hemoglobins I, II, III and IV. A: Hemoglobins from a normal mouse. B: Hemoglobins from a mouse kept in a low oxygen chamber for 24 hours.

c) sheep erythropoietin (Step IV)* 18 units per 0.5 ml of Tyrode's solution or 36 units per 1 ml of Tyrode's solution was added in 5 ml of normal pooled plasma: sheep erythropoietin effect.

3. 5 ml of iron-59 as ferrous chloride in 0.85 percent NaCl solution, a total of 4.5 μg of iron with an initial specific activity of 22.8 mc/mg Fe.

Each tube containing 2 ml of the incubation mixture was incubated under 95 percent N_2 and 5 percent O_2 for 0.5, 1, 3, or 6 hours at 37° C as described by Kraus *et al.*[9] At the end of the incubation time each mixture was centrifuged, the supernatant removed, and the cells washed three times with physiological saline. The bone marrow cells were hemolyzed in 2 percent pooled, normal mouse cyanmethemoglobin solution. The hemoglobin was fractionated by starch gel electrophoresis, all the gels were sectioned in the same manner and the sections counted in a well-scintillation counter. The percent distribution of iron-59 on the gel was calculated and that found in the four different hemoglobins recorded.

In Vivo Experiments. Mice were injected with iron-59-citrate, 1 μc per mouse. The control groups were kept in a normal environment and bled 24 or 48 hr later. The hemoglobins of the individual mice were prepared, fractionated and

* Allocated to this laboratory by the Hematology Study Section, USPHS.

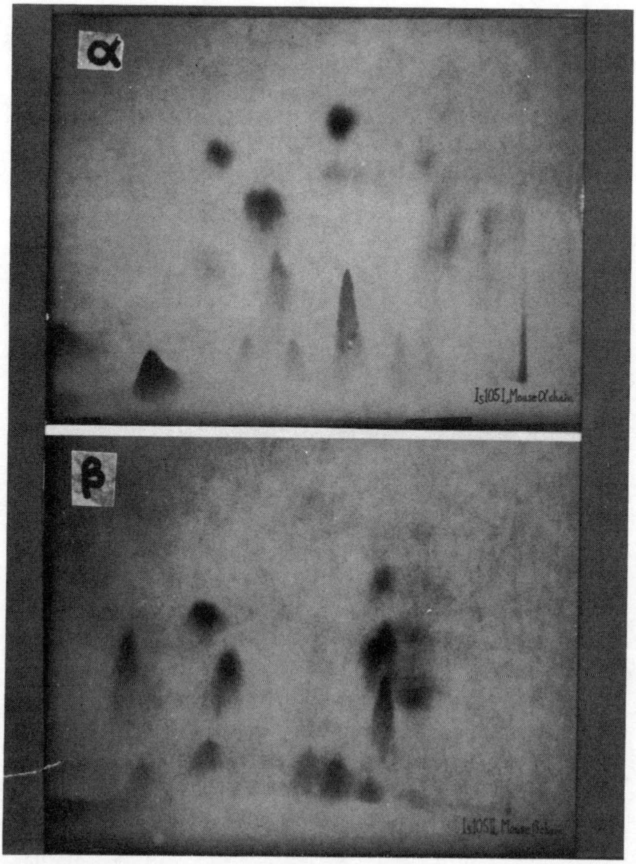

FIGURE 2. Fingerprints of the tryptic peptides of α and β chains from total Swiss mouse globin separated by countercurrent distribution.

the radioactivity evaluated. Other mice were placed in a low oxygen chamber (one-half atm) for 24 hr or 48 hr and then bled. The hemoglobins of the individual mice were treated in the same manner as the control group.

RESULTS

The starch gel fractionation of the diffuse hemoglobin of the Swiss mice into four hemoglobins is seen in FIGURE 1. The change in this pattern as a result of 24 hr in a low oxygen chamber at one-half atm may be compared to the normal.

The peptide maps of the isolated α and β chains of the total globin are seen in FIGURE 2. The identity of the four hemoglobins was established by tryptic digestion and by peptide maps. In FIGURE 3 the peptide maps of the four hemoglobins are compared to that of total mouse globin and the peptides which are not visible are indicated. Only peptide deletions were observed. No additional peptides, as compared to the total mouse globin, were found. Hemoglobin I appears to have lost mostly β chain peptides. Hemoglobin II is almost identical to total globin, there being only a few peptides missing. Hemoglobin III appears to be the same as total globin. Hemoglobin IV seems to have lost chiefly α pep-

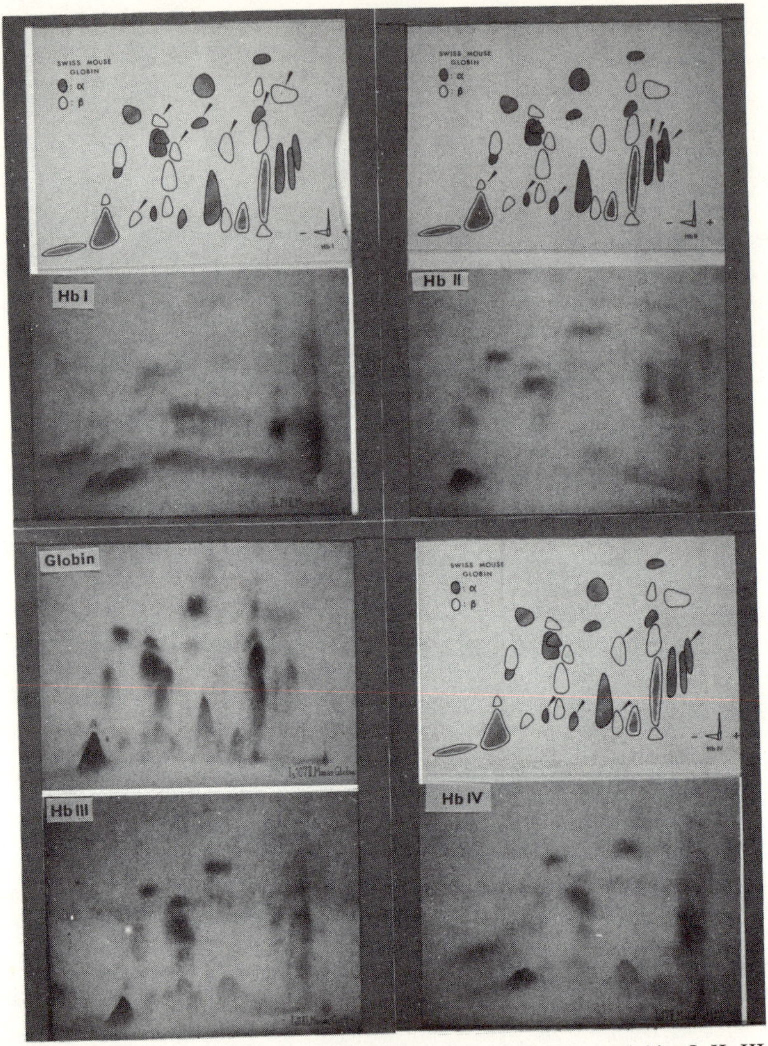

FIGURE 3. Fingerprints of the tryptic peptides of the isolated hemoglobins I, II, III and IV as compared to that of total globin. The differences are marked by arrows.

tides. The amino acid analyses of the α and β chains indicated that the α chain had more basic amino acids and fewer acidic amino acids than did the β chain. The peptide content of the different hemoglobins and the electrophoretic mobility of the hemoglobins agree with the charge differences found in the two polypeptide chains. A difference in the percent distribution of iron-59 in the hemoglobins was detected when normal bone marrow cells were incubated with normal plasma as compared to incubation with plasma containing erythropoietin (FIGURE 4). The plasma from the hypoxic mice after 12 hr in a low oxygen chamber appeared to depress the hemoglobin biosynthesis. Nevertheless, a change in the biosynthesis of the four hemoglobins was observed. The sheep

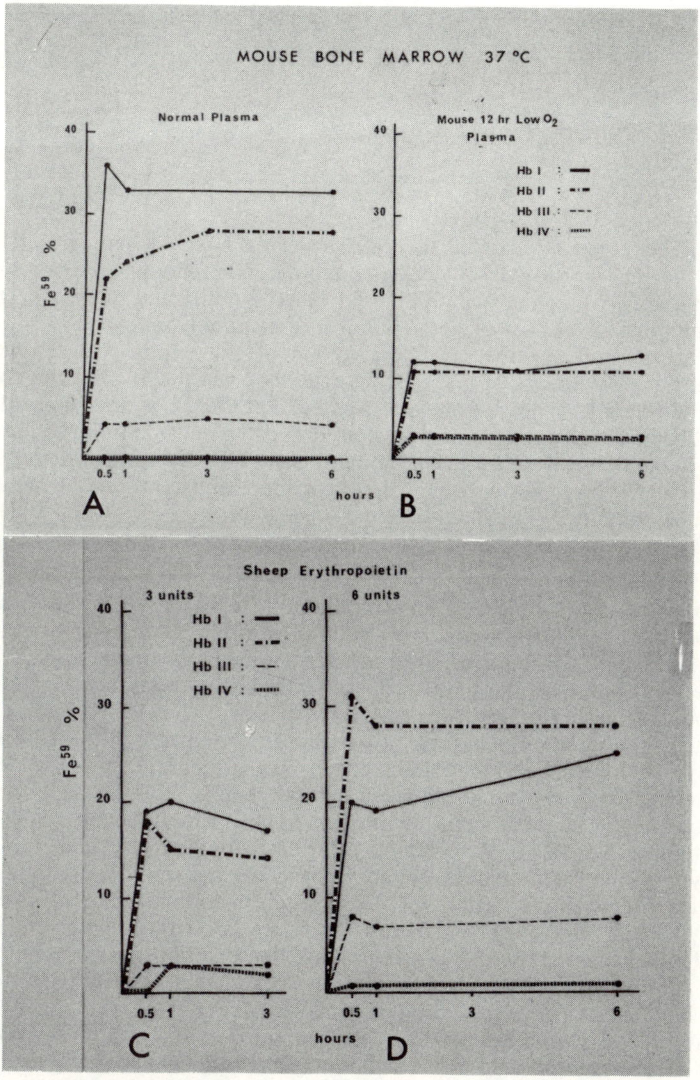

FIGURE 4. In vitro studies: The percent iron-59 distribution in hemoglobins I, II, III and IV following incubation of normal bone marrow cells in A: pooled normal plasma (average of three experiments); B: pooled plasma from mice kept in a low oxygen chamber for 12 hr; C: pooled normal plasma containing 3 units of sheep erythropoietin (Step IV) per tube; and D: pooled normal plasma containing 6 units of sheep erythropoietin (Step IV) per tube.

TABLE 1

IN VIVO HEMOGLOBIN BIOSYNTHESIS IN SWISS MOUSE AFTER STARCH GEL ELECTROPHORESIS

Hb	Percent ^{59}Fe Distribution			
	24 hr		48 hr	
	Normal	Low O_2	Normal	Low O_2
I	7	2	2	2
II	18	19	16	17
III	38	48	55	47
IV	14	8	9	8

erythropoietin (Step IV) added to normal plasma affected hemoglobin biosynthesis in normal bone marrow cells. Doubling the amount of erythropoietin doubled the biosynthesis of hemoglobin III (total globin) and increased synthesis of hemoglobin II over that of hemoglobin I (FIGURE 4).

The in vivo study of the peripheral blood of the hypoxic mice revealed a change in the biosynthesis of hemoglobin after 24 hr in the low oxygen chamber. At 48 hr no change from the normal was evident. In 24 hr the biosynthesis of hemoglobin in the hypoxic mice was altered and the cells containing the altered ratios of hemoglobin were found in the peripheral blood. Namely, hemoglobins I and IV were less radioactive while there was increased synthesis of hemoglobin III, and hemoglobin II remained the same (TABLE 1).

DISCUSSION

The in vitro effect of sheep erythropoietin (Step IV) upon biosynthesis of hemoglobins in normal bone marrow cells in normal plasma is clearly demonstrated. Increased amounts of erythropoietin appear to have a progressively greater effect upon the alteration of hemoglobin biosynthesis.

The pooled plasma taken from mice after 12 hr in the low oxygen chamber caused an altered hemoglobin biosynthesis but it also appeared to depress hemoglobin synthesis. The erythropoietin effect was present in spite of decreased biosynthesis. Since one ml of hypoxic plasma per incubation tube was used, nonerythropoietin impurity could be present in large amounts and could account for this finding. Further in vitro studies using erythropoietin isolated from plasma of the hypoxic mouse are planned to answer this question. In the 24-hour hypoxic mouse, erythropoietin is acting for 24 hr upon a compartment of cells which normally requires 48 to 60 hr for cells to differentiate from a precursor cell to a cell in the peripheral blood. Within this time hemoglobin biosynthesis is altered and the altered hemoglobin is found in the peripheral blood. After 48 hr no change from normal is seen.

Erythropoietin would appear to affect hemoglobin biosynthesis by increasing the rate of biosynthesis and if more than one hemoglobin is being synthesized, by altering the rates of the synthesis of the different hemoglobins.

SUMMARY

It has been established by electrophoretic mobility and peptide maps that the four hemoglobins found in the diffuse hemoglobin of the adult Swiss mouse are different.

In Vitro Study. A difference in the percent distribution of iron-59 in the hemoglobins was detected when normal bone marrow cells were incubated with normal plasma as compared to incubation with plasma containing erythropoietin. Increased amounts of sheep erythropoietin appeared to have a progressively greater effect upon the alteration of hemoglobin biosynthesis.

In Vivo Study. Peripheral blood of the hypoxic mice revealed a change in the biosynthesis of the four hemoglobins after 24 hr in the low oxygen chamber. After 48 hr little change from normal was seen.

Erythropoietin would appear to affect hemoglobin biosynthesis by increasing the rate of biosynthesis and if more than one hemoglobin is being synthesized, by altering the rate of the synthesis of the different hemoglobins.

References

1. Drabkin, D. L. 1946. Spectrophotometric studies. XIV. The crystallographic and optical properties of the hemoglobin of man in comparison with those of other species. J. Biol. Chem. **164**: 703–723.
2. Crosby, W. H., J. I. Munn & F. W. Furth. 1954. Standardizing a method for clinical hemoglobinometry. U. S. Armed Forces Med. J. **5**: 693–703.
3. Smithies, O. 1955. Zone electrophoresis of serum in starch gels: group variations in the serum proteins of normal human adults. Biochem. J. **61**: 629–641.
4. Boyer, S. H., D. C. Fainer & M. A. Naughton. 1963. Myoglobin: Inherited structural variation in man. Science **140**: 1228–1231.
5. Anson, M. L. & A. E. Mirsky. 1930. Protein coagulation and its reversal: the preparation of insoluble globin, soluble globin and heme. J. Gen. Physiol. **13**: 469–476.
6. Ingram, V. M. 1958. Abnormal human haemoglobins. I. The comparison of normal human and sickle cell haemoglobins by "fingerprinting." Biochim. Biophys. Acta. **35**: 539–545.
7. Baglioni, C. 1961. An improved method for fingerprinting of human hemoglobin. Biochim. Biophys. Acta. **48**: 392–396.
8. Hill, R. J. & L. C. Craig. 1959. Countercurrent distribution studies with adult human hemoglobin. J. Amer. Chem. Soc. **81**: 2272–2273.
9. Kraus, L. M., D. B. Morrison & A. P. Kraus. 1959. Abnormal human hemoglobins. I. Biosynthesis in vitro of ^{59}Fe-labeled human hemoglobin A and hemoglobin S. Blood **14**: 1103–1111.

APPLICATION OF THE IN VITRO ERYTHROPOIETIN SYSTEM TO THE STUDY OF HUMAN BONE MARROW DISEASE: POLYCYTHEMIA VERA

Sanford B. Krantz

*Argonne Cancer Research Hospital**
and the Department of Medicine, University of Chicago,
Chicago, Ill.

The development of a cell culture system[1] in which human marrow responds to the introduction of erythropoietin by increased hemoglobin synthesis has facilitated our ability to study many red cell diseases. Because this method allows separation of the marrow from the body for periods during which it can be studied directly, many of the common clinical disorders can be subjected to a more intensive biochemical investigation. It is now possible to trace the chemical handling of labeled precursors, and to measure the accumulation of metabolites in a number of disorders as a means of determining the metabolic defect responsible for the disease. Hitherto, alteration of the administered precursor or synthesized metabolites by other body tissues has served to hide much of this information from direct observation.

Since erythropoietin is believed to regulate erythropoiesis by initiating the differentiation of primitive stem cells into erythroblasts,[2–5] this system provides an especially good model for studying proliferative diseases of the red cell in which this control mechanism appears to have malfunctioned. Such a disease is polycythemia vera in which, while there is an overproduction of white cells and platelets as well as red cells, the latter may be singled out for study with this system. I shall report some preliminary experiments with polycythemia vera marrow, which show that this marrow does not respond in a normal way to the in vitro introduction of erythropoietin and that this relative lack of response to the hormone is not due to a plasma factor but to an intrinsic marrow cell defect.

Materials and Methods

The bone marrow cell suspension was prepared as previously described[1,6] but was also filtered through a sterile stainless steel mesh to remove loose bone particles, thereby producing a more uniform suspension. The dispersed cells were added to 35 × 10 mm tissue culture dishes (Falcon Plastics) in 0.8 ml of a medium which consisted of 60 percent NCTC 109, 20 percent newborn calf serum, and 20 percent human AB plasma or serologically compatible polycythemia vera plasma. ^{59}Fe was added in 0.1 ml of homologous AB plasma as a source of transferrin, and radioactive heme was extracted and counted as previously indicated.[6] In order to compare sequential experiments in which the plasma and marrow unlabeled iron might vary, the data are expressed as percent of control in the dose response experiments or percent of initial four-hour rate in the time course experiments. Sheep plasma erythropoietin (Step IV, lot K 103214A) was used throughout and was obtained from the United States Public Health Service Study Section on Hematology.

Results

When human marrow is placed into this in vitro system and treated with

* Operated by the University of Chicago for the United States Atomic Energy Commission.

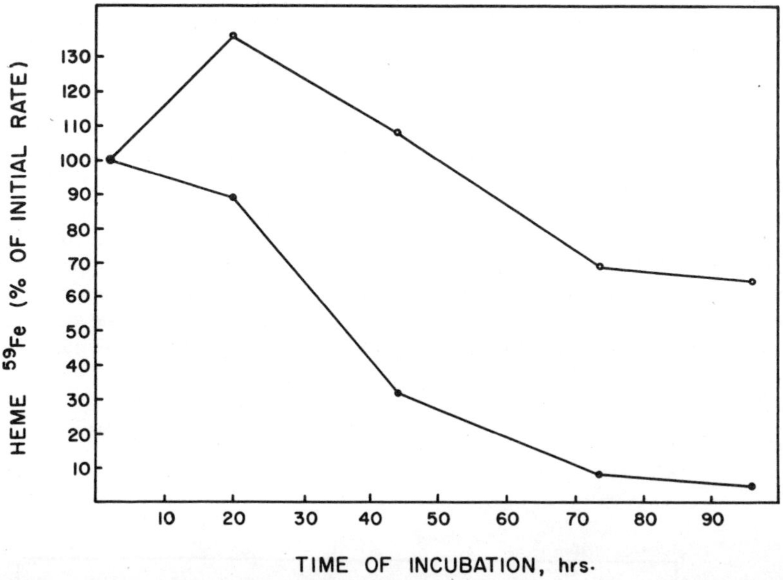

FIGURE 1. Erythropoietin effect on normal human marrow in vitro. The marrow was obtained from a 43-year-old female (hematocrit 41 percent). Twenty-eight hundred nucleated cells per cu mm and 108,000 red blood cells (RBC) per cu mm were present in each plate with 20 percent homologous AB plasma. ○ = erythropoietin, 0.3 units per ml. ● = no added erythropoietin. Each point is the mean of duplicates and indicates the middle of a four-hour incubation period with 0.49 μc of ^{59}Fe per ml.

erythropoietin, the rate of heme synthesis is maintained within 70 percent of the initial rate for up to 70 hr while the control rate falls progressively (FIGURE 1). A dose response experiment with normal human marrow shows a 500 percent stimulation of heme synthesis above the controls (FIGURE 2). These data provide a clear baseline for comparison of the response of diseased bone marrow to the hormone.

The effect of erythropoietin on the rate of heme synthesis by polycythemia vera marrow incubated in 20 percent of the patient's own plasma is shown in FIGURE 3. With this marrow the control rate of heme synthesis also falls progressively; here, however, the erythropoietin produces a much smaller stimulation than occurs with the normal marrow.

TABLE 1 shows the results of polycythemia vera marrow and normal marrow, incubated in neighboring dishes, treated simultaneously with erythropoietin, and then tested for heme synthesis. A marked difference in the two responses is again evident, showing that the response is not simply due to variations in material or conditions of incubation.

In order to find out whether this comparative lack of response to erythropoietin might be related to a different dose requirement of the hormone in this disease, a dose response experiment was performed on polycythemia vera marrow (FIGURE 4). This shows a graded but relatively small response to increasing amounts of the hormone, the maximum response at high concentrations being only 127 percent of the control. The fall in heme synthesis with very large doses of the

Step IV erythropoietin preparation has been noted before with rat marrow and is probably related to a contaminant in the preparation. This experiment demonstrates that polycythemia vera marrow follows a dose response pattern similar to that of normal marrow but with a much smaller response to all doses of the hormone.

The lack of a normal response of polycythemia vera marrow to erythropoietin could be due to a difference within the cell itself or to the presence of an inhibitor in the patient's plasma. This latter possibility was tested by incubating normal human marrow in polycythemia vera plasma. Samples of the same marrow tested with erythropoietin in normal human plasma (FIGURE 1) were treated with the hormone in polycythemia vera plasma. FIGURE 5 shows that a similar response was obtained: addition of the hormone resulted in a normal marked increase in heme synthesis despite the presence of the polycythemia vera plasma. No inhibitor of the hormone, therefore, is present in the polycythemic plasma.

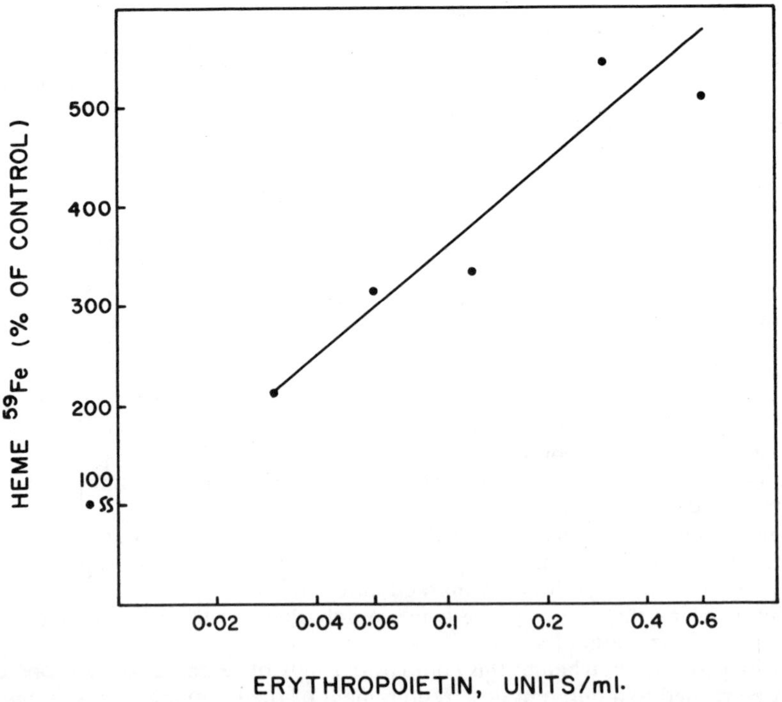

FIGURE 2. Erythropoietin dose response curve with normal human marrow in vitro. The marrow was obtained from a 25-year-old male (hematocrit 43 percent). Four hundred and eight nucleated cells per cu mm and 100,800 RBC per cu mm were present in each plate with 20 percent homologous AB plasma. After 46 hr of incubation, 0.55 μc ^{59}Fe was added and the cultures were terminated 24 hr later. Each point is the mean of triplicates.

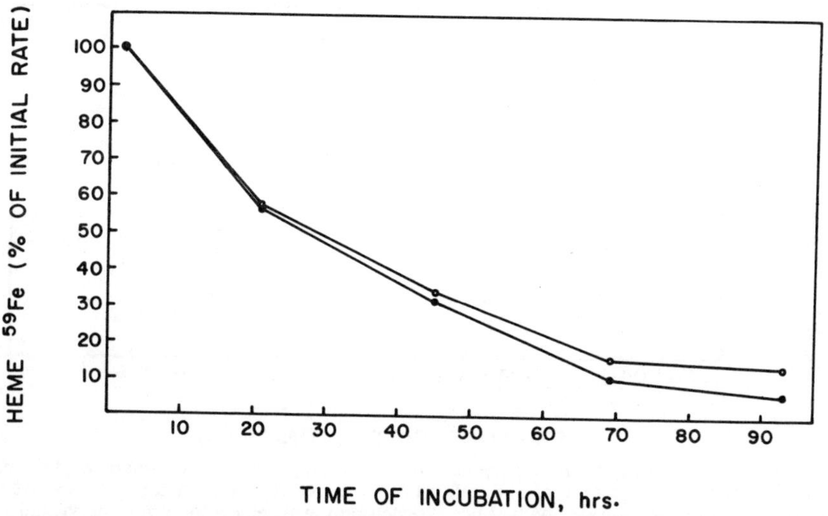

FIGURE 3. Erythropoietin effect on polycythemic vera marrow. The marrow was obtained from a 69-year-old female who had polycythemia vera for 10 years. When first seen, the white blood count (WBC) and RBC were elevated; the marrow was 100 percent cellular and splenomegaly was present. At the time of this marrow aspiration, no suppressive drugs had been administered for four years and the WBC was 6,300 and RBC 6.05 million cells per cu mm. The hemoglobin was 16.3 g percent. Each plate had 4,000 nucleated cells per cu mm and 280,000 RBC per cu mm in 20 percent of the patient's own plasma. ○ = erythropoietin, 0.3 units per ml. ● = no added erythropoietin. Each point is the mean of duplicates and indicates the middle of a four-hour incubation with 0.99 μc ^{59}Fe per ml.

TABLE 1

EFFECT OF ERYTHROPOIETIN ON NORMAL MARROW AND POLYCYTHEMIA VERA MARROW*

Sample	Treatment	Heme (Counts/Minute)
Normal marrow	Control	282
	Erythropoietin (0.3 units per ml)	842
Polycythemia vera marrow	Control	332
	Erythropoietin (0.3 units per ml)	388

* The polycythemic marrow was obtained from a 65-year-old male who had polycythemia vera treated only with phlebotomy for 1.5 years. When first seen, the hemoglobin was 20.6 g percent and the RBC was 7.06 million cells per cu mm. The bone marrow was 90 percent cellular with clumps of megakaryocytes present. Each plate had 1100 nucleated cells per mm^3 and 148,000 RBC per cu mm in 20 percent of the patient's own plasma.

The normal marrow was obtained from a 44-year-old male who had tuberculosis but normal blood counts. At the time of this marrow aspiration his WBC was 7500 cells per cu mm with a normal differential count and the hematocrit was 41 percent. Each plate had 1600 nucleated cells per cu mm and 440,000 RBC per cu mm in 20 percent of the above polycythemic patient's plasma. Both series were incubated simultaneously for 67 hr and then 0.62 μc ^{59}Fe was added for eight hr before terminating the cultures. Each set is the mean of triplicates.

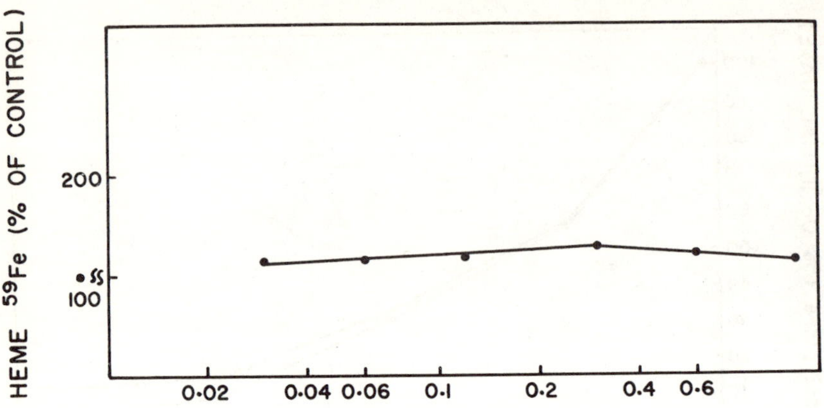

FIGURE 4. Erythropoietin dose response curve with polycythemia vera marrow. The marrow was obtained from a 66-year-old male who had polycythemia vera for 11 years. At the time this marrow was aspirated he had been treated only with phlebotomy for one yr and had a RBC of 7.65 million cells per cu mm; WBC was 12,900 cells per cu mm and platelet count was 955,100 cells per cu mm. Each plate had 2,100 nucleated cells per cu mm. and 372,000 RBC per cu mm in 20 percent of the patient's own plasma. After 46 hr of incubation 0.95 μc ^{59}Fe was added and the cultures were terminated 24 hr later. Each point is the mean of triplicates.

Discussion

These experiments demonstrate that polycythemia vera is characterized by a relative lack of marrow response to erythropoietin and that this characteristic is not due to an environmental or plasma defect but to an intrinsic marrow cell defect. Using animal assays, other investigators have already clearly demonstrated that subnormal levels of erythropoietin are present in the blood and urine of polycythemia vera patients.[7–9] Theoretically, erythropoietin could still cause the overproduction of red cells in this disease if the marrow were hypersensitive to low doses of the hormone. The experiments reported here with this in vitro system now show that no such hypersensitivity exists.

It might still be maintained that erythropoietin is consumed at a higher rate by the polycythemic marrow, thus maintaining a low blood level, or that the animal assays for the hormone are not valid for a newly mutated erythropoietin that is active only on human marrow. The former hypothesis can be discarded because of recent studies which show that hyperactive marrows do not decrease the blood half-life of injected hormone more than normal marrows do.[10,11] Again, it has been shown that normal rat marrow in vitro does not consume much of the erythropoietin present.[12] The data supplied by this in vitro method now make it unlikely that a new, species-specific erythropoietin is present since when polycythemia vera plasma is assayed on human marrow in vitro, it does not stimulate heme synthesis beyond the levels observed with normal plasma. Indeed the rate of heme synthesis is usually lower than that with normal plasma.[13] Thus erythropoietin is clearly not the cause of the overproduction of red cells in this disease.

Erythropoietin normally acts on primitive stem cells to promote differentiation into erythroblasts,[2–5] and this is believed to occur through the synthesis of new messenger RNA.[14] If erythropoietin production in the mouse is suppressed by

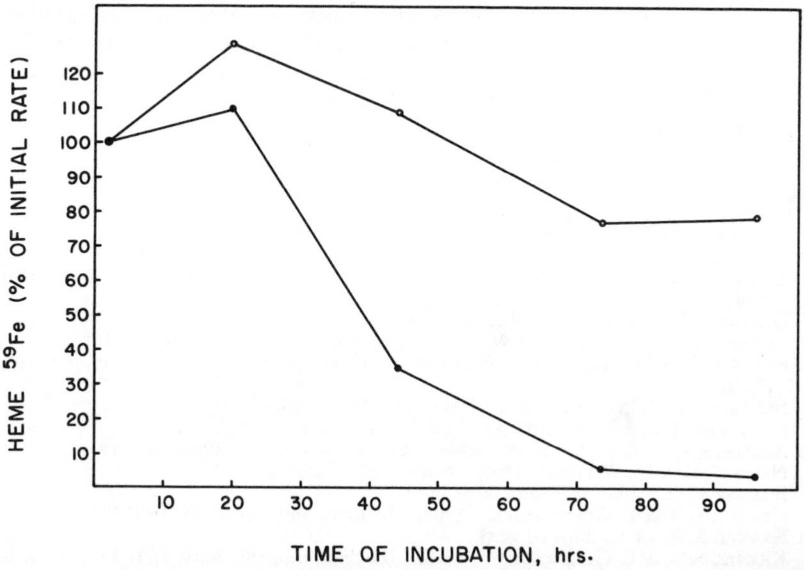

FIGURE 5. Erythropoietin effect on normal human marrow incubated in 20 percent polycythemia vera plasma. The marrow is a replicate specimen of the one described in FIGURE 1 and cell counts are the same. ○ = erythropoietin, 0.3 units per ml. ● = No added erythropoietin. The polycythemic plasma was obtained from a 68-year-old male who had polycythemia vera for three years. When first seen, the hemoglobin was 19.2 g percent and the hematocrit 68 percent. The bone marrow was 90 percent cellular and palpable splenomegaly was present. At the time this plasma was obtained he had been treated only with phlebotomy for six months and had a hemoglobin of 16.4 g percent, hematocrit of 59 percent and RBC of 7.43 million cells per cu mm. Each point is the mean of duplicates and indicates the middle of a four-hour incubation with 0.49 μc ^{59}Fe per ml.

hypertransfusion, then further differentiation ceases and no normoblasts can be found in the marrow.[2] Similarly, removal of the erythropoietin in vitro by transferring the cells to normal medium stops a further increase in hemoglobin synthesis above the controls.[12] Thus, the stem cells are normally inhibited from further differentiation in the absence of the hormone. This inhibitor acts like the "repressor" described by Jacob and Monod[15] and erythropoietin may be considered as analogous to the "de-repressor." An absence or malfunction of the repressor would produce an uncontrolled differentiation not very responsive to the de-repressor. Therefore, polycythemia vera is best viewed as a disease with an intrinsic defect in the specific stem cell repressor that is acted on by erythropoietin. Further investigation must now center on the repressor mechanism that ordinarily prevents this red cell overproduction unless the switch is turned by by erythropietin.

Summary

Human marrow in vitro shows a marked increase in heme synthesis when erythropoietin is added. Polycythemia vera marrow shows a much reduced response to the hormone. This is neither due to a different dose response nor to the presence of an inhibitor in polycythemic plasma because such plasma allows a normal marrow to respond normally to the hormone. The red cell overproduction in this disease cannot be caused by erythropoietin because the plasma does not contain increased amounts of erythropoietin and the cells are not hypersensitive to the low amounts present. The disease appears to be due, rather, to an intrinsic cell defect that may be a malfunction, or absence, of the specific stem cell repressor acted on by erythropoietin.

References

1. Krantz, S. B. 1965. Life Sciences **4**: 2393.
2. Jacobson, L. O., E. Goldwasser, L. F. Plzak & W. Fried. 1957. Proc. Soc. Exp. Biol. Med. **94**: 243.
3. Alpen, E. L. & D. Cranmore. 1957. *In* The Kinetics of Cellular Proliferation. F. S. Stohlman, Jr., Ed. : 290. Grune and Stratton. New York, N. Y.
4. Erslev, A. J. 1959. Blood **14**: 386.
5. Lajtha, L. G., R. Oliver & C. W. Gurney. 1962. Brit. J. Haematol. **8**: 461.
6. Krantz, S. B., O. Gallien-Lartigue & E. Goldwasser. 1963. J. Biol. Chem. **238**: 4085.
7. Noyes, W. D., B. M. Domm & L. C. Willis. 1962. Blood **20**: 9.
8. DeGowin, R. L. & C. W. Gurney. 1964. Arch. Int. Med. **114**: 424.
9. Adamson, J. W. & C. A. Finch. 1966. Trans. Assoc. Amer. Physicians **79**: 419.
10. Naets, J. P. & M. Wittek. 1965. Nature **206**: 726.
11. Bozzini, C. E. 1966. Nature **209**: 1140.
12. Krantz, S. B. & E. Goldwasser. 1965. Biochim. Biophys. Acta. **108**: 455.
13. Krantz, S. B. Unpublished work.
14. Krantz, S. B. & E. Goldwasser. 1965. Biochim. Biophys. Acta. **103**: 325.
15. Jacob, F. & J. Monod. 1961. Cold Spring Harbor Symp. Quant. Biol. **26**: 193.

IN VITRO STUDIES ON DNA SYNTHESIS OF BONE MARROW CELLS STIMULATED BY ERYTHROPOIETIN

Peter P. Dukes*

*Argonne Cancer Research Hospital***
and the Department of Biochemistry, University of Chicago,
Chicago, Ill.

Materials and Methods

Bone marrow cells from the femora and tibiae of six-to-eight-week-old male Sprague-Dawley rats were collected and incubated as described previously[1] in 35 mm × 10 mm plastic culture dishes in an atmosphere of 95 percent air and 5 percent CO_2. The incubation medium was 50 percent NCTC 109, 50 percent calf serum (heated for 20 min to 56° C.) containing 40 units penicillin and 50 μg streptomycin per ml. Where indicated, thymidine-free NCTC 109 was employed. Radioactive label was added as 0.05 or 0.5 μc of thymidine-methyl-^{3}H (6.7 μc/mmole) and 0.1 μc of glucosamine-1-^{14}C (2.5 mc/mmole).

After incubation the dishes were chilled for 10 min at 4° C. The cell suspensions were then washed over to and collected on cellulose ester membranes of 0.45 μ pore size and 47 mm diameter (Millipore HAWP 04700) with 6 ml of saline. For evaluation of total cell radioactivity the cells were then washed five more times on the filter with 1 ml portions of saline. The samples for the determination of acid insoluble radioactivity were prepared by lysing the washed cells on the filter with 10 ml 5 percent trichloroacetic acid (TCA), followed by a wash with 10 ml of a mixture of ethanol-water (1:1). In order to make sure that these samples actually reflected incorporation of ^{3}H-thymidine into cellular DNA, they were compared in one experiment (TABLE 1) with samples prepared from TCA-precipitated washed cells that had been incubated in 0.5 N NaOH at 37° C for 18 hr to hydrolyze the RNA and then reprecipitated with TCA and collected for counting on the filters. Both procedures yielded similar results with some loss in recovery of radioactivity in the latter.

The thoroughly dried filters were rolled into a cylinder, cell side in, and placed in glass vials containing 18 ml of a scintillation fluid (5 g 2,5 diphenyloxazole, 200 mg 1,4-bis-2-(5-phenyloxazolyl)-benzene in 1 liter toluene). Radioactivity was determined in a Packard Tricarb scintillation counter.

Erythropoietin (Step III, lot 137) was generously provided by the United States Public Health Service Study Section on Hematology. Hydroxyurea was bought from Nutritional Biochemicals Inc. Culture dishes were bought from Falcon Plastics Inc., medium NCTC 109 and thymidine-free NCTC 109 from Grand Island Biological Company Inc., and calf serum from Colorado Serum Co. Labeled thymidine and glucosamine were bought from the New England Nuclear Corporation.

Results

The rate of DNA synthesis in cultures decreased with time of incubation. (FIGURES 1–3). By 24 hr it was about 5 percent of the initial rate and by 50 hr, about 2.5 percent of the initial rate. During this period the rate rose and fell, suggesting partial synchrony of the cultures.

* Present address: Childrens Hospital of Los Angeles, Departments of Pediatrics and Biochemistry, University of Southern California, Los Angeles, Calif.

** Operated by the University of Chicago for the United States Atomic Energy Commission.

TABLE 1

ERYTHROPOIETIN EFFECT ON ^{3}H-THYMIDINE INCORPORATION RATE INTO ACID-INSOLUBLE MATERIAL OF BONE MARROW CELLS*

	Control dpm/hour	0.25 Units Erythropoietin dpm/hour	Ratio Erythropoietin/Control
Acid-insoluble prepared on filter	102010 (92400, 108140)**	122410 (108690, 134450)	1.20
Acid-insoluble after NaOH hydrolysis and reprecipitation	76930 (71220, 82290)	96780 (86950, 103240)	1.26

* 16.5 × 10^{6} cells per ml were incubated in 50 percent NCTC 109–50 percent calf serum medium. Erythropoietin was added at 0 time, 0.5 μc ^{3}H-thymidine was added for a one-hour period terminating at three hr and 30 min of incubation.

** Mean and range of quadruplicates.

TABLE 2

ERYTHROPOIETIN EFFECTS ON THE RATE OF INCORPORATION OF LABELED PRECURSORS IN TWO-DAY CULTURES OF MARROW CELLS

	Control	0.1 Units Erythropoietin from Start of Incubation	Difference from Control		0.1 Units Erythropoietin *from* 47 Hr of Incubation	Difference from Control	
	dpm*	dpm	dpm	%	dpm	dpm	%
Cell cultured in thymidine-free medium:							
1. ^{3}H-thymidine incorporation into acid-insoluble	1724 (1687, 1760)**	971 (710, 1336)	− 753	−44	1798 (1705, 1891)	+ 74	+ 4
2. ^{14}C-glucosamine incorporation into whole cells	4435 (4101, 4808)	5636 (5472, 5820)	+1201	+27	6462 (5686, 7504)	+2027	+46
3. ^{14}C-glucosamine incorporation into acid-soluble	2883 (2596, 3171)	1843 (1286, 2646)	−1040	−36	2724 (2416, 3034)	− 159	− 6
Cells cultured in thymidine-free medium containing 10^{-3} M hydroxyurea:							
1. ^{3}H-thymidine incorporation into acid-soluble	630 (438, 747)	878 (768, 1061)	+ 248	+39	838 (764, 930)	+ 208	+33
2. ^{14}C-glucosamine incorporation into whole cells	3760 (3344, 4078)	3594 (3473, 2708)	− 166	− 4	3383 (2932, 4052)	− 377	−10
3. ^{14}C-glucosamine incorporation into acid-soluble	1177 (914, 1341)	1550 (1207, 1766)	+ 373	+32	1681 (1389, 1852)	+ 504	+43

* Incorporation during a two-hour period terminating at 52 hr and 45 min of incubation. 0.05 μc ^{3}H-thymidine and 0.1 μc of ^{14}C-glucosamine were added.
** Mean and range of triplicates.

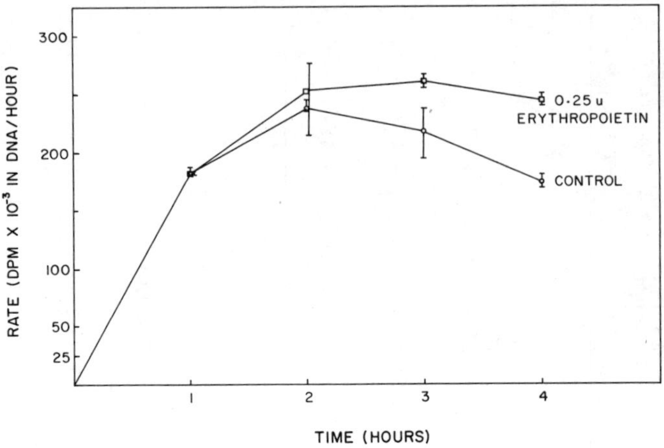

FIGURE 1. Erythropoietin effect on rates of ^{3}H-thymidine incorporation into acid insoluble material. 17.7 $\times$ 10^{6} cells per ml were incubated in 50 percent NCTC 109–50 percent calf serum medium. ^{3}H-thymidine (0.5 μc) was added for one-hour periods to the cultures. 0.25 units/ml erythropoietin was added to the samples indicated. Samples were run in triplicate; means and ranges are indicated.

The effect of erythropoietin added at various times during incubation and therefore, at various levels of DNA synthesis was investigated both with regard to DNA synthesis and to glucosamine incorporation.

When erythropoietin was added to the cultures at zero time, DNA synthesis was increased over the control level starting from the second-hour interval of incubation (FIGURE 1, TABLE 1). This increase was about 40 percent by four hours. A difference of this order of magnitude persisted to 24 hours. In effect, the decline of the DNA synthetic rate with time was retarded by the addition of erythropoietin.

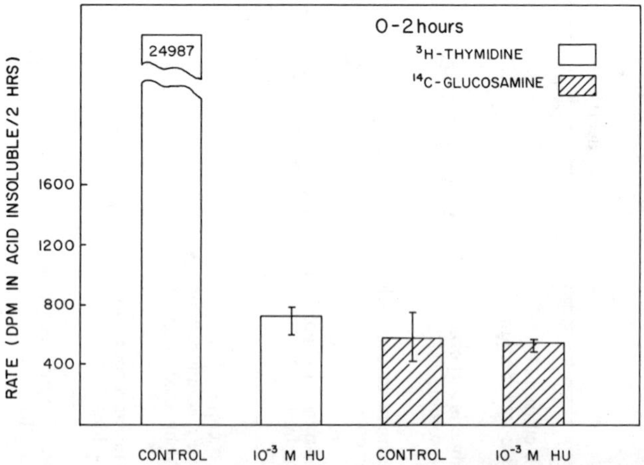

FIGURE 2. Effect of 10^{-3} M hydroxyurea on the rate of incorporation of ^{3}H-thymidine and ^{14}C-glucosamine into acid-insoluble material. 14.4 $\times$ 10^{6} cells per ml were incubated in 50 percent thymidine-free NCTC 109–50 percent calf serum medium. ^{3}H-thymidine (0.05 μc) and ^{14}C-glucosamine (0.1 μc) were added for the indicated two-hour interval of the incubation. Samples were run in quadruplicate; means and ranges are indicated.

In the period between 43 and 53 hr of incubation, this relationship was reversed; cultures that had received erythropoietin at zero time now showed DNA synthesis about 40 percent below that of controls (TABLE 2).

It has previously been reported that erythropoietin added at 0 time causes increased amounts of glucosamine to be incorporated starting between two and three hr of incubation.[2] An erythropoietin-stimulated constant rate of glucosamine incorporation is rapidly achieved and maintained for about 24 hours.

By 43 hr, when DNA synthesis in the samples with erythropoietin was depressed, glucosamine incorporation into acid-insoluble material had also fallen to a level below that of the controls. It must be pointed out, however, that total cellular label derived from glucosamine incorporation was still more than that of controls even after 53 hr of incubation in the presence of erthropoietin (TABLE 2).

When the hormone was added to the cultures after 18.3 hr of incubation, the same relationships were obtained as when it was added at zero time. After a slight rise during the zero- to two-hour period after erythropoietin addition, DNA synthesis and glucosamine incorporation attained a highly stimulated level by the four- to six-hour period.

Cells that had been incubated for 47 hr were no longer capable of responding to erythropoietin with increased DNA synthesis or glucosamine incorporation into acid-insoluble material although the total amount of glucosamine taken up from the medium (TABLE 2) was increased.

Hydroxyurea at a concentration of 10^{-3} M was added to the medium to reduce DNA synthesis by preventing the formation in the cells of deoxyribonucleotides from ribonucleotides.[3] Under these conditions, at the beginning of the incubation, DNA synthesis was reduced to 3 percent of its normal rate and ^{14}C-glucosamine incorporation into acid-insoluble material virtually unchanged (FIGURE 2).

After 24 hr of incubation, DNA synthesis in hydroxyurea-containing cultures was 25 percent of that of controls (FIGURE 3). The shift in the proportion of the rates was due to the sharp decline of DNA synthesis in the controls by 24 hr

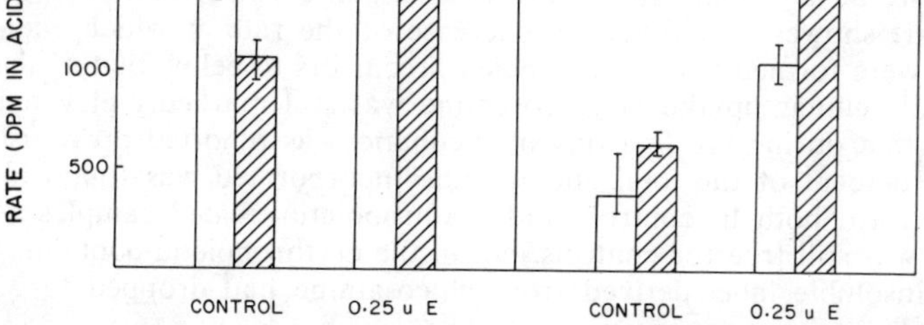

FIGURE 3. Effect of 0.25 units erythropoietin added at the start of the incubation on the rate of incorporation of ^{3}H-thymidine and ^{14}C-glucosamine into acid-soluble material of cells cultured with and without 10^{-3} M hydroxyurea. For details see legend to FIGURE 2.

of incubation at a time when there was little change in the hydroxyurea-treated cultures. Glucosamine incorporation in hydroxyurea-treated samples was at 60 percent of control rate. In the interval from 24 to 26 hr of culture the effect of erythropoietin added to the hydroxyurea-containing cultures was initially a 179 percent increase in the DNA synthetic rate and a 174 percent increase in the rate of glucosamine incorporation. These rate increases were larger than in cultures without hydroxyurea when expressed as percent changes but of a similar order of magnitude when expresed as incorporated radioactive label (FIGURE 3).

In the period between 51 to 53 hr of incubation the hydroxyurea-treated cells still responded to erythropoietin added at zero time with increased incorporation of ^{3}H-thymidine and ^{14}C-glucosamine into acid-insoluble material (TABLE 2).

After 18.3 hr of incubation, hydroxyurea-containing cultures responded to the addition of erythropoietin with an increased rate of DNA synthesis and glucosamine incorporation in the same manner as untreated cultures.

By 47 hr of incubation a marked difference had appeared between untreated and hydroxyurea-treated cultures. Only in the latter did the addition of erythropoietin cause an increase in rate of precursor incorporation into acid-insoluble materials (TABLE 2).

Discussion

This investigation was designed to shed some light on whether the rate of DNA synthesis in bone marrow cell cultures is in some way correlated with their response to erythropoietin as measured by the glucosamine incorporation assay. It turned out that the cultures displayed the same increment of glucosamine incorporation due to erythropoietin during the time of high initial rates of DNA synthesis and 24 hr later when much lower rates of DNA synthesis were observed. Addition of hydroxyurea to the cultures reduced the level of DNA synthesis initially to about 3 percent of the control, but the erythropoietin effect on glucosamine incorporation was only slightly reduced. A very low level of DNA synthesis in the cultures, which probably reflects the activity of a small number of cells, is therefore adequate to permit erythropoietin action.

It was found that during the first 24 hr all cultures increased their DNA synthesis after the addition of erythropoietin. This increase was easily measurable during the third hour of contact with the hormone, at about the same time as the effect on glucosamine incorporation became apparent. Addition of erythropoietin at the start of incubation, when DNA synthesis was falling rapidly, merely delayed the decrease of rate with time, but when DNA synthesis was already low at the time of addition, the subsequent increase in rate was no longer obscured by the overall tendency to decline.

After two days of incubation cultures to which erythropoietin had been added at the start showed a paradoxical decrease of the rate at which acid-insoluble products were formed from both labeled precursors to below that of the controls while total cellular uptake of glucosamine was still markedly elevated. It must be noted that during the first day of incubation, as reported previously,[1] about 60 to 70 percent of the total glucosamine incorporated was found in an acid-insoluble form both in controls and erythropoietin-treated samples. After two days this was still true for controls, but in the erythropoietin-containing samples the acid-insoluble label derived from glucosamine had dropped to 33 percent of the total.

The best explanation for this seems to be that in the continued presence of erythropoietin the cells were reduced in their capacity to synthesize the proper macromolecular acceptors for the labeled glucosamine or related carbohydrate moieties. Krantz and Goldwasser[4] have observed that with time bone marrow cells lose their ability to respond to erythropoietin with hemoglobin synthesis, and have suggested that exhaustion of an essential nutrient might be the cause. It is likely that the medium in our cultures also was exhausted of essential nutrients rather than that cell enzymes had declined in synthetic ability under the influence of erythropoietin since addition of the hormone after 47 hr of incubation neither decreased nor increased the subsequent rate of formation of acid-insoluble glucosamine products. Under these conditions total cellular incorporation of glucosamine label had risen so sharply that the acid-insoluble fraction was 42 percent of the total. The formation of the hypothetical acceptor, therefore, could not be accelerated to meet the demand created by erythropoietin action as it was during the first day of incubation, but on the other hand, neither was it directly depressed by erythropoietin.

The formation of DNA completely paralleled the formation of acid-insoluble compounds labeled with glucosamine after 47 hr of incubation so that a similar explanation is suggested. (^{3}H-thymidine label also increased in cells under the influence of erythropoietin when there was no change or a decrease in DNA synthesis.)† It is probable that exhaustion of a cofactor from the medium was to blame for the reduced DNA synthesis.

It is also possible that the increases in total cellular label incorporation that occurred at a time when there was no increase in the acid-insoluble fractions reflect the action of a factor contaminating the relatively impure Step III erythropoietin used in these experiments. Conceivably this action could even have been on cells different from the stem cells on which erythropoietin presumably acts, but in view of Hrinda and Goldwasser's recent demonstration of the effect of erythropoietin on Fe transport into the cells,[5] these possibilities seem less likely.

When hydroxyurea was added to the cultures, its direct effect was to restrict DNA synthesis to those few cells which had available scavenging pathways leading to DNA synthesis utilizing preformed deoxyribonucleosides. As an indirect consequence, the medium was still adequate during the second day of incubation to support such increased DNA synthesis as was demanded by erythropoietin action. Similarly, the blocking of many cells just prior to S-phase probably resulted in a lower consumption of some critical medium constituents by the survivors. Obviously, experiments are in order to explore these possible nutritional deficiencies in the culture media after two days of incubation.

It is interesting that those cells which are able to respond to erythropoietin are not seriously affected by hydroxyurea and can also survive adverse culture conditions better than the majority of the bone marrow cells. This was borne out by the fact that while cell numbers declined drastically during incubation, when they had fallen to 50 percent, the response of a culture in terms of the stimulated glucosamine incorporation rate was unchanged from its initial value.

It is concluded that in bone marrow cells increased DNA synthesis occurs within one to two hr after the addition of erythropoietin. Under favorable conditions this response, like the increased glucosamine incorporation into acid-insoluble stroma, persists up to 53 hr of incubation. It is assumed that erythropoietin acts on the stem cells during a limited part of their cell cycle to cause them to differentiate.[1,4] By 53 hr all stem cells should have passed through the cell cycle and should have been triggered out during their sensitive phase, thus permitting no further response unless their number was replenished by division. Preparation for such divisions would require additional DNA synthesis. One

† P. P. Dukes, unpublished observation.

would also expect a contribution to increased DNA synthesis per unit time from those cells triggered by erythropoietin to differentiate if their cell cycle was shorter than that of the undifferentiated stem cells. At the present time it seems equally possible that any one, or a combination, of these two processes could account for the observed increases in DNA synthesis in the erythropoietin-stimulated cultures.

Acknowledgment

The experiments were done with the able technical assistance of Leda Ellis.

References

1. Dukes, P. P. & E. Goldwasser. 1965. On the mechanism of erythropoietin-induced differentiation. III. The nature of erythropoietin action on ^{14}C-glucosamine incorporation by marrow cells in culture. Biochim. Biophys. Acta **108:** 447.
2. Dukes, P. P., F. Takaku & E. Goldwasser. 1964. In vitro studies on the effect of erythropoietin on glucosamine-1-^{14}C incorporation into rat bone marrow cells. Endocrinology **74:** 960.
3. Sinclair, W.K. 1965. Hydroxyurea: Differential lethal effects on cultured mammalian cells during cell cycle. Science **150:** 1729.
4. Krantz, S. B. & E. Goldwasser. 1965. On the mechanism of erythropoietin-induced differentiation. IV. Some characteristics of erythropoietin action on hemoglobin synthesis in marrow cell culture. Biochim. Biophys. Acta **108:** 455.
5. Hrinda, M. E. & E. Goldwasser. 1966. Facilitated iron entry into marrow cells: An induced permease like activity. Fed. Proc. **25:** 284.

STUDIES ON MITOTIC ACTIVITY IN VITRO AND KINETICS OF PROLIFERATION OF ERYTHROID CELLS FROM SPLENIC COLONIES IN IRRADIATED, MARROW-TRANSFUSED MICE

Y. Matoth

Tel Aviv University Medical School, Beilinson Hospital, Petah Tikva, Israel

Colonies of hemopoietic cells, produced in spleens of heavily irradiated and marrow-transfused mice, usually consist of one cell type: erythroid, myeloid or megakaryocytic. Pure erythroid colonies are most common. Important information on the kinetics of erythropoiesis can be obtained from the study of such erythroid colonies (or clones), which in the course of nine to ten days grow from a single cell to a population of several million. In addition, these colonies offer the opportunity of studying the behavior in vitro of a pure erythroid cell population.

Splenic colonies were produced in albino mice of a locally bred strain. The mice were given a radiation dose of 750 r, followed by transfusion of 36,000 isologous marrow cells. Cell suspensions aspirated from splenic colonies on the tenth post-transfusion day were used for cultures.

Cultures were done in plasma clots with colchicine added to the fluid phase. In general, a method previously described was followed.[1] Cell morphology was quite satisfactory in ten-hour cultures. There were fewer earlier forms and the cell population consisted largely of late normoblasts. The number of erythroid mitoses was not markedly increased in cultures from mice injected during life with an erythropoietically potent plasma. Similarly, there was no increase over control when plasma from anemic animals was added to the culture medium. Mitotic rates ranged between 3–4% in all cultures. These values are very low compared to results obtained in our previous work with marrow cultures, where the number of accumulated arrested mitoses following ten hours' incubation was in the range of 20–40% of cells capable of mitosis. In the present work modifications of the original method, necessitated by the small volume of material, have probably introduced limiting factors to an optimal proliferative activity of red cell precursors in vitro. No definite conclusions can, therefore, be drawn from the negative results.

Total and differential cell counts were done and mitotic indices determined on colony aspirates obtained on the seventh to 12th post-transfusion days. Total cell counts in pure erythroid colonies on the tenth day ranged between three and eight million.

To account for the growth of a colony from a single cell to several million, the following models were considered, in which 5×10^6 cells was taken to represent the average number of erythroid cells on the tenth post-transfusion day.

Multiplication by a Simple Geometrical Progression

The number of generations can easily be calculated as 22, and the average generation time as 10.8 hours. This figure is in good agreement with a generation time which can be calculated from mitotic indices determined for the erythroid cell population on the seventh through 12th days. Mitotic indices based on 5000 cell counts are summarized in TABLE 1. There is no definite trend in the day-to-day variation, which can be accounted for by statistical error. The mean value for the entire six-day period was 66. Assuming the mitotic time to be 45 min, a mean generation time of 11.4 hr can be calculated.

TABLE 1

MITOTIC INDICES IN ERYTHROID COLONIES 7–12 DAYS AFTER TRANSFUSION

Day	7	8	9	10	11	12
Erythroid mitoses/1000 cells capable of mitosis	45	64	50	76	97	66

For this model to be accepted, it has to be assumed that erythroid precursor cells retain their ability to divide for 10–12 days, during which period they undergo 22 divisions. Such an assumption is not in accord with widely held views on the kinetics of red cell proliferation. It is held that the generation time of erythroid cells remains constant even under stimulation.[2] Furthermore, it is assumed that after four to five generations, the erythroid cell reaches a stage of maturation where it becomes incapable of further division.[3]

Taking these assumptions into consideration, colony growth by a simple geometrical progression could be visualized as multiplication of stem cells for 18 generations, followed by simultaneous differentiation into erythroid cells, which then continue to divide for the ensuing four generations. Such an event would imply the emergence of a uniform cohort of erythroid cells advancing in age from day to day. This is not the case. Age distribution of the erythroid population remains fairly constant throughout the period of observation, as can be seen from TABLE 2. The day-to-day variation in early forms may be due to sampling error resulting from their small numbers. The larger compartments of intermediate and late normoblasts were affected to a much smaller degree by these fluctuation and remained fairly constant throughout the six-day period.

Colony Growth in Two Stages

Stem cells increase their numbers geometrically in the first stage while in the second they maintain their number and at the same time differentiate into erythroid cells, each of which undergoing up to four divisions. The generation time will vary with the length of the first stage (t_1). For a colony that has reached the size of 5×10^6 cells in ten days, the generation time (t_G) can be calculated from the formula

$$2^{\frac{t_1}{t_G}} \times 15 = 5 \times 10^6$$

whereby the figure 15 represents the total number of erythroid cells produced after three successive divisions of each stem cell in stage 2 (FIGURE 1). Assuming

TABLE 2

AGE DISTRIBUTION OF ERYTHROID CELLS IN SPLENIC COLONIES

Day	7	8	9	10	11	12
Proerythroblasts and early normoblasts	49	99	85	67	29	32
Intermediate normoblasts	560	659	639	633	584	641
Late normoblasts	391	242	276	300	387	327
Total	1000	1000	1000	1000	1000	1000

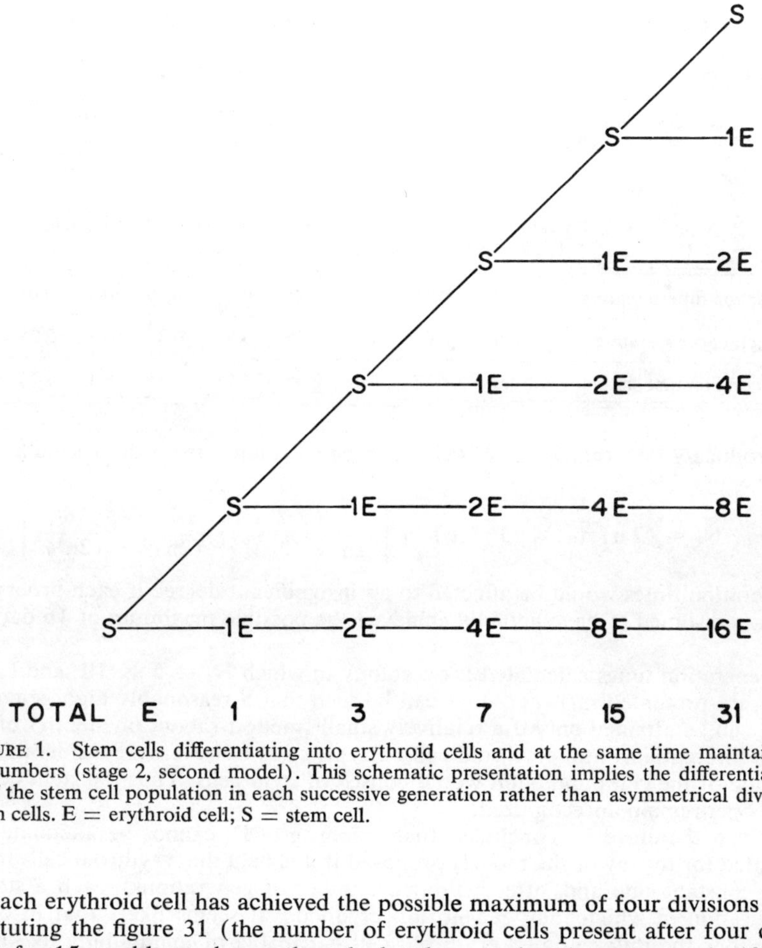

FIGURE 1. Stem cells differentiating into erythroid cells and at the same time maintaining their numbers (stage 2, second model). This schematic presentation implies the differentiation of half the stem cell population in each successive generation rather than asymmetrical division of stem cells. E = erythroid cell; S = stem cell.

that each erythroid cell has achieved the possible maximum of four divisions and substituting the figure 31 (the number of erythroid cells present after four divisions) for 15 would not change the calculated generation times to any significant degree.

Generation times calculated for different lengths of stage 1 are listed in TABLE 3. It can be seen that stage 1 cannot be much shorter than eight days since a generation time well under ten hr is unlikely in mammalian cells, in which each of the three periods of the cell cycle is known to last for several hours.[4] On the other hand, a late beginning of differentiation (stage 2) about the sixth or seventh day would not account for the predominantly erythroid population and for the presence of late normoblasts on the seventh day.

Simultaneous Proliferation and Differentiation of Stem Cells

A fraction (n) of the stem cell population proliferates, while the remaining fraction (1-n) differentiates into erythroid precursors, each of which producing a maximum of 16 daughter cells. In this model the generation time (t_G) will vary with the proportion of differentiating cells and assuming each proetrythroblast

TABLE 3

CALCULATED GENERATION TIMES FOR COLONY GROWTH IN TWO STAGES*

Stage 1, Days	2	3	4	5	6	7	8
Generation time, hours	2.62	3.93	5.25	6.55	7.86	9.17	10.48

* See text.

TABLE 4

VARIATION OF GENERATION TIME WITH VARYING FRACTIONS OF STEM CELLS DIFFERENTIATING INTO ERYTHROID CELLS

Fraction differentiating	0.4	0.35	0.3	0.25	0.2	0.15	0.1	0.05	0.01
Fraction proliferating	0.6	0.65	0.7	0.75	0.8	0.85	0.9	0.95	0.99
Generation time, hours	3.08	4.32	5.4	6.35	7.15	7.85	8.4	8.45	8.5

to produce an average of eight cells, can be calculated from the formula

$$N_t = (2n)^{\frac{t_1}{t_G}} \times (1 - n) \times \left[\frac{1}{2n} + \frac{2}{(2n)^2} + \frac{4}{(2n)^3} + \frac{8}{(2n^4)} \right]$$

Generation times would be affected to an insignificant degree if each proerythroblast is assumed to have actually achieved the possible maximum of 16 daughter cells.

Generation times calculated for a colony in which $N_t = 5 \times 10^6$ and $t = 10$ days are presented in TABLE 4. It can be seen that a reasonably high generation time can be attained only if a relatively small fraction (about one-tenth) of stem cells differentiates into erythroid cells. In this case, however, a considerable proportion of the cell population would consist of stem cells. Thus the stem cell can no longer remain unrecognized.

It can therefore be concluded that colony growth cannot be adequately accounted for by any of the models proposed if it is held that erythroid cells mature at a constant rate and, after a limited number of generations, reach a stage of maturation in which they can no longer divide. It seems likely that in certain situations the differentiated erythroid cell is capable of maintaining its kind by undergoing numerous divisions, thereby fulfiilling at least one criterion of a stem cell.

References

1. MATOTH, Y. & E. BEN-PORATH (ARKIN). 1959. Effect of erythropoietin on the mitotic rate of erythroblasts in bone marrow cultures. J. Lab. Clin. Med. **54**: 722.
2. ALPEN, E. L. & D. CRANMORE. 1959. Observations on the regulation of erythropoiesis and on cellular dynamics by ^{59}Fe autoradiography. *In* the Kinetics of Cellular Proliferation. F. Stohlman, Jr., Ed. : 290–300. Grune & Stratton. New York, N. Y.
3. LAJTHA, L. G. & R. OLIVER. 1960. Studies on the kinetics of erythropoiesis: a model of the erythron. *In* Haemopoiesis. a Ciba Foundation Symposium. : 289–313. J. & A. Churchill. London, England.
4. PRESCOTT, D. M. 1964. The normal cell cycle. *In* Synchrony in Cell Division. E. Zenthen, Ed. : 71–97. Interscience Publishers. New York, N. Y.

STUDIES ON THE CONTROL OF HEMOGLOBIN SYNTHESIS: NUCLEIC ACID SYNTHESIS AND NORMOBLAST PROLIFERATION IN THE PRESENCE OF ERYTHROPOIETIN*

Thomas F. Necheles,† Richard G. Sheehan** and Heidi J. Meyer

Blood Research Laboratory, New England Medical Center Hospitals and the Department of Medicine, Tufts University School of Medicine, Boston, Mass.

Previous reports from this laboratory[1] have indicated that the in vitro addition of erythropoietin to human bone marrow cell suspensions results in an increase in the rate of hemoglobin synthesis. Goldwasser *et al.*,[2,3] using rat bone marrow cell suspensions, reported that the stimulatory effect of erythropoietin on ^{59}Fe incorporation into heme was abolished by the addition of actinomycin, suggesting that the erythropoietin effect was mediated via changes in RNA synthesis. Other workers[4-6] have presented evidence that normoblast proliferation is increased in the presence of added erythropoietin. Perfusion of isolated limbs with erythropoietin-rich perfusate has provided evidence for an effect of erythropoietin beyond the stem cell stage.[7,8] It appeared logical, therefore, to correlate the effects of erythropoietin on hemoglobin synthesis, nucleic acid synthesis and normoblast proliferation, using the in vitro human bone marrow cell suspension previously developed in this laboratory.

Methods and Materials

Adult human bone marrow was obtained by aspiration from fasting young adult males and cells suspensions were prepared by the methods previously described.[1] Glycine-^{14}C (2.5 mc/mM)‡ was used as the radioactive label. Heme and globin were isolated by acid-acetone precipitation from the supernatant obtained by osmotic lysis. The cells and cellular debris remaining following momentary exposure to hypotonic solution were saved at $-20°$ C for isolation of the nucleic acids. A modification of the micromethod described by Kahan[9] was used to isolate total nonhemoglobin protein and total nucleic acids. Basically, this method consists of precipitation of the protein and nucleic acids by cold 0.3 N perchloric acid (PCA), separation onto a membrane filter§ (25 mm diameter, 0.45 μ pore size, HA), heating of the filter and precipitate at 60° C for nine min in 1.6 N PCA, and subsequent separation of precipitate (protein) and filtrate (nucleic acids). The nucleic acids were then autoclaved at 132° C for four hr and adsorbed on acid-washed charcoal¶ which was again separated on a membrane filter. The filters were mounted on steel planchets and counted in a Nuclear-Chicago low background automatic β-counter preset for 10,000 counts. Self-absorption was compensated for by using empirically derived correction curves. Results were calculated as millimoles of glycine incorporated into nonhemoglobin protein and total nucleic acids per nucleated cell present in the

* These studies aided with funds from U.S. Public Health Service Grant number CA 04168–08 from the National Cancer Institute.

† Assistant Professor of Pediatrics, established investigator of the American Heart Association.

** Trainee in Hematology under U.S. Public Health Service Graduate Training Grant number T1 AM 5210-07.

‡ Obtained from New England Nuclear Corporation, Boston, Massachusetts.

§ Millipore Filter Corporation, Bedford, Mass.

¶ Norite A-neutral decolorizing carbon. Fisher Scientific Co., Fairhaven, N. J.

TABLE 1

GLYCINE-^{14}C INCORPORATION IN THE PRESENCE OF ERYTHROPOIETIN

mM glycine incorporation/10^{13} nucleated precursors

	Heme			Globin			Total Protein			Nucleic Acids		
	Control	Erythropoietin	Percent	Control	Erythropoietin	Percent	Control	Erythropoietin	Percent	Control	Erythropoietin	Percent
2 hours	7.27	7.81	107	3.97	3.47	87	0.98	0.97	99	.058	.136	234
	7.52	9.04	120	4.78	8.15	171	0.60	0.89	148	.028	.118	421
	5.80	6.59	114	4.04	5.31	131	0.38	0.55	145	.030	.095	317
	6.86	7.81	114	4.26	5.64	130	0.65	0.80	131	.039	.116	324
		$0.1 > p > .05$			$.4 > p > .3$			$.3 > p > .2$			$p < .01$	
24 hours	41.2	58.3	142	29.3	41.7	142	4.83	7.17	148	.138	.287	208
	82.0	106.8	130	—	92.0	—	5.77	7.77	124	.098	.295	301
	43.5	52.8	121	49.0	75.0	153	3.48	5.94	171	.074	.236	319
	55.6	72.6	131	39.1	69.6	148	4.69	9.96	148	.103	.273	276
		$0.1 > p > .05$						$p < .01$			$.05 > p > .01$	
48 hours	62.6	74.8	119	51.3	70.3	137	7.41	10.58	143	.266	.538	202
	157.8	179.4	114	115.1	127.6	111	12.60	16.80	133	.101	.583	577
	61.7	62.2	101	62.7	84.8	135	5.32	10.11	190	.117	.301	257
	94.0	105.5	111	76.4	84.2	128	8.44	12.58	155	.161	.474	345
		$.4 > p > .3$			$.1 > p > .05$			$p < .01$			$0.1 > p > .05$	

original suspension. Preliminary trials demonstrated that added adenine-^{14}C resulted in no activity in the protein fraction and that protein labeled with isoleucine-^{14}C did not result in radioactivity in the nucleic acid fraction or in heme. Replicate samples from the same cell suspension agreed within 10 percent, as did samples obtained from the same individuals at intervals up to one year.

Cell proliferation was measured using (1) autoradiographs following pulse labeling with thymidine-^{3}H and (2) mitotic indices in the presence of colchicine. Cell suspensions were incubated with 1 μc/ml thymidine-methyl-^{3}H(1.9 c/mM)[11] for one hour at 37° C, the unincorporated label washed off, and the cells reincubated in nonradioactive incubation media with partially purified erythro-

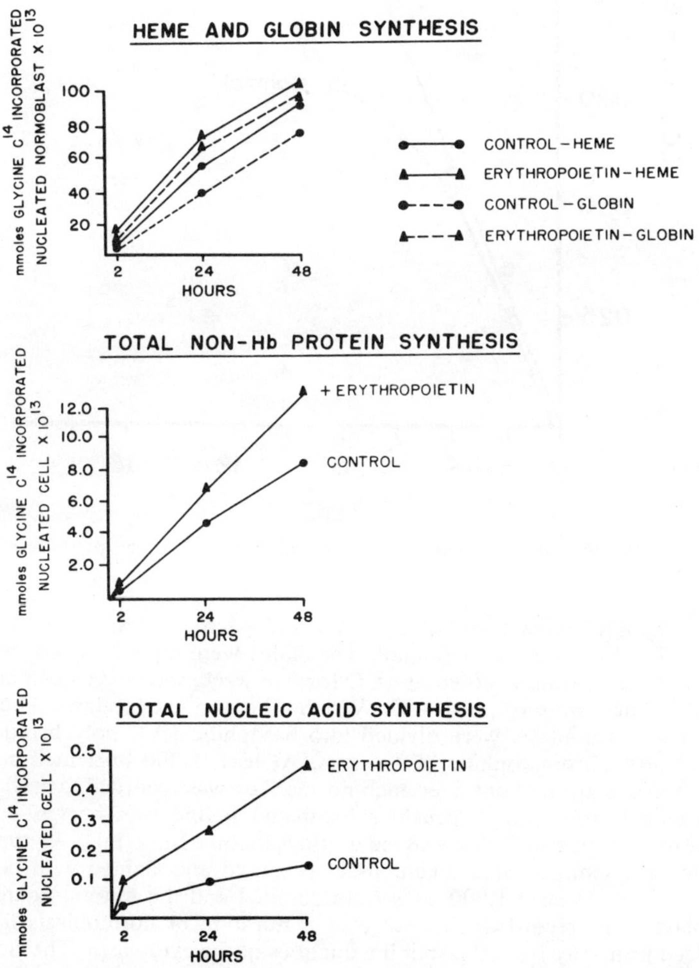

FIGURE 1. Glycine-^{14}C incorporation into hemoglobin, total nonhemoglobin protein and total nucleic acids isolated from human bone marrow cell suspensions incubated with erythropoietin.

[11] Obtained from New England Nuclear Corporation, Boston, Mass.

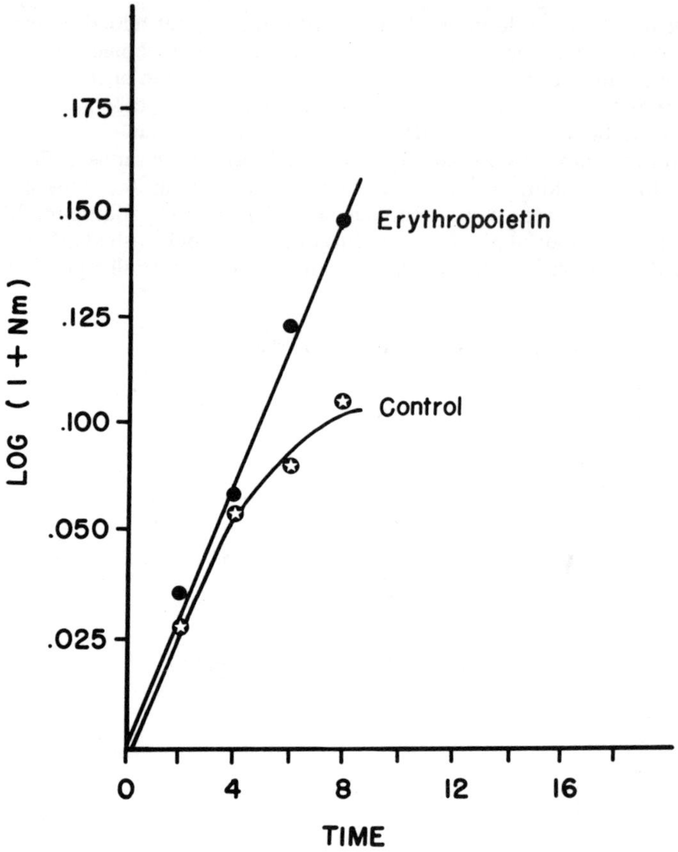

FIGURE 2. Mitotic indices of human normoblasts incubated in the presence of erythropoietin and colchicine.

poietin.* Samples were taken at 0, 2, 24 and 48 hr, slides prepared and immediately fixed in absolute methanol. The slides were dipped in Kodak NTB-2 nuclear track emulsion, exposed at 4° C for one week, then developed and fixed. Duplicate slides were stained with Wright-Giemsa and Ralph's hemoglobin stain.[10] The normoblasts were divided into basophilic (A), polychromatophilic (B), and orthochromatophilic (C) forms. At least 1,000 nucleated cells were counted and the grain count over each normoblast was recorded. Mitotic indices were obtained from cell suspensions incubated in the presence of colchicine (0.4 μg/ml)† with and without added erythropoietin (1unit/ml). At appropriate time intervals, samples were taken, slides prepared and stained with benzidine-Giemsa stain.[10] At least 1,000 cells were counted and the mitotic figures in the normoblast series recorded. The stage of maturation of normoblasts in mitosis was judged primarily from the staining qualities of the cytoplasm. The fraction of normoblasts in mitosis were recalculated using Puck's collection fraction:[11]

* Provided through the courtesy of Dr. F. Stohlman, Jr., St. Elizabeth's Hospital, Brighton, Mass.

† Obtained from Eli Lilly Company, Indianapolis, Ind.

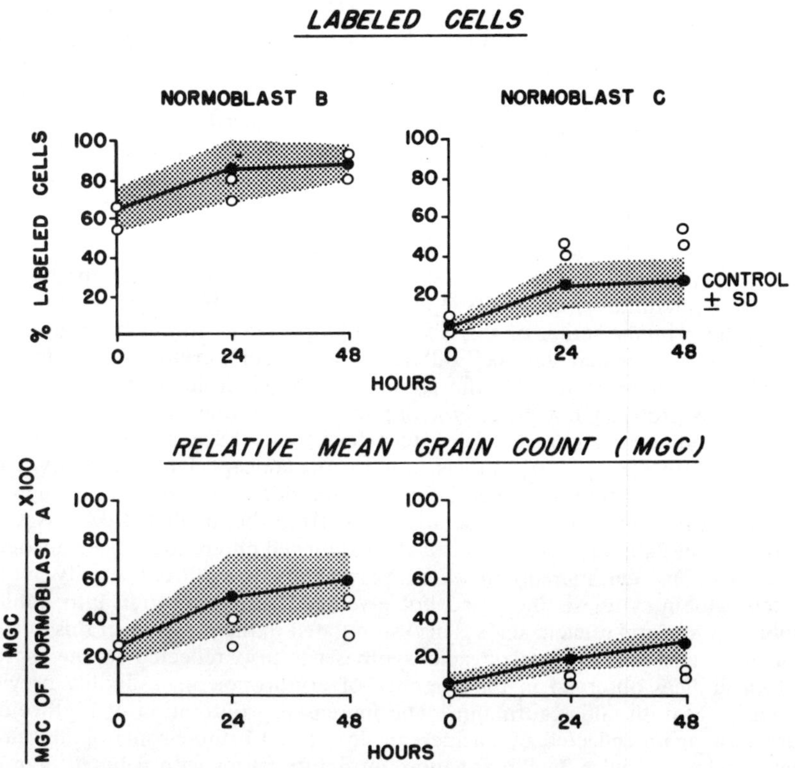

FIGURE 3. Percent labeling and mean grain count of labeled normoblasts following pulse labeling with thymidine-^{3}H and incubated with erythropoietin. Solid line is the mean of eight normal bone marrow cell suspensions, the shaded area encloses one standard deviation. The results from individual experiments using human erythropoietin are indicated by a circle (○).

Log (1 + Nm) where N_m = fraction in mitosis. Incubation for over 24 hr in the presence of colchicine led to the loss of mitotic forms.

Results

Incubation of human bone marrow cell suspensions with added erythropoietin leads to an increased rate of incorporation of glycine-^{14}C into heme, globin, and total protein (TABLE 1 and FIGURE 1). However, the largest and most consistent increase was found in the nucleic acid fraction where a significant increase in rate of glycine-^{14}C incorporation was observed as early as after two hr of incubation. This increase in de novo nucleic acid synthesis was paralleled by an increase in mitotic rate which was noted by two hr and was quite significant by six hr (FIGURE 2). Pulse labeling of early erythroid precursors with thymidine-^{3}H demonstrated that in control incubation there was a progressive appearance of the label in the more mature erythroid forms (FIGURE 3), indicating that maturation occurred under these conditions. The mean grain count of the labeled cells decreased in the more mature forms, reflecting intervening mitotic divisions. In the presence of erythropoietin a greater percentage of the orthochromatophilic forms were labeled and there was a concomitant decrease in the mean grain count over these cells. This again reflected an increased rate of proliferation in the presence of erythropoietin. In all of the control incubations, a few orthochromatophilic cells were noted in which the grain count was markedly higher than the mean grain count for that particular stage of maturation. It is felt that these heavily labeled cells represented cells that had matured without undergoing the usual number of mitotic divisions, the so-called "skipped-divisions" of Stohlman *et al.*[12] No increase in the relative number of such heavily labeled cells was observed in the presence of erythropoietin.

Discussion

It is well established that erythropoietin leads to an increase in the rate of hemoglobin synthesis, in vitro[12–14] as well as in vivo. However, whether or not this is the primary action of this hormone is less clear. In intact animals and in vitro systems in which stem cell differentiation occurs, erythropoietin is thought to act by inducing stem cell differentiation into erythroid precursors.[15,16] However, this is probably not the only action of this hormone. An effect on erythroid proliferation, as well as reticulocyte release, has been suggested by several workers.[7,8,17,18] The present studies support this concept. Under the in vitro conditions employed here, stem cell differentiation does not occur to any significant extent and basophilic normoblasts disappear from the incubated cell suspensions by the end of 24 hours. Despite this lack of stem cell differentiation, erythropoietin leads to a consistent increase in several parameters of erythroid activity. Not only is hemoglobin synthesis increased but glycine-^{14}C incorporation into nonhemoglobin protein and nucleic acids is also stimulated in the presence of this hormone. The increased rate of nucleic acid synthesis is also reflected in the increased mitotic indices observed in the presence of erythropoietin, a finding previously noted by Matoth and Kaufmann.[4] The increased proliferation of erythroid precursors is again reflected by an increase in labeled orthochromatophilic normoblasts following pulse labeling of more immature forms with tritiated thymidine, a finding similar to that recently reported by Powsner and Berman.[6] It is interesting to note that under the present conditions, no evidence could be found for increased rate of maturation without proliferation in the presence of erythropoietin.

These studies suggest that under these conditions, erythropoietin acts to induce nucleic acid synthesis from glycine-^{14}C and to stimulate normoblast proliferation. Associated with this increase in nucleic acid synthesis is a secondary increase in hemoglobin and nonhemoglobin protein synthesis.

Summary

Hemoglobin, nonhemoglobin protein and nucleic acid synthesis as well as normoblast proliferation and maturation were measured in human bone marrow cell suspensions. Addition of human erythropoietin to these cell suspensions led to an increase in practically all parameters measured. Thus, both nucleic acid synthesis, as measured by glycine-2-^{14}C incorporation, and cell proliferation, as reflected by mitotic indices, are increased by the end of two to six hr of incubation. Total protein and hemoglobin synthesis are increased by 24 to 48 hr of incubation. It is suggested that erythropoietin acts by inducing normoblast proliferation; protein and hemoglobin synthesis are increased only after more prolonged incubation.

Acknowledgments

The authors wish to acknowledge the skillful help and assistance of Mrs. Theresa A. Boles and Mrs. Paula A. Saltman.

References

1. NECHELES, T. F., R. G. SHEEHAN & H. J. MEYER. 1965. Effect of erythropoietin and oxygen tension on in vitro synthesis of hemoglobin A and F by adult human bone marrow. Proc. Soc. Exper. Biol. Med. **119**: 1207.
2. GALLIEN-LARTIGUE, O. & E. GOLDWASSER. 1965. On the mechanism of erythropoietin-induced differentiation. I. The effects of specific inhibitors on hemoglobin synthesis. Biochem. Biophys. Acta **103**: 319.
3. KRANTZ, S. B. & E. GOLDWASSER. 1965. On the mechanism of erythropoietin-induced differentiation. II. The effect on RNA synthesis. Biochem. Biophys. Acta **103**: 324.
4. MATHOTH, Y. & L. KAUFMANN. 1962. Mitotic activity of erythroblasts previously exposed to erythropoietin. Blood **20**: 165.
5. ROSSE, W. F. & C. W. GURNEY. 1959. Studies on erythropoietin. X. The use of bone marrow tissue culture in demonstrating erythropoietin. J. Lab. Clin. Med. **53**: 446.
6. POWSNER, E. R. & L. BERMAN. 1965. Effect of erythropoietin on erythroblast DNA synthesis in vitro. Blood **27**: 884 (abstract).
7. GORDON, A. S., J. LOBUE, B. S. DORNFEST & G. W. COOPER. 1962. Reticulocyte release from isolated perfused rat legs and femurs. *In* Erythropoiesis, Jacobson, L. O. and M. Doyle, eds. Grune and Stratton. New York : 321.
8. FISHER, J. W., B. L. ROH, C. COUCH & W. O. NIGHTINGALE. 1964. Influence of cobalt, sheep erythropoietin and several hormones on erythropoiesis in bone marrow of isolated perfused hind limbs of dogs. Blood **23**: 87.
9. KAHAN, F. M. 1960. Purification and measurement of microgram amounts of radioactive nucleic acids and proteins from animal cells in tissue culture. Anal. Biochem. **2**: 107.
10. RALPH, P. H. 1941. The histochemical demonstration of hemoglobin in blood cells and tissue smears. Stain Technology **6**: 105.
11. PUCK, T. T. & J. STEFFEN. 1963. Life cycle analysis of mammalian cells. I. A method for localizing metabolic events within the life cycle, and its application to the action of colecemide and sublethal doses of x-irradiation. Biophys. J. **3**: 379.
12. STOHLMAN, JR. F., G. LUCARELLI, D. HOWARD, B. MORSE & B. LEVENTHAL. 1964. Regulation of erythropoiesis. XVI. Cytokinetic patterns in disorders of erythropoiesis. Medicine **43**: 651.
13. ERSLEV, A. J. 1962. Effect of erythropoietin on the uptake and utilization of iron by bone marrow cells in vitro. Proc. Soc. Exper. Biol. Med. **110**: 615.
14. KRANZ, S. B., O. GALLIEN-LARTIGUE & E. GOLDWASSER. 1963. The effect of erythropoietin upon heme synthesis by marrow cells in vitro. J. Biol. Chem. **238**: 4085.
15. FILMANOWICZ, E. & C. W. GURNEY. 1961. Studies on erythropoiesis. XVI. Response to a single dose of erythropoietin in polycythemic mouse. J. Lab. Clin. Med. **57**: 65.
16. STOHLMAN, JR. F. 1961. Humoral regulation of erythropoiesis. VI. Mechanism of action of erythropoietin on the inucleated animal. Proc. Soc. Exper. Biol. Med. **107**: 751.
17. GALLAGHER, N. I., G. C. SEIFERT, J. L. CALLINAN, A. A. MAES & R. D. LANGE. 1963. Influence of erythropoietin on erythropoiesis in polycythemic rats. J. Lab. Clin. Med. **61**: 258.
18. STOHLMAN, JR. F., A. BELAND & D. HOWARD. 1963. The macrocytic response to erythropoietin. J. Clin. Invest. **42**: 984.

Part VIII. Subjects Related to the Physiology of Erythropoietin

THE EFFECT OF CARBON DIOXIDE ON ERYTHROPOIESIS

José Faura,* Clifford W. Gurney and Walter Fried†

Argonne Cancer Research Hospital‡ and the Departments of Medicine and Physiology, University of Chicago, Chicago, Ill.

Introduction

It has been demonstrated that under hypoxic conditions, due either to anemia[1–3] or to low pressure of O_2 in the inspired air,[4,5] erythropoietin is released into the plasma. Secondary polycythemia has been observed to occur in patients with hypoxia from various causes. Patients with pulmonary insufficiency, however, often fail to develop polycythemia to the degree that might be expected from the extent of their hypoxia.[6–9] Since carbon dioxide retention occurs in many patients with pulmonary disease, we became interested in the effect that carbon dioxide might have on the ability to respond to hypoxia and carried out the following experiments.

Methods and Materials

Six-to-eight-week-old CF No. 1 mice were used. To induce hypoxia, mice were kept in a lucite chamber 60 × 40 × 30 cm. The chamber had two openings: one was attached by a hose connection to the cylinder containing the desired gas mixture, the other was open to the room air. The gas was obtained from commercial sources in cylinders containing the appropriate mixture, and was delivered to the chambers at a flow rate of 6 l per minute. Erythropoietin assays were performed on 0.5 ml of the appropriate plasma, using the polycythemic mouse assay described by DeGowin *et al.*[10]

Results

The Effect of High Inspired PCO_2 on the rate of ^{59}Fe Incorporation into Red Blood Cells of Hypoxic Polycythemic Mice

The first experiment was designed to demonstrate the effect of high inspired PCO_2 on the rate of ^{59}Fe incorporation into red blood cells of hypoxic polycythemic mice. Plethora was induced by injecting the animals with 0.5 ml packed red cells on each of two consecutive days. Forty-eight hr after the last injection they were placed in the chamber at the desired gas mixture for eight hours. Forty hr later ^{59}Fe was injected i.v. Blood was withdrawn by cardiac puncture 72 hr later. The radioactivity in this blood was determined and expressed as a percentage of the injected dose.

The results are recorded in FIGURE 1. The animals exposed to an atmosphere containing 20 percent O_2 incorporated only 0.5 percent of the injected dose of iron, while animals exposed to an atmosphere containing 10 percent O_2, incorpo-

* National Institute of Health International Fellowship, No. 1–F05–TW–922–01.

† Postdoctoral Public Health Service Fellow, National Institute of Arthritis and Metabolic Diseases, No. F2–AM–20, 919–01A1. Present address: West Side Veterans Administration Hospital, 820 South Damen, Chicago, Ill.

‡ Operated by the University of Chicago for the United States Atomic Energy Commission.

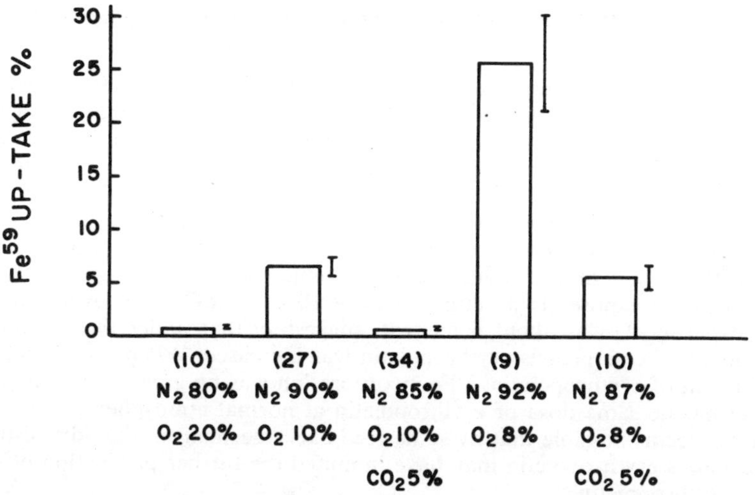

FIGURE 1. The effect of high inspired PCO_2 on the rate of ^{59}Fe incorporation into red blood cells of hypoxic polycythemic mice. Vertical lines along the tops of bars indicate ± 1 standard error of the mean. Numbers in parentheses indicate number of animals.

rated over 6 percent of the injected iron. If the gas mixture contained 5 percent CO_2 and 10 percent O_2, the erythropoietic response was abolished. Mice exposed to an atmosphere containing only 8 percent O_2 incorporated over 25 percent of the injected iron, whereas mice exposed to a mixture of 8 percent O_2 and 5 percent CO_2 incorporated less than 6 percent of the injected iron. These experiments indicate that high inspired PCO_2 somehow suppresses the ability to respond to hypoxia. To determine the mechanism of suppression, we next tested the effect of high inspired PCO_2 on the response of polycythemic mice to exogenous erythropoietin.

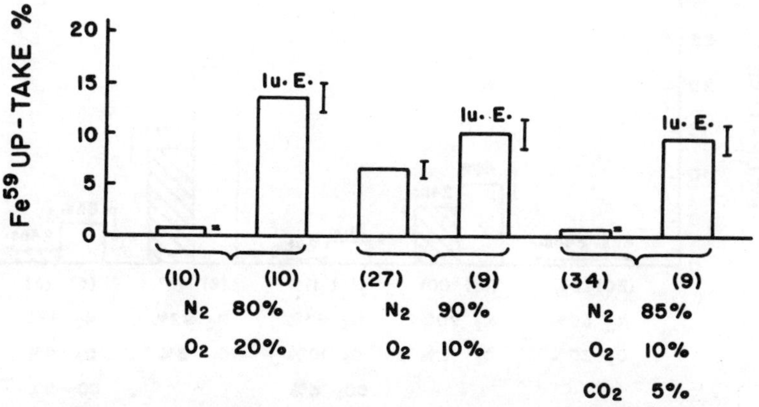

FIGURE 2. The effect of high inspired PCO_2 on the response of polycythemic mice to exogenous erythropoietin. Vertical lines along the tops of bars indicate ± 1 standard error of the mean. Numbers in parentheses indicate number of animals.

The Effect of High Inspired PCO_2 on the Response of Polycythemic Mice to Exogenous Erythropoietin

Polycythemic mice were prepared as in the previous experiment. Forty-eight hr after the last transfusion they received one unit of erythropoietin in saline solution and were then placed immediately in the chamber containing the desired gas mixture for eight hours. ^{59}Fe was injected 48 hr later and the 72-hour incorporation determined. The results are indicated in FIGURE 2.

Radioiron incorporation into the blood of animals exposed to an atmosphere containing 20 percent O_2 increased from less than 1 percent to over 13 percent after injection of 1 unit of erythropoietin. Compared with these figures, the ^{59}Fe uptake of mice exposed to an atmosphere of 10 percent O_2, as shown in the previous experiment, was about 6 percent, suggesting that under these conditions the amount of endogenous erythropoietin was increased. When these mice were given 1 unit of erythropoietin, ^{59}Fe incorporation was no greater than in control mice given the same dose of erythropoietin at normal atmosphere.

Thus it seems possible that by some feed-back mechanism, the administration of exogenous erythropoietin may have inhibited the further production of endogenous erythropoietin.

When mice were exposed to an atmosphere containing a mixture of 10 percent O_2 and 5 percent CO_2, ^{59}Fe incorporation was less than 1 percent and the injection of erythropoietin produced a response comparable to that observed in the two other groups. Thus a high inspired PCO_2 apparently does not inhibit the erythropoietic response to hypoxia by suppressing the ability to respond to erythropoietin.

The Effect of High Inspired PCO_2 on Erythropoietin Levels of Hypoxic Mice

The next experiment was designed to determine whether the production of erythropoietin is inhibited in the presence of 5 percent CO_2. Two groups of mice were exposed to each of the five different gas mixtures, some of them for eight hr and other for 24 hours. Immediately afterwards they were killed and the plasma

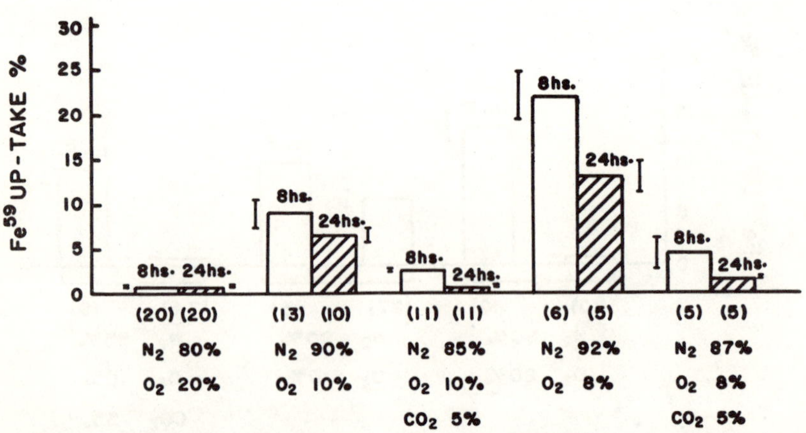

FIGURE 3. The effect of high inspired PCO_2 on erythropoietin levels of hypoxic mice. Vertical lines along the tops of bars indicate ± 1 standard error of the mean. Numbers in parentheses indicate number of animals.

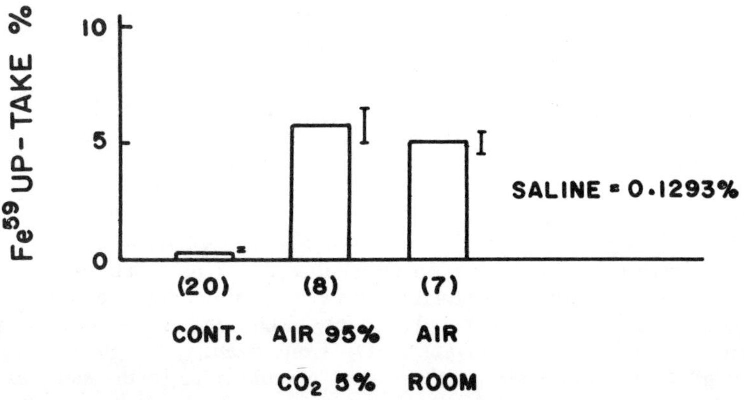

FIGURE 4. The effect of high inspired PCO_2 on erythropoietin levels of anemic mice. Vertical lines along the tops of bars indicate $\pm$ 1 standard error of the mean. Numbers in parentheses indicate number of animals.

was collected and assayed for erythropoietin activity. FIGURE 3 shows the results.

The plasma from mice exposed to an atmosphere containing 20 percent O_2 showed no detectable erythropoietin titer. Plasma from animals maintained in an atmosphere containing 10 percent O_2 for eight hr incorporated about 9 percent ^{59}Fe; that from mice in the same atmosphere for 24 hr about 6 percent. The plasma from mice exposed to 10 percent O_2 and 5 percent CO_2 for eight hr and 24 hr incorporated only 2 percent and 1 percent, respectively. Plasma from animals in an atmosphere containing 8 percent O_2 incorporated 22 percent and 13 percent if exposed for eight or 24 hours, respectively. Mice in an atmosphere of 8 percent O_2 and 5 percent CO_2 or similar periods incorporated 4 percent and 1 percent.

Erythropoietin titers were always less after 24 hr than after eight hr of exposure to hypoxia. This has previously been reported by others[11] and the reason remain unknown. The experiment also shows that plasma from animals exposed to hypoxia and CO_2 contains considerably less erythropoietin than does that of mice exposed to an identical degree of hypoxia without CO_2. This suggests that the presence of 5 percent CO_2 suppresses erythropoiesis by suppressing erythropoietin production.

The Effect on High Inspired PCO_2 on Erythropoietin Levels of Anemic Mice

We next investigated the effect of high inspired PCO_2 on the ability of anemic animals to produce erythropoietin. Mice were made anemic my removal of 0.5 ml of blood by cardiac puncture. Immediately thereafter one group was placed in an atmosphere containing 95 percent air and 5 percent CO_2, while the other group was maintained in room air. After eight hr both groups were sacrificed, and the plasma was collected and assayed for erythropoietin. FIGURE 4 shows that plasma from nonanemic mice causes less than 1 percent ^{59}Fe incorporation into red blood cells of assay mice. Plasma from anemic mice, maintained in either a normal atmosphere or one with 5 percent CO_2 added, resulted in over 5 percent incorporation. This indicates that 5 percent CO_2 was incapable of suppressing erythropoietin production in response to anemia.

Discussion

Carbon dioxide decreases the erythropoietic response to a decreased alveolar O_2 tension. It does not do so by affecting the ability to respond to erythropoietin but rather, by affecting the ability to produce erythropoietin. However, while CO_2 decreases the ability to respond to hypoxia produced by a decrease in the inspired PO_2, it does not affect the ability to respond to hypoxia induced by anemia.

There are several possible ways in which a high inspired PCO_2 may act to suppress erythropoietin production. A high plasma CO_2 tension may affect the organ of erythropoietin production either directly or by its effect on acid-base balance. This is an unlikely explanation of the action observed here since the plasma PCO_2 of anemic mice would probably be elevated to at least the same level as that of mice with a low alveolar PO_2. Consequently, a high inspired PCO_2 should affect erythropoietin production of anemic mice to the same extent as that of mice breathing a gas mixture containing 10 percent O_2. This was not observed.

Since erythropoietin production is at least partially regulated by the ratio of the O_2 demand to the O_2 supply, an increase in the O_2 supply should decrease the stimulus to erythropoietin production. A high inspired PCO_2 might affect the O_2 supply in several ways. High CO_2 tension is known to act locally as a potent capillary vasodilator. It is possible that perfusion of the organ responsible for erythropoietin production would thus be increased by a high plasma CO_2 content. This in turn would ameliorate the deficit in tissue O_2 supply. Again, however, one would expect this to occur in anemic mice as well as in those exposed to a decreased O_2 tension.

High PCO_2 also produces a shift of the hemoglobin O_2 dissociation curve, resulting in a tendency for O_2 to dissociate at lower O_2 tensions. Consequently, O_2 bound to hemoglobin becomes more easily available to the tissues. Once again, though, such an action might be expected to affect anemic mice as well as mice hypoxic for other reasons.

Carbon dioxide can increase the ventilatory rate of animals by its action in stimulating the respiratory centers. This increase in the ventilatory rate increases the alveolar O_2 tension. Unless the hemoglobin is already saturated, an increase in the alveolar O_2 tension will increase the amount of O_2 carried by the hemoglobin and consequently the amount delivered to the tissues. If erythropoietin is regulated by the ratio between O_2 supply and O_2 demand, an increase in the O_2 supply to the tissues should decrease the stimulus to erythropoietin production. The effect of PCO_2 on ventilation best explains our results. Since the O_2 saturation of the hemoglobin of mice exposed to a gas mixture containing only 10 percent O_2 would be about 83.5 percent, an increase in the alveolar O_2 tension would tend to increase the O_2 saturation of the hemoglobin and consequently would significantly increase the amount of O_2 carried to the tissues. In anemic mice breathing air, on the other hand, the hemoglobin would be nearly 100 percent saturated and the increase in the alveolar O_2 tension produced by hyperventilation would thus affect the blood O_2 only by a small increase in the dissolved O_2 of the plasma. The increase in the amount of O_2 carried to the tissues would therefore be extremely small and probably insufficient to affect erythropoietin production.

The findings presented here and the interpretations which we have offered do not explain why patients with pulmonary disease have less than the expected erythropoietic response to their hypoxia. Patients with high PCO_2 secondary to pulmonary disease have ventilatory obstruction and consequently the above explanation for the action of PCO_2 in suppressing erythropoiesis would not be pertinent. In fact, the findings reinforce some clinical data which suggest that high PCO_2's are not related to the suppressed erythropoietic response observed in patients with pulmonary disease.

Summary

High inspired PCO_2 suppresses the erythropoietic response to administration of gas mixture containing a low partial pressure of O_2. It does so by decreasing the production of erythropoietin. Five percent CO_2 in the inspired air of anemic mice does not impair their ability to produce erythropoietin.

We suggest that high inspired PCO_2 suppresses erythropoietin production by inducing hyperventilation, thereby increasing HbO_2 saturation and the delivery of O_2 to the tissues.

References

1. Borsook, H., A. Graybiel, G. Keighley & E. Windsor. 1954. Polycythemic response in normal adult rats to a nonprotein plasma extract from anemic rabbits. Blood **9:** 734–742.
2. Plzak, L., W. Fried, L. O. Jacobson & W. F. Bethard. 1955. Demonstration of stimulation of erythropoiesis by plasma from anemic rats using ^{59}Fe. J. Lab. Clin. Med. **46:** 671.
3. Piliero, S. J., P. T. Medici, B. Pansky, L. Luhby & A. S. Gordon. 1957. Erythropoietic-stimulating extracts from anemic human subjects. Proc. Soc. Exp. Biol. Med. **93:** 302.
4. Stohlman, F. L. & G. Brecher. 1957. Humoral regulation of erythropoiesis. III. Effect of exposure to stimulated altitude. J. Lab. Clin. Med. **49:** 890.
5. Mirand, E. A. & T. C. Prentice. 1957. Presence of plasma erythropoietin in hypoxic rats with or without kidney(s) and/or spleen. Proc. Soc. Exp. Biol. Med. **94:** 237.
6. Lemon, W. S. 1929. A study of effect of chronic pulmonary disease on volume and composition of blood. Ann. Intern. Med. **3:** 430.
7. Wilson, H. H., C. W. Borden & R. V. Ebert. 1951. Adaptation to anoxia in chronic pulmonary emphysema. A.M.A. Arch. Intern. Med. **88:** 581.
8. Hammersten, J. F., W. H. Whitcomb, P. C. Johnson & J. R. Lowell. 1958. The hematologic adaptation of patients with hypoxia due to pulmonary emphysema. Am. Rev. Tuberc. **78:** 391.
9. Gallo, R. C., W. Fraimow, R. T. Cathcart & A. J. Erslev. 1964. Erythropoietic response in chronic pulmonary disease. Arch. Intern. Med. **113:** 559–568.
10. DeGowin, R. L., D. Hofstra & C. W. Gurney. 1962. A comparison of erythropoietin bioassays. Proc. Soc. Exp. Biol. Med. **110:** 48–51.
11. Stohlman, Jr., F. & D. Howard. 1962. Humoral regulation of erythropoiesis. IX. The rate of disappearance of erythropoietin from the plasma. *In* Erythropoiesis. L. O. Jacobson and M. Doyle, Eds. : 120–124. Grune and Stratton, Inc. New York, N. Y.

THE PHYSIOLOGICAL SIGNIFICANCE OF AN ERYTHROPOIETIC INHIBITOR FACTOR APPEARING IN PLASMA SUBSEQUENT TO HYPERTRANSFUSION*

Walter H. Whitcomb and Margaret Moore

Veterans Administration Hospital, Oklahoma City, Okla.

Krzymowski and Krzymowska[1] reported the presence of an erythropoiesis-inhibiting factor in hypertransfused sheep, and Reynafarje *et al.*[2] noted that inhibitory activity existed in the plasma of polycythemic individuals residing at high altitude. We have reported the appearance of a factor in the plasma of hypertransfused mice, rabbits and sheep which blocks red cell iron incorporation in the assay mouse. Heat-flocculated plasma filtrates of hypertransfused sheep inhibited iron incorporation in three test systems, i.e., normal mice, mice exposed to hypoxia and mice receiving erythropoietin-rich preparations.[3]

The purpose of this report is to document the time of appearance of this inhibitory activity in hypertransfused animals and to suggest a mechanism for its action.

Material and Methods

Female Dorsett and Suffolk sheep weighing 26–45 kg were transfused daily with washed erythrocytes. Only sheep having type R cells and compatible on crossmatching were used. The blood of donor animals was cellected in 250 ml vacuum bottles containing 3 ml of a 1:1000 heparin solution as the anitcoagulant. Erythrocytes were separated by centrifugation, washed three times, and resuspended in 0.9% sodium chloride solution. The hematocrit of this suspension was adjusted to 80%.

The recipient sheep received daily transfusion of washed erythrocytes for three days for a total amount of packed cells varying from 22.2–43.9 ml/kg body weight.

Whole sheep plasma to be assayed was obtained from blood collected in heparinized syringes and centrifuged at 2700 rpm for 45 minutes. The plasma was stored at −18° C.

The sheep plasma filtrates to be assayed were prepared as follows: The blood was drawn in 250 ml vacuum containers with heparin as the anticoagulant and centrifuged. The plasma was removed and its pH adjusted to 5.5 by the addition of 1N HCl. It was then heated in a boiling water bath for sufficient time to bring the internal temperature to 95° C. for five minutes. The preparation was then centrifuged at 4° C. and the supernatant removed. The pH of the supernatant was adjusted to 7.0 by the addition of 1N NaOH. The volume of the supernatant was concentrated ten times by evaporation in a Buchler flash-evaporator at 40° C. The concentration procedure required approximately two hours. Two pools of concentrated sheep plasma filtrates were prepared, one from the plasma of normal sheep and the other from the plasma of hypertransfused sheep. Each pool was divided into 3 ml aliquots and stored in −18° C until used. A sample of each pool was analyzed for its content of porphyrin[4] and of heme.[5] Neither protoporphyrin nor heme was detected.

Mouse plasma to be assayed was obtained from two groups of 90 mice each. Each mouse in the first group was bled 0.4 ml of whole blood by cardiocentesis on

* This project was supported by NIH grant HE 09864–01 and the Veterans Administration Research Service, and with the assistance of Biostatistical Unit and Computer Facility (NIH grant FR–00005) of the University of Oklahoma Medical Center.

two consecutive days. The hematocrits of these animals were: 26 ± 0.6% at 24 hr, 30 ± 0.5% at 48 hr and 33 ± 0.6% at 72 hours. Each mouse in the second group received 0.8 ml of washed homologous erythrocytes on two consecutive days. Their hematocrits were 69 ± 1.6% at 24 hr, 70 ± 1.4% at 48 hr and 68 ± 1.1% at 72 hours. The hematocrits of normal mice serving as controls were 45 ± 0.5%. Each group was divided into three lots; one lot of 30 animals from each group was exsanguinated 24, 48 and 72 hr following the last procedure. Three pools of whole plasma were prepared and stored at −18° C. The first pool was anemic mouse plasma; the second, plethoric mouse plasma; and the third, a 50–50 mixture of the two. One ml aliquots of these three pools of whole mouse plasma was assayed in the plethoric hypoxic mouse.

The activity of whole plasma (sheep and mouse) was tested in plethoric hypoxic mice. Twenty-to-twenty-five-gram CF-1 female mice were used in the bioassay system. The assay developed by Cotes and Bangham[6] and De Gowin *et al.*[7] was modified as follows: Mice were injected s.c. with one mg of Imferon and maintained at reduced barometric pressure (0.5 atm) for 21 days. They were then returned to atmospheric air for three days. On the fourth day, a single s.c. injection of the test substance was given in a one ml volume. Immediately following this injection, the animals were exposed to 0.5 atm for eight hours. Forty-eight hr later, 0.5 μc of ^{59}Fe citrate in 0.5 ml saline was injected i.v. Forty-eight hr after the ^{59}Fe injection, red blood cell ^{59}Fe incorporation (RBC ^{59}Fe I) was estimated on a 0.2 ml sample of whole blood. The blood volume was assumed to be equal to 7% of the body weight and all animals having a hematocrit of less than 55% at the time of determining RBC ^{59}Fe incorporation were removed from consideration.

The activity of plasma filtrates was also assayed in normal CF-1 female mice. The mice were injected s.c. each day with 0.5 ml of the test substance. One group of 20 mice received plasma filtrate from normal sheep; another, plasma filtrate from hypertransfused sheep. Five mice from each group were exsanguinated after receiving injections for five, ten and 16 days, respectively. Twenty-four hr prior to exsanguination, each mouse received 0.5 μc of ^{59}Fe citrate in 0.5 ml of 0.9% saline i.v. At the time of exsanguination erythrocytes were enumerated using a Coulter electronic cell counter model B. Hemoglobin concentrations were measured by the cyanmethemoglobin method and hematocrits performed by the micro technique. Erythrocyte iron incorporation was measured in 0.5 ml samples of whole blood, assuming the blood volume to be 5% of the body weight. Estimates of total iron together with the ^{59}Fe uptake of the liver and spleen were made using a modification of the method of Leffingwell *et al.*,[8] in which the tissue is digested with sulphuric acid, and the iron complexed with orthophenanthroline and extracted with isoamyl alcohol. Total iron was measured spectrophotometrically and the colored complex introduced into a gamma radiation detection instrument. The proportion of erythroid, myeloid and lymphoid cells was estimated in bone marrow from the femoral shaft prepared on cover slips and stained with Wright's stain. The estimates of bone marrow cellularity were made without knowledge of the experimental stimulus.

Results

The first groups of experiments were designed to determine the time of appearance of inhibitor activity in the plasma of hypertransfused sheep. Sheep were transfused on the first, second and third days with packed erythrocytes sufficient to raise their hematocrit from 33–41% pretransfusion to 60–70% on the fourth

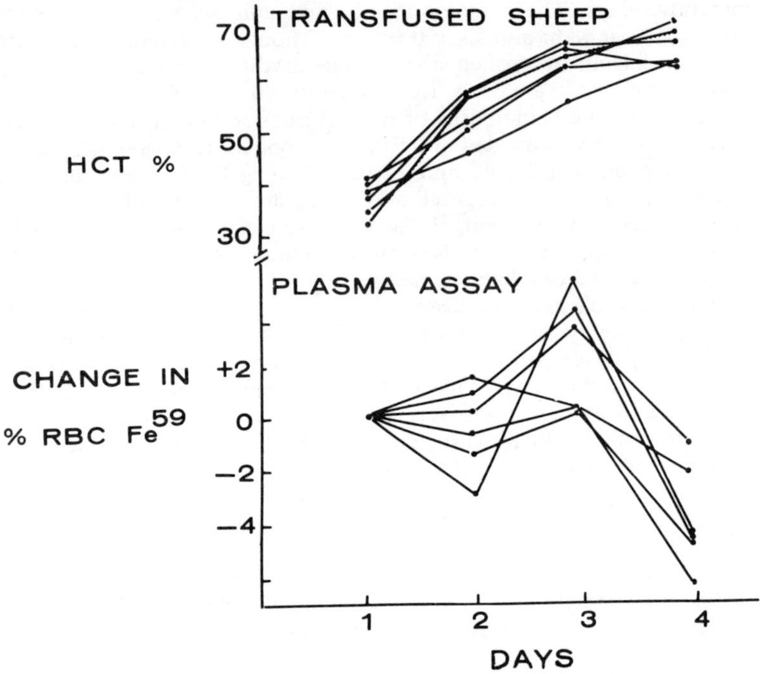

FIGURE 1. The effect of hypertransfused sheep plasma on RBC ^{59}Fe incorporation of plethoric hypoxic mice. Plasmas taken 24 hr after transfusions on the second, third and fourth days are compared to plasmas taken prior to transfusion on the first day. Results are expressed as the difference in percent RBC ^{59}Fe incorporation of assay mice. The hematocrits of the donor sheep are presented for comparison.

day. Whole plasma for assay was collected on the first, second, third and fourth days. The samples were always taken immediately before transfusion. This procedure allowed 24 hr for adaptation. All plasma samples from a given animal were assayed at the same time using the plethoric-hypoxic mouse system. The effect of posttransfusion plasma samples on the incorporation of ^{59}Fe into mouse erythrocytes is compared with the pretransfusion sample obtained on the first day. The results are expressed as the change in per cent ^{59}Fe erythrocyte incorporation. These results are presented in FIGURE 1. The pretransfusion plasmas (first day) did not alter the response of the assay mouse to hypoxia. Plasmas collected on the second day altered RBC ^{59}Fe Incorporation from −2.7% to +1.2%; on the third day, from +0.1% to +4.7%; and on the fourth day, from −1.0% to −6.2%. Thus, inhibitory activity was not consistently observed until 72 hr (fourth day) following the first transfusion.

The second group of experiments was designed to test the effect of repeated injections of plasma filtrate from hypertransfused sheep (HSPF) on erythropoiesis of normal mice at atmospheric pressure. The results of injecting HSPF were compared with those obtained from injecting similar quantities of filtrate from normal sheep (NSPF). The experimental design for these experiments is presented above. The results are presented in TABLE 1 and FIGURES 2, 3 and 4. In the Table the mean ($\bar{x}$), standard error of the mean (SEM), the variance (S^2), and

TABLE 1

EFFECT OF NORMAL AND POLYCYTHEMIC SHEEP PLASMA FILTRATES ON ERYTHROPOIESIS OF NORMAL MICE FOR PERIODS OF FIVE, TEN AND SIXTEEN DAYS*

	Day of Sacrifice		Normal Plasma Filtrate	Hyper-transfused Plasma Filtrate	Differ-ence	P Value < .05
Hemoglobin G %	5	$\bar{x}$ $S^2(N)$	13.2 ± 0.3 0.098 (5)	12.9 ± 0.3 0.087 (6)	−0.3	N.S.
	10	$\bar{x}$ $S^2(N)$	12.6 ± 0.3 0.503 (5)	13.3 ± 0.5 1.030 (5)	−0.7	N.S.
	16	$\bar{x}$ $S^2(N)$	13.6 ± 0.2 0.260 (5)	12.1 ± 0.3 0.409 (4)	−1.5	Sig.
Hematocrit %	5	$\bar{x}$ $S^2(N)$	40.0 ± 1.2 1.451 (5)	40.0 ± 1.0 0.967 (6)	0	N.S.
	10	$\bar{x}$ $S^2(N)$	38.6 ± 1.1 6.300 (5)	40.6 ± 2.3 7.300 (5)	+2.0	N.S.
	16	$\bar{x}$ $S^2(N)$	39.6 ± 0.4 0.800 (5)	34.8 ± 1.6 10.916 (4)	−4.8	N.S.
RBC × 10^6	5	$\bar{x}$ $S^2(N)$	8.21 ± 0.3 0.059 (5)	8.31 ± 1.0 0.945 (6)	+0.1	N.S.
	10	$\bar{x}$ $S^2(N)$	8.4 ± 1.0 0.534 (5)	8.28 ± 3.2 4.991 (5)	−0.12	N.S.
	16	$\bar{x}$ $S^2(N)$	9.08 ± 1.0 0.482 (5)	6.81 ± 0.8 0.255 (4)	−2.27	Sig.
WBC × 10^3	5	$\bar{x}$ $S^2(N)$	5.159 ± .688 0.474 (5)	6.028 ± .962 0.926 (6)	+.865	N.S.
	16	$\bar{x}$ $S^2(N)$	5.900 ± 0.7 2.604 (5)	7.185 ± 1.6 10.134 (4)	+1.285	N.S.
Normoblasts Femoral Marrow %	5	$\bar{x}$ $S^2(N)$	26.7 ± 1.0 3.083 (3)	21.2 ± 3.9 79.075 (5)	−5.5	N.S.
	10	$\bar{x}$ $S^2(N)$	21.7 ± 1.8 8.450 (5)	12.6 ± 1.7 13.925 (5)	−9.1	Sig.
	16	$\bar{x}$ $S^2(N)$	23.9 ± 1.5 12.050 (5)	11.4 ± 1.9 14.229 (4)	−12.5	Sig.
Granulocytes Femoral Marrow %	5	$\bar{x}$ $S^2(N)$	61.2 ± 6.1 110.333 (3)	66.8 ± 2.8 40.700 (5)	+5.6	N.S.
	10	$\bar{x}$ $S^2(N)$	68.5 ± 4.1 86.250 (5)	77.6 ± 2.9 43.675 (5)	+9.1	N.S.
	16	$\bar{x}$ $S^2(N)$	62.8 ± 2.5 31.200 (5)	73.8 ± 4.5 80.250 (4)	+11.0	N.S.
Lymphocytes Femoral Marrow %	5	$\bar{x}$ $S^2(N)$	13.2 ± 4.9 73.583 (3)	10.4 ± 3.0 45.550 (5)	−2.8	N.S.
	10	$\bar{x}$ $S^2(N)$	9.5 ± 2.7 36.808 (5)	11.7 ± 4.0 79.950 (5)	+2.2	N.S.
	16	$\bar{x}$ $S^2(N)$	12.8 ± 1.1 6.075 (5)	15.1 ± 4.4 77.395 (4)	+2.3	N.S.

TABLE 1 — Continued

	Day of Sacrifice		Normal Plasma Filtrate	Hyper-transfused Plasma Filtrate	Difference	P Value < .05
RBC Fe^{59}%	5	$\bar{x}$	12.0 ± 0.6	15.1 ± 1.6	+3.1	N.S.
		S^2(N)	0.331 (5)	2.643 (5)		
	10	$\bar{x}$	13.0 ± 0.5	10.6 ± 0.1	−2.4	Sig.
		S^2(N)	1.482 (5)	0.018 (5)		
	16	$\bar{x}$	11.5 ± 0.3	7.3 ± 0.1	−4.2	Sig.
		S^2(N)	0.412 (5)	0.066 (4)		
Liver Fe^{59} $\frac{\text{NCPM}}{\mu g \text{ Fe}}$	5	$\bar{x}$	2.48 ± 0.35	2.09 ± 1.85	−0.39	N.S.
		S^2(N)	0.497 (4)	0.059 (5)		
	10	$\bar{x}$	1.96 ± 0.61	2.76 ± 0.45	+0.82	N.S.
		S^2(N)	1.859 (5)	1.008 (5)		
	16	$\bar{x}$	2.88 ± 0.29	8.69 ± 0.77	+5.81	Sig.
		S^2(N)	0.426 (5)	2.325 (4)		
Spleen Fe^{59} $\frac{\text{NCPM}}{\mu g \text{ Fe}}$	5	$\bar{x}$	1.99 ± 0.59	1.85 ± 0.52	−0.14	N.S.
		S^2(N)	1.389 (4)	1.367 (5)		
	10	$\bar{x}$	0.84 ± 0.13	0.97 ± 0.20	−0.13	N.S.
		S^2(N)	0.910 (5)	0.196 (5)		
	16	$\bar{x}$	2.63 ± 0.19	1.91 ± 0.17	−0.72	N.S.
		S^2(N)	0.179 (5)	0.111 (4)		

* The observations were analyzed assuming that $\bar{x}$ has a normal distribution with unequal variances and using the formula

$$t' = \frac{\bar{x}_1 - \bar{x}_2}{\sqrt{\frac{S^2_{x_1}}{N_1} + \frac{S^2_{x_2}}{N_2}}}$$

where t′ is approximately equal to Student's t with degrees of freedom between $N_1 - 1$ and $N_2 - 2$.[10] Statistical significance was accepted if the p value was .05 or less.

the number of observations (N) are presented for each of the parameters measured on the fifth, tenth and 16th days. The following effects were observed.

Neither the total body weight nor the organ weights differed significantly in the mice receiving HSPF and those receiving NSPF. Both groups tolerated the experiment without weight loss. No significant differences were observed in hemoglobin, hematocrit, erythrocyte count and leukocyte count between the two groups receiving the plasma filtrates until the 16th day. On the 16th day there was a significant decrease in hemoglobin concentration and erythrocyte count in mice receiving HSPF for 16 days. Bone marrow examinations of the two groups revealed a significant decrease in normoblasts of the femoral marrow in mice receiving HSPF for ten days and for 16 days. The red cell incorporation of ^{59}Fe also showed a significant reduction in the mice receiving HSPF on the tenth and 16th days. The organ incorporation of ^{59}Fe showed a significant difference between the two groups only on the 16th day and only in liver counts.

The third group of experiments was designed to contrast the effects of normal plasma, anemic mouse plasma, plethoric mouse plasma and an equal mixture of anemic and plethoric plasmas on the rate of ^{59}Fe incorporation into erythro-

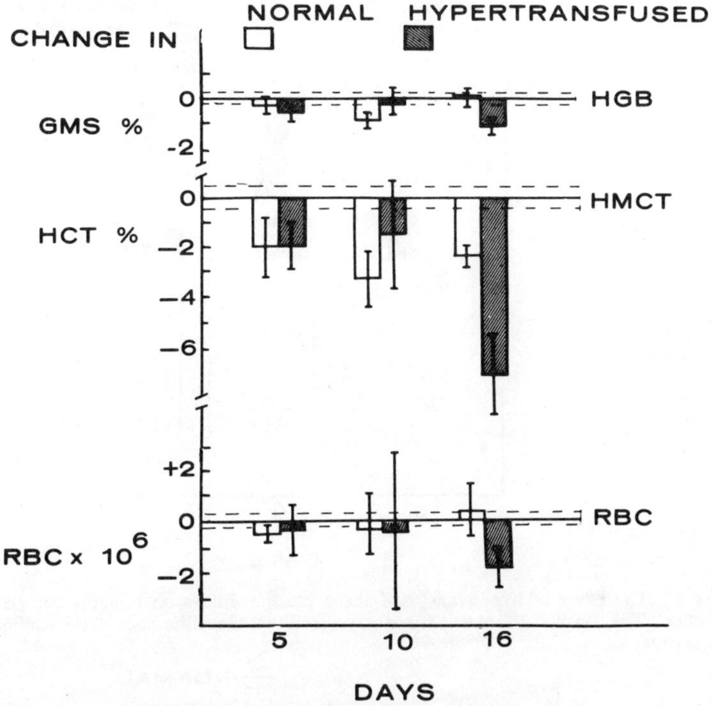

FIGURE 2. The effect of normal and hypertransfused sheep plasma filtrates on hemoglobin concentration, hematocrit and erythrocyte count of normal mice. The results (TABLE 1) are expressed as the differences observed from mice who did not receive filtrates.

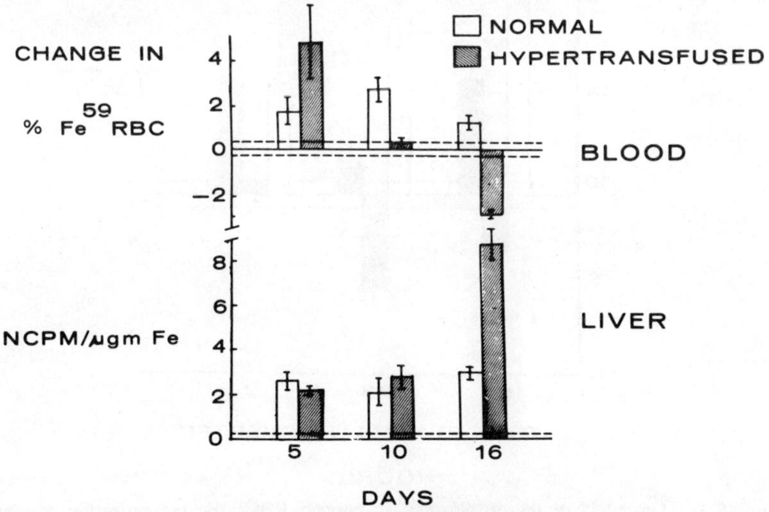

FIGURE 3. The effect of normal and hypertransfused sheep plasma filtrates on percent RBC ^{59}Fe incorporation and ^{59}Fe liver uptake in normal mice. The results (TABLE 1) are expressed as the differences observed from mice who did not receive filtrates.

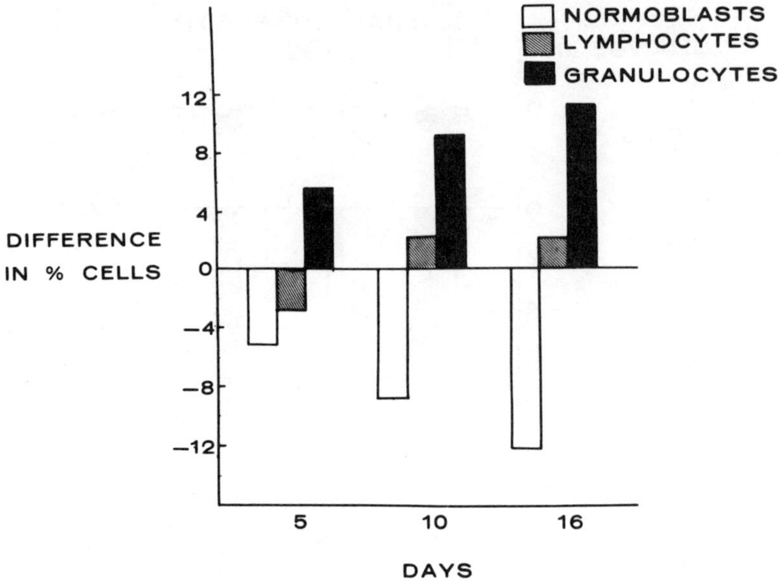

FIGURE 4. The effect of hypertransfused sheep plasma filtrate on marrow composition of normal mice. The results (TABLE 1) are expressed as the difference from animals who received normal sheep plasma filtrate.

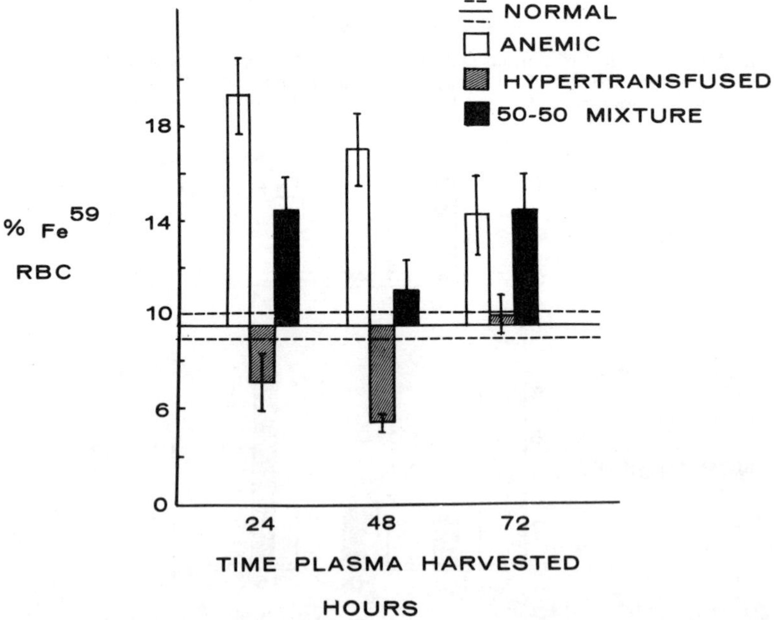

FIGURE 5. The effect of mouse plasmas on percent RBC ^{59}Fe incorporation of plethoric mice exposed to hypoxia. The results are expressed as the effect of plasmas from normal, anemic and hypertransfused animals on percent RBC ^{59}Fe incorporation of the assay mouse. A 50–50 mixture of the anemic and hypertransfused plasmas are presented for comparison.

cytes of the plethoric-hypoxic mouse assay system. The experimental design has been presented in the *Materials and Methods* section. The results of these experiments are illustrated in FIGURE 5. There is a marked stimulatory effect of anemic plasma which is maximal 24 hr after the phlebotomy and which decreases as the hematocrit in the bled animal recovers. Plasma from hypertransfused mice shows significant inhibition at 24 and 48 hr after transfusion but this inhibition disappears after 72 hours. The mixture of anemic and hypertransfused plasma effects a change in the incorporation of iron which appears to be an approximate summation of the two effects.

Discussion

In earlier experiments[3] the plasmas to be tested for inhibitory activity were empirically collected at a single point in time. The duration of time from the first transfusion to the collection of the plasmas was five days for mice, six days for rabbits and five days for sheep. The experiments reported here were designed to document the possible earlier appearance of this activity in hypertransfused sheep and mice and to obtain evidence for the mechanism of the depression of RBC ^{59}Fe incorporation.

In the first group of experiments the plasma collected from hypertransfused sheep 24 hr after the first transfusion exhibited a variable effect on RBC ^{59}Fe incorporation of the plethoric hypoxic mouse and the plasmas of three of the six animals collected at 48 hr augmented iron incorporation. All plasmas collected at 72 hr inhibited iron incorporation when compared to those plasmas taken prior to the initiation of transfusion. These data indicate that the inhibitory activity in the plasma of hypertransfused sheep appears at about 72 hr subsequent to the first transfusion and 24 hr subsequent to the third. Because the experiments were designed to achieve a venous hematocrit of 60–70% after the third transfusion, no comment can be made regarding the threshold at which this activity appears. The observation that plasmas of three of the six sheep collected at 48 hr augmented RBC ^{59}Fe incorporation is of interest. Erslev[9] has recently considered the problem of suboptimal oxygen transport in association with high hematocrits and high viscosity blood in rabbits. Although computed oxygen flow was decreased in normovolemic polycythemic animals, erythropoietin activity was not observed in the plasma when the polycythemic rat assay was employed.[9] One might postulate that oxygen transport is also suboptimal in sheep (transfused at the rate indicated in this report) for a brief period during which adaptation occurs and that this state is reflected in the augmentive activity of the plasma collected at 48 hours. Observations in our laboratory suggest that the plethoric mouse exposed to hypoxia may provide a more sensitive bioassay for erythropoietic activity than the plethoric mouse not exposed to hypoxia.

In the second set of experiments hypertransfused sheep plasma filtrate and normal sheep plasma filtrate, concentrated ten times, was given to normal mice for periods of five, ten and 16 days. These data suggest that the daily administration of concentrated hypertransfused sheep plasma filtrate to normal mice results in a decrease in the normoblasts of the femoral marrow and RBC ^{59}Fe incorporation by the tenth day and a decrease in hemoglobin concentration, hematocrit and erythrocytes by the 16th day, and that these events are accompanied by an increased uptake of ^{59}Fe in the liver. The hypertransfused sheep plasma filtrate used here was obtained from the same plasma which showed inhibitory activity in the plethoric hypoxic mouse.

These observations suggest that the factor blocking RBC ^{59}Fe incorporation in the plethoric hypoxic mouse mediates its effect on erythrocyte precursors.

This hypothesis is supported by the decreased cellularity in the marrow and the decreased incorporation of ^{59}Fe. This inhibition is observed before a fall in hemoglobin, hematocrit and RBC and the time interval is consistent with the normal maturation interval required by normoblasts.

This factor appears to have no influence on the leukocyte concentration of the peripheral blood and we assume that the change in marrow cellular composition is the result of decreased erythropoiesis with no decrease in granulopoiesis.

The third set of experiments indicates (FIGURE 5) that there is a wave of inhibition which reaches its peak 48 hr after the last transfusion and thereafter wanes. Earlier experiments using white Swiss mice indicated that inhibitor activity was present in plasma harvested at 72 hr and that the amount of inhibitory activity was proportional to the level of the hematocrit.[3] The results of mixing plasmas from anemic and plethoric mice indicate that the plasmas showing inhibitory activity when assayed alone also show inhibitory activity when assayed in combination with plasmas of anemic mice.

If endogenous inhibitory activity is present in the plasma of the hypertransfused mouse, one may postulate that exogenous erythropoietin must be present in an amount sufficient to overcome this inhibition in order to provide a stimulus to erythropoiesis. That the exposure of the plethoric mouse to eight hr of 0.5 atm may more than overcome this endogenous inhibition is suggested by: 1) the apparent inability of the plasma of the hypertransfused mouse to suppress RBC ^{59}Fe incorporation to less than 1% (FIGURE 5), and 2) by the observation that plasma from anemic animals and man, when assayed in the PHM system, exhibits an increase in RBC ^{59}Fe incorporation greater than the sum of that seen when assayed in the plethoric mouse, an increase apparently due to hypoxia.

The observations reported above are consistent with the hypothesis that the erythropoietic inhibitor factor(s), like erythropoietin itself, exerts its (their) influence on erythrocyte precursors. These data alone might be interpreted to indicate that inhibition is only the result of impaired maturation of the normoblast. This latter interpretation seems unlikely to us. In previous experiments[3] we showed that inhibition could be induced if given within 18 hr of the administration of active erythropoietin. If, however, the plasma showing inhibitory activity was given 24 and 40 hr after an injection of erythropoietin, inhibition was no longer demonstrable.

Summary

1. The plasma from sheep rendered polycythemic by transfusion inhibits the incorporation of ^{59}Fe into erythrocytes of the plethoric-hypoxic mouse assay system. This inhibition appears consistently at 72 hr following hypertransfusion.

2. Inhibition can be demonstrated in two assay systems, i.e., the plethoric-hypoxic mouse system, and in normal mice.

3. When concentrated plasma filtrates from hypertransfused sheep are given repetitively to normal mice, there is a fall in hemoglobin concentration and red cell count which is preceded by a decrease in the normoblastic composition of the marrow and a decrease in iron incorporation into red cells.

4. We propose the hypothesis that the inhibitory factor(s), like erythropoietin itself, exerts its (their) influence on erythrocyte precursor cells, perhaps as early as the stage of induction of the stem cell.

Acknowledgments

The authors wish to express their appreciation to Dr. Benjamin Rasmussen, Department of Animal Science, University of Illinois, Urbana, Ill., who provided the sheep RBC typing sera and to Dr. Sylvia Bottomley, Medical Service, Veterans Administration Hospital, Oklahoma City, Okla., for the chemical determinations of protoporphyrin and heme. The authors gratefully acknowledge the technical assistance of Mr. John V. Patmon.

References

1. Krzymowski, T. & H. Krzymowska. 1962. Studies on the erythropoiesis-inhibiting factor in the plasma of animals with transfusion polycythemia. Blood **19:** 38.
2. Reynafarje, C., J. Ramos, J. Faura & D. Villavicencio. 1964. Humoral control of erythropoietic activity in man during and after altitude exposure. Proc. Soc. Exp. Biol. Med. **116:** 649.
3. Whitcomb, W. H. & M. Z. Moore. 1965. The inhibitory effect of plasma from hypertransfused animals on erythrocyte iron incorporation in mice. J. Lab. Clin. Med. **66:** 641.
4. Schwartz, S., M. H. Berg, I. Bossenmaier & H. Dinsmore. 1960. Determination of porphyrins in biologic materials. Meth. Biochem. Anal. **8:** 280, 253.
5. Falk, J. E. 1964. Porphyrins and Metalloporphyrins. Elsevier Publishing Co. : 181.
6. Cotes, P. M. & D. R. Bangham. 1961. Bioassay of erythropoietin in mice made polycythemic by exposure to air at a reduced pressure. Nature **191:** 1065.
7. De Gowin, R., D. Hofstra & C. W. Gurney. 1962. A comparison of erythropoietin bioassays. Proc. Soc. Exp. Biol. Med. **110:** 48.
8. Leffingwell, T. P., G. S. Melville & R. W. Reiss. 1959. A semimicrotechnique for iron[59] beta determinations in biologic materials. J. Lab. Clin. Med. **53:** 622.
9. Erslev, A. J. 1966. The erythropoietic effect of hematocrit variation in normovolemic rabbits. Blood **27:** 629.
10. Cochran, W. G. & G. M. Cox. 1957. Experimental Design. 2nd Ed. : 100. John Wiley & Sons, Inc. London, England.

HUMORAL REGULATION OF THE ERYTHROPOIETIC DEPRESSION OF HIGH ALTITUDE POLYCYTHEMIC SUBJECTS AFTER RETURN TO SEA LEVEL*

César Reynafarje

Instituto de Biología Andina, Lima, Perú

When polycythemic subjects of high altitude are brought down to sea level, a decrease of red cells and a depression of the erythropoietic tissue occur. Although the mechanism of this phenomenon could be explained, at least in part, by a diminution of the erythropoietin secretion, we intended to see if there were also a humoral inhibitory factor responsible for the erythropoietic depression.

In previous observations we have found that plasma filtrates from high altitude natives brought to sea level injected into rats, previously stimulated in low pressure chambers (at 18,000 feet), produced less ^{59}Fe incorporation than in rats which were injected with normal sea level plasma. This effect was optimum when plasma from high altitude natives after seven to 20 days of residence at sea level was used.[1] After several experiments on this area we concluded that clear-cut positive results were obtained only when plasma from high altitude natives with a very high degree of polycythemia (hematocrit up to 70%) was used, and that the best assay method is the study of ^{59}Fe incorporation in rats previously stimulated in a low pressure chamber.

TABLE 1 shows the results of recent experiment in which 18 rats were submitted to a low pressure of 18,000 feet for 24 hr. Following this, six of these rats were injected with plasma filtrate from high altitude natives after nine days' residence at sea level. This filtrate was previously lyophilized and used in a concentration seven times greater than its original volume. The second group of six rats received plasma filtrate from a normal sea level subject. And the third group had saline. Each animal received 4 cc of the respective material, 2 cc simultaneously with 0.5 μc of ^{59}Fe and 2 cc four hr later. It was found that the ^{59}Fe incorporation in the blood obtained after 24 hr following the first injection in the group of rats which received the plasma filtrate from the high altitude native was about one-half that obtained in rats which received either plasma filtrate from normal sea level subjects or saline. The reticulocytosis was also significantly less in the group of rats which had plasma filtrate from the polycythemic natives. In the same manner, there were significantly less immature nucleated red cells in the bone marrow of the rats belonging to this group.

TABLE 2 shows a comparative study obtained in two groups of rats which received plasma filtrate from a high altitude native after nine days residence at sea level; one of the groups received the filtrate without concentration and the other received a seven-fold concentrate of it. Under the same experimental conditions described, the ^{59}Fe incorporation was three times less in the group receiving the concentrated plasma filtrate.

Pure plasma from a high altitude native after 11 days' residence at sea level also produced less ^{59}Fe incorporation in blood of rats stimulated by exposure to 19,000 feet, as compared with the effect of plasma from a normal sea level subject (TABLE 3).

Finally, we show the modifications in the amount of hemoglobin when normal rats were given daily doses of 1 cc of plasma filtrate from high altitude natives

* Partially supported by a grant from the U.S. Army (DA-ARO-49-092-65-G90).

TABLE 1

EFFECT OF PLASMA FILTRATE FROM HIGH ALTITUDE NATIVES AFTER NINE DAYS AT SEA LEVEL, PLASMA FROM NORMAL SEA LEVEL SUBJECTS AND SALINE IN RATS EXPOSED TO 18,000 FEET

	Natives Brought Down to Sea Level	Sea Level Subjects	Saline
^{59}Fe incorporation in Blood % (Mean ± S.E.)	18.8 ± 2.3	36.7** ± 3.2	40.0** ± 0.6
Reticulocytes % (Mean ± S.E.)	0.55 ± 0.16	1.22** ± 0.20	1.78** ± 0.18
Pronormoblast % (Mean ± S.E.)	0.81 ± 0.41	0.82 ± 0.31	1.41 ± 0.33
Basophilic normoblast (large) % (Mean ± S.E.)	0.98 ± 0.50	3.50* ± 0.84	3.55* ± 0.40
Basophilic normoblast (small) % (Mean ± S.E.)	5.98 ± 1.36	9.55* ± 0.54	11.48* ± 1.16
Policromatophilic normoblast % (Mean ± S.E.)	23.1 ± 2.6	24.5 ± 2.6	21.8 ± 3.0
Acidofil normoblast % (Mean ± S.E.)	68.9 ± 4.1	61.4 ± 4.1	61.5 ± 3.5
Number of rats	6	6	6

* P = 0.05. ** P = 0.01.

TABLE 2

COMPARISON OF THE EFFECT OF SIMPLE AND CONCENTRATED PLASMA FILTRATE FROM ALTITUDE NATIVES AFTER NINE DAYS AT SEA LEVEL ON STIMULATED RATS

	Plasma Filtrate without Concentration	Saline	Difference	Concentrated Plasma Filtrate (Seven Times)	Saline	Difference
^{59}Fe incorporation in blood (Mean ± S.E.)	29.0 ± 1.9	36.5 ± 5.7	− 7.5	18.8 ± 2.3	40.0 ± 0.6	−21.2
Number of rats	9	9		6	6	

TABLE 3

EFFECT OF TOTAL PLASMA FROM HIGH ALTITUDE NATIVES AFTER 11 DAYS OF RESIDENCE AT SEA LEVEL ON RATS EXPOSED TO 19,000 FEET

	High Altitude Native Plasma	Control (Sea Level Plasma)
^{59}Fe incorporation in blood %	35.7	50.0
(Mean ± S.E.)	± 3.5	± 4.5
Reticulocytes %	0.94	1.24
(Mean ± S.E.)	± 0.31	± 0.42
Number of rats	6	6

TABLE 4

EFFECTS OF PLASMA FILTRATE FROM HIGH ALTITUDE NATIVES AFTER TEN DAYS AT SEA LEVEL PLASMA FILTRATE OF SEA LEVEL SUBJECTS AND SALINE ON HEMOGLOBIN OF NORMAL RATS

	No. of Rats	Days of Treatment	Hb, g % (mean ± S.E.) Before Treatment	After Treatment	Mean Difference	P Value	Reticulocytes (%)
Plasma of high altitude natives	5	7	14.0±.25	13.5±.52	−1.5	/.05	2.6±.63
after ten days at sea level	5	14	16.2±.14	12.7±.99	−3.5	/.01	3.1±.85
Plasma of sea level subjects	5	7	15.5±.21	15.6±.18	+ .1		1.9±.45
	5	14	15.6±.22	15.3±.42	− .3		2.0±.50
Saline	5	7	15.9±.19	16.1±.26	+ .2		1.7±.48
	5	14	16.1±.17	16.4±.23	+ .3		2.1±.55

with ten days' residence at sea level. Hemoglobin diminished 1.5 percent after seven days and 3.5 percent after 14 days of this treatment. Plasma filtrate from sea level subjects, or saline, given at the same doses, did not produce modifications in the amount of hemoglobin (TABLE 4).

These experiments seem to indicate that an inhibitory humoral factor exists in the plasma of high altitude natives brought down to sea level that is one of the regulatory mechanisms of erythropoietic activity.

Krzymowsky and Krzymowsky[3] have described an inhibitory effect of plasma of sheep made polycythemic by transfusion. A possible plasma-depressing factor has also been suggested by Leaders *et al.*[3] who studied the effects of sheep erythropoietin on cell cultures, and by Maurice *et al.*[4] in rabbit splenic blood after splenic irradiation on nonirradiated rabbits. Recently, Whitcomb and Moore[5] have studied the effect of plasma from hypertransfused mice, sheep and rabbits. They concluded that an inhibitory factor is present in polycythemic plasma which is active against the erythropoietic stimulus of hypoxia, exogenous erythropoietin preparations, and that from normal mice. The degree of activity of the inhibitory factor is related to the administered doses.

Ramos *et al.*[6] in Brookhaven have studied urine and plasma extracts from hypertransfused patients, and from polycythemic rabbits after their removal from low pressure chambers. These extracts, injected into mice and rats, decreased erythrocyte ^{59}Fe incorporation, hemoglobin, hematocrit, and reticulocytes.

References

1. REYNAFARJE, C., J. RAMOS, J. FAURA & D. VILLAVICENCIO. 1964. Humoral control of erythropoietic activity in man during and after altitude exposure. Proc. Soc. Exp. Biol. Med. **116:** 649.
2. KRZYMOWSKY, T. & H. KRZYMOWSKY. 1962. Studies on the erythropoiesis inhibitory factor in plasma of animals with transfusion polycythemia. Blood **19:** 38.
3. LEADERS, F. E., A. A. WERDER & C. SCHIMIT. 1964. Erythropoietic-stimulating factor (ESF) as a stimulant of cell growth in vitro. Proc. Soc. Exp. Biol. Med. **115:** 658.
4. MAURICE, P. & A. JEANRENAUD. 1964. Erythropoietic depression due to splenic irradiation. Brit. J. Haemat. **10:** 327.
5. WHITCOMB, W. H. & M. Z. MOORE. 1964. Erythropietic inhibitory effect of plasma from hypertransfused animals. J. Lab. Clin. Med. **60:** 1017.
6. RAMOS, J., E. P. CRONKITE, M. L. GREEBERG, L. M. SCHIFFER & P. STRYCKMANS. 1965. To be published.

TWO HEREDITARY MOUSE ANEMIAS (Sl/Sl^d and W/W^v) DEFICIENT IN RESPONSE TO ERYTHROPOIETIN*

Seldon E. Bernstein, Elizabeth S. Russell and Geoffrey Keighley

The Jackson Laboratory, Bar Harbor, Me., and California Institute of Technology, Pasadena, Calif.

Introduction

Two different anemia-producing mutants in the mouse are of special interest to experimental hematologists concerned with control of erythropoiesis because of their particular responses to anoxia, erythropoietin and tissue transplant therapy. These mutations, although strikingly similar in their phenotypic manifestations, occurred spontaneously at loci in two different genetic linkage groups and we have reason to believe that members of the two allelic series act on two different parts of the hematopoietic system. Semidominant alleles at the steel (S1) locus in linkage group IV, and alleles at the W locus in linkage group XVII, show very similar pleiotropic effects on pigmentation, fertility, and blood-formation. Animals bearing double doses, either of mutant S1 alleles or of mutant W alleles, are all black-eyed, white sterile mice afflicted with severe macrocytic anemia. Of these anemias, the W series mutants have been the most thoroughly described, while steel series mutants have as yet been inadequately reported in the literature. We will neither examine the genetic features of either type of anemia in this paper nor present a comprehensive treatise on their pathology, physiology, histology, biochemistry, longevity, or breeding performance; for these, the reader is referred to review articles (Bernstein, 1963; Russell & Bernstein, 1966; Russell & Meier, 1966). Rather, we will present only that information which is directly applicable to our analysis of the hematopoietic responses of W/W^v and S1/S1^d anemic mice. A tabulation of selected characteristics of the mutants and their normal littermates is presented in TABLES 1 and 2 as a reminder to those who have examined previous literature on the subject, and as a starting point for those who have a different orientation.

The tabulation indicates that untreated W/W^v anemics and S1/S1^d anemics are phenotypically indistinguishable, except that the S1/S1^d anemia tends to be more severe, with lower mean hematocrit levels and higher relative and absolute numbers of reticulocytes. Even though the experienced investigator is unable to tell them apart, they still differ in some interesting and significant ways in their reactions to experimental manipulation. It is our intention, therefore 1) to describe several types of physiological experiments which we employed in our search for the steps in hematopoiesis that are deranged by the action of these genetic determinants; 2) to present information obtained thereby; and 3) to consider briefly the possible significance of these results.

Materials and Methods

Mice

W-Series Anemics. The genetically anemic WBB6F$_1$-W/W^v and littermate normal WBB6F$_1$-+/+ mice used in these experiments were young adults (two-

* Investigations at The Jackson Laboratory were supported in part by research grants HD 00254 from the National Institute of Child Health and Human Development, CA 01074 from the National Cancer Institute of the U.S. Public Health Service, and in part by Contract (AT30–1)–1800 from the U.S. Atomic Energy Commission. Investigations at the California Institute of Technology were supported by research grant HE 07683 from the U.S. Public Health Service to the Division of Biology, California Institute of Technology.

TABLE 1

SUMMARY OF ADULT CHARACTERISTICS OF TWO DIFFERENT HEREDITARY ANEMIAS

Name	Normals	W-Series Anemics	Steel-Series Anemics
Genotype	+/+	W/W^v	Sl/Sl^d
Condition	Normal	W–anemic	Steel Anemic
Genetic background	$WBB6F_1$ or $WCB6F_1$	$WBB6F_1$	$WCB6F_1$
Produced by crossing	WB +/+ × C57BL/6 +/+ or selecting from segregating litters	WB–W/+ × C57BL/6–W^v/+	WC–Sl/+ × C57BL/6–Sl^d/+
Pigmentation	All black	Black-eyed white	Black-eyed white
Fertility	Normal	Sterile	Sterile
Anemia	None	Severe macrocytic	Severe macrocytic

TABLE 2

HEMATOLOGICAL CHARACTERISTICS OF ADULT NORMAL MICE AND MICE WITH TWO DIFFERENT HEREDITARY ANEMIAS

Name	Normals	W-Anemics	Steel Anemics
Erythrocytes $\times 10^6/mm^3$	10.4	6.3	4.2
Hematocrit (%)	48.7	39.8	29.3
Mean cell volume (μ^3)	46.9	63.1	71.2
Reticulocytes (%)	2.5	3.5	9.1
Reticulocytes $\times 10^4/mm^3$	24.7	19.2	35.0
Leucocytes $\times 10^3/mm^3$	10.5	14.0	11.6
Marrow cellularity $\times 10^7$/femur	2.1	1.3	1.0
Colony-forming units/10^5 marrow cells	21	<1	22

to-four-month old) offspring produced at the Jackson Laboratory from crosses of WB/Re-W/+ × C57BL/6J-W^v/+ parents. Genotypes resulting from these matings were W/W^v, W^v/+, W/+, and +/+, all segregating in the same litter and for practical purposes genetically identical except for the W-gene substitution.

Steel-Series Anemics. These mice were produced by crossing WC/Re-Sl/+ with C57BL/6J-Sl^d/+ mice. Crosses of this sort yield Sl/Sl^d, Sl^d/+, Sl/+, and +/+ genotypes all congenic with the WCB6F_1-+/+ hybrid.

Normal Mice. Normal mice from inbred strain C57BL/6J were purchased from the Jackson Laboratory and used in some experiments as donors of cells employed in hypertransfusion plethorization and as erythropoietin assay animals. In all other experiments the +/+ genotype was selected from WBB6F_1 or WCB6F_1 litters segregating for steel or W anemics.

Tissues

Tissues for implantation were obtained from embryos or adults resulting from crosses of WC/Re-+/+ × C57BL/6J-+/+ or WB/Re-+/+ × C57BL/6J-+/+.

In the case of adult donors, nucleated cells were obtained from the femoral marrow cavity by flushing with saline. Four to 8 × 10^6 marrow cells were administered i. v. to appropriate recipients. The implantation of embryonic hematopoietic tissue involved the i.p. injection of a saline suspension of 8 × 10^6 nucleated cells obtained from the livers of 15½-day embryos.

Plethorization by Hypertransfusion. Mice were plethorized by hypertransfusion with red blood cells from C57BL/6J retired breeders. On three successive days 0.5 ml of an 80–90 percent suspension of red blood cells in saline were administered to each mouse by i.p. injection. Recipients with hematocrits in excess of 65% were used three to four days after the final injection of erythrocytes.

Plethorization by Hypoxia. In experiments carried out at the California Institute of Technology mice were made polycythemic by exposure to low oxygen tension in a tank maintained at a reduced pressure of 345 mm Hg (P_{O_2} = 72 mm Hg). Mice used for erythropoietic assays were usually exposed to hypoxia for ten days in the reduced pressure chamber.

Assays for Erythropoietin Activity or Response. Mice were first made polycythemic either by hypertransfusion or by hypoxia. Three to four days after the completion of plethorization they were injected with exogenous erythropoietin or the material to be assayed. Sixty hr later they were injected with 4–5 μc of ^{59}Fe citrate, and 24 hr later the radioactivity of a sample of the blood was determined using a gamma scintillation counter. Knowing the hematocrit, the total blood volume, the activity in serum, and the activity in whole blood, it was possible to calculate the percentage of ^{59}Fe that was incorporated in red blood cells.

Results

Erythropoietin Production and Response

Our first two attempts were to determine whether W/W^v anemics had low red cell numbers because they were deficient in their responses to erythropoietin, and to determine whether erythropoietin was produced by these mice. Results published elsewhere (Keighley *et al.*, 1966) show that W/W^v mice are good producers of this hormone, but very poor responders to this stimulus. FIGURE 1 (adapted from Keighley *et al.*, 1966) compares the responses to graded doses of erythropoietin of normal and W/W^v mice which had been made polycythemic by exposure for 18 days to reduced pressure. Note that roughly 150 times the dose required to initiate a response in normal mice is required to increase significantly ^{59}Fe uptake in W/W^v anemics.

Similar analyses of Sl/Sl^d anemic mice revealed that their serum contained significant concentrations of erythropoietin or an erythropoietin precursor which could be utilized by plethorized normal mice (TABLE 3, lines 3 & 4).

Injections of Sl/Sl^d or +/+ serum along with 2A-units of human urinary erythropoietin showed that presence of Sl/Sl^d serum in polycythemic normal mice does not prevent their response to exogenous erythropoietin (TABLE 3, lines 5 & 6). Thus steel anemics appear to produce erythropoietin in large amounts but do not appear to respond well to their own erythropoietic hormone and possibly to exogenous erythropoietin.

To examine the latter possibility, we plethorized Sl/Sl^d and +/+ mice and gave them graded doses of human urinary erythropoietin, (see FIGURE 1). We found that steel anemics were totally unresponsive to massive doses of exogenous erythropoietin (98 A-units). It is significant that more than one thousand times the minimal effective dose for normals was administered without effect.

Synthesis of Mosaics for Analysis of Gene Action

In 1956 we demonstrated that W series anemics could be permanently cured of their macrocytic anemia by injecting them with 4–8 × 10^6 histocompatible

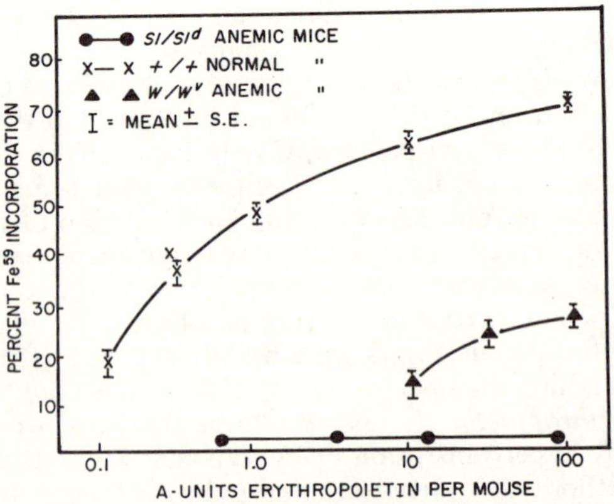

FIGURE 1. Response of plethorized normal (+/+) mice and two types of plethorized anemic mice (W/W^v and Sl/Sl^d) to injections of exogenous erythropoietin.

TABLE 3

ERYTHROPOIETIN LEVELS, ASSAYED IN PLETHORIZED NORMAL MICE AS 24-HOUR ^{59}Fe UPTAKE

Source	Trial 1 Percent ^{59}Fe Uptake	Trial 2 Percent ^{59}Fe Uptake
1. Plasma +/+ mice	0–1	0.4
2. Plasma W/W^v mice	4	—
3. Serum +/+ mice	0.2	0.4
4. Serum Sl/Sl^d mice	13	8.9
5. Serum +/+ mice + 2 A units EP	19	15.4
6. Serum Sl/Sl^d mice + 2 A units EP	21	16.7
7. Serum Sl/Sl^d mice plethorized seven days	0–0.5	<0.5
8. Serum W/W^v mice plethorized seven days	0–0.5	<0.5

hematopoietic cells obtained from the livers of 15½ day embryos (Russell *et al.*, 1956). We have since shown through studies of hemoglobin electrophoretic differences that the indigenous defective marrow is completely or nearly completely replaced by the implanted hematopoietic tissue (Russell & Bernstein, unpublished data). In our hands, however, this form of therapy has been totally ineffective for steel anemics. Typical degree and extent of success in therapy of W/W^v anemia and of failures in therapy of steel-series anemias obtained by this implantation technique are summarized in TABLE 4. We are happy to report that marrow cells from steel anemics also are effective in curing the W series anemic state. Indeed, W/W^v macrocytic anemics were permanently converted to normocytic normochromic individuals as a result of the implantation of either steel "stem cells" or normal (+/+) "stem cells." As a consequence of this form of implantation we have produced new mosaic types, namely +/+-implanted W/W^{v}s, and S1/S1^d-implanted W/W^{v}s, both types with normal blood values. Using these, it has been possible to conduct experiments aimed at ascertaining whether a given gene-determined defect was fixed within erythropoietic cells, or whether the blockage in erythropoietin utilization or response stemmed from some factor in their cellular environment.

Erythropoietin Response of Mosaic Mice

W/W^v anemics were inoculated i.v. with 8×10^6 histocompatible femoral marrow cells, from either normal mice or steel anemic mice. Forty-five to 90 days later, when implanted mice achieved normal blood values (red blood cells $= 9-10 \times 10^6$ per mm^3, or hematocrit $= 45-50\%$), they were plethorized by hypertransfusion with +/+ red blood cells to a hematocrit of 70+%, and injected with human urinary erythropoietin (63–37–1) obtained from Dr. Keighley's laboratory. Our results clearly indicated that +/+ cells residing in a W/W^v environment respond similarly to +/+ cells in a +/+ environment. S1/S1^d cells (originally erythropoietin-unresponsive) transplanted to a W/W^v environment dramatically display a normal response (see FIGURE 2). These findings are further evidence that the defect in W/W^v mice is intrinsic to the hematopoietic tissue, since W/W^v cellular environment is capable of supporting the normal growth, development and continued proliferation of normal and S1/S1^d stem cells and their differentiation products. In contrast, steel stem cells have no intrinsic defect, but appear to be suppressed or improperly stimulated by their usual

TABLE 4

EFFECTIVENESS OF HEMATOPOIETIC TISSUE TRANSPLANTS IN CURING SEVERAL TYPES OF HEREDITARY ANEMIAS

Tissue Donor	Type of Tissue	No. of Cells $\times 10^6$	Type of Recipient	Hematocrit Day 0	Hematocrit Day 30	Hematocrit Day 90	No. Treated	No. Cured
			W-Series					
$WCB6F_1$ +/+	EL*	4–8	$WCB6F_1$ W/W^v	36.5 ± 0.7	—	44.7 ± 0.5	19	16
$WBB6F_1$ +/+	EL	8	$WBB6F_1$ W/W^v	40.2	—	46.7	6	6
$WBB6F_1$ +/+	EL	8	$WCB6F_1$ W/W^v	38.9	—	46.7	12	12
$WBB6F_1$ +/+	AM**	1.7	$WBB6F_1$ W/W^v	37.7 ± 0.7	48.7 ± 0.7	—	15	14
C57BL/6+/+	AM	6.0	$WBB6F_1$ W/W^v	37.2 ± 1.9	47.8 ± 1.7	46.2 ± 1.2	6	6
$WCB6F_1$ Sl/Sl^d	AM	6.0	$WBB6F_1$ W/W^v	37.2 ± 2.0	42.2 ± 4.3	43.7 ± 2.9	5	3
$WCB6F_1$ Sl/Sl^d	AM	1.4	$WBB6F_1$ W/W^v	37.9 ± 0.5	49.1 ± 0.7	—	14	14
			Steel-series					
C57BL/6 +/+	EL	4–8	C57BL/6 Sl^d/Sl^d	30.2 ± 1.4	—	28.2 ± 0.9	7	0
C57BL/6 +/+	EL	4–8	$B6D2F_1$ Sl^d/Sl^d	29.8 ± 1.1	—	28.1 ± 1.6	19	0
C57BL/6 +/+	EL	50	$WCB6F_1$ Sl/Sl^d	31.1 ± 1.9	—	21.8 ± 1.3	6	0
$B6D2F_1$ +/+	EL	10	$B6D2F_1$ Sl^d/Sl^d	30.3 ± 1.8	—	30.5 ± 0.7	8	0
			Normal control					
None	—	—	$WCB6F_1$ +/+	48.3	—	—	—	—
None	—	—	$WBB6F_1$ +/+	49.4	—	—	—	—

* 15½-day embryonic liver cells administered i.p.
** Adult femoral marrow cells given i.v.

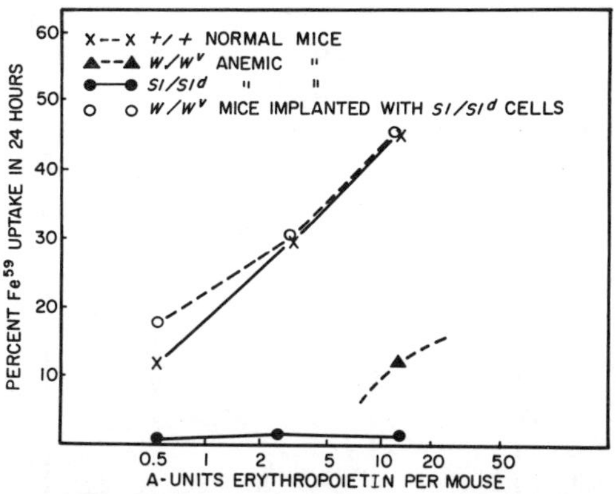

FIGURE 2. Response to erythropoietin of plethorized Sl/Sl^d anemic mice and plethorized W/W^v mice cured of their anemia by the implantation of Sl/Sl^d marrow cells.

cellular environment, for when these steel stem cells are transplanted to a W/W^v cellular environment, they respond in the fashion characteristic of normal stem cells.

Response of Different Genotypes to Anoxia

Many investigators have proposed that the increase in red cell mass which follows exposure to low levels of atmospheric oxygen is mediated by the production and utilization of erythropoietin. If this is true, one might be able to study still another step in the control of erythropoiesis, notably, the production of erythropoietin. In this connection we have established only the simple response to anoxia. We exposed steel anemics, W anemics, and normal mice to a mixture of 10% oxygen and 90% nitrogen for a period of nine days and followed the changes in hematocrit percentage and reticulocyte count. The data presented in FIGURE 3 show that previously unprepared normal and W/W^v mice exposed for a prolonged period to continuous low oxygen tension responded with parallel linear increases in hematocrit percentage with time. However, when previously untreated S1/S1^d mice were subjected to the same treatment, many of them (eight out of 12) died, apparently unable to tolerate sudden continuous exposure to this low level of oxygen tension. Those that survived showed slight but equivocal increases in hematocrit percentages.

Further tests, starting with intermittent exposures of +/+, W/W^v, and S1/S1^d mice to low oxygen tension, gave more conclusive results (FIGURE 4). Six normal, two W/W^v, and six S1/S1^d mice were subjected to low oxygen tension (P_{O_2}, 59–60 mm Hg) for six to eight hr on nine successive days, followed by 12–16 hr exposure on 16 successive days, and then were maintained constantly under low oxygen tension for another 25 days. All mice survived this 51-day course of hypoxic exposure, and all developed greatly increased hematocrit percentages. When exposure to hypoxia was discontinued, the hematocrit levels of all mice dropped rapidly and after 24 days, all hematocrit percentages were at or below pretreatment level.

Thus, it appears that although S1/S1^d mice have difficulty adapting to sudden exposure to constant hypoxia, hypoxia nevertheless induces a true erythropoietic response in both Sl/Sl^d and W/W^v mice. At present we have no evidence indicating whether the same, or a different, mechanism is involved in the responses of the two kinds of anemic mice.

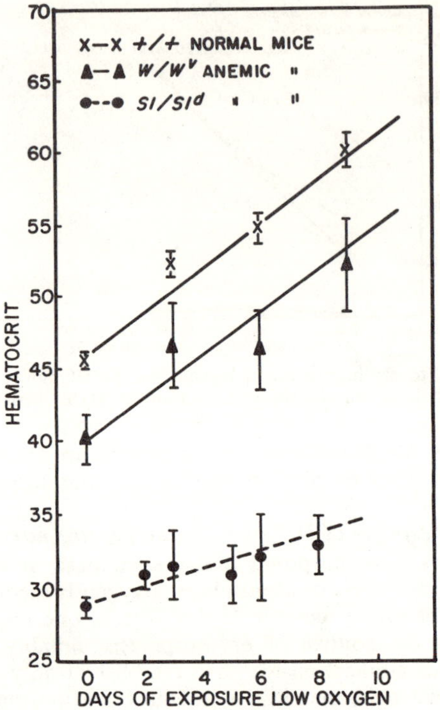

FIGURE 3. Differential response of mutants to continuous exposure to hypoxic anoxia (10% oxygen balance nitrogen).

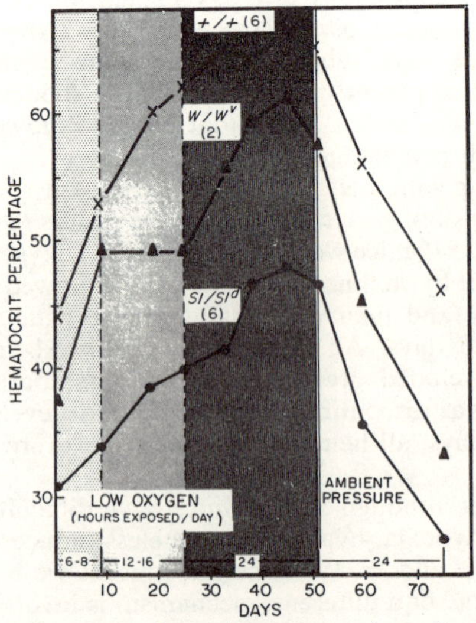

FIGURE 4. Response of anemic mutants to intermittent anoxia.

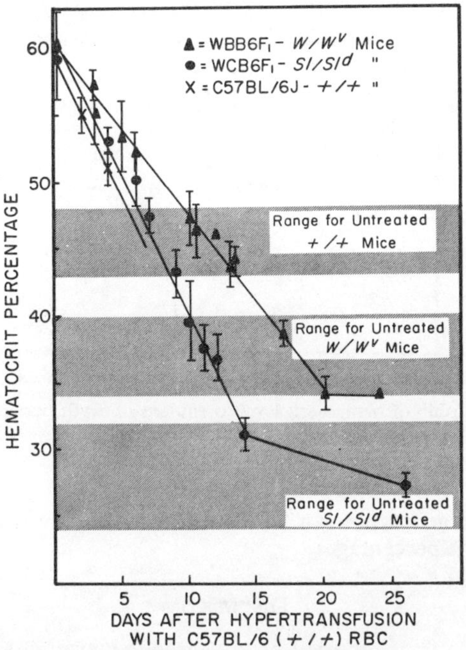

FIGURE 5. Decline in hematocrit following plethorization by hypertransfusion.

Relationship Between the Severity of Anemia and the Serum Content of Erythropoietin

In some of our investigations we were concerned with the possibility that the severity of the anemia may have some significant effect on the amount of erythropoietin found in the blood serum. In order to obtain a variety of hematocrit percentages for mice of any one genotype, mice were plethorized by the i.p. hypertransfusion of normal red blood cells until their hematocrit was 70+% and at intervals thereafter, as the plethoric state declined, hematocrit percentages were determined and serum samples taken for the analysis of erythropoietin content. Erythropoietin assays were performed in C57BL/6-+/+ mice, hypertransfused with C57BL/6-+/+ red blood cells.

It can be seen from the curves in FIGURE 5 that the rate of hematocrit decline for all genotypes was essentially the same. Indeed, all of the corrected ^{51}Cr T/2 values were the same. Even though the decay rates were the same, they did not level out at a normal hematocrit level of 45–59 percent. Instead, each mouse returned directly to the pretreatment level characteristic of its genotype.

In mice of all three genotypes, when hematocrit percentages were 40–80%, no erythropoietin was detected in the plasma (FIGURE 6). When the hematocrit level dropped below 40%, there was a more or less direct linear relationship between hematocrit and log of erythropoietin content. In a general way, the more anemic an animal, the greater was its content of serum erythropoietin, all other things being equal.

These observations are pertinent, especially to the analysis of the two anemias, and suggest that the differences in erythropoietin levels between nonstressed

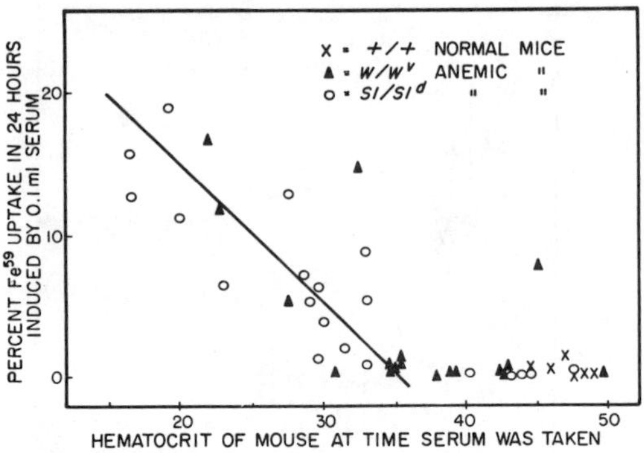

FIGURE 6. Relationship of hematocrit level to content of erythropoietin in serum, measured as percentage of Fe^{59} appearing in erythrocytes in 24 hours.

animals of the two genotypes can be related in the simple way to the differences in mean hematocrit percentages.

Discussion

In view of the findings reported here, we see that two amazingly similar genetically induced hematological abnormalities not only may be caused by different genetic determinants but also may have different cellular and physiological bases. In the one case, (W series), the basic defect appears to reside within the hematopoietic stem cell itself or within its immediate descendants. Other experiments have shown that their erythroid stem cell population is deficient (Till & McCulloch, 1964) and their blood-forming tissue is intrinsically defective in response to erythropoietin (Keighley *et al.*, 1962 & 1966). The W/W^v defect is apparently unrelated to the genotype of the rest of the body in which the cells reside, for normal hematopoietic cells transplanted to this environment behave in a normal fashion (Keighley *et al.*, 1962).

It is possible to speculate that although W/W^v stem cells always contain potential sources of energy and substrate for differentiation, under most conditions erythropoietin cannot enter these cells because of the nature of their cell surface (Keighley *et al.*, 1966). The positive erythropoietic response to low oxygen tension may result from alteration of some metabolic process within the cell membrane or cytoplasm.

In direct contrast to this, Sl/Sl^d anemics were found to contain normal numbers of stem cells per 10^6 nucleated marrow cells, and while they too are extremely resistant to erythropoietin, their nonreactivity to this hormone is a function of the local cellular environment. They performed normally in a W/W^v environment, known to support normal function of $+/+$ stem cells. One must postulate, therefore, either an inability on the part of the steel body to produce or transport essential substrates to these cells, or the inability of the steel body to activate erythropoietin. Certainly a low renal threshold for erythropoietin must be ruled out, with the findings of large amounts of this substance in the circulation.

It is safe to conclude that both steel and W anemics are unresponsive to erythropoietin and that two different facets of erythropoietin utilization are involved.

References

BERNSTEIN, S. E. 1963. Problems and potentialities of hematopoietic tissue transplants. Trans. New Eng. Surg. Soc. **44**: 76–83.

KEIGHLEY, G. H., E. S. RUSSELL & P. LOWY. 1962. Response of normal and genetically anaemic mice to erythropoietic stimuli. Brit. J. Haematol. **8**: 429–441.

KEIGHLEY, G. H., P. LOWY, E. S. RUSSELL & M. W. THOMPSON. 1966. Analysis of erythroid homeostatic mechanisms in normal and genetically anemic mice. Brit. J. Haematol. **12**: 461–477.

MCCULLOCH, E. A., L. SIMINOVITCH & J. E. TILL. 1964. Spleen-colony formation in anemic mice of genotype WW^v. Science **144**: 844–846.

MCCULLOCH, E. A., L. SIMINOVITCH, J. E. TILL, E. S. RUSSELL & S. E. BERNSTEIN. 1965. The cellular basis of the genetically determined hemopoietic defect in anemic mice of genotype Sl/Sl^d. Blood **26**: 399–410.

RUSSELL, E. S., L. J. SMITH & F. A. LAWSON. 1956. Implantation of normal blood-forming tissues in radiated genetically anemic hosts. Science **124**: 1076–1077.

RUSSELL, E. S. & S. E. BERNSTEIN. 1966. Blood and blood formation. *In* Biology of the Laboratory Mouse, 2nd ed. E. L. Green, ed. : 351–377. McGraw-Hill. New York.

RUSSELL, E. S. & H. MEIER. 1966. Constitutional diseases. *In* Biology of the Laboratory Mouse, 2nd ed. E. L. Green, ed. : 571–587. McGraw-Hill. New York.

MURINE VIRAL-INDUCED POLYCYTHEMIA*

E. A. Mirand

Roswell Park Memorial Institute, New York State Department of Health, and State University of New York at Buffalo, Buffalo, N. Y.

Studies have been carried out in our laboratory on a virus-induced murine leukemia which was reported by Dr. Charlotte Friend in 1957.[1,2] This virus-induced leukemia (FVA) is characterized by a rapid proliferation of the reticulum cells of the spleen and liver resulting in hepatosplenomegaly, accompanied by lymphocytosis, erythroblastosis, anemia, and progressive decrease in platelets (TABLE 1). During the course of our studies, we discovered that several of the Friend virus filtrates produced a polycythemic response (TABLE 2). One of these filtrates (FVP) has been passed through Ha/ICR Swiss and DBA/2 mice more than 72 times. It continues to induce a polycythemic response along with granulocytosis, an increase in platelets, and reticulum cell proliferation resulting in hepatosplenomegaly. Extensive studies have revealed that the virus is present in relatively high concentration in most tissues of infected mice (TABLE 3).

For several reasons we feel that we are working with a polycythemia-inducing virus (FVP) which may be a passenger virus and distinct from the virus originally reported by Dr. Friend, which we refer to as FVA, or Friend virus, which gives an anemic response.

Pregnant females infected with FVP (TABLE 4) develop Friend leukemia with polycythemia; however, their infected offspring (TABLE 5) develop Friend leukemia without polycythemia. With this biological technique, one can separate the polycythemic response from the anemic response. Subsequent passage of Friend virus filtrate obtained from such offspring (FVA) will not give a polycythemic response (TABLE 6).

Furthermore, we have studied various strains of Friend virus and find that only the Friend virus strain that produces a polycythemic response (FVP) is capable of initiating erythropoiesis in mice in a hypertransfused-polycythemic state (TABLE 7). The effect here is similar to that which occurs when erythropoietin is administered to hypertransfused-polycythemic animals. Also, the Friend virus that gives an anemic response (FVA) is incapable of initiating erythropoiesis in a hypertransfused-polycythemic state (TABLE 8). Like FVA, Rauscher virus, known to produce a marked erythropoietic response, does not initiate erythropoiesis in a hypertransfused-polycythemic state (TABLE 9).

The results of a study on the susceptibility of Swiss mice of various ages to FVA and FVP are given in TABLES 10 and 11, respectively. The data show that essentially 100% of the mice in each age group, in each experiment, developed the disease. The average time intervals from injection to the development of palpable spleens differ slightly for the different age groups, although the time to death lengthens as the age level of the mice at inoculation increases.

TABLE 12 illustrates the efficiency of FVP in inducing the disease in Swiss mice inoculated by various routes.

TABLE 13 shows the stability of FVP when subjected to physical and chemical treatments. The findings are similar to those which have been reported for most murine leukemia viruses.

* This investigation was supported in part by research grants AI-04506, CA–02728 and CA–07745 from the U.S. Public Health Service, National Institutes of Health, and the John A. Hartford Foundation, Inc.

TABLE 1

REPRESENTATIVE BLOOD COUNTS FROM FRIEND VIRUS (FVA) INFECTED HA/ICR MICE

Mouse Number	Days Post-infection	Spleen Weight (grams)	RBC 10^6	Hemato-crit	Hemoglobin grams/100 cc	Percent Erythroblasts No./200 Nucleated Cells	WBC 10^3
Infected mice							
1	19	2.35	5.30	32	8.2	2.5	55.5
2	19	2.10	4.85	30	7.1	3.5	30.8
3	20	1.85	6.72	35	10.1	2.0	62.0
4	21	3.10	6.39	34	9.8	3.0	101.2
5	22	3.50	3.85	30	5.8	6.0	48.0
6	24	1.46	5.41	36	6.3	8.0	65.0
7	30	4.20	6.01	35	6.9	4.0	86.8
8	32	3.45	3.75	31	5.2	10.5	57.8
9	36	1.63	5.85	33	6.1	12.5	125.2
10	40	3.25	5.52	36	7.1	12.0	145.0
11	45	1.95	6.01	34	8.2	18.0	45.0
12	55	2.45	4.58	29	5.3	18.5	87.0
Average		2.61	5.35	33	7.2	8.4	75.8
Noninfected mice							
1	0	0.14	9.2	43	13.5	0	3.5
2	0	0.15	9.8	44	14.8	0	5.8
3	0	0.11	7.4	42	12.5	0	5.3
Average		0.13	8.8	43	13.6	0	4.9

TABLE 2

REPRESENTATIVE BLOOD COUNTS IN INFECTED HA/ICR SWISS MICE INOCULATED WITH FRIEND VIRUS FILTRATE CONTAINING THE POLYCYTHEMIA VIRUS (FVP)

Mouse Number	Days Post-infection	Spleen Weight (grams)	RBC 10^6	Hemato-crit	Hemoglobin grams/100 cc	Percent Erythroblasts No./200 Nucleated Cells	WBC 10^3
Infected mice							
1	19	2.20	9.37	55	16.6	0	78.5
2	19	2.66	10.96	61	19.9	0	128.0
3	22	3.46	12.41	74	18.8	2.5	117.0
4	22	2.68	11.82	74	19.0	0	83.0
5	22	2.95	10.13	76	21.4	1.0	72.0
6	22	3.15	17.82	82	25.0	0	11.2
7	26	2.43	11.30	71	18.2	0	12.5
8	26	1.81	9.53	66	18.8	1.0	70.2
9	26	2.20	10.23	65	19.5	1.5	10.2
10	26	1.53	8.39	51	15.0	0	22.8
11	40	4.80	16.08	86	25.4	13.5	136.1
12	41	3.67	17.58	81	22.0	12.0	88.5
Average		2.80	12.13	70	19.9	2.6	69.2
Noninfected mice							
1	0	0.16	8.0	45	14.2	0	2.8
2	0	0.16	7.3	43	15.1	0	7.2
3	0	0.14	7.9	42	13.8	0	5.5
Average		0.15	7.7	43	14.4	0	5.2

TABLE 3

RELATIVE POTENCIES OF EXTRACTS OF VARIOUS TISSUES HARVESTED FROM HA/ICR SWISS MICE INJECTED AT 30 DAYS OF AGE WITH FRIEND VIRUS FILTRATE CONTAINING POLYCYTHEMIA VIRUS (FVP)*

Tissue	Dilution of Tissue Extract (log)	Positive Number	Total Percent	Average Time of Response		Number with Polycythemia
				Palpation (days)	Death (days)	
Spleen	−1	12/12	100	8	28.2	5
	−2	9/10	90	11	31.0	8
	−3	10/10	100	20	42.8	10
	−4	6/10	60	38	71.8	5
	−5	2/10	20	46	83.0	2
Plasma	−1	14/14	100	8.2	30.8	8
Liver	−1	10/10	100	11.2	34.2	6
Kidney	−1	10/10	100	14.3	40.5	7
Thymus	−1	8/10	80	18.3	42.5	6
Lung	−1	10/10	100	12.5	34.8	5
Brain	−1	6/10	60	18.5	43.0	5
Muscle	−1	7/14	50	22.4	50.5	6
Lymph nodes	−1	18/24	75	25.8	61.5	14
Bone marrow	−1	10/10	100	17.8	37.2	8

* Pools of tissue collected from 28 infected Ha/ICR Swiss mice 22 days postinoculation. All animals observed for a period of 362 days.

TABLE 4

RESPONSE OF PREGNANT FEMALES TO FRIEND VIRUS FILTRATE CONTAINING THE POLYCYTHEMIA VIRUS (FVP)

Pregnant Females	Days Post-infection	Spleen Weight (grams)	RBC 10^6	Hematocrit	Hemoglobin grams/100 cc	Percent Erythroblasts No./200 Nucleated Cells	WBC 10^3
A	15	1.35	8.38	52	14.9	0	35.2
B	18	1.85	9.01	65	17.0	0	21.7
C	18	0.95	8.25	62	18.2	1.5	45.5
D	20	1.10	12.08	71	18.0	0	50.3
E	20	1.45	11.85	69	16.5	0	62.0
Average		1.34	9.91	64	16.9	0.3	42.9

TABLE 5

RESPONSE OF OFFSPRING FROM MOTHERS INFECTED WITH FRIEND VIRUS FILTRATE CONTAINING THE POLYCYTHEMIA VIRUS (FVP)

Number Offspring* from Mother	Number Free of Disease	Number with Friend Leukemia	Number with Anemia	Number with Polycythemia
A — 8	6	2	2	0
B — 10	8	2	2	0
C — 7	7	0	0	0
D — 12	9	3	3	0
E — 8	5	3	3	0

* Offspring observed for 12 months.

TABLE 6

INFECTIVITY OF SPLENIC FILTRATES FROM OFFSPRING INFECTED WITH FRIEND LEUKEMIA VIA MATERNAL TRANSMISSION

Filtrate	Number Adult Mice Injected	Number with Friend Leukemia	Number with Anemia	Number with Polycythemia
Splenic filtrate B*				
Passage 1	12	10	10	0
2	10	9	9	0
3	10	10	10	0
4	10	8	8	0
5	8	8	8	0
Splenic filtrate E**				
Passage 1	14	12	12	0
2	8	8	8	0
3	12	11	11	0
4	10	10	10	0
5	9	8	8	0
6	11	11	11	0
7	12	10	10	0
8	13	12	12	0

* Spleens pooled from offspring from infected Mother B and passed consecutively for 5 ×.
** Spleens pooled from offspring from infected Mother E and passed consecutively for 8 ×.

TABLE 7

RESPONSE OF HYPERTRANSFUSED-POLYCYTHEMIC (HP) HA/ICR SWISS MICE TO FRIEND VIRUS CONTAINING THE POLYCYTHEMIA VIRUS (FVP)

Group	Days Postinfection	Average 24-Hour ^{59}Fe Uptake*			Average Spleen Weight* (grams)	Average Hematocrit*
		Femur	Blood	Spleen		
(A) Untreated control	7	0.50	24.7	2.0	0.11	42
FVP	7	0.43	25.7	4.2	0.75	43
HP	7	0.15	0.3	0.4	0.12	71
HP + FVP	7	1.9	1.9	1.1	0.18	74
(B) Untreated control	14	0.40	25.9	1.5	0.12	43
FVP	14	0.10	26.8	17.9	1.10	51
HP	14	0.10	0.3	0.5	0.14	75
HP + FVP	14	0.10	18.2	12.1	0.58	73
(C) Untreated control	28	0.48	29.9	1.8	0.15	42
FVP	28	0.08	27.0	13.7	2.38	68
HP	28	0.10	0.3	0.6	0.12	71
HP + FVP	28	0.09	29.3	14.5	1.06	79

* Average from minimum of five mice/group.

TABLE 8

RESPONSE OF HYPERTRANSFUSED-POLYCYTHEMIC (HP) HA/ICR SWISS MICE TO FRIEND VIRUS GIVING THE ANEMIC RESPONSE (FVA)

Group*	Average 24-Hour ^{59}Fe Uptake**			Average Spleen Weight (grams)**	Average Hematocrit**
	Femur	Blood	Spleen		
Untreated	0.55	25.8	1.7	0.15	42
FVA	0.25	27.4	7.8	0.89	37
HP	0.08	0.3	0.09	0.14	76
HP + FVA	0.10	0.5	0.14	0.29	74

* All data obtained 14 days after infection with Friend virus.
** Average from minimum of five mice/group.

TABLE 9

RESPONSE OF HYPERTRANSFUSED-POLYCYTHEMIC (HP) HA/ICR SWISS MICE TO RAUSCHER VIRUS

Group	Days Postinfection	Average 24-Hour ^{59}Fe Uptake*			Average Spleen Weight (grams)*	Average Hematocrit*
		Femur	Blood	Spleen		
(A) Untreated control	7	0.46	25.2	1.3	0.11	42
Rauscher virus	7	0.48	34.6	6.6	0.38	39
HP	7	0.12	0.2	0.5	0.13	74
HP + Rauscher virus	7	0.49	0.7	0.9	0.29	72
(B) Untreated control	14	0.51	28.2	2.1	0.15	42
Rauscher virus	14	0.30	25.0	15.5	1.13	40
HP	14	0.08	0.3	0.2	0.11	78
HP + Rauscher virus	14	0.17	0.4	0.5	0.41	73
(C) Untreated control	20	0.43	26.4	1.2	0.14	45
Rauscher virus	20	0.24	18.5	20.6	1.78	40
HP	20	0.09	0.4	0.2	0.10	71
HP + Rauscher virus	20	0.18	0.6	0.2	0.39	75
(D) Untreated control	28	0.47	25.3	1.8	0.13	43
Rauscher virus	28	0.27	19.8	10.0	1.89	35
HP	28	0.08	0.2	0.1	0.12	72
HP + Rauscher virus	28	0.17	0.6	1.2	0.29	67

* Average from minimum of five mice/group.

TABLE 10

SUSCEPTIBILITY OF HA/ICR SWISS MICE, INOCULATED AT VARIOUS AGES, TO FVP*

Age at Inoculation (Days)	Positive/Total		Average Time to		Number with Anemia	Number with Polycythemia
	Number	Percent	Palpable Spleens (Days)	Death (Days)		
1	30/30	100	6	24	30	0
3	20/20	100	7	25	20	0
7	12/12	100	5	25	10	0
14	12/12	100	8	26	11	0
21	8/8	100	10	29	8	0
28	9/10	90	9	30	7	0
42	8/10	80	13	39	8	0
49	6/10	60	16	43	6	0
56	12/12	100	13	46	12	0

* Animals received i.p. dilution of a standard virus preparation in amounts equivalent to 0.01 ml per gm of body weight.

TABLE 11

SUSCEPTIBILITY OF HA/ICR SWISS MICE, INOCULATED AT VARIOUS AGES, TO FRIEND VIRUS FILTRATE CONTAINING THE POLYCYTHEMIA VIRUS (FVP)

Age at Inoculation (Days)	Positive/Total		Average Time to		Number with Anemia	Number with Polycythemia
	Number	Percent	Palpable Spleens (Days)	Death (Days)		
1	12/12	100	5	28	0	5
3	10/10	100	6	24	0	4
7	12/12	100	5	28	0	7
14	10/10	100	4	31	0	4
21	9/10	90	7	33	0	6
28	10/10	100	5	29	0	5
42	8/10	80	11	35	0	7
49	10/10	100	12	39	0	10
56	12/12	100	9	41	0	10

* Animals received i.p. dilution of a standard preparation in animals equivalent to 0.01 ml per gm of body weight.

TABLE 12

EFFECT OF ROUTE OF INOCULATON ON RESPONSE OF HA/ICR SWISS MICE TO FRIEND VIRUS FILTRATE CONTAINING THE POLYCYTHEMIA VIRUS (FVP)*

Route of Inoculation	Number Mice	Positive (Percent)	Average Time of Response		Number with Polycythemia
			Palpable Spleens (Days)	Death (Days)	
Intraperitoneal	24	100	10	32.5	22
Intravenous	24	100	5	24.2	21
Intranasal	22	100	21	65.8	18
Intracerebral	24	63	48	135.3	15
Subcutaneous	24	100	11	38.0	20

* Each mouse was inoculated with 0.05 ml of a 10^{-1} dilution of standard pool. 32-day-old Ha/ICR Swiss mice of both sexes equally distributed among each group.

TABLE 13

STABILITY OF THE POLYCYTHEMIA VIRUS (FVP) IN HA/ICR SWISS MICE

Treatment	Positive/Total		Average Day of Response	
	Number	Percent	Palpable Spleens	Death
Experiment No. 1				
Untreated	20/20	100	10	39
Ether (10% overnight at 4° C)	0/12	0	—	—
Formalin (1:200)	0/20	0	—	—
Lyophilization (1 day)	12/12	100	12	37.8
4° C (39 days)	9/10	90	15	43
−70° C (6 months)	24/24	100	22	46.5
Experiment No. 2				
Untreated	12/12	100	9	32.4
28° C (120 min)	10/10	100	14.8	39.0
37° C (60 min)	18/24	75	18.6	49.3
56° C (30 min)	0/24	0	—	—

A 1:10 extract in 0.05 M K-citrate of infected spleen purified by differential centrifugation was used for the various treatments and for subsequent inoculation into mice. 30-day-old Ha/ICR Swiss mice were used as recipients. Same pool of virus was used for each experiment.

There was no significant loss of potency following incubation of FVP $10^{-1.4}$ and $10^{-2.4}$ log dilution) with antisera prepared in rabbits against the Moloney and Rauscher leukemogenic viruses (TABLE 14). The antisera prepared against FVA and FVP, however, produced similar decreases in induction of disease in mice inoculated with various dilutions of FVP. The results of this study indicate a lack of antigen similarity between FVP and the Moloney and, perhaps, Rauscher (see $10^{-1.4}$ log dilution) viruses, but a similarity between FVP and FVA. Attempts are being made to produce more potent antisera against FVP so that we can distinguish FVP from FVA.

Investigation of the levels of plasma and urine erythropoietin in FVP-infected mice at various intervals following injection was carried out. There was no detectable increase in the level of erythropoietin in either the plasma or urine (TABLE 15). This is similar to what we see in human polycythemia vera.

TABLE 14

IMMUNOLOGICAL RELATIONSHIP TO OTHER MURINE LEUKEMIC VIRUS

Polycythemia Virus (FVP) Mixed with:*	Log Dilution of Virus (Percent Positive) −1.4	−2.4	(Average Day to Palpation) −1.4	−2.4	(Average Day to Death) −1.4	−2.4
Saline	100	100	11	18	34	46.8
FVA antiserum (anemic response)	32.1	20.8	23.5	37.8	68	96.5
FVP antiserum (polycythemic response)	25.8	12.5	30.2	54.8	74.3	105.8
Moloney virus antiserum	100	100	12.8	21.4	39.8	52.3
Rauscher virus antiserum	84.5	46.8	17.5	32.1	45.8	65.3

The data tabulated 358 days postinoculation.

* Equal parts of saline or rabbit antiserum diluted 1:12 were mixed with the dilution of viruses indicated. Mixtures allowed to stand at room temperature for 120 minutes and then inoculated i.p. into groups of 24 30-day-old Ha/ICR Swiss mice.

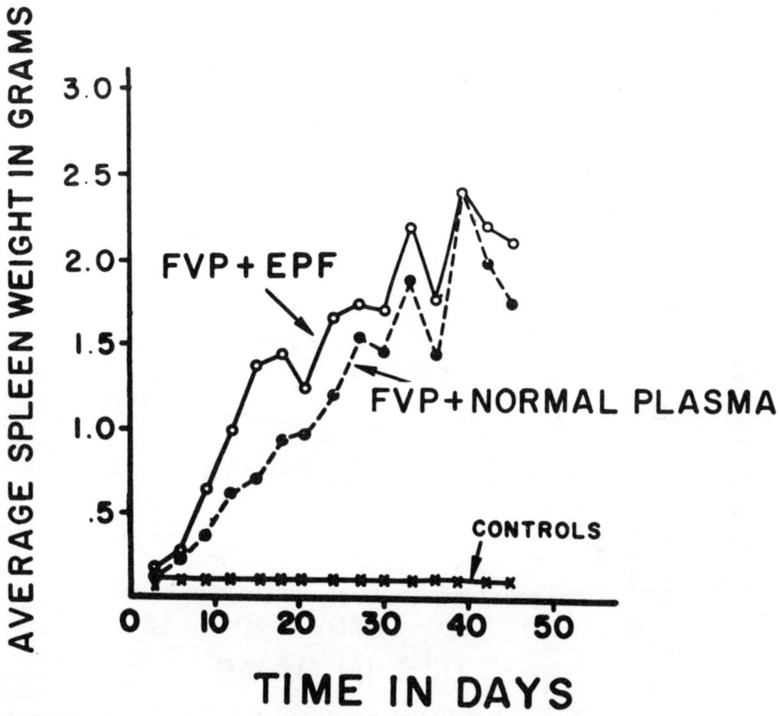

FIGURE 1. Effect of FVP (Friend virus with polycythemic response) and erythropoietin on spleen weight of Ha/ICR Swiss mice. Controls received erythropoietin alone.

Since we know that this virus induces a marked erythropoietic response, the influence of exogenous erythropoietin on the pattern of the disease was studied. Erythropoietin was injected i.p. for three days prior to the injection of the polycythemia virus and daily thereafter for 48 days. Infected mice given erythropoietin developed splenomegaly earlier than untreated infected mice (FIGURE 1). Also, the polycythemic response developed much sooner as indicated by the high hematocrit levels which occurred as early as ten days after infection compared with 20 days in controls (FIGURE 2).

An interesting fact about the murine viral polycythemia is that it is spleen-dependent. There is a direct relationship between the increase in spleen weight and increase in hematocrit (FIGURE 3). However, the RBC and hematocrit levels are not elevated in splenectomized infected mice (FIGURES 4 & 5) and the administration of erythropoietin to infected splenectomized mice does not induce polycythemia.

It is hoped that this murine virus-induced polycythemia, which may have similarities to polycythemia vera in the human, will provide a model system in which to study factors responsible for the abnormal proliferation of red blood cells. It is interesting that the polycythemia virus is capable of initiating erythropoiesis in a hypertransfused-polycythemic state in the same way that exogenous erythropoietin does. Studies are in progress to determine whether this virus initiates erythropoiesis by stimulating erythropoietin-producing cells to produce erythropoietin or whether it stimulates erythropoiesis directly.

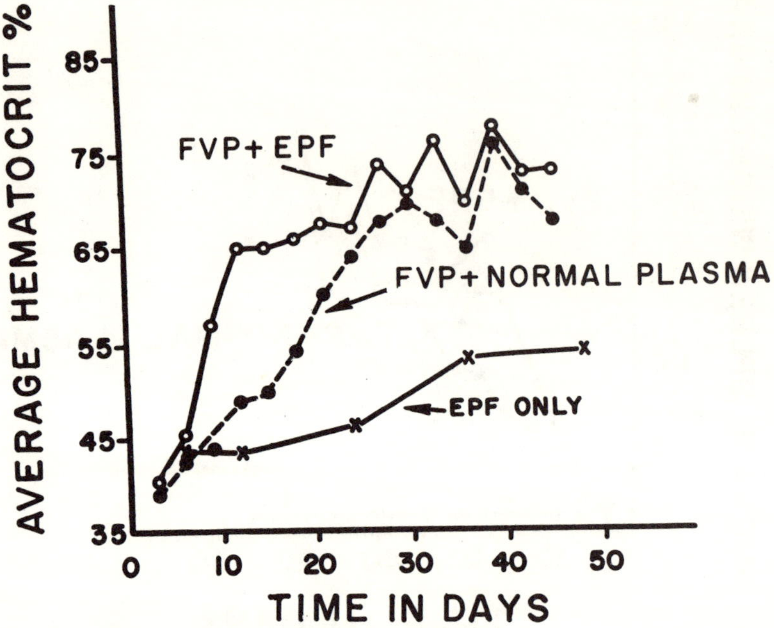

FIGURE 2. Effect of FVP (Friend virus with polycythemic response) and erythropoietin on hematocrit values in Ha/ICR Swiss mice.

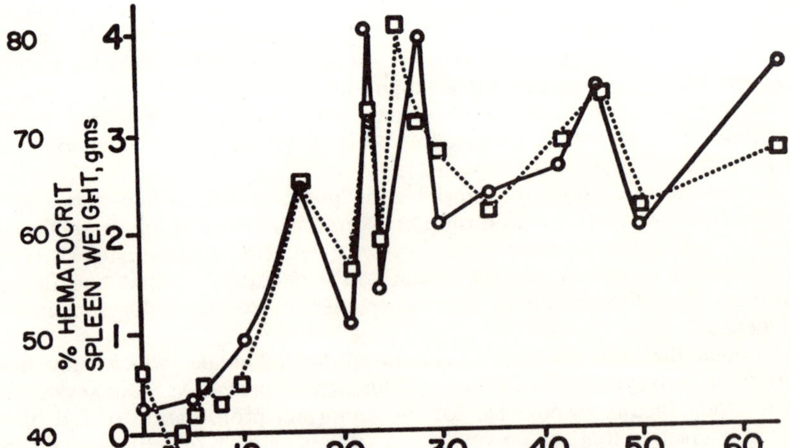

FIGURE 3. Increase in spleen weight (dotted circle), and hematocrit values (square) in Swiss mice at intervals (days) following inoculation with FVP (Friend virus with polycythemic response, 10^{-1}).

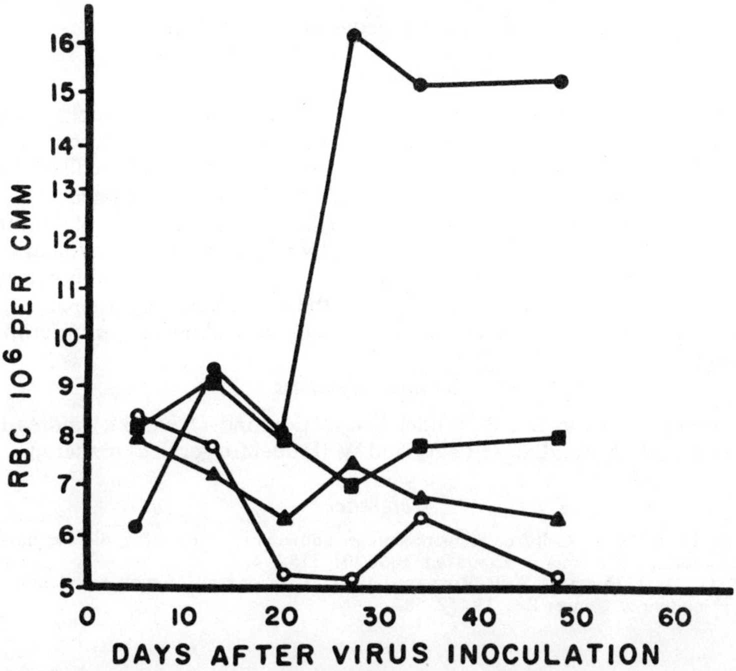

FIGURE 4. Effect of splenectomy on development of polycythemia in FVP (Friend virus with polycythemic response, 10^{-1}) infected Swiss mice. Solid circle = virus-infected non-splenectomized mice; solid square = uninfected splenectomized; solid triangle = virus-infected mice splenectomized three days prior to virus inoculation; circle = virus-infected mice splenectomized four days after virus inoculation.

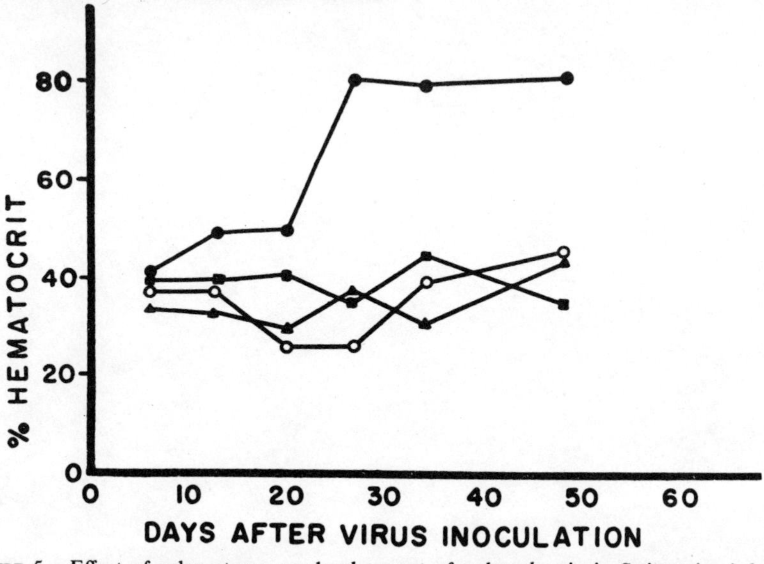

FIGURE 5. Effect of splenectomy on development of polycythemia in Swiss mice infected with FVP (Friend virus with polycythemic response, 10^{-1}). Solid circle = virus infected non-splenectomized mice; solid square = uninfected splenectomized mice; solid triangle = virus-infected mice splenectomized three days prior to virus inoculation; circle = virus-infected mice splenectomized four days after virus inoculation.

Summary

A murine viral polycythemia is reported. The polycythemia-inducing virus discussed herein appears to be a passenger virus and distinctly different from the leukemia virus originally published by Dr. Friend. It must be recalled that Dr. Friend never observed a polycythemia with the virus she isolated. The polycythemic-inducing virus, unlike other murine viruses capable of stimulating erythropoiesis, can initiate erythropoiesis in hypertransfused-polycythemic mice. Administration of exogenous erythropoietin will accelerate the usual polycythemic response one observes in mice infected with the virus. This might be an excellent experimental animal system in which to study the abnormal proliferation of hemopoietic cells.

Acknowledgments

We extend thanks to Dr. P. Trudel and to Edmund Dywinski, Andres Bulba, Joyce Jividen, A. Mirand, C. O'Leary and W. Trudel for services rendered.

References

1. FRIEND, C. J. 1957. Cell-free transmission in adult Swiss mice of a disease having the character of a leukemia. J. Exp. Med. **105:** 307–318.
2. METCALF, D., J. FURTH & R. F. BUFFETT. 1959. Pathogenesis of mouse leukemia caused by Friend virus. Cancer Res. **19:** 52–58.

PART IX. CLINICAL AND PATHOLOGICAL CONDITIONS RELATED TO ERYTHROPOIETIN PRODUCTION

ERYTHROPOIETIN PRODUCTION IN FETAL HYPOXIA AND IN ANEMIC UREMIC PATIENTS

Per Haavardsholm Finne
Pediatric Research Institute, University Hospital, Oslo, Norway

Since the introduction of premature delivery in the treatment of erythroblastosis and intrauterine transfusions in selected cases, the need for methods to evaluate the condition of the fetus has increased. Previous investigations have shown that erythropoietin is transferred from the fetus to the amniotic fluid (Halvorsen & Finne, 1963; Finne, 1964). In the present work an attempt has been made to correlate the degree of anemia (hypoxia) to the erythropoietin levels in cord blood and amniotic fluid.

Cord blood was collected immediately after delivery and amniotic fluid was collected by transabdominal amniocentesis before term or by rupturing the membranes during delivery. The erythropoietin content was determined using transfusion-induced polycythemic mice as recipients and the ^{59}Fe incorporation into red cells as parameter. One ml amniotic fluid and one half ml plasma was injected s.c. on two consecutive days.

Erythropoietin levels in cord blood from anemic erythroblastotic infants were significantly elevated and a correlation was found between capillary hemoglobin in the newborn infant and the cord blood erythropoietin content (FIGURE 1). An abrupt rise in plasma erythropoietin levels was found when the fetal hemoglobin had dropped below 11–13 g. The variations found in plasma erythropoietin levels in different infants with the same hemoglobin value may to some extent be the result of factors other than anemia which contribute to the fetal hypoxia since both anemic and hypoxic hypoxia may stimulate fetal erythropoietin production. Differences in fetal ability to compensate for tissue hypoxia by increased cardiac output may also play some role.

The erythropoietin levels in the amniotic fluid show a similar correlation with fetal anemia. In cases with capillary hemoglobin below 10–11 g, high levels of erythropoietin may be found as a sign of fetal hypoxia. However, in many cases, even with a milder degree of anemia, a slight increase in erythropoietin was found. By concentration of amniotic fluid from normal pregnancies erythropoietic activity was also found.

The erythropoietin assays in amniotic fluid do not allow an accurate prediction of the fetal hemoglobin level. Rather, they reflect the clinical condition of the fetus with regard to the tissue oxygenation. The cases demonstrated can be divided into two groups: the most important one consists of cases with markedly elevated amniotic fluid erythropoietin content, in which the tissue oxygenation is highly insufficient, due to fetal anemia. In these cases the capillary hemoglobin was 10–11 g or below. In the second group, which consists of cases with only small amounts of erythropoietin detectable in the amniotic fluid, capillary hemoglobin was above 10–11 g (FIGURE 2).

Repeated erythropoietin assays in amniotic fluid from *Rhesus* immunized pregnancies may demonstrate the increase in fetal hypoxia as pregnancy and hemolysis of fetal blood proceeds (FIGURE 3). An elevated erythropoietin level means that the fetus was suffering from a severe hypoxia and in danger. The prognosis in

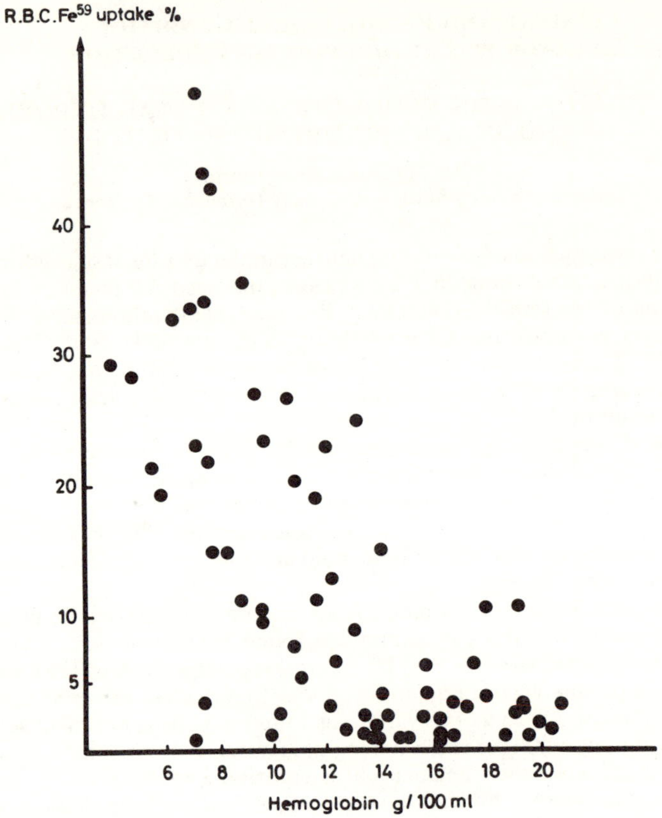

FIGURE 1. The ^{59}Fe uptake in polycythemic mice injected with plasma (0.5 ml × 2 s.c.) from erythroblastotic infants. Rise in erythropoietin levels was found when hemoglobin dropped below 11–13 g/100 ml.

such cases is dubious. The figures attached to the letters indicate the capillary hemoglobin at delivery.

The rise in erythropoietin levels in cord blood and amniotic fluid may be mainly due to the fetal anemia per se, but placental disturbances may also be a contributory factor. Edema of the placenta may be found in severe erythroblastosis and cardiac circulatory failure due to anemia may also contribute to the tissue hypoxia and thus cause an increase in fetal erythropoietin production.

The erythropoietin in amniotic fluid was transferred from fetal plasma through the urine, and a correlation between erythropoietin content in fetal plasma, urine and amniotic fluid was found (TABLE 1).

Other causes of fetal hypoxia, such as preeclampsia, postmaturity and diabetes may also increase fetal erythropoietin production, and even in such cases antenatally erythropoietin assays in amniotic fluid may reveal fetal hypoxia. As demonstrated in FIGURE 4, erythropoietin levels in normal newborn infants were higher than in premature infants, suggesting less available oxygen for the fetus at term than at an earlier stage of gestation (statistical significant difference $p<0.001$). In postmature infants with gestational age beyond 42 weeks cases

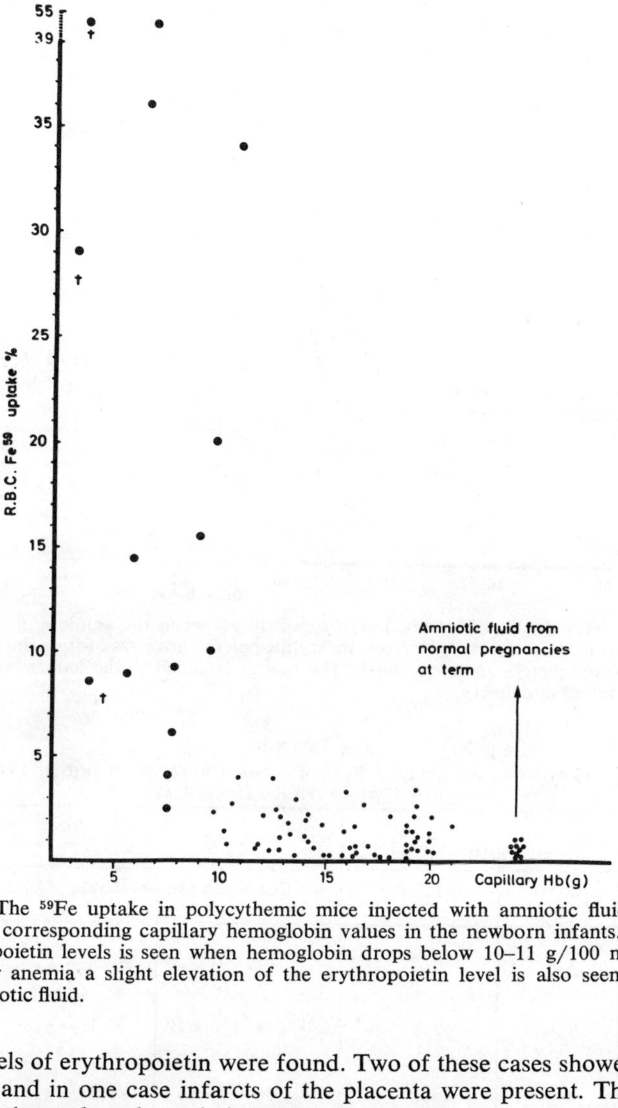

FIGURE 2. The ^{59}Fe uptake in polycythemic mice injected with amniotic fluid (1 ml × 2 s.c.) and the corresponding capillary hemoglobin values in the newborn infants. An abrupt rise in erythropoietin levels is seen when hemoglobin drops below 10–11 g/100 ml. In many cases of milder anemia a slight elevation of the erythropoietin level is also seen, compared to normal amniotic fluid.

with high levels of erythropoietin were found. Two of these cases showed signs of dysmaturity, and in one case infarcts of the placenta were present. The greatest frequency of elevated erythropoietin levels were found in the preeclamptic group, indicating the high risk of intrauterine hypoxia, especially when the mothers suffered severe preeclampsia. In this group the incidence of dysmaturity and placental infarctions was high. Also, in amniotic fluid, increased erythropoietin levels could be demonstrated. The high erythropoietin levels in this group confirms the work of other investigators, who found reduced oxygen saturation in cord blood and elevated hemoglobin and red cell values (Walker & Turnbull, 1953). Although placental infarctions were present in many cases in this group, there were cases without gross placental changes in which increased erythropoietin levels could also be demonstrated. In two infants of diabetic mothers erythropoietin levels in amniotic fluid were increased. These infants died in utero.

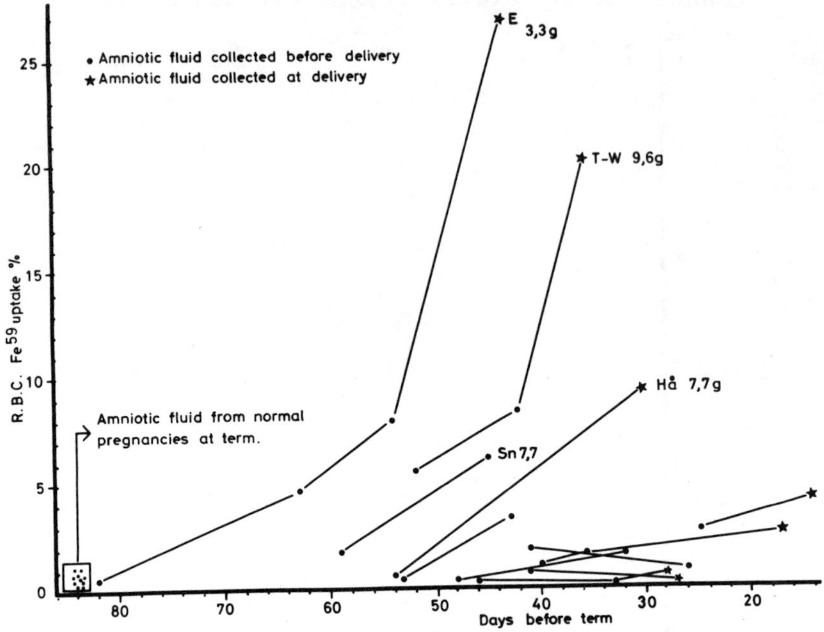

FIGURE 3. The results of repeated erythropoietin assays in the amniotic fluid in some Rh-immunized women. A marked increase in erythropoietin level was found in cases in which the fetuses were severely anemic at birth. The figures attached to the letters indicate capillary hemoglobin values at delivery.

TABLE 1

ERYTHROPOIETIN LEVELS IN FETAL PLASMA, URINE AND AMNIOTIC FLUID IN SOME CASES WITH RH-IMMUNIZATION*

NAMF	Hemoglobin g/loo ml		Fe^{59} uptake o/o (± s.e.)		
	Cord	Capillary	Cord plasma	Amniotic fluid	Urine
Ha	3.5	5.8	19.3 ± 2.9 (5)	14.1 ± 2.4 (5)	22.8 ± 2.9 (2)
Bæ	4.4	7.5	3.5 ± o.2 (5)	4.1 ± o.6 (3)	2.6 ± o.4 (7)
Pe	-	1o.7	26.8 ± 3.3 (6)	34.2 ± 3.8 (5)	26.0 (1)
My	8.3	12.1	3.3 ± o.3 (3)	1.2 ± o.1 (4)	1.o ± o.1 (3)
Vi	12.1	14.1	4.4 ± o.6 (2)	1.o ± o.1 (5)	1.6 ± o.1 (5)

Number of mice in parentheses

* A correlation is found between levels in plasma, urine and amniotic fluid, which makes it likely that erythropoietin in the amniotic fluid is derived from the urine.

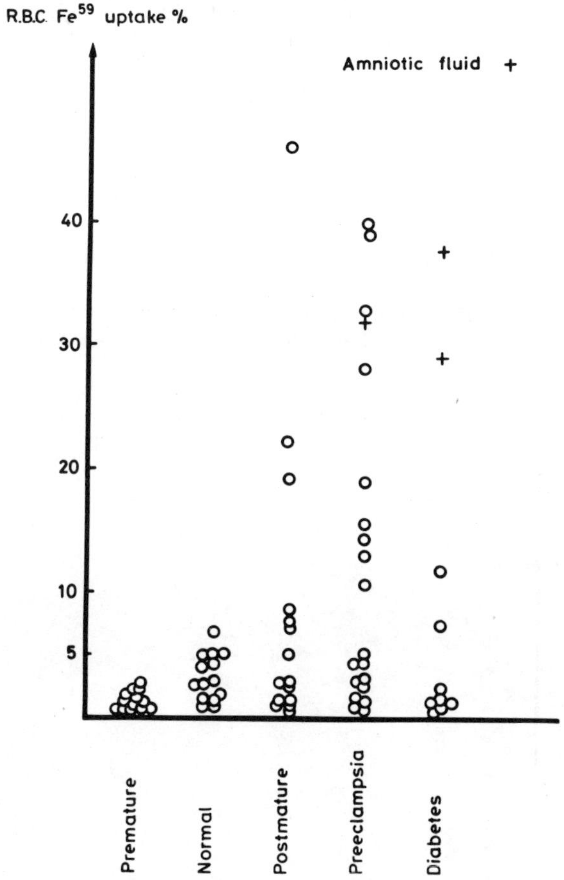

FIGURE 4. The ^{59}Fe uptake in polycythemic mice injected with plasma (0.5 ml × 2 s.c.) from normal, premature and postmature infants and infants born of diabetic and preeclamptic mothers. In several cases markedly elevated erythropoietin levels were found, indicating fetal hypoxia.

The presented findings indicate that the fetus, at least from the 32nd week of gestation, reacts to hypoxia with increased erythropoietin production, that erythropoietin also plays a role in red cell production during intrauterine life and that erythropoietin levels in cord blood and amniotic fluid may serve as an indicator of fetal hypoxia. In anemic erythroblastotic infants extramedullary erythropoiesis is greatly increased. This finding, together with the raised erythropoietin levels in these cases, indicates that erythropoietin also stimulates fetal extramedullary red cell production.

The previous findings of easily demonstrable amounts of erythropoietin in urine from healthy male adults (Finne, 1965) suggest a method to evaluate erythropoietin production in cases with presumably low production. Twenty-four-hour urine was collected from normal male adults, from uremic anemic patients and from three patients suffering from aplastic anemia. The urine samples were dialyzed against distilled water for 48 hr at 4° C, and then freeze-dried. The yield from each urine sample was dissolved in 10 ml saline and injected s.c. into polycythemic mice in doses of 1 ml on two consecutive days. All the normal adults investigated had hemoglobin values above 13.9 g. In the uremic patients the hemoglobin values varied between 6.5 and 9 g. Blood urea concentration was above 100 mg/100 ml in all of these patients. The aplastic anemic patients had hemoglobin levels between 4 and 7 g.

The results of the assays are shown in FIGURE 5. Erythropoietic activity was demonstrated in the urine from all the normal adults, but great variations were found in the amounts of erythropoietin excreted. The demonstration of erythropoietin in urine from normal persons indicates that erythropoietin acts during physiological conditions, and not just in emergency situations. The data also seem to indicate either that there is no renal threshold for erythropoietin excretion, or that this threshold is so low that erythropoietin is also excreted under normal conditions.

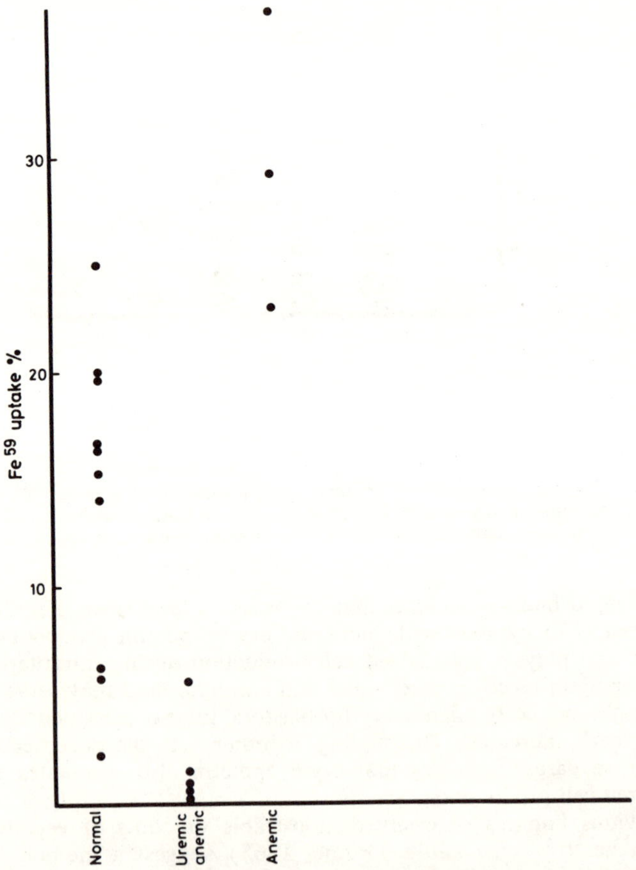

FIGURE 5. The ^{59}Fe uptake in polycythemic mice injected with urine concentrate from normal adults, anemic uremic patients and patients with aplastic anemia. The 24-hour urine sample was concentrated by freeze-drying; the yield was dissolved in 10 ml saline. One ml was then injected s.c. into polycythemic mice on two consecutive days. Slight or no erythropoietic activity was found in urine from anemic uremic patients.

In the anemic uremic group only slight or no erythropoietic activity was demonstrable in the urine. The small amounts of erythropoietin found in urine from these patients, combined with the anemia, suggest that deprivation of erythropoietin production because of renal damage is concerned with the development of the anemia, although reduced erythropoietin production may not be the only factor.

In the patients with aplastic anemia great erythropoietin excretion was found, indicating raised erythropoietin production as a response to the anemia. As long as the only way of assaying erythropoietin is by its biological activity and not by chemical quantitation, the easy method of concentration by dialysis and freeze-drying is most suitable for the purpose of quantitating urinary erythropoietin excretion. Further, it is suggested that studying the 24-hour urinary excretion of erythropoietin may be a better way of estimating the erythropoietin production than by merely assaying the plasma erythropoietin level.

References

FINNE, P. H. 1965. Erythropoietin in concentrates of urine from healthy persons. Brit. Med. J. **1**: 697–699.

FINNE, P. H. 1964. Erythropoietin levels in the amniotic fluid, particularly in Rh-immunized pregnancies. Acta Pediat. Scand. **53**: 269–281.

HALVORSEN, S. & P. H. FINNE. 1963. Transfer of erythropoietin to amniotic fluid in Rh-immunized pregnant women. Brit. Med. J. **1**: 1132–1134.

WALKER, J. & P. N. TURNBULL. 1953. Hemoglobin and red cells in the human foetus and their relation to the oxygen content of the blood in the vessels of the umbilical cord. Lancet **2**: 312–318.

HUMAN ERYTHROPOIESIS FOLLOWING KIDNEY TRANSPLANTATION

George C. Hoffman

Department of Clinical Pathology, Cleveland Clinic Foundation, Cleveland, Ohio

The clinical evidence for a relationship between the kidney and erythropoiesis has come mainly from two sources: studies of the anemia of renal disease, and the occasional association between erythrocytosis and various renal lesions. More recently, the inability of anephric man to elaborate normal amounts of erythropoietin[1] and the restoration of this function following successful renal transplantation has been demonstrated.[2,3] These findings add support to the thesis that the kidney plays an important role in the production or activation of erythropoietin. The hematologic changes that occurred in a group of patients who underwent renal transplantation form the basis for this report.

One hundred and five patients received 120 renal transplants at the Cleveland Clinic before February, 1966. All of these patients had reached the terminal stage of irreversible renal disease and required repeated hemodialysis to maintain life. Bilateral nephrectomy was performed in 103 patients and they remained anephric for a few days or weeks before receiving a transplant. Splenectomy was performed in 73 of these patients. Azothioprine* and prednisone† were given as immunosuppressant drugs to all patients; actinomycin C‡ and local irradiation to the graft were also used in some cases.

During the chronic nephritic and anephric stages, erythropoiesis was inadequate and all patients required weekly transfusions of one or two units of blood in order to maintain a blood hemoglobin content above 6 g/100 ml. A plasma erythropoietin assay was negative in the five patients tested. However, there is evidence that erythropoiesis had not entirely ceased. Reticulocytes could always be observed in the peripheral blood although their number was rarely above 2 percent. Erythroid precursors were present, but in reduced numbers, in the bone marrow of three anephric patients in whom it was studied. The iron (^{59}Fe) turnover and its incorporation into red blood cells were reduced to approximately 40 percent of normal in two anephric patients.

Erythropoiesis was not significantly stimulated by hemodialysis during either the chronic nephritic stage or the anephric stage. However, some improvement following dialysis in a group of uremic patients had been reported by Kurtides *et al.*[4]

Erythropoiesis improved in over 80 percent of patients after successful renal transplantation. One result of this improvement was an increase in blood hemoglobin content (FIGURE 1). However, more striking than this increase, which is not significant in all instances, is the fact that blood transfusions were seldom required to maintain the hemoglobin level. Of the four patients whose blood hemoglobin content decreased after renal transplantation, two subsequently improved and their hemoglobin level rose above 13 g/100 ml. Almost continuous hemorrhage from the gastrointestinal tract occurred in the third patient; the

* Imuran®, supplied through the courtesy of Burroughs Wellcome & Co. (U.S.A.) Inc., Tuckahoe, N. Y.

† Meticorten®, supplied through the courtesy of Schering Corporation, Bloomfield, N. J.

‡ Sanamycin®, supplied through the courtesy of FBA Pharmaceutical, Inc., New York, N. Y.

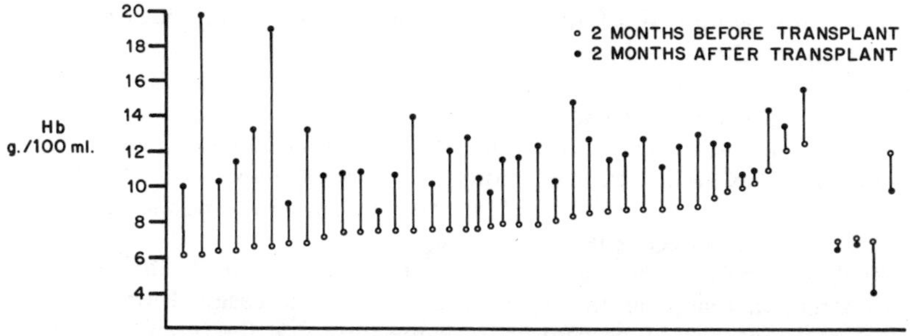

FIGURE 1. The change in blood hemoglobin content following renal transplantation in 43 patients in whom the grafted kidney functioned for at least two months.

fourth patient had oxaluria and the grafted kidney was rapidly damaged by oxalate deposition. The results of serial erythropoietin assays such as those performed by Denny *et al.*[3] indicate that the transplanted kidney is able to play its part in the production of this hormone. We found a high plasma erythropoietin level in one patient seven weeks after renal transplantation when he suffered a severe hemorrhage.[2] This finding shows that a patient with a transplanted kidney is able to respond to the stimulus of hemorrhage.

The improvement in erythropoiesis that occurred following successful renal transplantation was not related to the presence or absence of the spleen. No significant difference was observed between the response in patients receiving a graft from a living donor and that seen in patients receiving a cadaver kidney except that the increase in hemoglobin was delayed in the latter group. This delay may be related to the transient acute tubular necrosis that occurs in approximately 75 percent of transplanted cadaver kidneys. Although no striking reticulocytosis was noted immediately following transplantation, an increased reticulocyte count, occasionally as high as 10 percent, was usually found sometime during the first

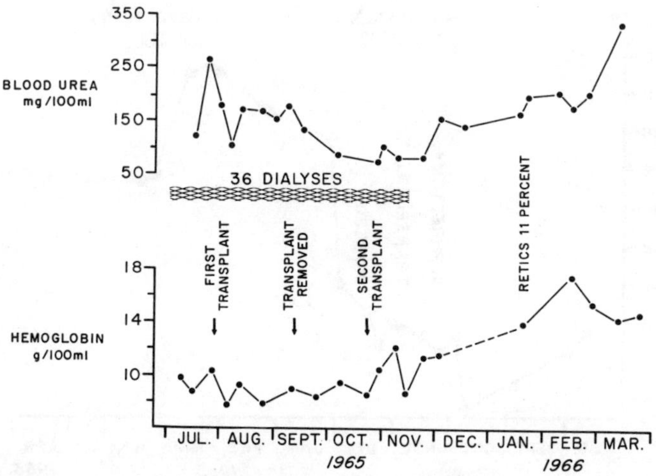

FIGURE 2. An outline of the progress of a patient who had a satisfactory hematologic response following a second renal transplant despite an increased blood urea content.

few months following operation. This contrasts with the reticulocytopenia found in the chronic nephritic and anephric stages.

In general, all transplanted kidneys that functioned normally as excretory organs were associated with a normal blood hemoglobin content. Conversely, when the transplanted kidney exhibited poor excretory function, some degree of anemia usually developed. Judging from these two extremes, there appears to be a correlation between excretory function and erythropoietic function in the transplanted kidney. However, there is a group of patients in which a dissociation between these functions can be seen. In one patient (FIGURE 2) the blood hemoglobin content increased as the blood urea content increased. Furthermore, the reticulocyte count was 11 percent at the same time that the blood urea was 170 mg/100 ml.

On rare occasions, the blood hemoglobin content may increase above the normal limits after renal transplantation (FIGURES 3 & 4). The first patient (FIGURE 4) received a cadaver kidney, but his spleen was not removed. Diuresis occurred three weeks after transplantation and was followed by a rapid rise in blood hemoglobin content to 22 g/100 ml. At this time, the white blood cell count and the platelet count were normal and the arterial oxygen saturation was 96.5 percent. The finding of a total blood volume of 105 ml/kg with a red cell mass of 59 ml/kg indicates that this was an absolute and not a relative erythrocytosis. When the blood hemoglobin content was at its greatest, renal excretory function was somewhat impaired as shown by a creatinine clearance of 29 ml/minute. It seems likely that this impairment was associated with an increase in blood viscosity because the creatinine clearance increased to 60/ml min after five venisections had reduced the blood hemoglobin content to 16 g/100 ml. This patient's hemoglobin has remained normal and the transplanted kidney has functioned well for more than 18 months. A plasma erythropoietin assay performed when the blood hemoglobin content was at its maximum resulted in a 1 percent ^{59}Fe uptake and a 0.7 percent reticulocyte count in the hypertransfused mouse. These figures are higher than those obtained with normal plasma but the result

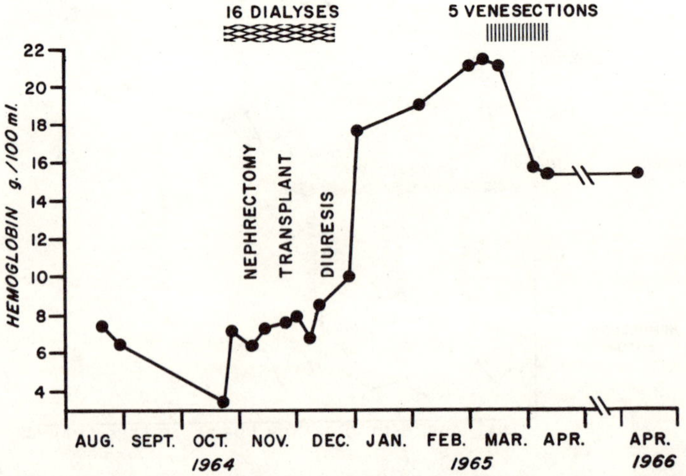

FIGURE 3. An outline of the progress of a patient in whom erythrocytosis developed following renal transplantation.

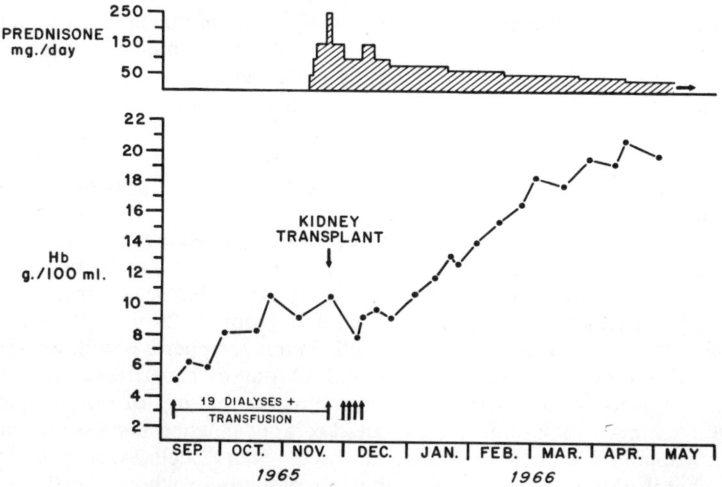

FIGURE 4. An outline of the progress of a second patient in whom erythrocytosis developed following renal transplantation.

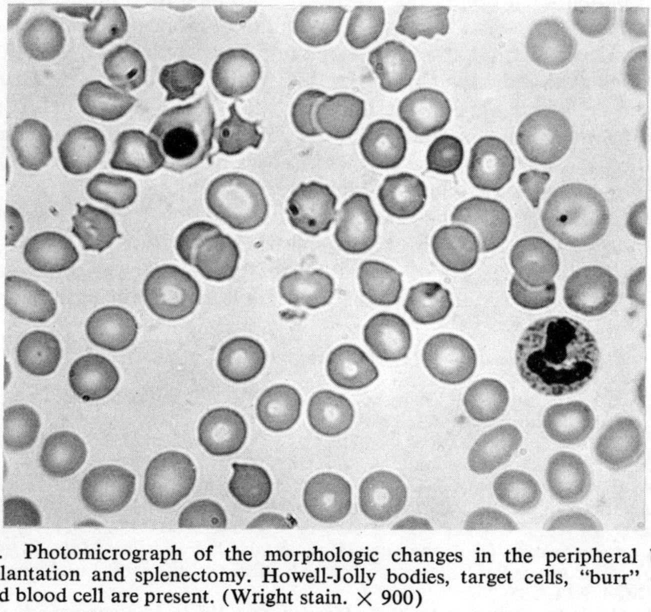

FIGURE 5. Photomicrograph of the morphologic changes in the peripheral blood after renal transplantation and splenectomy. Howell-Jolly bodies, target cells, "burr" cells and a nucleated red blood cell are present. (Wright stain. × 900)

is equivocal. Nies *et al.*[5] demonstrated erythropoietin in amounts nine times greater than normal in the urine of a similar patient. It seems likely that the development of an absolute erythrocytosis after renal transplantation is due to excessive production of erythropoietin and may be considered as another example of inappropriate erythropoietin production, the subject of a paper by Gallagher and Donati elsewhere in this Annal. In a second example of an abnormal increase in blood hemoglobin content (FIGURE 5) the rise was more gradual and at its height the total red cell mass was 42 ml/kg with a plasma volume of 37 ml/kg. These figures represent the upper and lower limits of normal, respectively. Thus, the erythrocytosis in this case was, at least in part, relative.

Several morphologic abnormalities may be found in the peripheral blood following renal transplantation; these include Howell-Jolly bodies, target cells, "burr" cells, and nucleated red blood cells (FIGURE 5). Despite the complex and variable therapeutic regimens employed in these patients, it is possible to offer an explanation for most of these changes. Howell-Jolly bodies and target cells are invariably found in the peripheral blood following splenectomy. It was hoped that the number of "burr" cells or nucleated red blood cells might be of some value in assessing graft function or in predicting rejection. However, these cells also appear to be related to splenectomy. Thus, in a group of 29 patients who underwent splenectomy, 24 had many "burr" cells in the peripheral blood, while "burr" cells were absent or very rare in the blood of a group of 15 patients whose spleens were not removed. Since "burr" cells are one of the features of microangiopathic hemolytic anemia,[6] they might be expected to appear when the vascular damage in the transplanted kidney is severe. However, "burr" cells were prominent in the peripheral blood of only two of the five patients in whom the transplanted kidney showed advanced vascular changes. A relationship to splenectomy was also found in the number of nucleated red blood cells in the peripheral blood. A group of 15 patients whose peripheral blood contained more than three nucleated red blood cells per 100 white blood cells had all undergone splenectomy. However, the spleen had been removed from only 12 out of a group of 27 patients with less than four nucleated red blood cells per 100 white blood cells. Macrocytosis of the red blood cells and hypersegmentation of the nuclei of the neutrophils were seen following renal transplantation in approximately one-third of the patients. In three patients, a megaloblastic erythroid series was found in the bone marrow. These changes appear to be related to the dose of azothioprine.

The results of renal transplantation in man provide further evidence of the important role of the kidney in erythropoiesis. Furthermore, this erythropoietic function can be transplanted, is operative in the denervated organ, and is unrelated to the excretory function of the kidney, at least in some cases.

References

1. NATHAN, D. G., E. SCHUPAK, F. STOHLMANN, JR. & J. P. MERRILL. 1964. Erythropoiesis in anephric man. J. Clin. Invest. **43:** 2158–2165.
2. MCMAIN, P. B., G. C. HOFFMAN, S. NAKAMOTO & W. J. KOLFF. 1965. Erythropoiesis and renal hemotransplantation. Canad. M. A. J. **93:** 241–244.
3. DENNY, W. F., W. J. FLANIGAN & C. F. ZUROSKI, III. 1966. Serial erythropoietin studies in patients undergoing renal hemotransplantation. J. Lab. Clin. Med. **67:** 386–397.
4. KURTIDES, E. S., W. A. RAMBACH, H. L. ALT & F. DEL GRECO. 1964. The effect of hemodialysis on erythrokinetics in the anemia of uremia. J. Lab. Clin. Med. **63:** 469–479.
5. NIES, B. A., R. COHN & S. L. SCHRIER. 1965. Erythremia after renal transplantation. New Eng. J. Med. **273:** 785–788.
6. BRAIN, M. C., J. V. DACIE & D. O'B. HOURIHANE. 1962. Microangiopathic haemolytic anaemia: The possible role of vascular lesions in pathogenesis. Brit. J. Haemat. **8:** 358–374.

THE ERYTHROPOIESIS-STIMULATING FACTORS PRODUCED BY TUMORS

Thomas A. Waldmann, Wendell F. Rosse
and Richard L. Swarm

Metabolism Branch, National Cancer Institute, National Institutes of Health, Bethesda, Md., and the Department of Pathology, University of Cincinnati College of Medicine, Cincinnati, Ohio

Erythrocytosis has been noted in man in association with various tumors and cysts including renal tumors,[1–8] renal cysts,[4,9,10] cerebellar hemangioblastomas.[7,11–15] hepatomas,[7,16–19] uterine fibromas,[5,20,21] pheochromocytomas,[22,23] and virilizing tumors of the ovary and adrenal.[23,24] Patients with this association have an elevated total red cell mass and usually have a normal white blood cell count, platelet count and arterial oxygen saturation. In the majority of these patients, resection of the tumor results in a remission of the erythrocytosis. In certain cases extracts of the tumor or cysts have been shown to contain erythropoiesis-stimulating activity.[4–8,14,15,19,22,25] Thus, the association of erythrocytosis and tumors appears to be secondary to the production of an erythropoiesis-stimulating factor by the tumors.

The Assay of Cyst Fluid, Tumor Tissue or Serum from Patients with Polycythemia for Erythropoiesis-Stimulating Activity

In the present study serum, cyst fluid or a saline extract of tumor from 44 patients with polycythemia and associated tumors was assayed for erythropoietin using the transfused polycythemic mouse assay system.[26] Female NIH strain mice weighing 18–22 g were injected i.p. on the first and second days of the assay with 0.7 ml of an 80 percent suspension of homologous red blood cells. On the fifth day an additional 0.5 ml of this suspension was given. On the fifth and sixth days 0.5 ml of serum or the saline extract of 0.5 g of tumor was injected s.c. into each of six to eight mice. Saline was injected into eight mice as a negative control. On the seventh day, 0.5 μc of ^{59}Fe citrate were injected i.p. On the ninth day the mice were bled by decapitation into tared bottles which were then re-weighed. The radioactivity due to ^{59}Fe was determined in a well-type gamma ray spectrometer. The percent incorporation of isotope into 1 ml of peripheral blood was determined by comparison with an appropriate standard. The results of the assays of cyst fluids and tumor tissue extracts are shown in FIGURE 1. Fluid from 11 out of 14 renal cysts and two out of two cystic cerebellar hemangioblastomas from patients with associated polycythemia had significantly elevated erythropoiesis-stimulating activity. Similarly, the saline extract of one out of three hypernephromes, one out of two pheochromocytomas and one out of two hepatomas had erythropoiesis-stimulating activity. Erythropoietin was demonstrated in only 27 percent of 26 sera from patients with renal tumors, renal cysts, cerebellar hemangioblastomas, pheochromocytomas or hepatomas and associated erythrocytosis.

Physical and Chemical Properties of Erythropoiesis-Stimulating Factors Produced by Tumors

Erythropoietin assays, as presently performed, detect erythropoiesis-stimulating activity but are not specific for any one substance. We have therefore per-

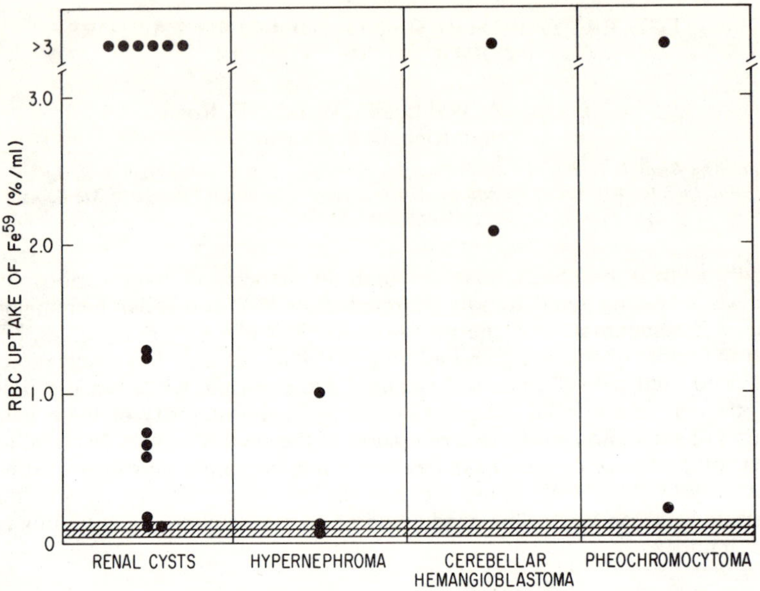

FIGURE 1. The assay of cyst fluid or tumor tissue from patients with polycythemia for erythropoiesis-stimulating activity. The mean value ± one standard deviation for saline-injected controls is shown by the cross-hatched area.

formed a number of studies to determine the chemical relationship of the erythropoiesis-stimulating factor formed in response to anemia and anoxia to that found in renal cysts and cerebellar hemangioblastoma cyst fluid.[27] The four materials containing erythropoiesis-stimulating activity studied were: (1) anemic serum: serum from a patient with aplastic anemia; (2) anoxic serum: serum from a patient with erythrocytosis secondary to transposition of the great vessels and anoxia; (3) renal cyst fluid obtained from a single unilocular renal cyst from a patient with mild polycythemia; and (4) cerebellar hemangioblastoma cyst fluid aspirated from a cerebellar cyst in a patient who had polycythemia. Each of the erythropoietically active materials was incubated with twice crystallized trypsin of bovine pancreatic origin. Controls for each incubation were treated identically except that saline instead of trypsin was added to the mixture. In each case erythropoiesis-stimulating activity, as estimated by subsequent bioassay, was completely destroyed by incubation with trypsin, whereas the control preparations were not affected (TABLE 1).

In order to determine whether removal of sialic acid inactivated the erythropoiesis-stimulating activity, each of the materials was incubated with sialidase of clostridial origin free of nonspecific proteolytic activity. The reaction was carried out according to the method described by Blumberg and Warren.[28] Incubation with sialidase destroyed all biological activity in each of the erythropoiesis-stimulating preparations (TABLE 1). Thus, the four erythropoiesis-stimulating factors are similar in their requirement of intact protein structure and sialic acid for biologic activity. The electrophoretic mobility of the active materials was studied with preparative zonal electrophoresis with a dilute barbital buffer at pH 8.6. Geon® (polyvinyl chloride particles) and Pevicon® (polyvinyl chloride,

TABLE 1
A COMPARISON OF SOME CHEMICAL PROPERTIES OF ERYTHROPOIESIS-STIMULATING FACTORS FROM DIFFERENT SOURCES

	Percent Incorporation ^{59}Fe in 1 ml of Blood of Transfused Mouse			
Source of Erythropoietin	Without Enzyme	With Trypsin	With Sialidase	With Antibody to Erythropoietin
Anemic serum	5.62	0.11	0.16	0.13
Anoxic serum	2.05	0.08	0.08	0.07
Cerebellar hemangioblastoma cyst fluid	7.46	0.06	0.19	0.09
Renal cyst fluid	1.55	0.07	0.07	0.03
Saline control	0.10			

polyvinyl acetate copolymer particles) in equal amounts were used as a supporting medium. The samples were applied in a narrow groove cut in the matrix. A current of 50 mamp was applied for 18 hours. The Geon Pevicon blocks were then divided into 1 to 4 cm segments, cut perpendicularly to the direction of the electromotive force. The protein was eluted with normal saline and the eluates were tested for erythropoiesis-stimulating activity. Erythropoiesis-stimulating activity of each of the materials migrated as an α_2-globulin.

The molecular weight of each of the preparations was studied by the radiation inactivation technique of Lea.[29] Using this technique the molecular weight of the active site of molecules can be determined from the curve of decline of biologic activity following exposure to graded doses of high energy electrons. It was shown that the erythropoiesis-stimulating factors present in renal cyst fluid, cerebellar hemangioblastoma cyst fluid and anemic serum were comparable in size with a molecular weight of the active site of from 27,000 to 37,000. Thus, these studies suggest that the biologically active material in each of the preparations was a mucoprotein of α_2 mobility with a molecular weight of approximately 30,000.

An antibody prepared in rabbits to a partially purified human urinary erythropoietin prepared by a modification of the method of Schooley and Garcia[30] was incubated in vitro with each of the active preparations. In each case the erythropoiesis-stimulating activity, as determined by subsequent bioassay, was completely neutralized following incubation in vitro with the antibody to erythropoietin (TABLE 1). A comparable incubation with normal rabbit serum or with serum of rabbits that had been immunized with normal human urine did not affect the biological activity of these preparations. Thus, it appears likely that the polycythemia associated with renal and cerebellar lesions is secondary to the production of erythropoietin by the tumors.

Studies on the Polycythemia Associated with Adrenal Cortical Carcinomas

Although in the majority of cases tumors associated with polycythemia produce an erythropoietin-like substance, the adrenal cortical and ovarian tumors associated with polycythemia may produce nonerythropoietin factors that stimulate erythropoiesis. In our studies, saline extracts of two adrenal cortical tumors

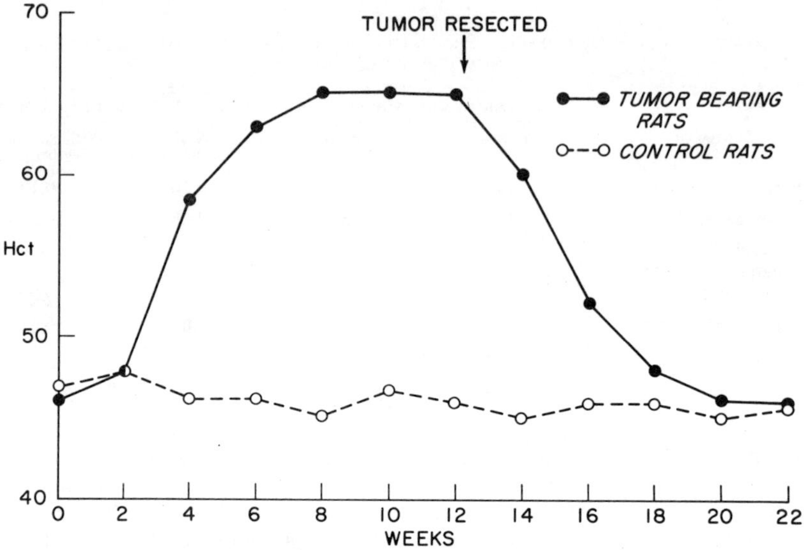

FIGURE 2. The hematocrit of Osborn Mendal rats transplanted with adrenal cortical tumor No. 494 of Snell and Stewart.

from patients with erythrocytosis and the sera from three such patients were negative when assayed for erythropoietin. In order to study the pathogenesis of polycythemia associated with such endocrine tumors, the erythropoiesis associated with adrenal cortical tumors of rats was examined. Osborn Mendel rats bearing i.m. or s.c. transplants of the adrenal cortical tumor no. 494 of Snell and Stewart[31] were shown to have marked erythrocytosis.[32] The hematocrit of the rats rose rapidly following transplantation of the tumor (FIGURE 2). The hematocrit of 25 animals (97 determination) with tumors greater than 10 × 10 × 10 mm, but less than 50 × 30 × 40 mm in size ranged from 53.8 to 82, with a mean of 62.7. Control animals studied stimultaneously had a hematocrit of 47±3.

The blood volume of groups of 10 tumor-bearing and control animals was estimated with ^{51}Cr-labeled isologous red blood cells. The total red cell volume was increased approximately 100 percent in both male and female tumor-bearing animals while the plasma volumes were comparable to those of controls (TABLE 2). Thus, the elevated hematocrit of tumor-bearing animals reflected a true increase in the total red cell volume and was not due to a decreased plasma volume.

TABLE 2

RED CELL VOLUME OF RATS WITH VIRILIZING ADRENAL CORTICAL TUMORS

	Red Cell Volume cc/kg*	Plasma Volume cc/kg
Female controls	24±1	31±4
Females with tumors	46±12	31±7
Male controls	25±1	29±2
Males with tumors	54±13	29±6

* Mean ± 1 standard deviation.

Transfusion of normal animals with red blood cells inhibits endogenous erythropoietin production and consequently inhibits red cell synthesis. Isologous red blood cells were transfused into tumor-bearing rats to determine if the erythropoiesis of such animals was still under physiological control. Groups of six control animals and animals bearing small adrenal cortical tumors with minimal hematocrit elevations were infused i.p. with packed red cells (hematocrit 80) equivalent to 5 percent of their body weight in divided doses over a two-day period. Five days after the initial transfusion 0.5 μc of ^{59}Fe citrate were injected i.p. into the transfused animals and into six nontransfused control animals and six nontransfused tumor-bearing animals. The uptake of ^{59}Fe into the peripheral red cells 16 hr following the injection of the radioiron was determined. The blood volume of each of the animals was determined before sacrifice, using isologous ^{51}Chromium-labeled red cells. The rate of iron incorporation into circulating red cells of control animals was markedly inhibited to 18 percent of preinfusion levels by the red cell infusions (FIGURE 3), while the erythropoiesis of tumor-bearing animals was not significantly affected by these transfusions. Thus, the erythropoiesis of animals with even small tumors was not responsive to this normal physiological-controlling mechanism.

Following resection of the tumors there was a rapid decline in the hematocrit (FIGURE 2), with a return to normal red cell volume by eight weeks following the procedure. None of the animals had a recurrence of the tumor and the normal hematocrit values were maintained for the length of the observation period, which lasted two to six months. Since no red cells were produced by the tumors, these studies suggested that the tumor was producing an erythropoiesis-stimulating factor. Saline extracts of tumor homogenates and sera from tumor-bearing animals were, however, negative when assayed for erythropoietin. Thus, the tumor probably acts by producing nonerythropoietin erythropoiesis-stimulating factors.

Polycythemia of the magnitude observed in the rats with adrenal cortical tumors could not be produced by the injection of 100 mg of testosterone enanthate per rat twice a week for six weeks, or by the injection of 100 mg of testosterone enanthate bi-weekly, and 20 units of ACTH daily to rats for six weeks. Following

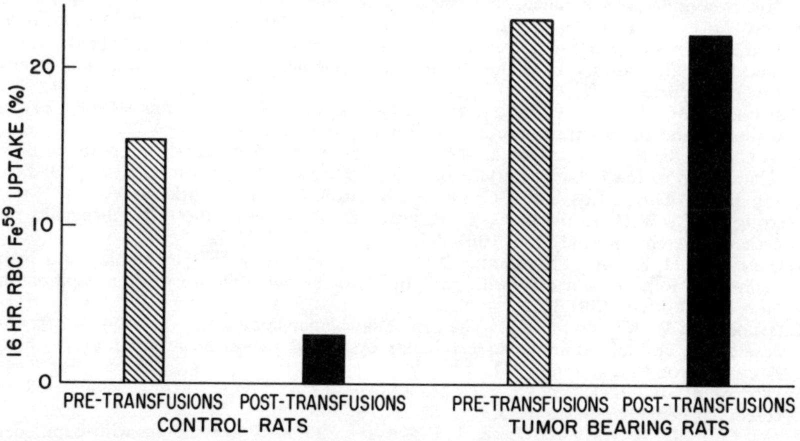

FIGURE 3. The 16-hour incorporation of ^{59}Fe into circulating red cells of nontransfused control, transfused control, nontransfused tumor-bearing and transfused tumor-bearing rats. The erythropoiesis of tumor-bearing animals was not inhibited by transfusions in contrast to the marked inhibition of erythropoiesis of transfused control animals.

treatment with these pharmacological doses of testosterone and ACTH for six weeks there was only a 10 percent increase in the hematocrit and an approximately 30 percent increase in the red cell volume expressed in ml per kg. Thus, although the polycythemia associated with adrenal cortical tumors of rats and man appears to be secondary to the production of an erythropoiesis-stimulating factor by the tumor, the chemical nature of this factor requires further study.

Summary

Erythrocytosis has been noted in association with a variety of tumors. Erythropoiesis-stimulating activity has been detected in the cyst fluid, saline extracts of the tumor tissue or the plasma from patients with polycythemia and associated tumors. The biological activity of renal and cerebellar hemangioblastoma cyst fluid and the erythropoietin from anemic and anoxic serum were shown to be associated with an α_2 mucoprotein with a molecular weight of approximately 30,000. Each of these materials was completely inactivated following incubation in vitro with an antibody to erythropoietin. Thus, the erythrocytosis seen in patients with renal and cerebellar cysts appears to be secondary to the secretion of erythropoietin by these lesions. Erythrocytosis has also been noted in association with adrenal cortical tumors in man and rats. The pathogenesis of the association of polycythemia with these tumors requires further study.

References

1. Bliss, T. L. 1929. Basal metabolism in polycythemia vera. Ann. Internal Med. **2:** 1155.
2. Lawrence, J. H. & W. G. Donald, Jr. 1959. Polycythemia and hydronephrosis or renal tumors. Ann. Intern. Med. **50:** 959.
3. Damon, A., D. A. Holub, M. M. Melicow & A. C. Uson. 1958. Polycythemia and renal carcinoma: Report of ten new cases, two with long hematologic remission following nephrectomy. Amer. J. Med. **25:** 182.
4. Gurney, C. W. 1960. Erythremia in renal disease. Trans. Ass. Amer. Physicians **73:** 103.
5. Hewlett, J. S., G. C. Hoffman, D. A. Senhauser & J. D. Battle, Jr. 1960. Hypernephroma with erythrocythemia: Report of a case and assay of the tumor for an erythropoietic-stimulating substance. New Eng. J. Med. **262:** 1058.
6. Korst, D. R., E. P. Frenkel, L. Cousineau & E. E. Muirhead. 1962. Erythropoietin studies in human renal abnormalities. Correlative renal explant attempts in the rat and dog. *In* Erythropoiesis. L. O. Jacobson and M. Doyle, Eds. : 374. Grune and Stratton, Inc. New York, N. Y.
7. Donati, R. M., J. M. McCarthy, R. D. Lange & N. I. Gallagher. 1963. Erythrocythemia and neoplastic tumors. Ann. Intern. Med. **58:** 47.
8. Lange, R. D. & N. I. Gallagher. 1962. Clinical and experimental observations on the relationship of the kidney to erythropoietin production: *In* Erythropoiesis. L. O. Jacobson and M. Doyle, Eds. : 361. Grune and Stratton, Inc. New York, N. Y.
9. Nixon, R. K., W. O'Rourke, C. E. Rupe & D. R. Korst. 1960. Nephrogenic polycythemia. Arch. Internal Med. **106:** 797.
10. Gardner, F. H. & J. G. Freymann. 1958. Erythrocythemia (polycythemia) and hydronephrosis: Report of a case with radioiron studies, with recovery after nephrectomy. New Eng. J. Med. **259:** 323.
11. Cramer, F. & W. Kimsey. 1952. The cerebellar hemangioblastomas; review of fifty-three cases, with special reference to cerebellar cysts and the association of polycythemia. Arch. Neurol. Psychiat. **67:** 237.
12. Ward, A. A., Jr., E. L. Poltz & L. M. Knopp. 1956. "Polycythemia" associated with cerebellar hemangioblastoma. J. Neurosurg. **13:** 248.
13. Starr, G. F., C. F. Stroebel, Jr. & T. P. Kearns. 1958. Polycythemia with papilledema and infratentorial vascular tumors. Ann. Intern. Med. **48:** 978.
14. Waldmann, T. A., E. H. Levin & M. Baldwin. 1961. The association of polycythemia with a cerebellar hemangioblastoma: The production of an erythropoiesis-stimulating factor by the tumor. Amer. J. Med. **31:** 318.

15. RACE, G. J., J. W. FINNEY, J. T. MALLAMS & G. A. BALLA. 1964. Hematopoietic stimulating effect of a cerebellar hemangioblastoma. J. Am. Med. Assoc. **187:** 150.
16. MCFADZEAN, A. J. S., D. TODD & K. C. TSANG. 1958. Polycythemia in primary carcinoma of the liver. Blood **13:** 427.
17. KAN, Y. W., A. J. S. MCFADZEAN, D. TODD & S. C. TSO. 1961. Further observations on polycythemia in hepatocellular carcinoma. Blood **18:** 592.
18. DAVIDSON, C. S. & B. CASTLEMAN. 1964. Liver failure and polycythemia. New Eng. J. Med. **270:** 627.
19. BROWNSTEIN, M. H. & H. S. BALLIARD. 1966. Hepatoma associated with erythrocytosis: Report of eleven new cases. Amer. J. Med. **40:** 204.
20. THOMSON, A. P. & F. G. W. MARSON. 1953. Polycythemia with fibroids. Lancet **2:** 759.
21. MENZIES, D. H. 1961. Fibromyomata and polycythaemia. J. Obstet. Gynaecol. Brit. Commonwealth **68:** 505.
22. WALDMANN, T. A. & J. E. BRADLEY. 1961. Polycythemia secondary to a pheochromocytoma with production of an erythropoiesis stimulating factor by the tumor. Proc. Soc. Exp. Biol. Med. **108:** 425.
23. GARDNER, F. H. June 1962. Polycythemia. Disease-A-Month: : 1.
24. GORDON, A. S. 1959. Hemopoietine. Physiol. Rev. **39:** 1.
25. PENINGTON, D. G. 1965. Polycythemia in neoplastic diseases. Proc. Roy. Soc. Med. **58:** 488.
26. ROSSE, W. F., T. A. WALDMANN & D. E. HOUSTON. 1962. Erythropoietin assays using $iron^{59}$ incorporation into blood and spleen of the polycythemic mouse. Proc. Soc. Exp. Biol. Med. **109:** 836.
27. ROSSE, W. F. & T. A. WALDMANN. 1964. A comparison of some physical and chemical properties of erythropoiesis-stimulating factors from different sources. Blood **24:** 739.
28. BLUMBERG, B. S. & L. WARREN. 1961. The effect of sialidase on transferrins and other serum proteins. Biochim. Biophys. Acta **50:** 90.
29. LEA, D. E. 1955. Actions of Radiations on Living Cells. 2nd Ed. University Press. Cambridge, England.
30. SCHOOLEY, J. C. & J. F. GARCIA. 1962. Immunochemical studies of human urinary erythropoietin. Proc. Soc. Exp. Biol. Med. **109:** 325.
31. SNELL, K. C. & H. L. STEWART. 1959. Variations in histologic pattern and functional effects of a transplantable adrenal cortical carcinoma in intact, hypophysectomized, and newborn rats. J. Nat. Cancer Inst. **22:** 1119.
32. SWARM, R. L., T. A. WALDMANN & W. F. ROSSE. 1963. Polycythemia in rats transplanted with an adrenal cortical carcinoma. Fed. Proc. **22:** 665.

PRODUCTION, UTILIZATION AND EXCRETION OF ERYTHROPOIETIN: I. CHRONIC ANEMIAS. II. APLASTIC CRISIS. III. ERYTHROPOIETIC EFFECTS OF NORMAL PLASMA*

Denman Hammond, Nomie Shore and Nasser Movassaghi

Division of Hematology, The Children's Hospital of Los Angeles and The Department of Pediatrics, School of Medicine, University of Southern California

In the years after 1950 when interest in the humoral control of erythropoiesis was rekindled, the state of erythropoietin was surveyed in a variety of clinical hematologic disorders. This led to the observation that increased erythropoietin activity was often, but not always, found in the serum of individuals with a variety of types of anemia.[1–4]

During these years, few attempts were made to relate the erythropoietin activity to the severity of anemia, except that, in general, it was recognized that when anemia was severe, erythropoietin activity was usually found to be increased. It was reported that no consistent correlation could be drawn between severity of anemia and erythropoietin activity.[1] It was also demonstrated that at times erythropoietin could be found in the urine of anemic patients although in lesser concentration than in their serum.[1,5]

Erythropoietin Production in Chronic Anemias

For several years our laboratory has been interested in the physiology of erythropoietin in hematologic disorders. In 1960 we reported the study of 20 patients with congenital hypoplastic anemia and our failure to discover that any of these could be ascribed to a deficiency of erythropoietin.[6] This study, however, demonstrated a direct relationship between the erythropoietin activity in the serum and the severity of anemia at the time of sampling (FIGURE 1). A similar relationship was found for erythropoietin activity in the urine of these patients.

Subsequently we reported that such a relationship also was found in patients with thalassemia major.[7] Patients with this type of chronic hemolytic anemia appeared to have less erythropoietin activity in serum and urine than patients with hypoplastic anemia at all comparable degrees of anemia which were studied (FIGURE 2).

These early studies were done using the starved rat assay. Gordon *et al.* had reported similar observations in patients with thalassemia major using a rat assay[8] and have confirmed the earlier observations employing a polycythemic mouse assay.[9]

Details of the polycythemic mouse assay employed for the studies reported here and data on its sensitivity and control are given in the APPENDIX.

In consideration of the marked difference in erythropoiesis that exists between hypoplastic and hemolytic anemias and the higher levels of erythropoietin found in congenital hypoplastic anemia in contrast to thalassemia major, our data supported the concept that erythropoietin was consumed or inactivated in exerting its erythropoietic effect.[7]

Further clinical support for this theory was found when we compared the rate of disappearance of endogenous erythropoietin following transfusion of patients

* Supported by U.S.P.H.S. funds from research grant AM 04048, postgraduate training grant 2T1 HD 48, Clinical Research Center grant FR–86 and funds from the Medical Research Committee of Delta Delta Delta.

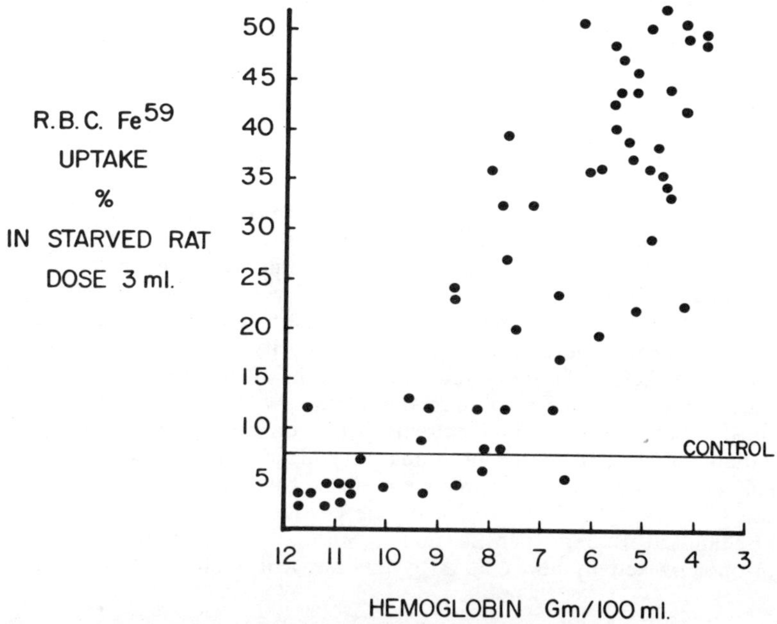

FIGURE 1. The relationship between serum erythropoietin activity and hemoglobin concentration in 22 patients with congenital hypoplastic anemia. Each of the 63 points represents the mean value from assay of a single sample in a group of five rats. Control represents the mean value plus one standard deviation obtained when using plasma from normal nonanemic adults.

with hypoplastic and chronic hemolytic anemias and noted more rapid disappearance of erythropoietin in patients with greater erythroid activity of the bone marrow.[10]

Small numbers of patients with sickle cell anemia have been reported to have elevated erythropoietin activity when severely anemic but not consistently so.[1,3,5,11] Our studies of such patients again demonstrate a relationship between erythropoietin activity and severity of anemia. FIGURE 3 shows this relationship with respect to serum erythropoietin as determined by assay in polycythemic mice. This represents assays of 48 specimens from 31 patients. Increased erythropoietin activity was found in the serum of all patients with a hemoglobin concentration of 9.5 g/100 ml or less, and progressively increased activity was found as the anemia became more severe. The activity in urine showed a similar relationship. We have not found as high an activity in sickle cell anemia as in hypoplastic anemia even when the anemia is severe.

Our interest in the relationship between the level of anemia and erythropoietin production has continued, stimulated by the desire to identify potential sources of human erythropoietin for use in research. The most consistently rich source of human erythropoietin thus far has been the urine of patients with congenital hypoplastic anemia. Such patients, however, are not numerous.

Early reports of erythropoietin in serum and urine of patients with iron deficiency anemia indicated that activity was not significantly increased unless the anemia was severe.[12–14] Data on erythropoietin production and excretion in iron deficiency anemia are still quite limited.

FIGURE 4 shows the results of assays on serum specimens from 49 children with iron deficiency anemia whose hemoglobin concentration varied between 9.5 and 2.4 g/100 ml. In these patients the activity was invariably elevated and increased progressively in proportion to the severity of the anemia. Very high activity was found in several patients, activity as high as that found in patients with hypoplastic anemia of comparable hemoglobin concentration.

Studies of erythropoietin excretion in the urine of these patients revealed the same relationship of erythropoietin activity to severity of anemia. All patients had significantly increased urinary erythropoietin when the hemoglobin concentration was below 10 g/100 ml. Patients with hemoglobin concentration below 6 g/100 ml had progressively increased urinary erythropoietin activity as the anemia became more pronounced. The majority of these yielded between 25 and 60% uptake of ^{59}Fe into circulating red cells of the exhypoxic polycythemic mouse given a dose of 0.8 ml of unmodified urine.

Thus, it would appear that patients with iron deficiency anemia provide a potentially important source of human erythropoietin for use in research. A patient with iron deficiency anemia whose urine gave an RBC ^{59}Fe uptake of 25% by the assay reported here would excrete erythropoietin equivalent to 1800 to 2000 Standard B units per 24 hours. Since many such patients had urine erythropoietin activity above 50% by this assay, it is obvious that patients with

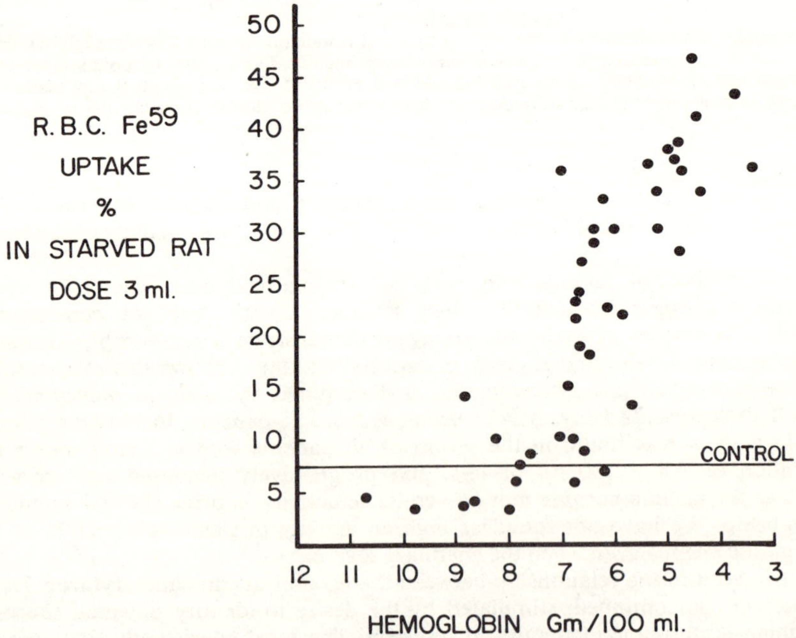

FIGURE 2. The relationship between serum erythropoietin activity and the hemoglobin concentration in thalassemia major. Forty-three samples from 16 patients are shown. Each point represents the mean value obtained from the assay of a group of five rats. Control represents the mean value plus one standard deviation obtained when using plasma from normal nonanemic adults.

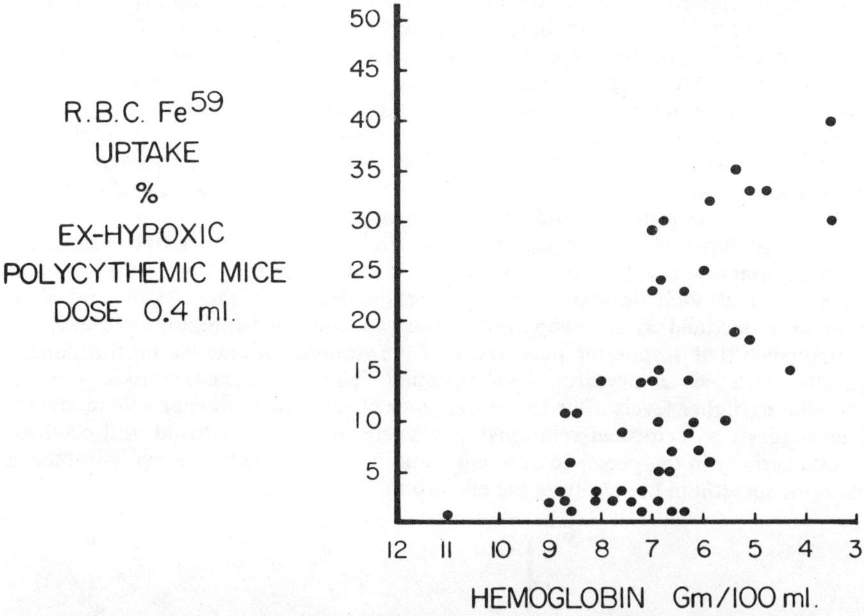

FIGURE 3. The relationship between serum erythropoietin activity and the hemoglobin concentration in 31 patients with homozygous sickle cell anemia. Each of the 48 points represents the mean value obtained from assay of a group of five mice. The control value for this assay using plasma from normal nonanemic adults is 0.7 ± 0.2%.

severe iron deficiency anemia excrete urine which has sufficient erythropoietin content to provide a widely available and easily recovered source of human erythropoietin for laboratory use.

Erythropoietin and Erythropoiesis in Aplastic Crisis

Studies on the physiology of erythropoietin and its relationship to bone marrow activity have been extended to patients with chronic hemolytic anemia having acute aplastic crisis. FIGURE 5 illustrates the hematologic events in a 14-year-old girl with sickle cell anemia who was studied during an aplastic crisis and spontaneous recovery. Her hemoglobin concentration was 5 g/100 ml, reticulocyte count was zero and the bone marrow showed normal cellularity but only 2.8% erythroid elements. At this time both her serum and urine showed increased erythropoietin as assayed in the polycythemic mouse.

The first hematologic evidence of bone marrow recovery was a marked increase in leukocyte count from 9,040 to 71,100/mm^3 on the sixth day. At that time a bone marrow aspirate revealed marked hypercellularity with 62% erythroid cells. A pronounced normoblastemia and reticulocytosis ensued which was followed by a gradual rise in hemoglobin. Erythropoietin in serum and urine decreased during the first seven days, particularly from the fifth to seventh day, although the hemoglobin concentration did not change during that time. This was a period during which a marked increase in marrow erythroid activity occurred. Interestingly, the erythropoietin levels rebounded between the seventh and ninth days and ultimately declined again to normal values by the 13th day as erythropoiesis continued sufficient to increase the hemoglobin to 8.7 g/100 ml.

We have observed this type of cyclic fluctuation of erythropoietin on several occasions when studying patients in aplastic crisis. FIGURE 6 illustrates five such cases. They were superimposed so day zero represents the lowest level of erythropoietin reached during the initial fall. The hemoglobin concentration of these five patients was between 3.5 and 7 g/100 ml at the start of the experiment. Reticulocyte count in all patients was less than 0.5%. All had decreased erythroid tissue in marrow aspirates and all had elevated erythropoietin activity. Before the hemoglobin values rose significantly, the erythropoietin activity declined. As bone marrow erythropoiesis became markedly hypercellular, erythropoietin levels reached their lowest values but rebounded to higher levels and then ultimately declined as erythropoiesis continued and the hemoglobin rose.

It appears that despite the persistence of the stimulus of anemia, erythropoietin activity declined as erythropoiesis resumed following aplastic crisis, but rebounded to higher levels after the initial wave of marrow erythropoietic recovery. This suggests a reciprocal relationship between marrow erythroid and erythropoietin activity in the presence of anemia and illustrates the homeostatic influence of erythropoietin in maintaining the erythron.

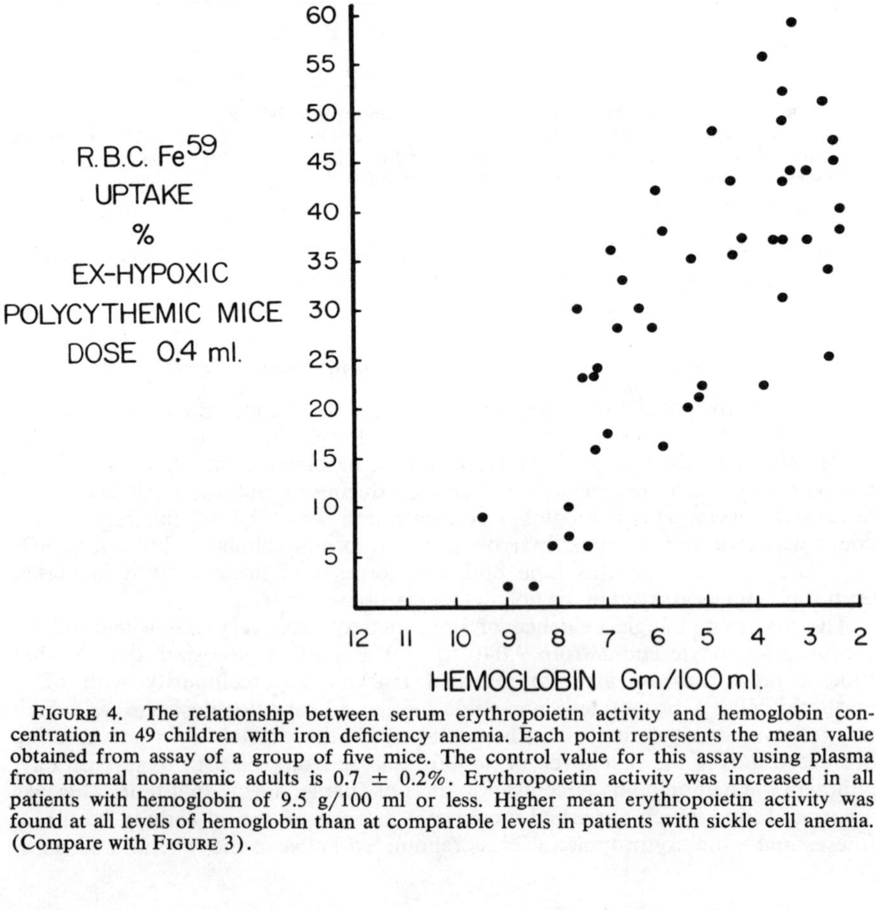

FIGURE 4. The relationship between serum erythropoietin activity and hemoglobin concentration in 49 children with iron deficiency anemia. Each point represents the mean value obtained from assay of a group of five mice. The control value for this assay using plasma from normal nonanemic adults is 0.7 ± 0.2%. Erythropoietin activity was increased in all patients with hemoglobin of 9.5 g/100 ml or less. Higher mean erythropoietin activity was found at all levels of hemoglobin than at comparable levels in patients with sickle cell anemia. (Compare with FIGURE 3).

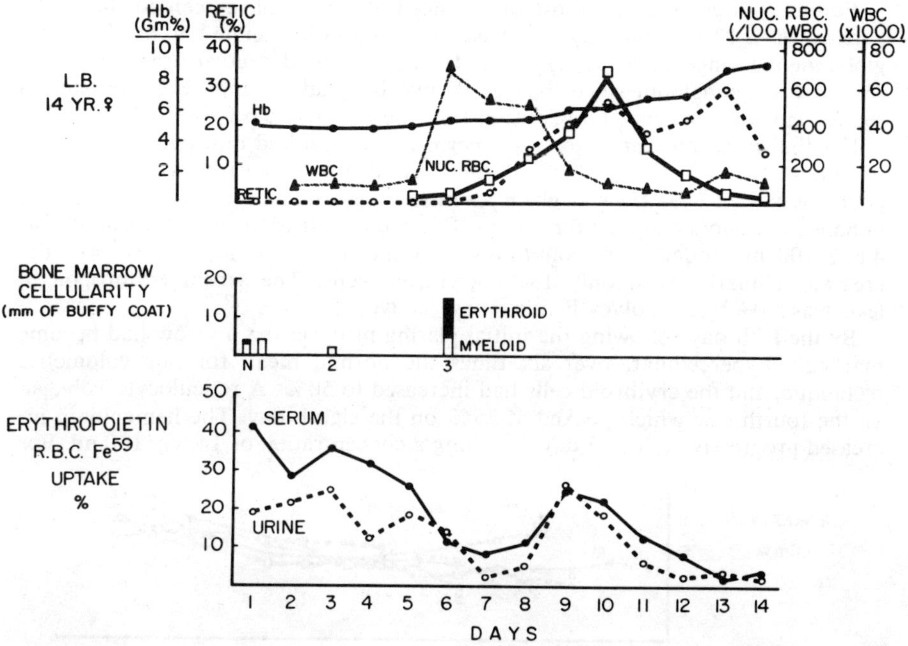

FIGURE 5. Hematologic response and erythropoietin activity in a patient with sickle cell anemia recovering from an acute aplastic crisis. Marrow cellularity represents the measurement of the nucleated cell layer of 1 ml of marrow aspirate centrifuged in a hematocrit tube. Marrow cellularity and the proportion of nucleated cells in the erythroid series is shown on each of three occasions as compared to normal values for this technique. Erythropoietin values represent the mean RBC ^{59}Fe uptake in 48 hr in groups of five exhypoxic polycythemic mice given a total dose of 0.4 ml of serum or 0.8 ml of unmodified urine.

Erythropoietic Effect of Normal Plasma in Hypoplastic Anemia

In 1962 we reported that the administration of normal human plasma to a patient with congenital erythroid hypoplasia repeatedly brought about increased erythropoiesis, as judged by increased reticulocyte count and increased marrow erythroid tissue, despite the presence of high levels of endogenous erythropoietin.[15] Such patients rarely have a reticulocyte count over 1% and, characteristically, have a bone marrow showing specific erythroid hypoplasia. The serum erythropoietin activity of the patient reported ranged between 30 and 50% by the starved rat assay.

The patient developed reticulocytosis between 4 and 6% on three separate occasions when given fresh plasma, and on one occasion, when the marrow was compared before and after treatment, the cellularity doubled and erythroid cells increased from 13 to 66%. Thereafter, the patient ceased requiring transfusions for a period of many months.

Since then, we have repeated the experiment in eight patients with chronic hypoplastic anemia using fresh normal plasma and various plasma fractions. Some patients have a definite increase in erythropoiesis and others appear to be unresponsive.

FIGURE 7 illustrates the most pronounced effect we have seen to date. The patient was a 12-year-old boy who has had hypoplastic anemia and hypogammaglobulinemia since prior to age two. He has required regular transfusions to sustain his hemoglobin since the age of two but had an apparent spontaneous remission with a prolonged transfusion-free interval on one occasion.

For the six months prior to this experiment he required repeated transfusions of sedimented red cells totalling 25 units. He characteristically had reticulocyte counts less than 1%. He was given 25 ml/kg fresh human plasma from normal nonanemic donors daily for three days. Prior to the infusions his hemoglobin was 4.6 g/100 ml, reticulocyte count was zero and a marrow aspirate showed decreased cellularity with only 1.4% erythroid cells. The serum erythropoietin level was 35% by the polycythemic mouse assay.

By the fifth day following the initial plasma infusion the marrow had become markedly hypercellular, over six times the normal mean for our volumetric technique, and the erythroid cells had increased to 50%. A reticulocytosis began on the fourth day which peaked at 25% on the eighth day. The hemoglobin increased progressively for 35 days reaching a concentration of 14.6 g/100 ml. For

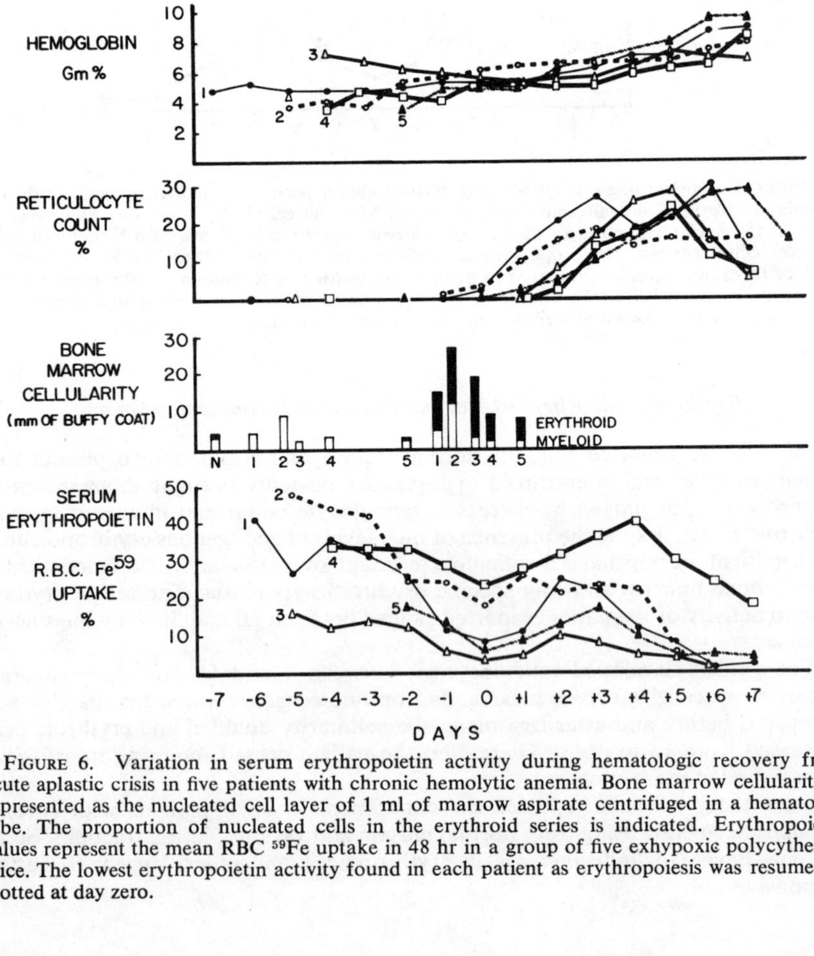

FIGURE 6. Variation in serum erythropoietin activity during hematologic recovery from acute aplastic crisis in five patients with chronic hemolytic anemia. Bone marrow cellularity is represented as the nucleated cell layer of 1 ml of marrow aspirate centrifuged in a hematocrit tube. The proportion of nucleated cells in the erythroid series is indicated. Erythropoietin values represent the mean RBC ^{59}Fe uptake in 48 hr in a group of five exhypoxic polycythemic mice. The lowest erythropoietin activity found in each patient as erythropoiesis was resumed is plotted at day zero.

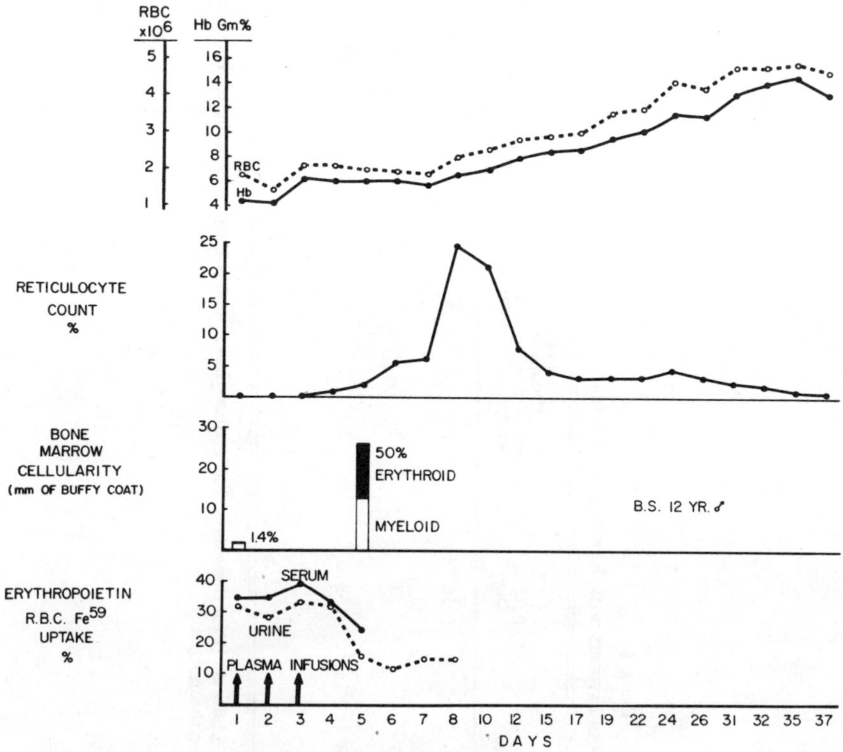

FIGURE 7. The erythropoietic effects of plasma administered to a patient with chronic hypoplastic anemia. Fresh plasma from a normal nonanemic adult was given i.v. in a dose of 25 ml/kg daily for three days. Marrow cellularity was determined by measuring the nucleated cell layer of 1 ml of marrow centrifuged in hematocrit tube. Erythropoietin values represent the mean RBC ^{59}Fe uptake in 48 hr of a group of five exhypoxic polycythemic mice given a total dose of 0.4 ml of serum or 0.8 ml of unmodified urine.

the following 60 days the hemoglobin declined gradually to 10 g/100 ml but in the next 15 days declined rapidly to 5.5 g/100 ml. The serum and urine erythropoietin, both initially above 30%, fell as marrow erythropoiesis increased but were not followed throughout the experiment.

TABLE 1 shows the most pronounced erythropoietic effects of plasma in each of four patients who have responded to this treatment repeatedly and to treatment with certain plasma fractions. Despite elevated erythropoietin activity, the patients had erythroid hypoplasia, reticulocytopenia and anemia. In response to plasma there was reticulocytosis peaking in seven to 16 days, an increase in marrow cellularity and sometimes pronounced increase in marrow erythroid cells. Four other similar patients have failed to show an erythropoietic response to this treatment.

Patients with specific erythroid hypoplasia may have the same clinical and hematologic findings but which result from different causes. Some such patients may spontaneously resume erythropoiesis and have a remission for prolonged periods or even permanently. Others respond partially or completely to cortico-

TABLE 1

EFFECT OF PLASMA INFUSION IN PATIENTS WITH HYPOPLASTIC ANEMIA*

Patient	Age/Sex	Serum Erythropoietin % Uptake	Retic. %		Peak at Day	Marrow Cellularity		Marrow Erythroid %	
			Before	After		Before	After	Before	After
G. H.	12 yr M	25	1.6	6.4	16	3	6	13	62
P. B.	6 yr F	40	0.0	5.3	7	1	6	3	26
B. S.	12 yr M	33	0.0	24.8	8	2	26	1	50
D. N.	4 yr M	35	0.2	3.0	7	7	10	5	9

* Each was given 25 ml/kg fresh plasma from normal nonanemic adults daily for three days. Each patient has responded similarly on up to five occasions. Four additional patients failed to show a detectable increase in erythropoiesis.

steroid therapy while others remain refractory and require repeated transfusions throughout their lifetime. Another differing characteristic is the ability of some to respond to a factor in normal plasma despite a high level of endogenous erythropoietin to which they do not respond.

We previously postulated that the factor in the plasma and urine of these patients which stimulates erythropoiesis in the intact assay animal may be a functionally inactive erythropoietin in the human, or that these patients may lack a component of normal plasma which has an essential role in activating, protecting, or transporting erythropoietin.[15] Some support for our speculations about these patients has since been found.

Kuratowska *et al.*[16] reported finding a factor in the perfusate of isolated hypoxic rabbit kidneys which was erythropoietically inactive when injected s.c. into fasted rats, unless it was preincubated with normal plasma or alpha globulins. The material was erythropoietically active when injected i.v. even without preincubation. They hypothesized that the renal factor formed a complex with proteins, activated a precursor of erythropoietin in plasma or was activated by an activator present in alpha globulin fractions.

Goldwasser has indicated that with progressive purification of erythropoietin from sheep plasma, instability and loss of activity may be prevented by the addition of albumin.[17] Lowy and Keighley have found that concentrated preparations of erythropoietin from the urine of patients with hypoplastic anemia have considerable activity in the region of albumin after electrophoresis in acrylamide gel.[18] Gardner *et al.*[19] have recently reported the enhanced erythropoietic effect of rabbit serum on an erythropoietin fraction from the urine of a patient with hypoplastic anemia. These observations illustrate the apparent affinity of erythropoietin for certain plasma proteins and their protective or potentiating effect on erythropoietin.

Contrera *et al.*[20,21] have reported the extraction of two erythropoietic factors from the kidneys of hypoxic rats. One is derived from the plasma trapped in the renal vasculature and resembles plasma erythropoietin. The other is identified upon differential centrifugation, with the light mitochondrial fraction of kidney cells. It is erythropoietically inactive unless previously incubated with normal rat serum. They hypothesize that the renal factor is an enzyme which produces erythropoietin by its action on a particular serum protein or that it functions as an erythropoietin precursor which must be complexed with a serum factor to become physiologically active.

Our demonstration of the enhancement of erythropoiesis by administering normal plasma to a patient unresponsive to his own high level of erythropoietin[15] indicated that in the human, some plasma component is required for activation, transport or utilization of erythropoietin.

In view of these numerous observations, it seems apparent that the mechanism of action of erythropoietin in stimulating erythropoiesis is more complex than was thought to be the case several years ago. It should be recognized, moreover, that since measurement of erythropoietin at present depends upon assay in animals, it is difficult to distinguish between erythropoietic factors present in the material being assayed and those that may be contributed by the assay animal. Two substances producing a similar erythropoietic effect when injected into a prepared assay animal may nonetheless be materials of different nature interacting with different factors present in the animal. They may stimulate erythropoiesis by the same, or by a different, mechanism.

Patients with specific marrow erythroid hypoplasia, particularly those of congenital origin, present unique opportunities for study of this phenomenon in man. Experiments are in progress to determine which fractions of plasma produce the erythropoietic effects and the fate of endogenous erythropoietin incident to plasma administration.

Final clarification of all substances that are essential for the action of erythropoietin may not be obtained until its precise biochemical nature is known. Meanwhile, further study of erythropoietin enhancement by plasma and the search for activating, transporting and inhibiting systems related to erythropoietin should be helpful in providing an ultimate understanding of the role of erythropoietin in maintaining the erythron.

Acknowledgments

We would like to acknowledge the competent technical assistance of Mr. Charles Greene and Mr. Curtis Polk in these studies.

Appendix

Erythropoietin Assay Methodology and Standardization

Virgin female $B_6D_2F_1$ mice, specific pathogen-free, and weighing 18–22 g are placed in a hypobaric chamber and maintained at ½ atmospheric pressure for eight hr daily for 14 days.

On the fourth and fifth days after return to normal atmospheric pressure, they are given an i.p. injection of 0.2 ml of the material to be assayed. On the sixth day, 0.2 μc of ^{59}Fe Cl in phosphate buffer, pH 3.5, is injected into the tail vein. Forty-eight hr later a sample of blood is obtained by cardiac puncture. Heparinized blood, 0.5 ml, is placed in a glass vial, hemolyzed by addition of 3 ml distilled water and its radioactivity determined in a well type gamma scintillation counter. A portion of blood is also used for duplicate determinations of hematocrit by the micro method. Animals with hematocrit below 52% are discarded from the experiment.

The RBC ^{59}Fe uptake is calculated as a percentage of the total dose administered using a formula in which the blood volume is assumed to be 7% body weight.

Groups of five mice are used for assay of each specimen. Each assay procedure includes a group of mice given injections of pooled normal nonanemic human plasma as a negative control and a group given injection of a laboratory standard of pooled plasma from rabbits made anemic with phenylhydrazine. In experiments in this laboratory involving 250 mice and extending over a period of 12 months, the mean RBC ^{59}Fe uptake for the negative control pool of normal human plasma was $0.7 \pm 0.2\%$, and for the anemic rabbit plasma laboratory standard was $32.0 \pm 4.9\%$. Saline controls averaged $0.3 \pm 0.2\%$.

Information on the standardization of this assay in terms of the International Reference preparation of Erythropoietin (Standard B) is presented elsewhere.[22]

References

1. Piliero, S. J., P. T. Medici, B. Pansky, A. L. Luhby & A. S. Gordon. 1956. Erythropoietic-stimulating effects of plasma extracts from anemic human subjects. Proc. Soc. Exper. Biol. Med. **93:** 302.
2. Prentiss, T. C. & E. A. Mirand. 1957. Studies of plasma erythropoietic factor in anemic human patients. Blood **12:** 993.

3. Gurney, C. W., E. Goldwasser & C. Pan. 1957. Studies on erythropoiesis. VI. Erythropoietin in human plasma. J. Lab. Clin. Med. **50:** 534.
4. Gordon, A. S. 1959. Hemopoietine. Physiol. Rev. **39:** 1.
5. Winkert, J., A. S. Gordon, P. T. Medici, S. J. Piliero, A. L. Luhby & M. Tannenbaum. 1958. Erythropoietic-stimulating activity of urine from anemic human subjects. Proc. Soc. Exper. Biol. Med. **97:** 191.
6. Hammond, D. & G. Keighley. 1960. The erythrocyte-stimulating factor (ESF) in serum and urine in congenital hypoplastic anemia. A. M. A. J. Dis. Child. **100:** 466; 1962. Proc. VIII Int. Cong. Hemat. : 999. Tokyo, Japan.
7. Hammond, G. D., A. Ishikawa & G. Keighley. 1962. Relationship between erythropoietin and severity of anemia in hypoplastic and hemolytic states. *In* Erythropoiesis. L. O. Jacobson & M. Doyle, Eds. : 351. Grune & Stratton. New York, N. Y.
8. Winkert, J. W. & A. S. Gordon. 1960. Biological assay of human urinary erythropoietic-stimulating factor (ESF). Proc. Soc. Exper. Biol. Med. **104:** 713.
9. Gordon, A. S., A. H. Weintraub, J. F. Camiscoli & J. F. Contrera. 1964. Plasma and urinary levels of erythropoietin in Cooley's anemia. Ann. N. Y. Acad. Sci. **119:** 561.
10. Hammond, G. D. & A. Ishikawa. 1962. The rate of disappearance of erythropoietin following transfusion of severely anemic patients. *In* Erythropoiesis. L. O. Jacobson & M. Doyle, Eds. : 128. Grune & Stratton. New York, N. Y.
11. Jones, B. & W. G. Klingberg. 1960. A study of erythropoietin in two types of hemolytic anemia – erythroblastosis fetalis and sickle cell anemia. J. Ped. **56:** 752.
12. Van Dyke, D. C. 1960. Sources and properties of human urinary erythropoietin. *In* Haemopoiesis. Ciba Foundation Symposium. : 397. Churchill. London, England.
13. Gallagher, N. I., J. M. McCarthy & R. D. Lange. 1960. Observations on erythropoietic-stimulating factor (ESF) in the plasma of uremic and nonuremic anemic patients. Ann. Int. Med. **52:** 1201.
14. Van Dyke, D. C., M. Layrisse, J. H. Lawrence, J. F. Garcia & M. Pollycove. 1961. Relation between severity of anemia and erythropoietin titer in human beings. Blood **18:** 187.
15. Hammond, G. D. 1962. *In* Erythropoiesis. L. O. Jacobson & M. Doyle, Eds. : 270. Grune & Stratton. New York, N. Y.
16. Kuratowska, Z., B. Lewartowski & B. Lipinski. 1964. Chemical and biologic properties of an erythropoietin-generating substance obtained from perfusates of isolated anoxic kidneys. J. Lab. Clin. Med. **64:** 226.
17. Goldwasser, E. & C. Kung. 1966. On the purification and properties of sheep plasma erythropoietin. Ann. N. Y. Acad. Sci. This Annal.
18. Lowy, P. & G. Keighley. 1966. Fractionation of erythropoietin from anemic and normal urine. This Annal.
19. Gardner, E., C.-S. Wright, J. P. Lewis & R. R. Moore. 1966. Potentiation of purified erythropoietin with serum proteins. Clin. Res. **14:** 90 (Abstract).
20. Contrera, J. F., A. S. Gordon & A. H. Weintraub. 1965. Extraction of an erythropoietin-producing factor from a particulate fraction of rat kidney. American Society of Hematology. Blood **26:** 885 (Abstract).
21. Contrera, J. F. & A. S. Gordon. 1966. Production of erythropoietin by a particulate fraction of kidney. This Annal.
22. Shore, N. A., N. Movassaghi & D. Hammond. 1966. Quantitative estimation of erythropoietin. This Annal.

INAPPROPRIATE ERYTHROPOIETIN ELABORATION

Neil I. Gallagher and Robert M. Donati

Radioisotope Laboratory, St. Louis Veterans Administration Hospital and the Department of Internal Medicine, St. Louis University School of Medicine, St. Louis, Mo.

INTRODUCTION

Erythrocytosis as an unusual complication of tumors or renal disease has been documented in an increasing number of reports.[1–3] In selected instances an apparent causal relationship between uterine myomata, cerebellar hemangioblastoma, renal carcinoma, renal cysts, renal adenoma, hydronephrosis or pheochromocytoma and associated erythrocytosis has been suggested because of remission of the erythrocytosis following surgical extirpation or radiologic obliteration of the lesion.[1–3] Moreover, elevations of plasma erythropoietin levels have been described in patients with erythrocytosis in association with tumors or renal abnormalities.[1–9] Extracts obtained from certain of these pathologic tissues had erythropoietic-stimulating potential when bioassayed in a sensitive system. Inappropriate erythropoietin production by the neoplasm or pathologically altered renal tissue provides an explanation for this association.

In this laboratory we have evaluated erythropoietin production in a number of patients with neoplastic and nonneoplastic diseases and associated erythrocytosis. Patients with nonneoplastic diseases included those with hydronephrosis, renal tuberculosis and renal cysts. In the neoplastic group, patients with hepatocellular carcinoma, renal carcinoma, cerebellar hemangioblastoma, uterine myoma and adrenal adenoma, both medullary and cortical, have been evaluated. Plasma erythropoietin levels and renin activity have also been measured in patients with unilateral renal artery stenosis and hypertension. This report summarizes our general experience, details observations in a patient with an aldosterone-secreting adrenal adenoma and erythrocytosis, and outlines the experimental attempts to clarify this relationship.

MATERIALS AND METHODS

Patient Studies

The erythropoietic-stimulating activity of plasma or cyst fluid was determined by bioassay in starved rats,[10] polycythemic rats[10] or polycythemic mice by a modification of[11] or by the bioassay of Cotes and Bangham.[12] Graded doses of plasma obtained from a patient with erythrocytosis and an adrenal adenoma prior to and following surgery were assayed in polycythemic mice.[12]

Five patients with hypertension were evaluated with determination of plasma renin activity[13] and plasma erythropoietin activity.[11] In one instance plasma samples were obtained before and after the infusion of angiotensin II similarly to the manner of Kaplan and Silah.[14]

Animal Studies

Female Sprague-Dawley rats weighing 180–200 g previously fed a diet of Purina laboratory chow* were starved for 96 hr and allowed water ad libitum. In one experiment, test material was injected i.p. 24 and 48 hr after the initiation of

* Iron content 275 ppm. Sodium content 0.9%.

TABLE 1

RESULTS OF ERYTHROPOIETIN ASSAY OF PATIENTS WITH ERYTHROCYTOSIS

Diagnosis	No. Patients	No. Positive Plasma EP	No. Positive Cyst Fluid EP
Renal tuberculosis	1	0	
Renal cysts	4	3	2
Hydronephrosis	3	2	
Renal carcinoma	5	4	
Uterine myoma	1	0	
Pheochromocytoma	1	0	
Hepatic carcinoma	1	1	
Cerebellar hemangioblastoma	5	3	3
Adrenal adenoma	1	1	

starvation. In another experiment injections were given 48 and 72 hr after starvation was begun. The test materials given were angiotensin II,** 200 μg; renin,† 1500 μg; aldosterone,†† 2 μg; 0.9% saline solution or an extract of plasma from rabbits rendered anemic by phenylhydrazine administration.[10] Eighteen hr prior to the completion of the experiment, 1 μc ^{59}Fe/1 μg ^{56}Fe citrate was administered via the tail vein. Eighteen hr later blood was obtained by cardiac puncture and the radioactivity of an aliquot determined in a well-type scintillation counter. Percent red blood cell ^{59}Fe incorporation was then determined using 5% total body weight as the blood volume.[10]

To determine the effects of increased endogenous production of renin, angiotensin and aldosterone, a sodium-deficient diet§ and water were offered ad libitum to 20 female Sprague-Dawley rats weighing 180–200 g. A similar number of rats were given Purina laboratory chow and water. Hemoglobins and microhematocrits were determined on each animal prior to the initiation of the diet. After three weeks' maintenance on these diets, hemoglobin concentration, microhematocrits and red blood cell mass were determined by ^{59}Fe-tagged homologous red blood cells.[15]

Female Sprague-Dawley rats weighing 180–200 g were maintained on a diet of Purina laboratory chow with water allowed ad libitum. One group of animals received 0.9% saline solution i.p. at 0 and 12 hr, the other group received 1 mg polythiazide¶ i.p. at the same time intervals. One-half of the saline-injected group was exposed to 0.5 atm pressure for a period of eight hours. All animals were killed at 32 hr by exsanguination under light ether anesthesia, the plasma harvested and the kidneys removed. Subsequently, plasma was prepared after the manner of Helmer[13] and bioassayed for renin activity.[16] Plasma erythropoietin levels were determined[12] and the renal juxtaglomerular granularity index determined by the method of Hartroft and Hartroft.[17]

** Procured as Hypertensin®, Ciba, Lot 262400A.

† Procured as hog renin from Dr. H. M. Perry, St. Louis, Mo.

†† Procured as Aldosterone®, Ciba, Lot E 6403.

§ Sodium Deficient Test Diet, procured from Nutritional Biochemicals Corporation, Cleveland, Ohio, Iron content 475 ppm. Sodium content, not measurable.

¶ Procured as Renese® (I.M.) from Chas. Pfizer and Co. Inc., N. Y., N. Y. Lot No. 2X–282–02–EPD.

Results

Patient Results

The number of erythrocythemic patients studied, the diagnoses and the results of erythropoietin assay are presented in TABLE 1. Polycythemia vera was excluded by the absence of splenomegaly, leukocytosis and thrombocytosis. All of these patients demonstrated erythrocytosis as manifested by the peripheral hematocrit elevation and an elevation in measured red blood cell mass. Since these patients were evaluated over a period of six years, the assay procedures varied and the results are therefore tabulated only as the number of patients demonstrating increased erythropoietic-stimulating activity in the plasma or cyst fluid. The patients with uterine myoma, renal tuberculosis or pheochromocytoma demonstrated no elevation of the plasma erythropoietin levels. Three out of four patients with renal cysts and erythrocytosis had increased plasma erythropoietin levels, and in two of these the renal cyst fluid was also positive. Two out of three patients with erythrocytosis and hydronephrosis had elevated plasma erythropoietin levels, and four out of five patients with renal carcinoma and erythrocytosis had positive plasma assays. Single patients with erythrocytosis and hepatic carcinoma or adrenal adenoma had elevated plasma erythropoietin. Of five patients with erythrocytosis and cerebellar hemangioblastoma, one had increased erythropoietic activity in the plasma alone, two in the plasma and cyst fluid, and one in the cyst fluid alone.

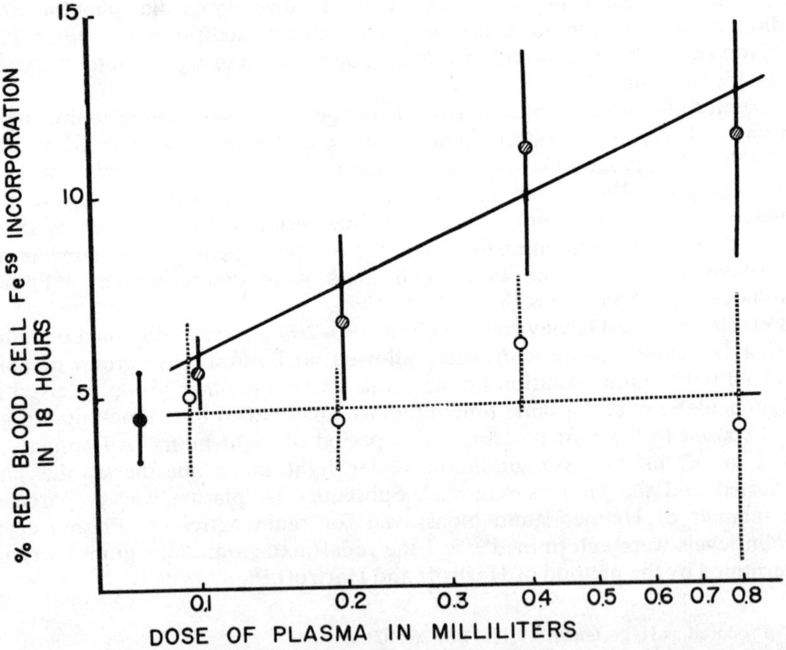

FIGURE 1. Plasma erythropoietin bioassay. The saline control is indicated by the closed circle. Presurgical plasma is indicated by the cross-hatched circles and the solid line. Postsurgical plasma is indicated by the open circles and the interrupted line. Each point represents the average of determinations in each of five mice, the standard deviation is indicated by the vertical lines.

TABLE 2

PLASMA RENIN AND ERYTHROPOIETIN ASSAYS IN HYPERTENSIVE PATIENTS

Diagnosis	Renin ng/ml	% 18 Hr ^{59}Fe RBC Inc. ± S.D.
Saline		4.8 ± 1.1
Normal	10.9	6.2 ± 0.6
Hypertension*	16.0	6.9 ± 1.8
Hypertension**	7.5	6.1 ± 2.1
Malignant hypertension	46.0	7.6 ± 1.0
Malignant hypertension	43.0	7.1 ± 0.8
Renal artery stenosis	50.0	30.2 ± 2.4
Renal artery stenosis	46.0	11.2 ± 1.8

* Before angiotensin II infusion.
** After angiotensin II infusion.

Results of the dose response assay of plasma obtained from a patient with erythrocytosis prior to and following surgical removal of an aldosterone-secreting adrenal adenoma are presented in FIGURE 1. The presurgical plasma was erythropoietically active and the postsurgical plasma was not.

The results of renin and erythropoietin assays of plasma from hypertensive patients are presented in TABLE 2. These patients were not erythrocythemic by the criteria of hematocrit, hemoglobin or red blood cell count. However, the red blood cell mass was not measured. Plasma erythropoietin was not elevated in patients with benign or malignant hypertension, and the renin levels were normal in the former while elevated in the latter. In addition, the infusion of angiotensin II into a hypertensive patient produced no alteration of the plasma erythropoietin levels. In the two instances of unilateral renal artery stenosis both the plasma renin and plasma erythropoietin levels were increased.

Animal Results

The results of the first animal experiments are presented in TABLE 3. The percent red blood cell ^{59}Fe incorporation was not increased over control values by the administration of angiotensin II, renin or aldosterone, while the known erythropoietic stimulus of anemic rabbit plasma induced an approximate sixfold increase.

TABLE 3

PERCENT 18-HOUR RED BLOOD CELL ^{59}FE INCORPORATION

	Assay Material Injected 24 and 48 hr	Assay Material Injected 48 and 72 hr
Assay material saline	4.1 ± 1.5 (5)*	5.8 ± 2.3 (5) t
Angiotensin II, 200 μg	4.5 ± .4 (5) N.S.**	5.1 ± 2.4 (5) N.S.**
Renin, 1500 μg	2.7 ± .4 (5) N.S.**	6.4 ± 1.8 (5) N.S.**
Aldosterone, 2 μg	3.9 ± 1.5 (5) N.S.**	5.4 ± 2.0 (5) N.S.**
Phenylhydrazine anemic rabbit plasma	32.2 ± .6 (5) .001**	30.4 ± .8 (5) .001**

* Number of animals in each group.
** P value determined by students "t" test.

TABLE 4

HEMATOLOGICAL ALTERATION ON THREE-WEEK SALT-FREE DIET AND REGULAR DIET

	No. Rats	Hct vol, % ± S.D.	Red Cell Mass, ml/100 g Body Wt
Regular diet			
before	10	40.5 ± 1.4	
after	10	45.0 ± 1.6	2.12 ± 3.5
Na-free diet			
before	10	40.5 ± 1.5	
after	10	45.5 ± 2.5	1.96 ± .28

TABLE 5

EFFECT OF POLYTHIAZIDE OR HYPOXIA ON PLASMA RENIN OR ERYTHROPOIETIN AND RENAL JUXTAGLOMERULAR GRANULARITY INDEX (JGI)

	Renin ng/100 ml ± S.D.*	Erythropoietin % 48 Hr RBC ^{59}Fe Inc. ± S.D.*	JGI ± S.D.*
Control	668 ± 101	1.0 ± 0.4	21.5 ± 3.5
Polythiazide	1479 ± 597	1.0 ± 0.6	22.0 ± 4.0
Hypoxia	189 ± 62	13.6 ± 3.4	32.0 ± 5.5

* Five animals.

Pertinent hematologic data resulting from sodium deprivation is presented in TABLE 4. No alteration in hemoglobin concentration, hematocrit, or red blood cell mass was observed in animals on sodium free diets when compared to the rats on the liberal sodium diet.

The effect of polythiazide or hypoxia on the plasma renin and erythropoietin levels as well as the renal juxtaglomerular granularity index is tabulated in TABLE 5. Polythiazide produced an increase in the plasma renin level with no alteration in the plasma erythropoietin level or the renal juxtaglomerular granularity index, whereas hypoxia produced a diminution of the plasma renin levels and elevations of the plasma erythropoietin titers and renal juxtaglomerular index.

DISCUSSION

Erythrocytosis has been observed in patients with several types of malignant and nonmalignant tumors. These patients are not easily categorized within the usual classification of polycythemia since abnormalities in leukopoiesis and thrombopoiesis have not been found and arterial oxygen saturation has been normal. Hematologic remission following surgical or radiologic extirpation of the tumor has indeed suggested a causal relationship.[1–3] In addition, erythrocytosis has been noted in patients with neoplastic and nonneoplastic renal disease. The demonstration that erythropoiesis is regulated, in part, by a humoral factor, erythropoietin, and the subsequent demonstration of elevated plasma and tissue erythropoietin levels in these patients[1–3] has suggested that the mechanism by which the erythrocytosis is produced is that of augmented erythropoietin production, either by the altered tissue per se, by the production of a trophic substance, or alternatively, by diminished erythropoietin degradation.

Renal Erythrocytosis

The association of accelerated erythropoiesis and erythrocytosis with certain renal lesions including hydronephrosis, carcinoma, cysts, adenoma and sarcoma has been well documented. Remission of the erythrocytosis following excision of the renal lesions suggests that the renal lesions either produced or stimulated the production of an erythropoietic factor with resultant erythrocytosis. A basis for this hypothesis is clearly provided by many experimental observations[18–23] indicating that erythropoiesis is regulated by the erythropoietic hormone, erythropoietin, and that the kidney is probably the site of formation.

The accumulated evidence supports the contention that the kidney is an important site of erythropoietin production. The hypothesis that increased erythropoietin production was the mechanism responsible for the erythrocytosis associated with renal lesions is supported by the demonstration of elevated plasma erythropoietin levels in plasma, tumor extracts or renal cysts fluid.[1–3] We have evaluated erythropoietin levels in patients with renal tuberculosis, renal cysts, hydronephrosis and renal carcinoma. The patient with renal tuberculosis demonstrated no increased plasma activity. Of the four patients with renal cysts, three had elevated plasma erythropoietin levels, and two of these demonstrated augmented erythropoietic-stimulating activity when the renal cyst fluid was bioassayed. (TABLE 1). Of the three patients with hydronephrosis, two demonstrated augmented plasma erythropoietic-stimulating activity, and four out of five patients with renal carcinoma had elevated plasma erythropoietin levels (TABLE 1). The mechanism by which the anatomic changes in the kidney initiate erythropoietin production is unknown but demonstration of erythropoietic activity in the plasma or cyst fluid of patients with renal lesions and erythrocytosis is consistent with the hypothesis that this erythrocytosis is due to inappropriate production of erythropoietin.

Neoplastic Erythrocytosis

In the single instances of uterine myoma and pheochromocytoma with associated erythrocytosis, plasma erythropoietic-stimulating activity was not demonstrable.

In contrast plasma erythropoietic activity was elevated in the patient with hepatic carcinoma. Erythrocytosis has been reported so frequently in such patients that the presence of erythrocytosis in patients with liver disease should suggest the diagnosis of hepatoma.[7] Erythropoietin levels have been reported as elevated[3–8] or not elevated[5] in such patients.

Recently, many investigators have suggested that erythropoietin may be produced in other organs besides the kidney.[24–27] Hepatic production has been emphasized by Reissman.[26] It is therefore possible that in patients with hepatic carcinoma and erythrocytosis there is hypertrophy of a usual endocrine hepatic function either by the neoplasm or alternatively, by the intervening normal hepatic tissue which may be metabolically altered due to tumor infiltration. This clinical situation seems analogous to that of renal lesions and erythrocytosis mediated through augmented erythropoietin production.

Four out of the five cases of cerebellar hemangioblastoma with associated erythrocytosis studied demonstrated increased erythropoiesis-stimulating activity, one in the plasma alone, two in both the plasma and the cyst fluid, and one in the cyst fluid alone. These findings are in agreement with other reports.[1,3,9] Hypotheses advanced as explanations for the association of erythrocytosis and cerebellar hemangioblastoma have been that 1) the tumor serves as a site of extramedullary erythropoiesis; 2) depression of the respiratory center secondary to increased intracranial pressure produces altered pulmonary ventilation with resultant hypoxemia; 3) stimulation of a mesencephalic erythropoietic center results from altered intraventricular pressure; or finally, 4) there is production of a humoral erythropoietic-stimulating substance by the tumor.[9] If the tumor is a site of extramedullary erythropoiesis, it should concentrate radioiron; the studies of Waldmann *et al.*[9] failed to demonstrate radioiron localization in a cerebellar hemangioblastoma. Stimulation of the medullary respiratory center or an erythropoietic regulatory center by the increased intraventricular pressure seems unlikely since hemangioblastomas constitute only six percent of cerebellar tumors[28] and yet are unique in their association with erythrocytosis. Furthermore, the demonstration of elevated plasma and cyst fluid erythropoietin levels supports the concept that the tumor is producing erythropoietin. Inappropriate elaboration of hormones by nonendocrine tissues has been described in other clinical situations.[29] The morphological similarities between cerebellar hemangioblastoma and renal carcinoma and the concomitant occurrence of both tumors in the same patient suggest an alternate possibility that the cerebellar hemangioblastoma may have a primordial endocrine capacity that manifests itself by regression.

Of particular interest is the patient with erythrocytosis and an aldosterone-secreting adrenal adenoma. Plasma erythropoietin levels were elevated prior to surgical removal of the adenoma and normal after surgery (FIGURE 1). Clinical remission of the erythrocytosis and diminution of the elevated plasma erythropoietin levels following surgical extirpation of the adenoma suggest the existence of a causal relationship between the adenoma and the erythrocytosis. Urinary aldosterone levels which were also elevated prior to surgery returned to normal following surgery, and the hypertension was partially controlled. Although the consensus is that erythropoietin is produced by the kidney, there is no agreement as to the specific renal site. The juxtaglomerular site has many proponents. Hirashima and Takaku[30–31] produced unilateral renal ischemia by the application of a metal ring to the renal artery of rats with resultant augmentation of erythropoiesis and an increase in the plasma erythropoietin. Increased granularity of the juxtaglomerular cells followed application of the constricting ring. They then correlated the granularity of the juxtaglomerular cells with the intensity of the erythropoietic response in several situations. Animals stimulated by bleeding or hemolysis from phenylhydrazine administration showed hypergranularity of the juxtaglomerular cells. Conversely, transfused polycythemic rats with diminished erythropoiesis were noted to have decreased granularity of the juxtaglomerular cells. Goldfarb and Tobian[32–33] have confirmed this indirect evidence that erythropoietin is secreted by the juxtaglomerular cells of the kidney. The juxtaglomerular cell is also the site of production of the renal enzyme, renin, important in the regulation of aldosterone production. Evidence suggesting that erythropoietin is produced in the juxtaglomerular apparatus and the similarity between the renin-angiotensin-aldosterone mechanism and the erythropoietin activator-substrate-erythropoietin mechanism described by Kuratowska *et al.*[34] warrant comparison of the two systems. Alterations in juxtaglomerular granularity have been reported in clinical and experimental situations in which there is increased renin or increased erythropoietin production. Increased juxtaglomerular granularity has also been noted when there is augmented production of renin. The interrelationship of renin, angiotensin II and aldosterone in regulation of arterial pressure and fluid balance has been established.[35–37] Thus, a possible explanation for the coincidence of increased juxtaglomerular granularity and augmented erythropoietic-stimulating activity is that renin, angiotensin or aldosterone exert a direct or indirect erythropoietic effect. Fisher and Crook[38] and Piliego and Rossini[39] have reported that angiotensin II has erythropoietic activity. Bilsel *et al.*[40] were unable to confirm these results. In this laboratory, attempts to demonstrate erythropoietic activity in animals by the exogenous administration of renin, angiotensin II or aldosterone were unsuccessful (TABLE 3). Furthermore, stimulation of the renin-angiotensin-aldosterone system in experimental animals by salt deprivation failed to produce any alteration in red blood cell mass. (TABLE 4). These results suggest that aldosterone does not exert an erythropoietic-stimulating effect and that the elevated plasma erythropoietin levels demonstrated in the patient with an aldosterone-secreting adrenal adenoma were not related to elevated plasma aldosterone.

Augmentation of erythropoietin production has been demonstrated following renal artery constriction[41–42] or renal perfusion with blood maintained at a low oxygen tension.[43-45] However, other investigators have been unable to confirm these results.[46] Recent clinical reports have suggested that erythrocytosis may accompany unilateral renal artery stenosis in man. Luke *et al.*[47] described a 54-year-old male patient with unilateral renal artery stenosis, hypertension and erythrocytosis and speculated that the altered kidney was producing erythropoietin as well as renin. Erythrocytosis characterized by a hematocrit reading in excess of 54 percent in males and 51 percent in females was found in 11 percent of 121 patients with hypertension reported by Frochlich *et al.*[48] These same investigators found hematocrit elevation in 18% of the patients with hypertension and renal arterial stenosis and in only three percent of the patients with essential hypertension, and concluded that the association of erythrocytosis with hypertension should suggest renal artery stenosis.

None of the patients with hypertension studied had elevated hematocrits. However, the two patients with renal artery stenosis and hypertension demonstrated elevated plasma renin and plasma erythropoietin levels (TABLE 5). The two patients with malignant hypertension and high renin levels had no elevation of erythropoietin levels. One patient demonstrated the expected alteration of plasma renin without a concomitant change in plasma erythropoietin following the administration of angiotensin II. The patient with an aldosterone-secreting adrenal adenoma and erythrocytosis had elevated plasma erythropoietin levels and presumably low plasma renin.[49] (FIGURE 1). These clinical observations supply evidence for separate and distinct secretion of renin and erythropoietin.

Administration of polythiazide to experimental animals produced elevation of plasma renin levels without alteration of the juxtaglomerular granularity index or the plasma erythropoietin levels. (TABLE 5). Hypoxia produced a diminution of plasma renin and an elevation of plasma erythropoietin. These results provide additional evidence for separation of the erythropoietic and hypertensive functions of the renal juxtaglomerular apparatus. Further studies are needed in order to delineate the relationship of the juxtaglomerular apparatus to the secretion of erythropoietin.

SUMMARY

The results of plasma or cyst fluid bioassay for erythropoietin in patients with tumors or renal abnormalities and associated erythrocytosis are presented. Erythropoietin levels were not increased in single patients with renal tuberculosis, uterine myoma and pheochromocytoma. Three out of four patients with renal cysts, two out of three patients with hydronephrosis, four out of five patients with cerebellar hemangioblastoma, and single patients with hepatic carcinoma or aldosterone-secreting adrenal adenoma demonstrated elevated erythropoietin levels. In addition, plasma from hypertensive patients was bioassayed for erythropoietic-stimulating activity and renin. Two patients with unilateral renal vascular disease and hypertension had elevated plasma renin and erythropoietin levels. Two patients with malignant hypertension and elevated plasma renin levels had normal plasma erythropoietin levels. The relationship of the renal juxtaglomerular apparatus, renin, angiotensin II, aldosterone and erythropoietin is discussed. Animal experiments are described in which renin, angiotensin II or aldosterone demonstrated no erythropoietic activity. Polythiazide administration produced elevated plasma renin levels without alteration of plasma renin or renal juxtaglomerular granularity whereas hypoxia depressed plasma renin levels and augmented renal juxtaglomerular granularity and plasma erythropoietin levels in rats.

Acknowledgments

We would like to express our thanks to Dr. Charles Kuhn, of the Department of Pathology, Washington University School of Medicine, St. Louis, Mo. for determining the renal juxtaglomerular granularity index, and to Dr. Jacques Bourgoignie, of the Hypertension Section of the Department of Internal Medicine, Washington University School of Medicine, St. Louis, Mo. for the plasma renin assays.

References

1. Lange, R. D. & V. Pavlovic-Kentera. 1964. Progress in Hematology. IV. Grune & Stratton. New York, N. Y.
2. Donati, R. M., R. D. Lange & N. I. Gallagher. 1963. Nephrogenic erythrocytosis. Arch. Int. Med. **112:** 960–965.
3. Donati, R. M., J. M. McCarthy, R. D. Lange & N. I. Gallagher. 1963. Erythrocythemia and neoplastic tumors. Ann. Int. Med. **58:** 47–55.
4. Bitterman, W. 1964. High plasma erythropoietin activity associated with prostatic carcinoma. J. Urol. **92:** 537–539.
5. Lehman, C. J., A. J. Erslev & R. M. Myerson. 1963. Erythrocytosis associated with hepatocellular carcinoma. Amer. J. Med. **35:** 439–442.
6. Libre, E. P. & P. T. Rodilosso. 1965. Hepatoma with dysproteinemia and erythrocythemia. Arch. Int. Med. **115:** 48–52.
7. Brownstein, M. H. & H. S. Ballard. 1966. Hepatoma associated with erythrocytosis. Amer. J. Med. **40:** 204–210.
8. Nakao, K., K. Kimura, Y. Miura & F. Takaku. 1966. Erythrocytosis associated with carcinoma of the liver. Amer. J. Med. Sci. **251:** 161–165.
9. Waldmann, T. A., E. H. Levin & M. Baldwin. 1961. The association of polycythemia with a cerebellar hemangioblastoma. Amer. J. Med. **31:** 318–323.
10. Gallagher, N. I., D. Q. Hagan, J. M. McCarthy & R. D. Lange. 1961. Response of starved rats and polycythemic rats to graded doses of erythropoietin. Proc. Soc. Exp. Biol. Med. **106:** 127–130.
11. Mann, D. L., M. L. Sites, R. M. Donati & N. I. Gallagher. 1965. Erythropoietic-stimulating activity during the first ninety days of life. Proc. Soc. Exp. Biol. Med. **118:** 212–214.
12. Cotes, P. M. & D. R. Bangham. 1961. Bioassay of erythropoietin in mice made polycythaemic by exposure to air at a reduced pressure. Nature (Lond.) **191:** 1065–1067.
13. Helmer, O. M. 1957. Differentiation between two forms of angiotonin by means of spirally cut strips of rabbit aorta. Amer. J. Physiol. **188:** 571.
14. Kaplan, N. M. & J. G. Silah. 1964. The effect of angiotensin II on the blood pressure of humans with hypertensive disease. J. Clin. Invest. **43:** 659–669.
15. Gibson, II, J. G., S. Weiss, R. D. Evans, W. C. Peacock, J. W. Irvine, Jr., W. M. Good & A. F. Kip. 1946. Measurement of circulating red cell volume by means of two isotopes of iron. J. Clin. Invest. **106:** 616–626.
16. Bourgonie, J., F. Catanzaro & H. M. Perry. Unpublished method.

17. Hartroft, P. M. & W. S. Hartroft. 1955. Studies on renal juxtaglomerular cells. II. Correlation of the degree of granulation of juxtaglomerular cells with the width of the zona glomerulosa of the adrenal cortex. J. Exp. Med. **102:** 205–212.
18. Jacobson, L. O., E. Goldwasser, W. Fried & L. F. Plzak. 1957. Role of the kidney in erythropoiesis. Nature (Lond.) **179:** 633.
19. Reichlin, M. & W. J. Harrington. 1960. Studies on erythropoietin. I. Demonstration of erythropoietin in normal plasma. Blood **16:** 1298.
20. Van Lessen, H. G., M. Stefanini & F. E. Smith. 1958. Erythrocytosis after unilateral partial ligation of renal vein in dogs. Clin. Res. **6:** 193.
21. Mitus, W. J., P. Galbraith & M. Gollerkeri. 1962. Experimental renal erythrocytosis. Trans. Internat. Soc. Hematol.
22. Naets, J. P. 1960. The role of the kidney in erythropoiesis. Acta. Clin. Belg. **15:** 361.
23. Suki, W. & A. Grollman. 1960. Role of the kidney in erythropoiesis. Amer. J. Physiol. **199:** 629–632.
24. Rosse, W. F. & T. A. Waldmann. 1962. The role of the kidney in the erythropoietic response to hypoxia in parabiotic rats. Blood **19:** 75.
25. Erslev, A. J. 1958. Erythropoietic function in uremic rabbits. Arch. Int. Med. **101:** 407.
26. Reissman, K. R. 1962. Erythropoiesis. L. O. Jacobson & M. Doyle, Eds. Grune & Stratton. New York, N. Y.
27. Jacobsen, E. M., A. K. Davis & E. L. Alpen. 1956. Relative effectiveness of phenylhydrazine treatment and hemorrhage in the production of an erythropoietic factor. Blood **11:** 937.
28. Cushing, H. & P. Bailey. 1928. Tumors Arising From Blood Vessels of the Brain. Malformations and Hemangioblastomas. Charles C. Thomas. Springfield, Ill.
29. Lipsett, M. D., W. D. Odell, L. E. Rosenberg & T. A. Waldmann. 1964. Humoral syndromes associated with nonendocrine tumor. Ann. Int. Med. **61:** 733–56.
30. Hirashima, K. & F. Takaku. 1962. Experimental studies on erythropoietin: II. The relationship between juxtaglomerular cells and erythropoietin. Blood **20:** 1.
31. Takaku, F., K. Hirashima & K. Nakao. 1962. Studies on the mechanism of erythropoietin production. I. Effect of unilateral constriction of the renal artery. J. Lab. Clin. Med. **59:** 815.
32. Goldfarb, B. & L. Tobian. 1962. The interrelationship of hypoxia, erythropoietin, and the renal juxtaglomerular cell. Proc. Soc. Exp. Biol. Med. **111:** 510–511.
33. Goldfarb, B. & L. Tobian. 1963. Relationship of erythropoietin to renal juxtaglomerular cells. Proc. Soc. Exp. Biol. Med. **112:** 65.
34. Kuratowska, Z., B. Lewartowski, & B. Lipinski. 1964. Chemical and biologic properties of an erythropoietin generating substance obtained from perfusates of isolated anoxic kidneys. J. Lab. & Clin. Med. **64:** 226–237.
35. Hartroft, P. M. & W. S. Hartroft. 1953. Studies on renal juxtaglomerular cells. J. Exp. Med. **97:** 415.
36. Slater, J. D. H., B. H. Barbour, H. H. Henderson, A. G. T. Casper & F. C. Bartter. 1963. Influence of the pituitary and renin-angiotensin system on the secretion of aldosterone, cortisol and corticosterone. J. Clin. Invest. **42:** 1504.
37. Tobian, L., J. Thompson, R. Twedt & J. Janeek 1958. The granulation of juxtaglomerular cells in renal hypertension, desoxycorticosterone and post-desoxycorticosterone hypertension, adrenal regeneration hypertension, and adrenal insufficiency. J. Clin. Invest. **37:** 660.
38. Fisher, J. W. & J. J. Crook. 1962. Influence of several hormones on erythropoiesis and oxygen consumption in the hypophysectomized rat. Blood **19:** 557.
39. Piliego, N. & P. Rossini. 1963. I fattori emodinamici efficienti sulla secrezione renale di eritropoietina. Nota IV: L'aumento dell'eritropoietina dopo infusione di angiotensina II sintetica. Rass. Fisiop. Cl. Ter. **35:** 688–693
40. Bilsel, V. C., J. E. Wood & R. D. Lange. 1963. Angiotensin II and erythropoiesis. Proc. Soc. Exp. Biol. Med. **114:** 475.
41. Hansen, P. 1964. Polycythaemia produced by constriction of the renal artery in a rabbit. Acta Path. Microbiol. Scand. **60:** 465–472.
42. Hansen, P. 1964. Demonstration of erythropoietin in urine and in kidney extracts from rabbits with experimental constriction of the left renal artery. Acta Path. Microbiol. **61:** 514–520.
43. Kuratowska, Z., B. Lewartowski & E. Michalak. 1961. Studies on the production of erythropoietin by isolated perfused organs. Blood **18:** 527.
44. Fisher, J. W., R. Schofield & D. D. Porteous. 1965. Effects of renal hypoxia on erythropoietin production. Brit. J. Haemat. **11:** 382–388.

45. Reissman, K. R. & T. Nomura. 1962. Erythropoiesis. L. O. Jacobson & M. Doyle, Eds. Grune & Stratton. New York, N. Y.
46. Cooper, G. W. & M. R. Nocenti. 1961. Unilateral renal ischemia and erythropoietin. Proc. Soc. Exp. Biol. Med. **108:** 546.
47. Luke, R. G., A. C. Kennedy, W. B. Stirling & G. A. McDonald. 1965. Renal artery stenosis, hypertension and polycythaemia. Brit. Med. J. **1:** 164–166.
48. Frohlich, E. D., R. C. Tarazi, H. P. Dunstan, R. W. Gifford & I. H. Page. 1965. Polycythemia in hypertension: Another clue to renal arterial disease. Clin. Res. **13:** 554.
49. Conn, J. W., E. L. Cohen & D. R. Rovner. 1964. Suppression of plasma renin activity in primary aldosteronism. J.A.M.A. **190:** 213.

ERYTHROCYTE PRODUCTION AND METABOLISM IN ANEPHRIC AND UREMIC MEN*

David G. Nathan, Laurence H. Beck, Constantine L. Hampers and John P. Merrill

Richard C. Curtis Hematology Laboratory and Department of Medicine, Peter Bent Brigham Hospital, and the Department of Medicine, Harvard Medical School, Boston, Mass.

Some of the data presented in this Annal suggest that in man total absence of renal tissue does not inhibit erythropoiesis more markedly than does severe uremia itself. We will present more confirmatory evidence of this statement, as well as some studies of the metabolism of uremic erythrocytes, which have led us to a general hypothesis regarding the pathogenesis of uremia.

Three years ago we presented erythrokinetic investigations of four patients made anephric in preparation for renal transplantation.[1] These studies revealed decreased erythropoiesis, with maximal RBC ^{59}Fe uptakes in the range of 35 to 70%. However, these patients were able to maintain hemoglobin levels of from 7–9 g percent. Furthermore, a sharply increased erythropoietic effort occurred in one patient who became hypoxic while in the anephric state. These results were interpreted as indications that in humans, in contrast to dogs, a basal rate of erythropoiesis exists which does not require the presence of kidneys, and that an augmented erythropoietic effort can occur without the participation of erythropoietin of renal origin.

We have now studied an additional three anephric patients. The results are shown in FIGURE 1. Two patients showed decreased plasma ^{59}Fe clearance rates and all three had depressed effective erythropoiesis, with maximal RBC ^{59}Fe uptake ranging from 31 to 44%.

One patient was studied just prior to nephrectomy and again in the anephric state (FIGURE 2). There was little difference between the two studies, indicating that the presence or absence of kidneys had no effect on erythropoiesis in this patient. It should be emphasized, however, that total nephrectomy in a patient with chronic renal disease may reduce renal mass very little. For example, the average combined renal weight in these three totally nephrectomized patients was 157 g, some of which was accounted for by fibrous scar tissue.

When bone marrow smears from these anephric patients and from several other uremic patients were examined, an abnormality of maturation was evident which, although quite variable in degree, was present in almost all cases. This is shown in FIGURE 3. Granulocyte precursor nuclei were elongated and twisted, an abnormality that is correlated with increased Arneth counts in the peripheral blood. Red cell precursors have suggestive megaloblastic changes, with poor clumping of chromatin. Since several of these patients were on chronic dialysis programs, the suggestion was made that folic acid stores were depleted through dialysis. Serum folate levels were, indeed, low in some cases, but these measurements did not correlate with the degree of abnormality in morphology.[2]

The findings suggest that the uremic state itself tends to depress maturation of bone marrow precursors. Lack of renal erythropoietin is not a satisfactory ex-

* These clinical studies were carried out in the Clinical Research Center of the Harvard Medical School and the Peter Bent Brigham Hospital supported by a grant (8M01–FR–03) from the National Institutes of Health, Public Health Service, United States Department of Health, Education, and Welfare; supported in part by the United States Public Health Service grant AM–00965–11 and by a grant from the John A. Hartford Foundation.

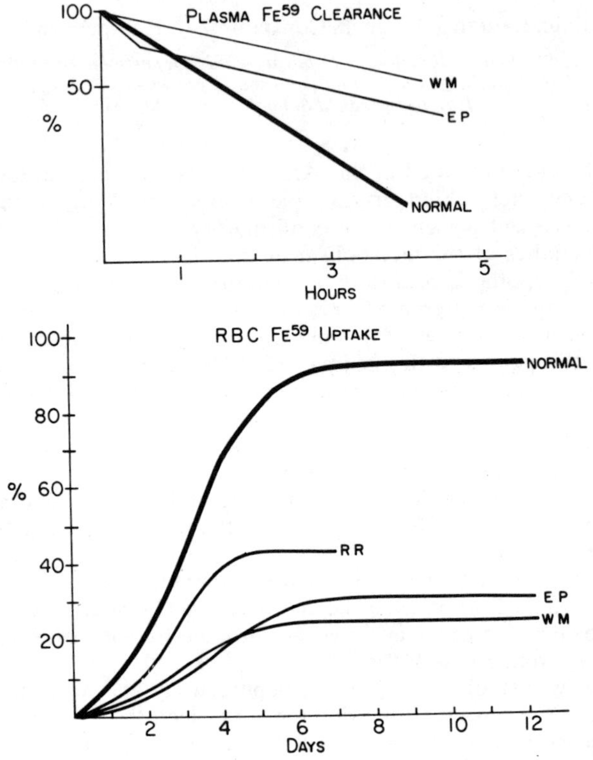

FIGURE 1. The rate of disappearance of ^{59}Fe from the plasma and the appearance of ^{59}Fe in the red cells of three anephric patients. Normal values are shown as heavy lines.

planation for such depression. Perhaps a circulating toxin, retained in uremia, is responsible. There is evidence in the literature for a suppressive effect of uremic plasma upon bone marrow precursor cells.[3,4]

We have not yet studied the effect of uremic plasma on marrow precursors, but we have examined the metabolism of the uremic erythrocytes of 15 patients in autologous plasma. Our measurements have included erythrocyte, potassium flux, ATP stability, and glycolysis. We were particularly interested in uremic erythrocytes because of their bizarre morphology, as shown in FIGURE 4. Note the spicules and helmet shapes in this smear of a patient with uremia.

Potassium flux was measured with ^{42}K and is the same in normal and uremic red cells, the potassium influx averaging 1.7 mEq/l cells/hour in each case. This continence of internal potassium is of interest in view of the bizarre morphology seen. ATP content is much higher in the uremic, than in the normal erythrocyte, averaging 2215 μmole/l cells in the uremic, compared with 1378 μmole/l cells in the normal. This is consistent with the recent work of Welt.[5] Associated with the high ATP content is an elevated glycolytic rate in uremic red cells. Uremic red

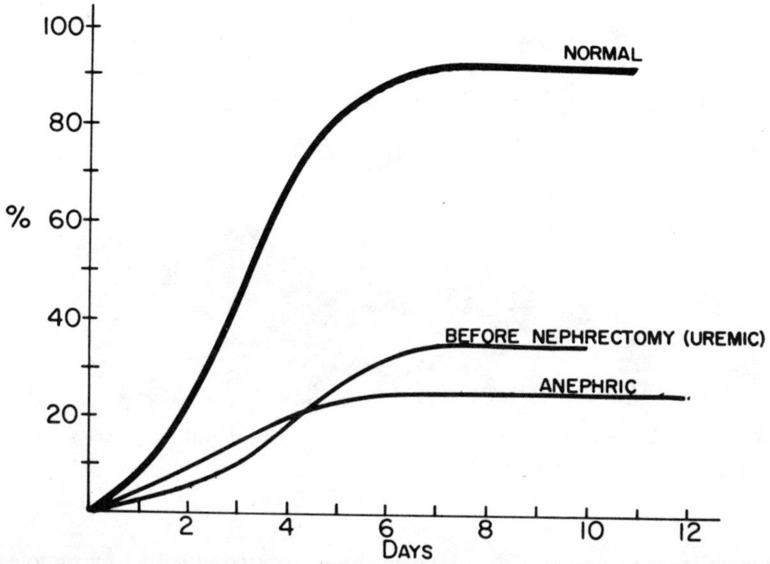

FIGURE 2. The rate of appearance of ^{59}Fe in the red cells of a uremic patient before and after nephrectomy.

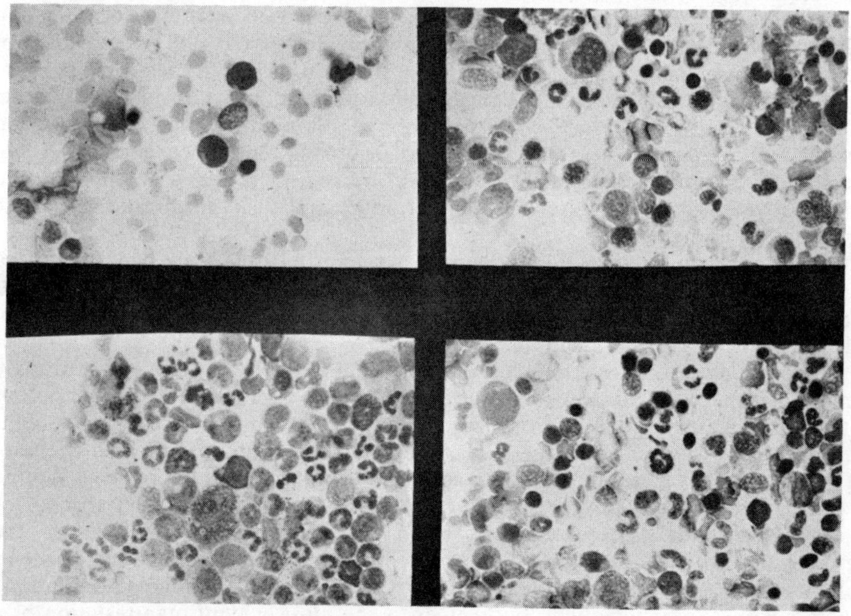

FIGURE 3. Bone marrow smears of anephric and uremic patients under treatment with hemodialysis. Erythroblasts are present. The granulocyte nuclei are twisted, elongated and multilobed.

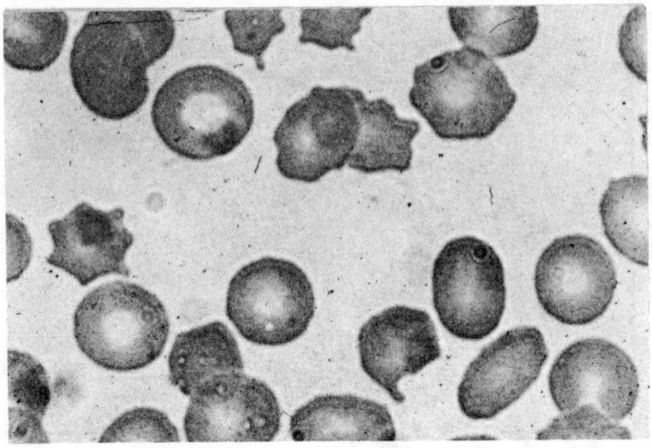

FIGURE 4. Peripheral smear of a severely uremic patient with an intact spleen. Note the numerous spicule and helmet forms.

cells utilize 2.33 mmole glucose/l cells/hour, compared with 1.69 mmole/l cells/hour in normal cells. Lactate production averages 4.47 mmole/l cells/hour in the uremic, and 3.32 mmole/l cells/hour in the normal red cell. These differences are significant.

The elevated glycolytic rate can not be attributed to a younger cell population since there was no correlation between the glycolytic rate and reticulocyte count. On the other hand, the glycolytic rate roughly increased with the severity of kidney disease. The latter is estimated as a function of serum creatinine concentration. Since serum phosphate concentration tends to rise with increasing renal disease, it was thought that glycolysis might be stimulated by the elevated intracellular phosphate concentration observed in uremia. Increased phosphate concentration is known to stimulate glycolysis.[6] Indeed, there was a definite correlation between glycolytic rate and the serum phosphate concentration in these patients.

In an effort to confirm this hypothesis, uremic red cells have been incubated in a plasma-like buffer with a normal phosphate concentration. Preliminary results indicate that the uremic red cell consumes glucose at a normal rate when placed in a normal phosphate medium.

These studies of uremic red cells do not reveal the presence of a retained toxin in the plasma of uremic patients. But a number of well-documented observations strongly suggest that one or more toxins must be attacking several organ systems in the uremic state. Lymphopenia and monocytopenia are common in uremia.[7] The thymus shows marked atrophy, and cellular immunity is depressed.[8] Wound healing is often markedly prolonged in uremic patients, with virtual absence of granulation tissue.[9] These examples represent rapidly proliferating tissues, the growth or turnover rates of which are depressed in the uremic state. It seems likely, therefore, that the suppression of erythropoiesis in the marrow by uremic factors is not a specific effect, but, rather, is the most evident manifestation of a total body suppression of active cell populations by noxious factor(s) retained in the plasma of uremic individuals.

References

1. Nathan, D. G., E. Schupak, F. Stohlman, Jr. & J. P. Merrill. 1964. Erythropoiesis in anephric man. J. Clin. Invest. **43:** 2158.
2. Hampers, C. L., R. Streiff, D. G. Nathan, D. Snyder & J. P. Merrill. 1967. Megaloblastic hematopoiesis in chronic renal failure. New Eng. J. Med. **276:** 551.
3. Markson, J. L. & J. B. Rennie. 1956. The anaemia of chronic renal insufficiency. The effect of serum from azotaemic patients on the maturation of normoblasts in suspension cultures. Scot. Med. J. **1:** 320.
4. Markson, J. L. & J. M. Moore. 1962. The anaemia of chronic renal insufficiency: autoradiographic studies in normoblasts cultured in uraemic serum. Brit. J. Haemat. **8:** 414.
5. Welt, L. G., J. R. Sachs & T. J. McManus. 1964. An ion transport defect in erythrocytes from uremic patients. Trans. Assoc. Amer. Phys. **77:** 169.
6. Rose, I. A., J. V. B. Warms & E. L. O'Connell. 1964. Role of inorganic phosphate in stimulating the glucose utilization of human red cells. Biochem. Biophys. Res. Comm. **15:** 33.
7. Jensson, O. 1958. Observations on the leukocyte blood picture in acute uremia. Brit. J. Haemat. **4:** 422.
8. Wilson, W. E. C., C. H. Kirkpatrick & D. W. Talmage. 1965. Suppression of immunologic responsiveness in uremia. Ann. Int. Med. **62:** 1.
9. Schreiner, G. E. & J. F. Maher. 1961. Uremia. Charles C. Thomas. : 375. Springfield, Ill.

FETAL AND NEONATAL ERYTHROPOIESIS*

G. Lucarelli, A. Porcellini, C. Carnevali, A. Carmena** and F. Stohlman, Jr.

Institute de Semeiotica Medica, Universita di Parma, Parma, Italy

and

St. Elizabeth's Hospital, Tufts Medical School, Boston, Mass.

The regulation of red cell production in the adult animal has been shown to be governed, at least in part, by oxygen-dependent erythropoietin production by the kidney. In rodents the degree of dependency on renally produced erythropoietin approaches the absolute.[1] Thus the nephrectomized rat or mouse has almost complete suppression of red cell production. Changes in the oxygen supply-demand relationship have been shown to have a profound effect upon the rate of erythropoiesis. It is to be noted, however, that such perturbations in high order mammals[2,3] do not produce as marked a change in red cell production as that in the rodent. The question has been raised as to whether regulation of erythropoiesis in fetal and neonatal life is the same as that for the "adult"[4] To answer this question, the evolution of the erythron and its regulation have been studied in the fetal and neonatal rat, which is a relatively immature animal in comparison with human beings at birth, and in the guinea pig, an animal in which the degree of maturity at birth approaches that of the human being. These data will be briefly summarized and are reviewed extensively elsewhere.[5]

Fetal Erythropoiesis in the Rat

As in all mammals erythropoiesis in the rat develops in three stages: the yolk sac, hepatic, and myeloid. Erythropoiesis in the rat is predominantly hepatic at birth. After birth there is an explosive increase in the erythroid activity of the bone marrow. To illustrate this, sections of fetal liver and bone marrow are shown in FIGURES 1 and 2, and are compared with that of the six-day-old newborn in FIGURE 3. During the period of hepatic red cell formation three distinct morphologic compartments may be identified (FIGURE 4). The first is that of an undifferentiated cell of about 30–50 μ in diameter, which frequently occurs in a syncytium and has a "foamy," pale, basophilic cytoplasma, and a leptochromatic nucleus with large nucleoli.[1] This, we feel, serves as the stem cell for the erythroid compartment; later in fetal life this cell can be seen differentiating into the hepatic cells. The second compartment is that of a primitive cell but one in which there is more basophilia of the cytoplasm, less vacuolization, more condensed nuclear chromatin, and somewhat smaller nucleoli. This has the appearance of a cell oriented toward erythroid differentiation, or the so-called Ferrata cell. Lastly, there are the clearly identifiable erythroid elements.

Hypertransfusion of the mother results in the shutdown of erythropoiesis that is characteristic of the adult rat. It has been shown, however, that this has little effect on red cell formation in the fetus.[6,7] Starvation of the adult rat also produces a profound suppression of red cell production, but as is shown in TABLES 1 and 2, fetal erythropoiesis is unaffected by maternal starvation.

Neonatal Erythropoiesis

Values for the peripheral blood of the rat at birth and during the neonatal

* Supported in part by grants HE–07542 and HTS–5600 from the National Heart Institute.

** Supported in part by the Consejo Nacional Investigaciones Cientificas, Argentina.

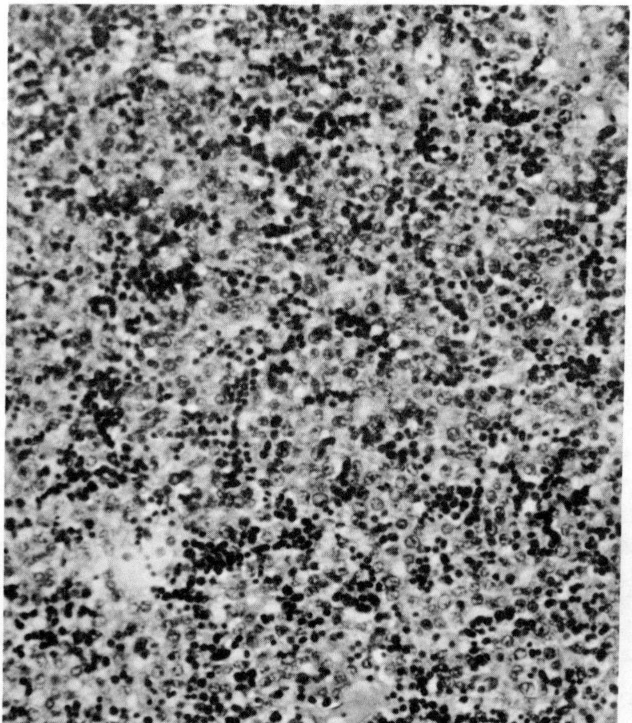

FIGURE 1. A section of the fetal liver from a 15-day-old rat. The parenchymal organization is not yet complete. Note intense erythropoietic activity.

period are given in TABLE 3. It is to be noted that there is hypochromia in the face of striking macrocytosis. This type of cell is not seen in the adult where microcytosis invariably precedes hypochromia.[8] As previously mentioned, there is an explosive increase in erythropoiesis in the bone marrow after birth and a concomitant decrease in hepatic red cell production (FIGURE 5). The bone marrow of the newborn rat, like the fetal liver, is characterized by three compartments, the syncytial cell, the Ferrata cell, and the differentiated erythroid elements. As the animal matures, there is a gradual decrease in the frequency of syncytial cells until the cell is rarely seen in adult life (TABLE 4).

Effects of Perturbation of Erythropoiesis in the Neonatal as Compared with the Adult Rat

It has been extensively documented that in the adult rodent hypoxia or anemia will stimulate red cell production, whereas nephrectomy, hypertransfusion and starvation suppress erythropoiesis. These effects are thought to be the results of changes in erythropoietin production by the kidney, which serves as a principal regulator of erythropoiesis in the adult. In contrast erythropoiesis in the newborn animal is relatively little affected by these perturbations. The effect of bilateral nephrectomy on red cell production is shown in FIGURE 6. After 48 hr in the adult there is a marked decrease in red cell precursors; those present are late polychromatophilic forms. Seventy-two hr after nephrectomy few erythroid elements are seen. In the newborn prior to the tenth day of life, nephrectomy does not affect red cell production. Thereafter there is a gradual transition to the adult type response (FIGURE 6). That the continued production of red cells in the newborn animal is not the result of absorption of maternal erythropoietin has been proven in studies in which the mother was hypertransfused.[4] This resulted in the predictable decrease in maternal erythropoiesis but the red cell production in the nursing nephrectomized animal was unaffected.

Starvation suppresses erythropoiesis in the adult, but the response is quite different in the newborn animal (TABLES 5–7). Not only does there appear to be

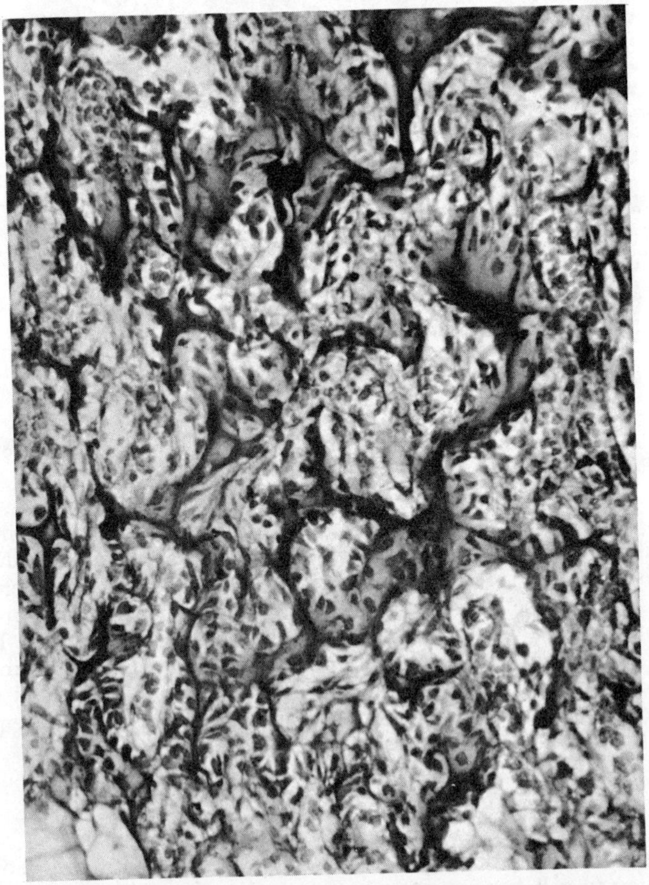

FIGURE 2. Section of the femur from an 18-day-old rat fetus. The bone marrow cavity is devoid of erythropoietic activity.

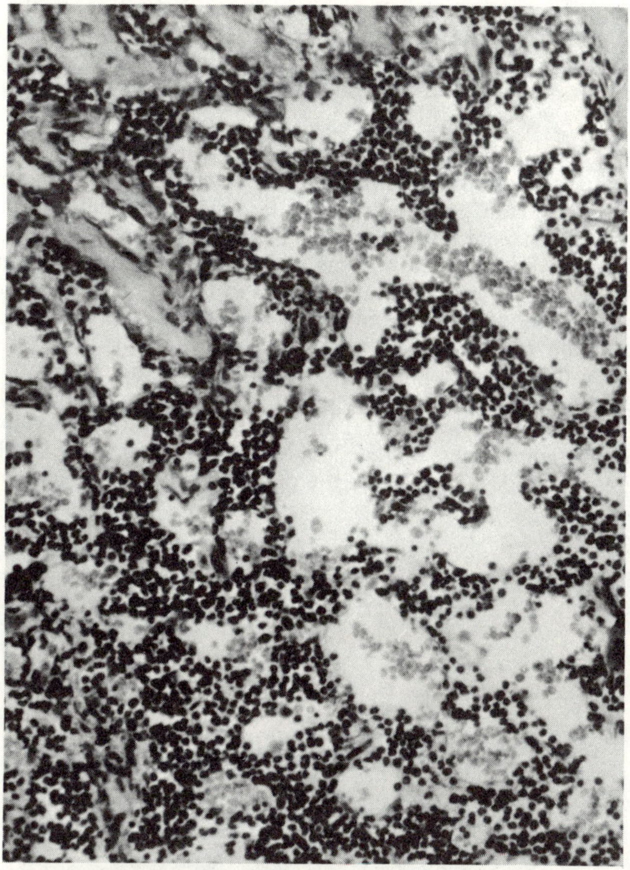

FIGURE 3. Intense erythropoietic activity in a section of the femur from a six-day-old rat.

no suppression of red cell production after starvation, but also in a substantial number of animals starved prior to the tenth to 15th day of life, the percentage of erythroid elements in the bone marrow appears to be somewhat greater than in litter mate controls. This appears to be due to an accumulation of cells in metaphase (FIGURE 7). The metaphase accumulation appears to be limited to the erythroid elements and the primitive undifferentiated cell. Myeloid and megakaryocytic metaphase accumulation has not been seen. The cause of metaphase accumulation is at the moment unknown, but it is clear that many cells escape the "block" since red cell production, as evaluated by their reticulocyte count, did not fall. After the 15th day of life the reaction to starvation gradually changes to that observed in the adult animal.

The pattern of response to hypoxia, a potent stimulus to erythropoiesis in the adult, also demonstrates the difference in the regulatory mechanism for neonatal and adult red cell production in the rat.[9] In animals exposed to 0.4 atm between the ninth and 16th day of life there was little stimulation of red cell production (TABLES 8 & 9). Those exposed between the 17th and 24th days of life had a questionable increase in red cell production, as judged from the hematocrit, reticulocyte count and the percent of erythroid elements in the bone marrow. Exposure between the 25th and 32nd days of life produced a more striking increase in erythropoiesis, but it was still not of the magnitude seen in adult animals.

The Guinea Pig

It is clear from the above that in fetal and newborn rats regulation of red cell production differs from that observed in the adult. To study the possible effect of maturity of animals at birth on the regulation of red cell production, erythropoiesis in the newborn guinea pig was evaluated. The guinea pig at birth has a hematocrit slightly higher than that observed in the adult animal (TABLE 10). In all other respects, however, the red cell values are not too dissimilar from those of the adult; the red cells are normocytic and the reticulocyte count is only slightly greater than in the adult. As the animal grows, there is a fall in hematocrit and between the 20th and 30th days of life, an increase in red cell production associated with reticulocytosis and return of hematocrit to adult values. The bone marrow of the guinea pig, unlike that of the rat, is actively erythropoietic at birth. There is a modest increase in the percentage of erythroid elements during

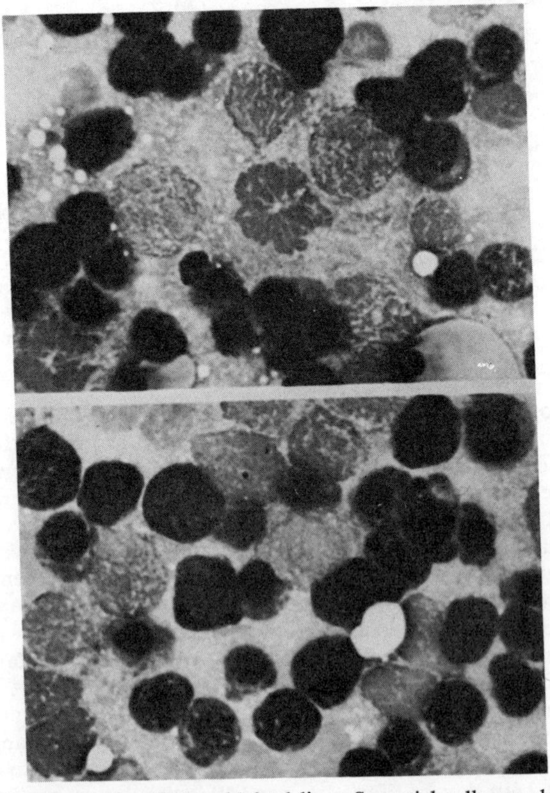

FIGURE 4. Imprint smear of a 15-day-old fetal liver. Syncytial cells are shown above and erythroid cells of all stages of maturation below.

TABLE 1

THE EFFECT OF STARVATION ON THE PREGNANT RAT AND FETUS*

	Normal	Starved 120 Hr
	Mother	
Hemoglobin	14.0	14.0
Hematocrit	40.0	42.0
Reticulocyte	2.7	0.1
Percent red cell precursors	26.0	5.0
	Fetus	
Undifferentiated cells	34.0	37.0
Ferrata cells	2.0	3.0
Erythroid percursors	61.0	59.0
Pronormoblasts	5.0	4.0
Basophilic normoblasts	17.0	15.0
Polychromatophilic normoblasts	39.0	40.0
Megaloblasts	2.0	1.0
Myeloid cells	1.0	1.0
Megakaryocytes	0.1	0.1
Erythroid mitotic index	6.0	7.0
Retic (peripheral blood)	90.0	90.0

* Peripheral blood and bone marrow values of a normal pregnant rat and one which was starved between the 12th and 17th days of life. Fetal values refer to average values from three fetuses from each mother. The fetal differentials were done on liver imprints.

TABLE 2

THYMIDINE LABELING OF ERYTHROID CELLS IN THE PREGNANT RAT*

	Percent Labeled Cells Normal	Percent Labeled Cells Fasted	Percent Labeled Mitosis Normal	Percent Labeled Mitosis Fasted
Undifferentiated cells	70	80	100	100
Ferrata cells	88	84	—	—
Pronormoblasts	96	99	100	100
Basophilic normoblasts	89	95	100	100
Polychromatophilic normoblasts	58	59	100	100

* The labeling index and labeled mitotic index from the liver imprint of fetuses from normal and starved mothers. The mothers were starved between the 12th and 17th days of life; 1 mc/g of thymidine was given to the mother four hr prior to sacrifice. The values represent the mean of 15 fetuses from three mothers.

TABLE 3

MEAN PERIPHERAL BLOOD VALUES FOR SIX ANIMALS ± 1 SE AT VARIOUS AGES IN THE RAT

Age Days	Weight g	Hematocrit %	Hemoglobin g/100 ml	MCV* μ^3	MCHC* %	Reticulocytes %
1	6.7 ± 0.16	34 ± 1.3	10.2 ± 0.4	136 ± 2.2	30 ± 0.3	89 ± 0.7
5	13.7 ± 0.48	29.3 ± 0.7	8.3 ± 0.4	107 ± 2.9	28.7 ± 1.0	45 ± 2.9
10	21 ± 0.81	30.3 ± 0.6	8.6 ± 0.4	89 ± 1.8	27.7 ± 0.8	29 ± 2.3
20	47 ± 2.7	32.5 ± 1.3	9.5 ± 0.5	67 ± 2.3	29.3 ± 0.97	22 ± 1.5
30	84 ± 3.9	40 ± 0.1	12.2 ±	63 ± 1.1	31 ± 0.1	6.6 ± 1.5
40	123 ± 10.1	42.4 ± 0.6	13.9 ± 0.3	61.5 ± 1.3	33 ± 0.4	3.7 ± 0.44
67	153 ± 4.4	44.0 ± 1.1	14.4 ± 0.3	55.3 ± 0.8	33 ± 0.3	2.3 ± 0.26

* MCV = mean corpuscular volume; MCHC = mean corpuscular hemoglobin concentration. (Reprinted from G. Lucarelli *et al.*, Journal of Clinical Investigation, Vol. 43, No. 11,

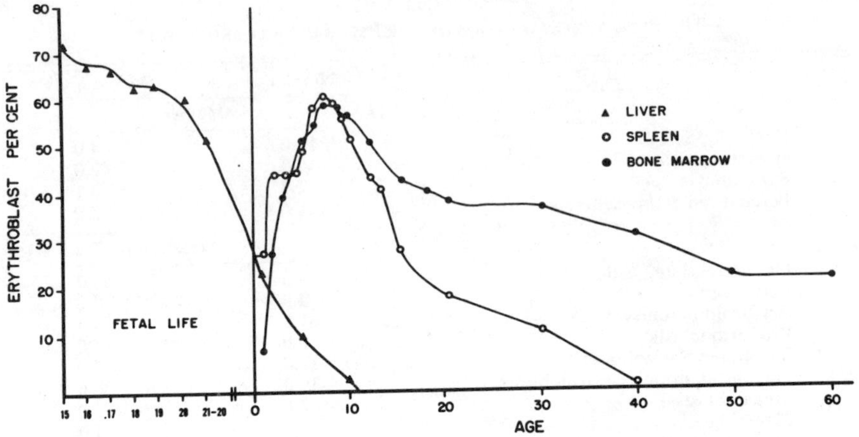

FIGURE 5. The percentage of nucleated red cell precursors with age in the liver, spleen, and bone marrow of the rat. Fetal values are based on the mean of eight animals per point; splenic and liver values of the newborn are the mean of six animals per point; the bone marrow values in the newborn represent the mean of 8–14 animals for each point (reproduced by courtesy of the Journal of Clinical Investigation **43:** 2198, 1964).

the first three days of life, but the percentage (~20%) is much less than that of the rat. The primitive undifferentiated syncytial type of cell is not seen in the guinea pig. Rather, there is an undifferentiated "reticulum" cell such as that seen after the 30th day in the rat. On about the 15th day there is a further increase in erythroid elements followed by a return to adult levels after the 30th day. This precedes the aforementioned reticulocytosis and increase in hematocrit. Unlike the neonatal rat the newborn guinea pig responds to starvation with a suppression

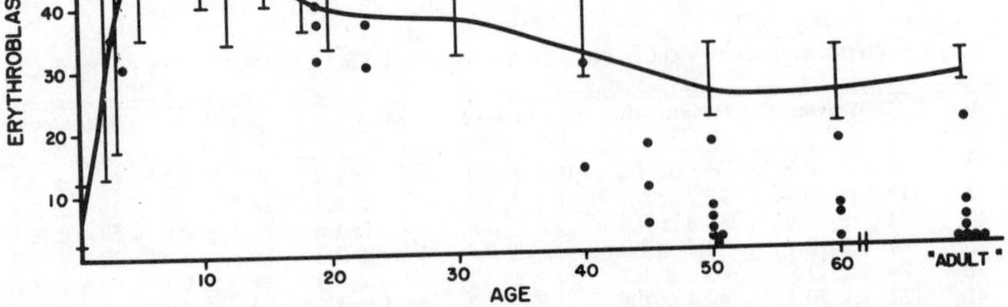

FIGURE 6. The effect of nephrectomy on the percentage of nucleated red cells in the bone marrow. The line represents the normal average with the range indicated by the bars. Each point represents a nephrectomized animal. (Courtesy of the Journal of Clinical Investigation **43:** 2195, 1964).

TABLE 4

RELATIVE NUMBERS OF NUCLEATED CELLS IN THE NORMAL RAT*

No. of Animals	Age days	Primitive	Mononuclear	Myeloid	Lymphoid	Erythroid	Prn	BN	PN	MI (red)
9	1	9	2	70	12	6	2	3	1	4
		1–26	2–4	46–86	4–18	3–12	1–4	1–10	2–11	1–12
7	3	14	2	36	5	43	7	15	22	5
		7–26	2–5	3–7	4–19	17–70	3–13	6–29	3–27	1–7
6	5	15	2	22	9	52	4	14	34	5
		12–18	1–4	14–41	5–15	35–61	3–7	7–20	24–35	3–7
8	8	7	3	17	14	59	9	21	29	5
		5–12	1–6	12–20	6–19	43–64	6–16	15–28	23–34	3–7
7	10	8	3	21	14	54	10	18	26	4
		5–14	2–6	13–25	7–25	40–69	6–14	12–24	14–35	2–5
5	15	5	4	26	23	42	8	14	20	4
		3–10	3–9	17–44	11–36	40–47	3–11	12–26	13–24	2–4
6	20	6	6	25	23	40	8	14	18	3
		4–9	2–11	15–47	6–32	32–50	4–10	9–19	14–23	2–4
4	32	2	2	42	15	39	5	12	22	2
		1–3	2–3	41–50	12–18	32–43	5–5	10–12	14–24	1–3
8	43	3	3	41	18	35	5	10	20	3
		1–4	1–6	23–51	10–25	28–43	3–7	9–14	14–23	1–5
4	60	6	5	46	17	26	4	7	15	2
		4–8	3–6	45–50	12–24	20–32	2–4	5–8	12–16	0–4

* The age refers to the day of sacrifice. The average value for each class is given above with the range below. Primitive cells during the first 30 days of life are a syncytial type of cell described in the text; thereafter, they are reticulum cells. Complete agreement on distinguishing hemocytoblasts (Ferrata) and lymphoblasts could not be achieved; accordingly, these are classified as mononuclear cells. The total percentage of nucleated red cells is given under erythroid; the cells are further subdivided into prn, pronormoblast; BN, basophilic normoblast; PN, polychromatophilic normoblasts and the rare orthochromatic normoblast. The values for the latter are given as percent of the total nucleated marrow population. The mitotic index (MI) refers to the red cell elements. (Reprinted from G. Lucarelli *et al.*, Journal of Clinical Investigation, Vol. 43, No. 11, 1964).

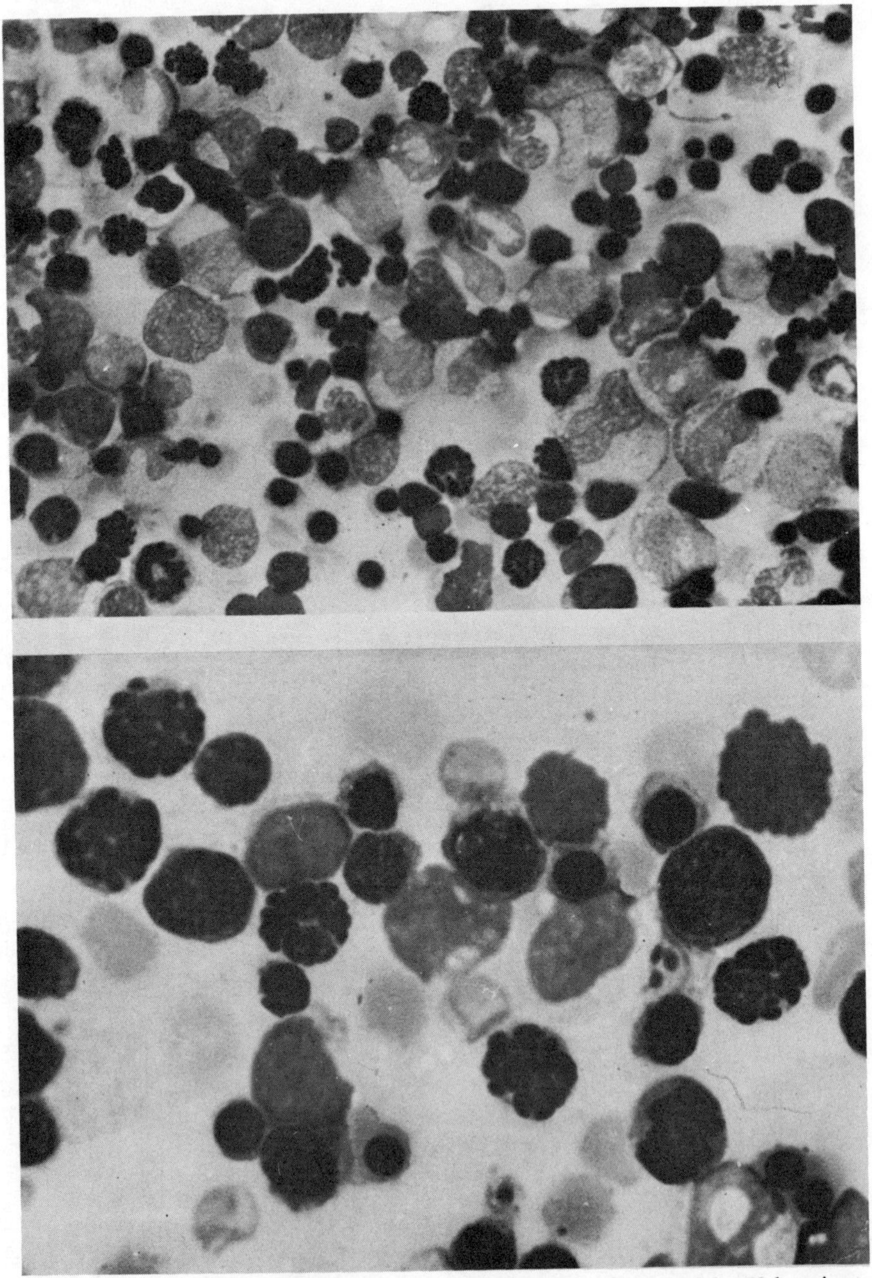

FIGURE 7. Bone marrow from a 14-day-old rat. The animal was starved for 72 hr prior to sacrifice. There is an increased number of mitotic figures in the erythroid series, all of which appear to be in metaphase.

TABLE 5

THE EFFECT OF 48 HOURS' STARVATION ON ERYTHROPOIESIS*

No. of Animals	Age Days	Primitive	Mono-nuclear	Myeloid	Lymphoid	Erythroid	Prn	BN	PN	MI (red)	Retic
6	10	9 (1.2)	1 (0.3)	18 (1.7)	12 (1.7)	57 (3.2)	12 (1)	18 (1.2)	27 (2.8)	7 (1.7)	33 (5)
5	15	6 (0.9)	4 (0.3)	22 (2)	32 (4.5)	39 (2.7)	9 (0.4)	13 (1.3)	17 (1.7)	2 (0.4)	18 (3.6)
4	20	6 (0.7)	3 (0.4)	28 (0.8)	17 (1.3)	43 (0.9)	7 (1)	17 (0.8)	19 (1)	3 (0.4)	12 (1.2)
5	30	5 (1.2)	3 (0.9)	47 (4.4)	32 (2.5)	13 (2)	2 (0.4)	3 (0.9)	8 (0.1)	1 (0.7)	7 (1.1)
5	Ad.	3 (0.5)	4 (0.76)	60 (1.46)	28 (2.8)	6 (1)	1 (0.2)	1 (0.26)	3 (0.67)	0 (0)	1.2 (0.2)

* The bone marrow differentials and peripheral reticulocyte counts in animals starved for 48 hr prior to sacrifice. The age refers to the age on the day of sacrifice. Values are given as mean ±1 SE. Cells are classified as in TABLE 4.

TABLE 6

THE EFFECT OF 72 HOURS' STARVATION ON ERYTHROPOIESIS*

No. of Animals	Age Days	Primitive	Mono-nuclear	Myeloid	Lymphoid	Erythroid	Prn	BN	PN	MI (red)	Retic
9	10	11 (1.3)	0.8 (0.6)	20 (3)	11 (2.8)	55 (7.4)	9 (1)	13 (1.4)	33 (5.7)	8 (1.7)	32 (4.3)
5	15	11 (1.5)	3 (0.7)	24 (1.6)	16 (3.5)	45 (3.5)	10 (1.1)	15 (1.4)	20 (1.3)	4 (0.7)	19 (2.1)
5	20	6 (1.2)	2 (0.8)	32 (3.9)	9 (0.7)	49 (6.2)	11 (1)	16 (2)	22 (4.2)	2 (0.3)	11 (1.3)
5	30	3 (0.7)	3 (1.2)	53 (3.8)	25 (2.3)	11 (1.7)	2 (0.5)	3 (0.6)	6 (1)	2 (0.6)	2 (0.5)
6	Ad.	3 (1)	6 (0.44)	59 (4.8)	26 (3.8)	6 (0.92)	1 (0.2)	2 (0.28)	3 (0.8)	0 (0)	0.2 (0.4)

* The bone marrow differentials and peripheral reticulocyte counts in animals starved for 72 hr prior to sacrifice. The age refers to the age on the day of sacrifice. Values are given as mean ±1 SE. Cells are classified as in TABLE 4.

TABLE 7

THE EFFECT OF 96 HOURS' STARVATION ON ERYTHROPOIESIS*

No. of Animals	Age Days	Primitive	Mono-nuclear	Myeloid	Lymphoid	Erythroid	Prn	BN	PN	MI (red)	Retic
4	10	10 (1.7)	2 (0.4)	16 (2.6)	3 (0.7)	68 (3.3)	10 (1.7)	19 (1.2)	39 (0.9)	4 (0.9)	28 (3.9)
4	15	7 (1)	1 (0)	23 (0.9)	8 (0.9)	58 (3.5)	8 (1.2)	14 (1.2)	36 (3.3)	4 (0.5)	20 (7.5)
4	20	4 (1.1)	1 (0.5)	51 (4.1)	13 (1.7)	26 (3.5)	7 (1.4)	10 (1.9)	9 (1.2)	1 (0)	9 (1.1)
4	30	3 (0)	2 (0.4)	60 (4.5)	30 (3.3)	6 (0.9)	1 (0.5)	1 (0.4)	4 (0.4)	0.0 (0)	0.9 (0.2)
16	Ad.	2 (0.36)	1 (0.23)	64 (0.83)	30 (0.4)	3 (0.42)	0.5 (0.1)	1 (1.8)	1.5 (0.25)	0 (0)	0.1 (0.2)

* The bone marrow differentials and peripheral reticulocyte counts in animals starved for 96 hr prior to sacrifice. The age refers to the age on the day of sacrifice. Values are given as mean ±1 SE. Cells are classified as in TABLE 4.

TABLE 8

EFFECT OF HYPOXIA IN THE NEWBORN RAT*

	Newborn Age						Adult			
	16 Days		24 Days		32 Days		Male		Female	
Numbr of Rats	Cont 5	Exp 12	Cont 7	Exp 14	Cont 8	Exp 12	Cont 6	Exp 7	Cont 6	Exp 6
Hematocrit	30 ± 1.2	30 ± 0.6	36 ± 0.9	39 ± 1.3	38 ± 1.1	50 ± 0.6	45 ± 0.9	55 ± 0.5	42 ± 0.9	53 ± 0.4
Reticulocyte	14 ± 0.3	17 ± 0.7	16 ± 1.6	23 ± 3.3	8 ± 0.6	14 ± 0.7	3.9 ± 0.6	14.9 ± 0.7	2.2 ± 0.2	12.6 ± 0.7
Erythroid precursors	40 ± 4.5	47 ± 1.8	41 ± 1.8	45 ± 1.6	31 ± 0.9	45 ± 1.4	38 ± 3.2	74 ± 5.1	20 ± 1.8	71 ± 2.7
MCV (μ^3)	63	64	62	62	58	73	51 ± 0.9	56 ± 2.0	52 ± 1.7	59 ± 0.6
^{59}Fe Inc.			58 ± 3.3	71 ± 2.7	64 ± 1.9	79 ± 4.9	23 ± 1.0	31 ± 1.9	22 ± 1.9	31 ± 2.4

* Rats were exposed to 0.4 atm for six hr a day for seven days; days refer to day of sacrifice. Values given are mean ± 1 SE. MCV = mean corpuscular volume; ^{59}F Inc. = 20-hour iron incorporation value. (Reprinted from A. Carmena *et al.*, Proceedings of the Society for Experimental Biology and Medicine, Vol. **121**: 652–655, 1966).

TABLE 9

EFFECT OF HYPOXIA ON NEWBORN ERYTHROPOIESIS*

Age (days)	16		24		32		Adult	
No. of animals	5 Control	12 Exp. Alt.	7 Control	14 Exp. Alt.	8 Control	12 Exp. Alt.	7 Control	8 Exp. Alt.
Primitive	8 (0.6)	9 (0.7)	8 (0.9)	10 (0.6)	6 (0.6)	10 (0.9)	5 (0.2)	12 (0.3)
Mononuclear	3 (0.6)	2 (0.3)	3 (0.3)	1 (0)	3 (0.4)	1 (0)	3 (0.1)	1 (0.3)
Lymphoid	13 (2.7)	10 (1.2)	14 (1)	11 (0.8)	17 (1)	7 (0.6)	16 (1.4)	11 (0.8)
Myeloid	35 (2.4)	31 (2.1)	33 (2.2)	33 (1.4)	41 (1.4)	37 (1)	47 (1.7)	35 (2)
Erythroid	40 (4.5)	47 (1.8)	41 (1.2)	45 (0.8)	31 (0.9)	45 (1)	26 (1.3)	40 (2.4)
Pronormoblast	6 (1.4)	7 (0.6)	5 (0.6)	6 (0.3)	4 (0.6)	6 (0.4)	4 (0.3)	6 (0.3)
Basophilic normoblast	11 (0.3)	13 (0.4)	10 (0.4)	13 (0.5)	7 (0.5)	15 (0.7)	7 (0.2)	13 (1)
Polychromatophilic normoblast	23 (2.8)	27 (1.6)	26 (1.4)	26 (1)	19 (0.3)	24 (0.9)	15 (0.2)	21 (1.7)
Erythroid mitotic index	3 (0.5)	3.7 (0)	3 (0)	3 (0)	3 (0)	4 (1.7)	2.7 (0.2)	3 (0.3)

* Bone marrow differentials on newborn and adult animals exposed to altitude as compared to control animals of a similar age. The animals were exposed at 0.4 atm for seven days prior to sacrifice. The age refers to the age at the time of sacrifice. Values are given as mean ± 1 SE.

TABLE 10

PERIPHERAL BLOOD VALUES FOR THE GUINEA PIG*

No. of Animals	Age Days	Hematocrit	Hemoglobin	RBC	Retic. %	MCV	MCHC
22	1	48 (1)	14 (0.2)	529 (20)	3.3 (0.5)	91 (3.3)	29 (0.5)
9	3	48 (2.5)	13 (0.6)	504 (29)	3.0 (0.6)	95 (1.7)	27 (0.5)
10	5	39 (1.3)	13 (0.5)	445 (16)	1.4 (0.1)	88 (3.5)	33 (1.3)
11	10	35 (0.9)	12 (0.5)	447 (19)	1.7 (0.6)	78 (1.7)	34 (0.8)
5	15	35 (0.9)	13 (0.7)	432 (20)	1.6 (0.3)	81 (2)	37 (1.7)
7	20	34 (0.6)	11 (0.3)	376 (14)	6.4 (2)	90 (2.6)	32 (1)
5	30	38 (0.8)	11 (0.3)	417 (7.2)	4.8 (1)	91 (1.7)	29 (0)
56	Adult	37 (0.9)	11 (0.6)	436 (8.2)	2.3 (0.3)	85 (1.3)	30 (0.3)

* The peripheral blood values of the guinea pig related to age. The values are given as mean ± 1 SE. MCV refers to mean corpuscular volume, MCHC refers to mean corpuscular hemoglobin concentration, RBC refers to red blood cells.

TABLE 11

BONE MARROW DIFFERENTIALS IN THE GUINEA PIG*

No. of Animals	Age Days	Primitive	Mononuclear	Myeloid	Lymphoid	Erythroid	Prn	BN	PN	MI (red)	Others
18	1	6 (0.7)	1 (0.3)	37 (1.4)	41 (2.0)	12 (2.2)	1 (0.2)	1 (0.3)	10 (1.7)	0.7 (0)	0.3 (0)
9	3	13 (1.0)	1 (0.2)	30 (2.0)	34 (1.7)	21 (1.4)	1 (0.2)	3 (0.1)	17 (1.0)	3.4 (0.4)	0.1 (0)
10	5	12 (1.5)	3 (0.1)	33 (3.6)	35 (2.4)	20 (2.2)	2 (0.1)	4 (0.1)	14 (1.4)	1.3 (0.3)	0.1 (0)
7	10	9 (1.7)	1 (0)	30 (2.2)	39 (1.0)	20 (1.4)	1 (0.2)	3 (0.4)	16 (1.0)	3.0 (0.3)	0.1 (0)
7	15	10 (1.0)	1 (0.1)	34 (3.9)	24 (1.7)	31 (4.0)	3 (0)	6 (0)	22 (2.6)	3.0 (0.9)	0.1 (0)
7	20	10 (1.0)	1 (0)	36 (2.6)	20 (2.0)	31 (1.4)	1 (0)	5 (0.1)	25 (1.0)	3.0 (0.8)	0.2 (0)
5	30	10 (0.2)	2 (0)	30 (1.7)	30 (1.4)	28 (1.0)	3 (0.2)	4 (0.1)	21 (1.7)	2.0 (0.6)	0.1 (0)
56	Adult	10 (0.5)	1 (0)	41 (1.4)	23 (0.8)	23 (1.0)	1 (0)	3 (0)	19 (1.0)	2.0 (0.4)	0.3 (0)

* The bone marrow differential in the guinea pig. Cells are classified as shown in TABLE 4. Values are given as mean ± 1 SE.

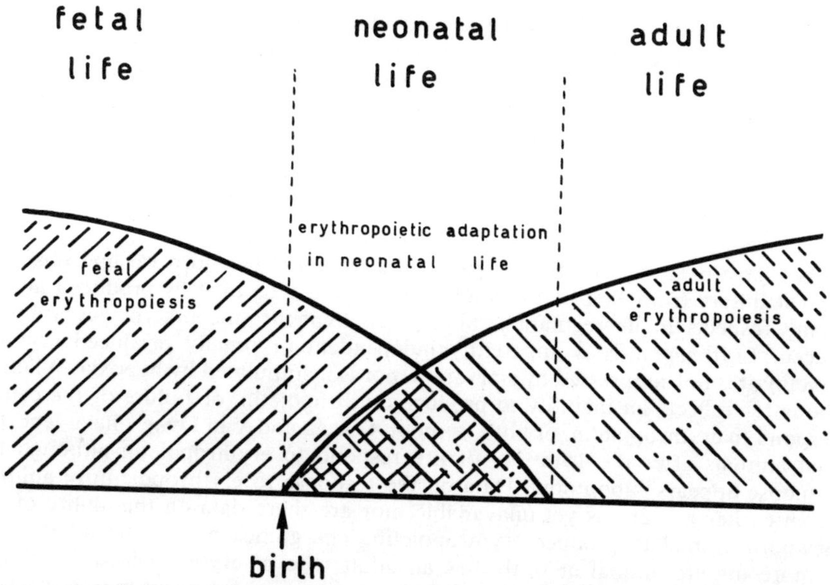

FIGURE 8. Schematic representation of the transition of rat's erythropoiesis from the fetal type to the adult type.

TABLE 12
EFFECT OF STARVATION ON ERYTHROPOIESIS IN THE GUINEA PIG*

	72 Hours			96 Hours
Age (days)	3	5	10	Adult
No. of animals	5	6	5	26
Hematocrit	47 (1.7)	46 (0.8)	42 (0.7)	41 (1)
Hemoglobin	12 (0.8)	14 (0.3)	12 (0.3)	12 (0.1)
RBC ($\times 10^{-6}$)	5.3 (.21)	5.2 (.12)	4.6 (2.7)	4.8 (.15)
Retic.	0.1 (0)	0.6 (0.3)	0.6 (0.2)	1.4 (0.2)
MCV	87 (3.8)	88 (1)	89 (5.7)	83 (2)
MCHC	25 (2.8)	29 (0.7)	28 (0.7)	30 (0.8)
Bone Marrow Differentials				
Primitive cells	8 (0.7)	8 (1)	12 (0.8)	7 (0.2)
Mononuclear	1 (0.3)	1 (0)	2 (1)	0.1 (0)
Lymphoid	45 (2.9)	40 (2.4)	44 (1.4)	30 (1.7)
Myeloid	44 (3.2)	44 (2.4)	32 (1.7)	51 (0.1)
Erythroid	3 (0.4)	6 (0.6)	4 (1.4)	8 (1.7)
Pronormoblast	0 (0)	0.0 (0)	0 (0)	0.4 (0)
Basophilic normoblast	1 (0)	0.5 (0)	0 (0)	1.0 (0)
Polychromatophilic normoblast	2 (0)	5.5 (0.4)	4 (1.7)	6.6 (1.4)
Erythroid mitotic index	0 (0)	0 (0)	0.0 (0)	0.3 (0)
Unclassified	0.2 (0)	0.1 (0)	0.6 (0)	0.3 (0)

* The effect of starvation on erythropoiesis and the bone marrow in the guinea pig. Age refers to the age at the time of sacrifice, the animals having been starved for 72 or 96 hr prior to sacrifice. Values are given as mean ± 1 SE. Cells are classified as in TABLE 4.

of erythropoiesis much the same as that seen in the adult (TABLES 11 & 12). Although nephrectomy and hypoxic stimulation have not as yet been studied in the guinea pig, it seems resasonable to suggest, in view of the effects of starvation, that these perturbations will also evoke a response in the newborn guinea pig similar to those seen in the adult.

Discussion

We have examined erythropoiesis in the fetal and newborn rat and observed that it differs from that of the adult, both in the type of cells produced and in many respects in its regulation. Short-lived hypochromic macrocytes are produced. Erythropoiesis is apparently independent of renally produced erythropoietin; it is not suppressed by starvation, nor is it stimulated by hypoxia. Whether the latter reflects an inability to produce erythropoietin, or failure of the cell to respond to erythropoietin, or both, is moot. Garcia and Van Dyke[10] have reported that animals after the 15th day of life respond to erythropoietin although the response appears suboptimal. Data on the response to erythropoietin in animals at an earlier age are as yet unavailable; nor are there data on the ability of the newborn animal to produce erythropoietin. The guinea pig on the other hand, a more mature animal at birth, has an adult type of erythropoiesis, both with respect to the type of cell produced and in its response to perturbations such as starvation.

The most striking difference between the rat and the human being or guinea pig at birth is the degree of maturity. In the human being there is active bone marrow erythropoiesis whereas the bone marrow of the rat is almost devoid of erythroid elements at birth. In fact the degree of development of the erythron in the rat is similar to that seen in the fifth or sixth month of gestation in the human being. At this time there is a transition from the hepatic to bone marrow erythropoiesis. It is therefore tempting to suggest that neonatal erythropoiesis in the rat is similar to that seen in the latter trimester of pregnancy in humans. By analogy then, it might be suggested that fetal erythropoiesis in man is not governed by the same regulators as in the adult. This may provide an explanation (as previously discussed) for certain congenital hypoplastic anemias and a basis for the understanding of the control of cell production in thalassemia.

In the rat fetal liver a primitive syncytial-type cell was present together with differentiating erythroid elements. A similar cell was seen during the early bone marrow phase of erythropoiesis at a time when red cell production did not respond to the adult regulatory mechanisms. It is perhaps noteworthy that in the starved neonatal rat metaphase accumulation was seen only among erythroid elements and the primitive cell. As the animal matured, there was a gradual transition to the adult type of regulation, which is graphically depicted in FIGURE 8. Coincident and parallel to this change was the decrease in frequency with which the primitive undifferentiated cell was seen. These correlations suggest that, in fact, this primitive undifferentiated cell, which may occur in a syncytium, serves as the stem cell for erythroid elements during the hepatic and early bone marrow phase of erythropoiesis. We would like to suggest that this is the case, that differentiation of this cell is independent of adult mechanisms, and that after birth there is a gradual transition in the rat from a fetal to an adult type of red cell production. In animals which are more mature at birth, e.g. the guinea pig and human beings, this transition occurs during intrauterine life.

Summary

Data have been presented to indicate that erythropoiesis in the fetal and neonatal rat is governed differently from that in the adult. The change in the type of regulation of red cell production in the rat is temporally correlated with the presence of a primitive-type cell that occurs in a syncytium and has been previously described. In animals more mature at birth the transition has already occurred and as a consequence, the newborn animals have an adult-type regulation of red cell production. The guinea pig is an example of a more mature animal and data are presented on the effects of perturbation of red cell formation in this animal.

References

1. JACOBSON, L. O., E. GOLDWASSER, W. FRIED & L. F. PLZAK. 1957. Role of kidney in erythropoiesis. Nature (London) **179:** 633.
2. NATHAN, D. F., E. SHUPACK, F. STOHLMAN, JR. & J. P. MERRILL. 1964. Erythropoiesis in anephric man. J. Clin. Invest. **43:** 11.
3. FLIEDNER, T. M., F. STOHLMAN, JR. & E. P. CRONKITE. Unpublished data.
4. LUCARELLI, G., D. HOWARD & F. STOHLMAN, JR. 1964. Regulation of erythropoiesis. XV. Neonatal erythropoiesis and the effect of nephrectomy. J. Clin. Invest. **43** (II).
5. LUCARELLI, G., C. CARNEVALI, A. PORCELLINI, V. RIZZOLI, L. FERRARI, D. HOWARD & F. STOHLMAN, JR. L'emopoiesi fetale e neonatale nel ratto. Haematologica. In press.
6. LUCARELLI, G., D. HOWARD & F. STOHLMAN, JR. Unpublished observations.
7. JACOBSON, L. O., E. K. MARKS & E. O. GASTON. 1959. Studies on erythropoiesis. XII. The effect of transfusion-induced polycythemia in the mother on the fetus. Blood **14:** 644.
8. STOHLMAN, F., JR., G. LUCARELLI, D. HOWARD, B. MORSE & B. LEVENTHAL. 1964. Regulation of erythropoiesis. XVI. Cytokenetic patterns in disorders of erythropoiesis. Medicine **43:** 6.
9. CARMENA, A., G. LUCARELLI, C. CARNEVALI & F. STOHLMAN, JR. 1966. Regulation of erythropoiesis. XIX. Effect of hypoxia on erythropoiesis in the newborn animal. Proc. Soc. Exp. Biol. Med. **2:** 121.
10. GARCIA, J. F. & D. C. VAN DYKE. 1961. Response of rats of various ages to erythropoietin. Proc. Soc. Exp. Biol. Med. **106:** 585.

ERYTHROPOIETIN AND THE POLYCYTHEMIAS*

John W. Adamson
and
Clement A. Finch

From the Department of Medicine, University of Washington, Seattle, Wash.

Erythropoiesis in man is regulated by erythropoietin. This humoral substance provides the means whereby tissue needs for oxygen influence the level of circulating erythrocytes. The usual cause of polycythemia is a decreased oxygen supply to tissues leading to increased erythropoietin output and increased erythropoiesis. However, there is good evidence that disorders in erythropoietin production itself or abnormal marrow activity may also result in elevated red cell levels. In the following discussion, these disorders are examined through the relationship of erythropoietin to erythropoiesis in polycythemic states in man.

The method used in these studies is a modification[1] of the polycythemic mouse assay previously described,[2–4] and features the injection of concentrates of human urine into mice previously made polycythemic by exposure to reduced atmospheric pressure. With the addition of a protein depletion diet, endogenous erythropoiesis, as measured by the incorporation of radioactive iron into newly formed red cells, is reduced to negligible levels ($0.02 \pm 0.01\%$ utilization). Concentrates of urine are prepared from collections stored at $-12°$ C. The thawed specimens are placed in a dialysis membrane and dialyzed in the cold against a high molecular weight material, polyethylene glycol. Following dialysis, urine sediment is removed by centrifugation, washed with saline, and the supernatants combined and stored frozen for use in the assay. In all patients studied, urine was collected in 24-hour lots or over consecutive six-hour intervals. Estimation of erythropoietin excretion was made by comparing the degree of erythropoiesis induced by the urinary concentrates to dilutions of erythropoietin Standard B. Activity, as measured in this assay, is, by definition, erythropoietin. In the studies to be reported, the regulation of erythropoiesis appears explainable on the basis of a single substance.

Control studies undertaken characterized the erythropoietin excretion of normal subjects in both the basal state and in response to limited phlebotomy. Daily erythropoietin output in 19 control subjects averaged 3.8 ± 2.3 Standard B units per day and increased as expected in seven individuals subjected to limited bleeding (FIGURE 1). With reduction in hematocrit of only 3 to 7 points, average erythropoietin excretion increased by 53 percent.

In the first group of patients studied, polycythemia represented a disorder of oxygen supply to tissue. In six individuals with either cardiac or pulmonary disease, daily erythropoietin excretion varied over a wide range (2.4 to 420.0 units). Again controlled phlebotomy in these patients produced easily demonstrable increases in plasma and urinary erythropoietin levels. In the one patient with hypoxic polycythemia and normal basal erythropoietin excretion, controlled bleeding was attended by a markedly exaggerated increase in erythropoietin output exceeding any of the responses seen in the similarly challenged normals (FIGURE 1).

* Investigation supported in part by U.S. Public Health Service research grant no. 5 F2 AM 29, 375–02, 5–R01–HE 06242 and training grant no. TI–AM–5130. A portion of this work was conducted through the Clinical Research Center Facility of the University of Washington supported by the National Institutes of Health (grant FR–37).

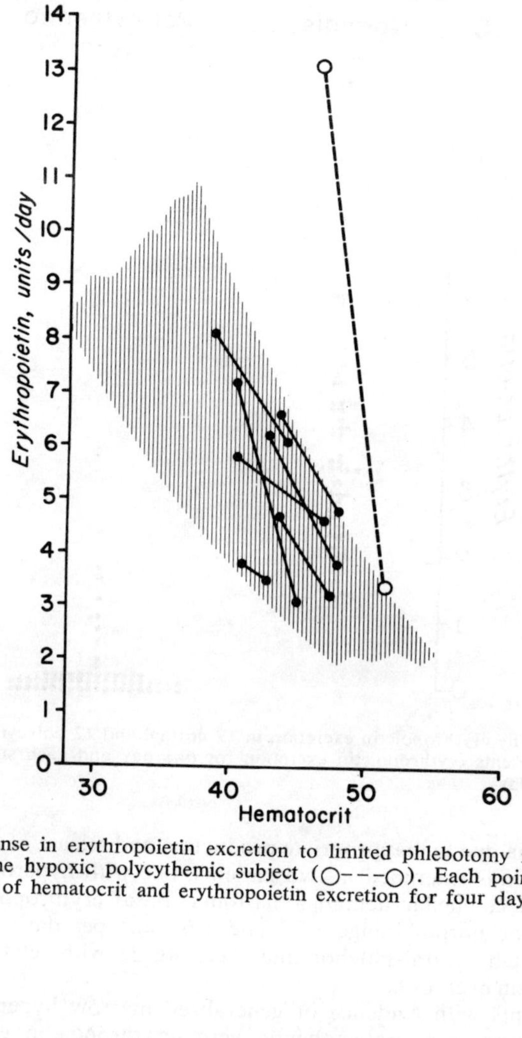

FIGURE 1. Response in erythropoietin excretion to limited phlebotomy in seven normal (●——●) and one hypoxic polycythemic subject (○- - -○). Each point on the graph represents the mean of hematocrit and erythropoietin excretion for four days' duration.

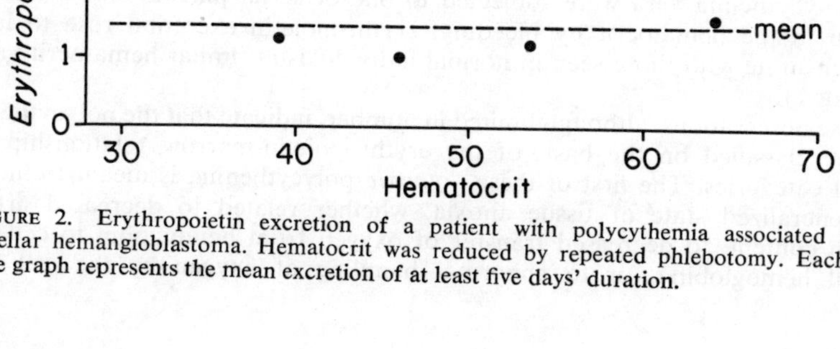

FIGURE 2. Erythropoietin excretion of a patient with polycythemia associated with a cerebellar hemangioblastoma. Hematocrit was reduced by repeated phlebotomy. Each point on the graph represents the mean excretion of at least five days' duration.

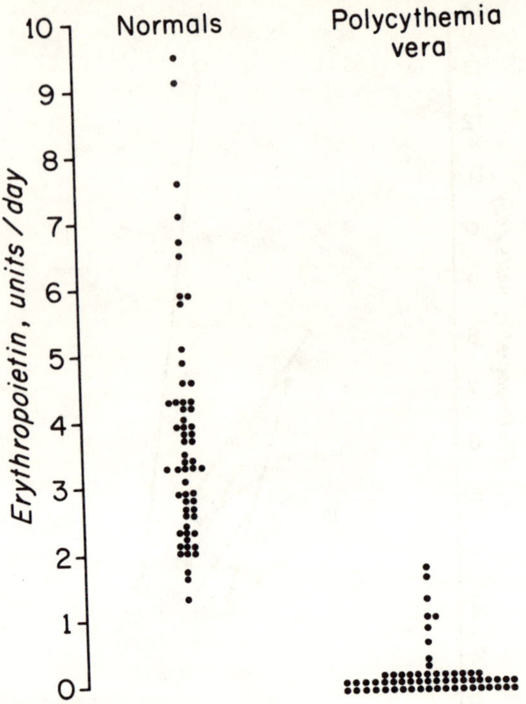

FIGURE 3. Daily erythropoietin excretion in 19 normal and 12 polycythemia vera subjects. Each point represents erythropoietin excretion for one day and each subject is represented by at least three days.

Polycythemia due to inappropriate production and release of an erythropoietin-like substance was examined in two patients, one with hypernephroma and one with recurrent cerebellar hemangioblastoma. Basal erythropoietin excretion in both was in the normal range (2.9 and 1.6 units per day). One patient was followed through several phlebotomies (FIGURE 2) with relatively little change in erythropoietin excretion.

In 12 patients with evidence of generalized marrow hyperproliferation who fulfilled the criteria of polycythemia vera, erythropoietin excretion was undetectable in ten, and so reduced in the others as to clearly separate them from normal (FIGURE 3). That the response of the erythropoietin mechanism was still functional was demonstrated by a series of experiments in which seven patients with polycythemia vera were subjected to one or serial phlebotomies. With reduction in the hematocrit by bleeding, erythropoietin excretion rose to levels commensurate with those seen in normal individuals at similar hematocrit values (FIGURE 4).

These observations, although limited in number, indicate that the polycythemias may be classified on the basis of the erythropoietin-marrow relationship into several categories. The first of these, *hypoxic* polycythemia, is meant to include any generalized state of tissue anoxia, whether related to decreased arterial oxygen content, to decreased transfer of oxygen from hemoglobin to cell (abnormal hemoglobin), or to abnormal handling of oxygen by the cell itself

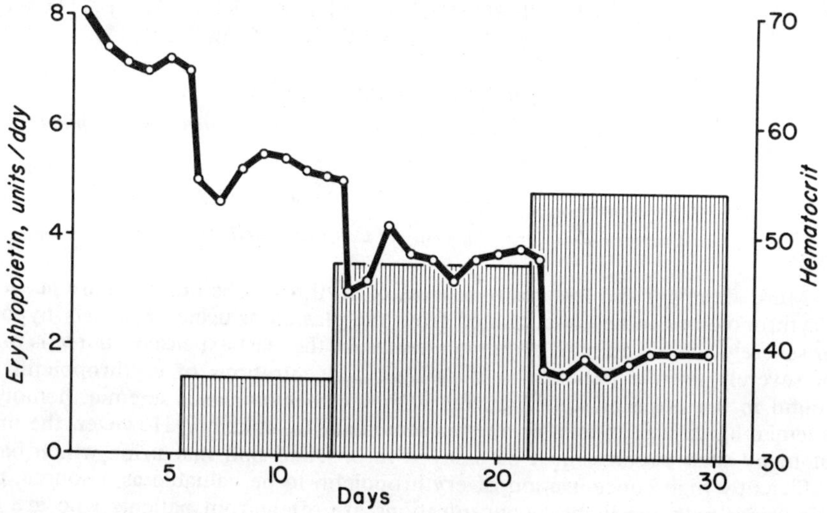

FIGURE 4. Relationship of daily erythropoietin excretion (shaded area) to hematocrit values in a patient with polycythemia vera subjected to three exchange phlebotomies. Erythropoietin excretion was undetectable for the first six days of the study.

(hypothetical). In hypoxic polycythemia, urinary erythropoietin is usually elevated but may be normal. If normal values are found, an exaggerated response to lowering of the hematocrit may be expected, and the urinary erythropoietin values will exceed those of the normal at any given hematocrit level. The second general mechanism leading to polycythemia is autonomous erythropoietin production. This may be considered a part of a larger pathophysiologic picture reflecting the production of biologically active materials by neoplasms. Here, erythropoietin is released by a variety of tumors and apparently not subject to physiologic control. It is postulated that in this disorder there will be a constant erythropoietin output over a wide range of hematocrit values, increasing only when significant anemia is induced and tumor secretion of erythropoietin becomes reinforced by erythropoietin output from the kidney. The third category is polycythemia due to autonomous erythropoiesis. The most reasonable interpretation of the data is that red cell production by the marrow is an independent phenomenon and that the output of erythropoietin has been suppressed by the increased red cell concentration.

References

1. ADAMSON, J. W., R. ALEXANIAN, C. MARTINEZ & C. A. FINCH. 1966. Erythropoietin excretion in normal man. Blood **28:** 354.
2. COTES, P. M. & D. R. BANGHAM. 1961. Bioassay of erythropoietin in mice made polycythemic by exposure to air at reduced pressure. Nature **191:** 1065.
3. DE GOWIN, R. L., D. HOFSTRA & C. W. GURNEY. 1962. The mouse with hypoxia-induced erythremia, an erythropoietin bioassay animal. J. Lab. Clin. Med. **60:** 842.
4. WEINTRAUB, A. H., A. S. GORDON & J. F. CAMISCOLI. 1963. Use of the hypoxia-induced polycythemic mouse in the assay and standardization of erythropoietin. J. Lab. Clin. Med. **62:** 743.

COLLECTION OF ERYTHROPOIETIN FROM URINE OF PATIENTS WITH ANEMIA SECONDARY TO HOOKWORM*

Abraham Gutnisky and Luis Malgor

Facultad de Medicina, Universidad Nacional del Nordeste, Corrientes, Argentina

and

Mary Lou Nohr and Donald Van Dyke

Donner Laboratory, University of California, Berkeley, Calif.

More abundant and less costly sources of erythropoietic hormone are needed.[1] Erythropoietin can be concentrated from the plasma or urine of acutely hypoxic or severely anemic animals or human beings;[2–6] the least expensive source is urine of severely anemic patients.[7–9] Very high concentrations of erythropoietin are found in the urine of some patients with severe hypoplastic anemia, hemolytic anemia, blood loss anemia or anemia secondary to leukemia. However, the urine of many such patients must be assayed in order to find that urine which has a sufficiently high concentration of erythropoietin to be valuable as a source, and the urines with the highest concentrations are often from patients who are terminal and therefore only temporary sources and very few in numbers. This study of the erythropoietin extract of a large number of patients with severe anemia secondary to hookworm was undertaken in an attempt to find a more reliable and inexpensive source of human urinary erythropoietin.

Materials and Methods

The people of the province of Corrientes in northern Argentina are severely infected with *Necator americanus*.[10] The capital city, Corrientes, serves a large rural population and its hospitals continually receive patients with hematocrits below 20% and hemoglobin below 6 g/100 ml. Two of the main hospitals were provided with freezers and glass bottles and the medical staff was requested to freeze immediately on voiding all urine of patients with hemoglobin under 6 g/100 ml. Collection of urine was continued until the patient's hemoglobin rose to 6 g/100 ml as a result of therapy. The frozen urine was transported daily to a large storage freezer at the Erythropoietin Collection Center in the Department of Physiology of the School of Medicine, Northeast University, Corrientes, Argentina.

The urine was thawed, an aliquot removed for assay as unmodified urine, and the remainder processed by the collodion adsorption method,[11] the yield from each patient being assayed separately. All samples were assayed by the starved rat assay,[12] using rats of the Wistar strain. Extracts with similar erythropoietic activity were combined to form large batches and re-assayed by the starved rat assay and by the ex-hypoxic mouse assay.[13]

Results

The results from nine months' collection are reported in this paper. During that time 127 patients were studied, 49 of which had their urine collected, pro-

* This work was carried out at the Facultad de Medicina, Universidad Nacional del Nordeste, Corrientes, Argentina, with the assistance of scientific personnel from Donner Laboratory of Medical Physics, University of California, Berkeley, Calif., and was funded in part by the Consejo Nacional de Investigaciones Cientificas y Tecnicas of Argentina (grant 1991), by the Comite de Investigaciones Medicas de Corrientes, Argentina, and by the United States Atomic Energy Commission.

TABLE 1

ERYTHROPOIETIN FROM URINE OF SEVERELY ANEMIC PATIENTS IN CORRIENTES, ARGENTINA

Diagnosis	Hgb. g/100 ml	Hct. %	Retic. %	Activity/mg IRP Units*	% recovery	Total Units Obtained IRP Units
			Hemoglobin 1–2 g/100 ml			
Hookworm	1.9	7.5	4.6	7.4	—	1,154
Hemolytic anemia	1.9	8.0	5.0	16.9	—	10,849
Hookworm	1.4	11.0	3.5	8.5	—	6,460
Hookworm	2.0	15.0	3.0	43.7	54	33,080
Hookworm	1.7	6.0	5.4	0		
Leukemia	1.7	5.0	0.9	20	42	7,060
			Hemoglobin 2–3 g/100 ml			
DeGugliemo's syndrome	2.6	8.0	1.4	9.1	41	4,076
Hookworm	2.7	11.0	10.0	33.3	58	14,585
Hookworm	2.5	11.0	2.5	4.2	—	2,461
Hookworm	2.4	12.0	7.0	34.3	—	49,597
Hookworm, tuberculosis	2.8	14.0	10.0	18.8	—	18,912
Hookworm	2.2	15.0	2.4	13.2	—	6,481
Hookworm	2.2	10.0	2.8	13.2	—	6,481
Hookworm	2.6	14.0	4.0	2.6	—	969
Hookworm	2.8	11.0	3.1	9.5	—	8,512
Hookworm	2.4	14.0	—	10.7	—	4,173
Hookworm	2.9	11.0	2.5	13.2	95	6,481
Hookworm	2.2	10.0	3.4	12.2	—	4,758
Hookworm	2.8	12.0	—	6.7	66	2,546
Hookworm	2.4	9.0	—	6.7	—	2,546
Leukemia	2.6	11.0	4.0	1.2	—	1,046
Hookworm	2.4	8.0	9.0	7.6	—	4,425
Hookworm	2.6	12.0	3.1	75.0	—	10,500
Hookworm	2.6	14.0	2.0	16.8	—	3,427
			Hemoglobin 3–4 g/100 ml			
Hookworm	3.3	14.0	2.0	6.1	37	4,617
Hemolytic anemia	3.1	9.0	10.0	2.8	—	5,465
Hookworm	3.2	16.0	2.0	13.2	—	6,481
Hookworm	3.3	15.0	8.8	4.4	37	1,707
Hookworm	3.7	15.0	13.0	5.6	—	3,628
Hookworm	3.1	13.0	13.5	5.6	—	3,628
Blood loss	3.7	15.0	14.0	28.0	—	61,936
Hookworm	3.4	19.0	—	3.0	—	4,806
Hookworm	3.5	21.0	—	7.6	—	6,064
Hookworm	3.3	19.0	2.4	7.6	—	6,064
Hookworm	3.5	18.0	—	8.5	—	6,460
Hookworm	3.6	12.0	3.6	12.2	54	4,758
Hookworm	3.9	14.0	3.8	8.5	—	6,460
Hookworm	3.4	17.0	2.4	13.0	—	9,711
Hookworm	3.2	15.0	6.2	7.6	—	6,232
Hookworm	3.7	12.0	1.6	6.7	—	2,546
Hookworm	3.3	13.0	—	14.7	—	5,336
Hookworm	3.3	16.0	3.4	6.6	59	3,187
Hookworm	3.7	19.0	2.3	8.3	79	3,046
			Hemoglobin 4–5 g/100 ml			
Aplastic anemia	4.3	20.0	—	5.6	—	3,628
Hemolytic anemia	4.8	27.0	—	2.6	—	969
Hookworm	4.6	19.0	2.0	7.6	—	6,064
Hookworm	4.4	22.0	3.2	12.3	—	4,514
Hookworm	4.8	22.0	—	6.7	—	2,546
Hemolytic anemia	4.1	14.0	3.5	10.9	—	2,217

* International Reference Preparation, previously Standard B, obtained from the Medical Research Council of Great Britain.

cessed and assayed. Of these, 40 had severe anemia secondary to hookworm, one had acute hemorrhage from a duodenal ulcer, one had aplastic anemia, four hemolytic anemia, two leukemia, and one deGugliemo's syndrome. Of the 49 patients processed, only one with anemia secondary to hookworm had insufficient erythropoietin to be useful. In the first part of the study, the unmodified urine, as well as the extract, was assayed in order to determine efficiency of extraction by the collodion adsorption method. As can be seen from TABLE 1, recovery varied from 29% to 95%, (average 55%), and activity of the extract from the urine of patients ranged from 1.2 to 75 units* per mg of dry, soluble powder. From two patients three separate collections were made, when the hemoglobin was 1–2, 2–3, and 3–4 g/100 ml (TABLE 2).

In the nine month period of working we collected 31,100 g of soluble extract with an average activity of approximately 12.5 Standard B units per mg or a total of 378,500 Standard B units.

TABLE 2

ERYTHROPOIETIN FROM URINE OF TWO ANEMIC PATIENTS (HOOKWORM) DURING TREATMENT

	Patient	Hgb. g/100 ml	Hct. %	Retic. %	Activity/mg IRP Units*
First Study	A	1.9	8.0	5.0	16.9
	B	2.0	15.0	3.0	43.7
Second study	A	3.4	19.5		3.0
	B	3.0	14.0	7.2	33.7
Third study	A	4.8	27.0		2.6
	B	4.1	20.0		5.6

* International Reference Preparation.

Discussion

This and a previous study[14] demonstrate that the urine from patients with hemoglobin below 6 g caused by hookworm infestation very frequently contains a high concentration of erythropoietin. At very low hemoglobin concentration there was no direct correlation between severity of anemia and erythropoietin recovery. Frequently, more erythropoietin was recovered from the urine of patients with hemoglobin of 3–4 g/100 ml than from those with hemoglobin of 1–2 g/100 ml (FIGURE 1).

By collecting in a heavily infested area such as Corrientes, Argentina, one can obtain an abundant supply of erythropoietically active urine. The present experience indicates that if one limits processing to patients with hookworm and hemoglobin below 6 g, preliminary assay of the urine and even assay of the individual extracts may not be necessary unless one wishes to separate the very active from the moderately active. By eliminating the need for assay of the extract from each donor, one is able to reduce the cost of preparation very greatly. If methods can be developed which provide more quantitative recovery, the cost of producing erythropoietin could be further reduced since recovery by the method used averaged 55%.

* Compared to Standard B, recently established as the International Reference Preparation, obtained from the Medical Research Council of Great Britain.

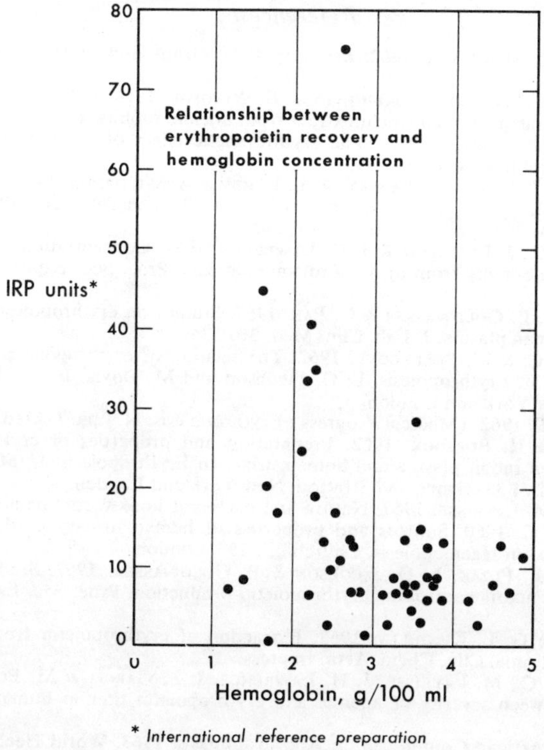

FIGURE 1. Relationship between erythropoietin recovery and hemoglobin concentration, using erythropoietin from urine of severely anemic patients.

It is estimated[15] that one-fourth of the world's population is infected with ancylostoma, particularly in warm, humid regions, although how many are severely anemic is not known, and it is not likely that this age-old scourge of mankind will be eliminated in the near future. In these studies it was found that the establishment of an erythropoietin collection center has created interest in and focused attention on the severity of the problem in this community and has contributed to improved patient care.

Summary

More abundant and less costly sources of erythropoietic hormone are needed. It has been found that the urine of patients with severe anemia (less than 6 g hemoglobin) caused by hookworm consistently contains a high concentration of erythropoietin. The specific activity of the material collected was from 1.2 to 75 units per mg with an average activity of 12.5 units per mg. It is believed that this is the least costly, most reliable and most abundant source of erythropoietin available at present.

Acknowledgments

The authors are indebted to Dr. Geoffrey Keighley of the California Institute of Technology, and to Dr. Denman Hammond of the Children's Hospital of Los Angeles, for the ex-hypoxic mouse assays.

References

1. JACOBSON, L. O., M. DOYLE. 1962. Erythropoiesis. Grune and Stratton. New York and London.
2. BORSOOK, H., A. GRAYBIEL, G. KEIGHLEY & E. WINDSOR. 1954. Polycythemic response to normal adult rats to a nonprotein extract from anemic rabbits. Blood **9:** 734.
3. HODGSON, G. & J. TOHA. 1954. The erythropoietic effect of urine and plasma of repeatedly bled rabbits. Blood **9:** 299.
4. PILERO, S. J., P. T. MEDICI, B. PANSKY, A. L. LUHBY & A. S. GORDON. 1956. Erythropoietic-stimulating effects of plasma extract from anemic human subjects. Proc. Soc. Exper. Biol. Med. **93:** 302.
5. VAN DYKE, D. C., J. F. GARCIA & J. H. LAWRENCE. 1957. Concentration of highly potent erythropoietic activity from urine of anemic patients. Proc. Soc. Exper. Biol. Med. **96:** 541.
6. GURNEY, C. W., E. GOLDWASSER & C. PAN. 1957. Studies on erythropoiesis. VI. Erythropoietin in human plasma. J. Lab. Clin. Med. **50:** 534.
7. VAN DYKE, D. C. & M. POLLYCOVE. 1962. The relation of erythropoietin to anemia and polycythemia in Erythropoiesis. L. O. Jacobson and M. Doyle, Eds. : 340. Grune and Stratton. New York and London.
8. STOHLMAN, JR. F. 1962. (Medical Progress) Erythropoiesis. N. Eng. J. Med. **267:** 342, 348.
9. LOWY, P. H. & H. BORSOOK. 1962. Preparation and properties of erythropoietin concentrates from rabbit plasma and human urine. In Erythropoiesis. L. M. Jacobson and M. Doyle, Eds. : 33. Grune and Stratton. New York and London.
10. ROCHE, M. & M. LAYRISSE. 1967. Nature and causes of hookworm anemia. In press.
11. VAN DYKE, D. C. 1960. Sources and properties of human urinary erythropoietin. Ciba Found. Symp. on Haemopoiesis. Churchill. : 397. London.
12. FRIED, W., L. F. PLZAK, L. O. JACOBSON & E. GOLDWASSER. 1957. Studies on erythropoiesis. III. Factors controlling erythropoietin production. Proc. Soc. Exper. Biol. Med. **94:** 237.
13. LOWY, P. H. & G. L. KEIGHLEY. 1967. Extraction of erythropoietin from human urine and rabbit plasma. Clin. Chem. Acta. In press.
14. VAN DYKE, D. C., M. LAYRISSE, J. H. LAWRENCE, J. F. GARCIA & M. POLLYCOVE. 1961. Relation between severity of anemia and erythropoietin titer in human beings. Blood **18:** 187.
15. CCTA/WHO African Conference on Ancylostomiasis. 1963. World Health Organization technical report series 255.

HIGH HEMATOCRIT IN HYPERTENSION AND ITS RELATIONSHIP WITH RENAL ARTERIAL DISEASE

Edward D. Frohlich and Robert C. Tarazi

Research Division, Cleveland Clinic, Cleveland, Ohio

We have been intrigued by the association of high hematocrit or hemoglobin with hypertension,[1] and have recently re-examined the problem by studying the incidence of elevated hematocrit in 301 hypertensive and normotensive patients with and without renal arterial disease.[2] We define high hematocrit as 54 percent or more in men and 51 percent or more in women. Our findings demonstrated a significantly higher incidence of "polycythemia" in patients with renal arterial disease ($p < .01$). High hematocrit was also found to be more prevalent in hypertensive patients with unilateral renal atrophy due to ischemia rather than to parenchymal disease ($p < .02$). When we compared the association of high hematocrit and renal arterial disease in either normotensive or hypertensive patients with peripheral atherosclerosis, we found a significantly higher incidence of high hematocrit in patients with renal arterial disease ($p < .02$) regardless of the presence of elevated blood pressure. These findings, summarized in TABLE 1, suggest that if an unexplained elevated hematocrit is found in a hypertensive patient, or in a normotensive patient with peripheral atherosclerosis, renal arterial disease should be considered. Perhaps these observations offer some explanation for the syndrome described by Felix Gaisböck in 1905.[3] We are presently exploring the role of erythropoietin in renal arterial disease with Dr. George Hoffman.

TABLE 1

INCIDENCE OF HIGH HEMATOCRIT

	Renal Arterial Disease	No Renal Arterial Disease
Hypertensives	19%	3%
Hypertension and unilat. renal atrophy	25%	4%
Peripheral atherosclerosis	24%	7%

References

1. GAISBÖCK, F. 1922. Die Polyzythämie. Ergebn. Inn. Med. Kinderheilk. **21:** 204.
2. TARAZI, R. C., E. D. FROHLICH, H. P. DUSTAN, R. W. GIFFORD, JR. & I. H. PAGE. 1966. Hypertension and high hematocrit: another clue to renal arterial disease. Amer. J. Cardiol. **18:** 855.
3. GAISBÖCK, F. 1905. Die Bedeutung der Blutdruckmessung für die ärztliche Praxis. Deutsch. Arch. Klin. Med. **83:** 363.

RENAL ERYTHROPOIETIN EXCRETION AS A FUNCTION OF ACID BASE BALANCE

Diana Marver and Clifford W. Gurney

Argonne Cancer Research Hospital and the Departments of Medicine and Physiology, University of Chicago, Chicago, Ill.*

It has been known for some time that erythropoietin is excreted in the urine of severely anemic patients.[1,2] The exact relationship between the plasma and urine levels of this hormone is not clear. Previous reports have indicated that the urinary titer is somehow related to the concentration of erythropoietin in the plasma, the plasma concentration being several fold greater than the urinary concentration.[3,4] In other studies, Van Dyke *et al.* have noted that there is great variability in the ratio of urinary erythropoietin to plasma erythropoietin and that the amount in the urine does not appear to be in direct proportion to the severity of the anemia.[5] They further reported that relatively few severely anemic patients produce sufficient quantities of erythropoietin in their urine to make urinary purification worth the cost and effort.[6] Our own experience in this area has been that patients do vary in the degree to which they excrete erythropoietin. In several instances, patients with plasma titers as high as 3–6 units/ml excreted only a slight or undemonstrable amount in their urine. Of these, a few were found to produce substantial amounts of this hormone in their urine during a subsequent hospital admission, although their plasma levels were comparable on both occasions.

The present study attempts to elucidate one of the factors which may determine the renal threshold and magnitude of erythropoietin excretion.

Methods

After obtaining a baseline plasma and 24-hour urine sample, several anemic patients were given either 6 g T.I.D. of $NaHCO_3$ or 3 g T.I.D. of NH_4Cl per day. In all but one patient, blood samples were drawn at the same hour each day throughout the study and the plasmas were frozen. Urine specimens were added to a bedside refrigerated bottle containing about 0.1 percent phenol as a preservative. The volume and pH of the pooled urine samples were measured upon completion of each 24-hour collection, and an aliquot of each was immediately frozen. Erythropoietin assays, sensitive enough to determine 0.05 units of erythropoietin, were carried out in the hypertransfused mouse, using a single, 1 ml injection of unconcentrated urine or plasma.[7] All urine and plasma fractions collected during a single study were assayed at the same time. The resulting percent ^{59}Fe incorporation was translated into units of erythropoietin using a Standard B reference curve assayed in our laboratory. The Standard B material, prepared from human urine, was provided by Mary Cotes and D. R. Bangham of the Division of Biological Standards, National Institutes of Medical Research, Mill Hill, London.

Results

The first patient (H.B.) was a 53-year-old farmer with myelofibrosis. At the time of admission, his hemoglobin was 7.5 g and his hematocrit, 22 percent. This patient had previously been observed to excrete consistently small amounts of erythropoietin, although his circulating levels prior to transfusion therapy were

* Operated by the University of Chicago for the United States Atomic Energy Commission.

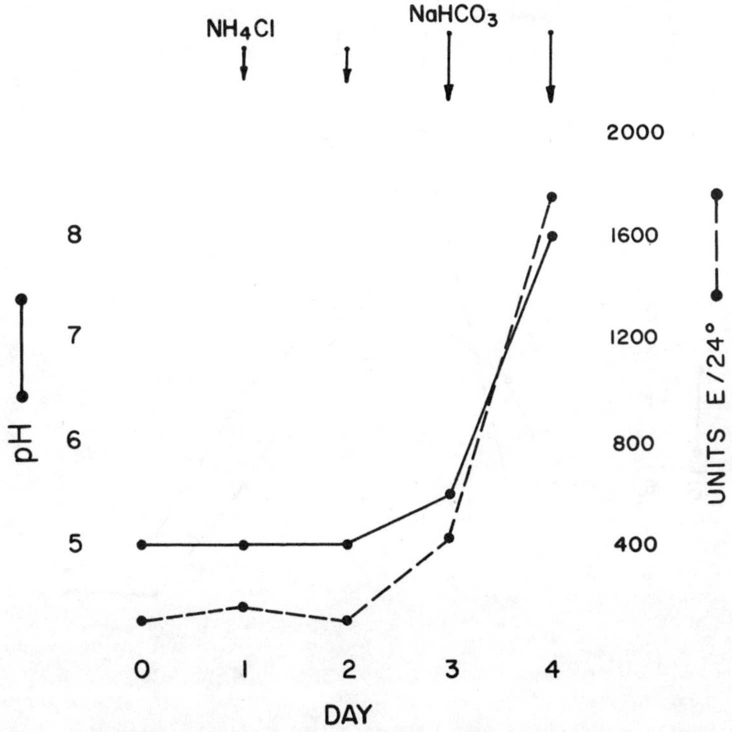

FIGURE 1. Daily change of urine pH (•——•) and units of erythropoietin excretion/24 hr (•— — —•) in a patient administered NH_4Cl for two days followed by $NaHCO_3$ for two days. Day 0 represents baseline values.

usually quite high. The results are shown in FIGURE 1. The 24-hour excretion of erythropoietin was not affected by NH_4Cl administration, but increased 17-fold as his urine pH increased to 8.0. The observed rise during $NaHCO_3$ administration was not the result of changes in urine volume, but rather of urinary erythropoietin concentration; therefore, the percent ^{59}Fe incorporation per ml urine, which is not presented in FIGURE 1, was equally as dramatic, rising from 2 percent to 30 percent per ml during this period. The same phenomenon was seen in this patient during a second hospital admission, at which time his hemoglobin was 6.7 and his hematocrit, 21 percent. On this occasion, the order of NH_4Cl and $NaHCO_3$ administration was reversed, as seen in FIGURE 2. The figure indicates the approximate "clearance" of erythropoietin per minute rather than the total 24-hour excretion. In order to calculate rough clearance data, it was assumed that the plasma concentration of erythropoietin did not vary significantly between each 24-hour specimen assayed. This assumption is supported by the fact that over the seven-day period of this particular study, the daily mean plasma concentration was 0.36 ± 0.07 unit/ml.

The second patient was an 18-year-old boy with a hypoplastic anemia of eight years' duration whose hemoglobin and hematocrit at the time of admission were 5.4 g and 16 percent, respectively. Although this patient had excreted moderate amounts of erythropoietin during previous admissions, alkali effectively increased

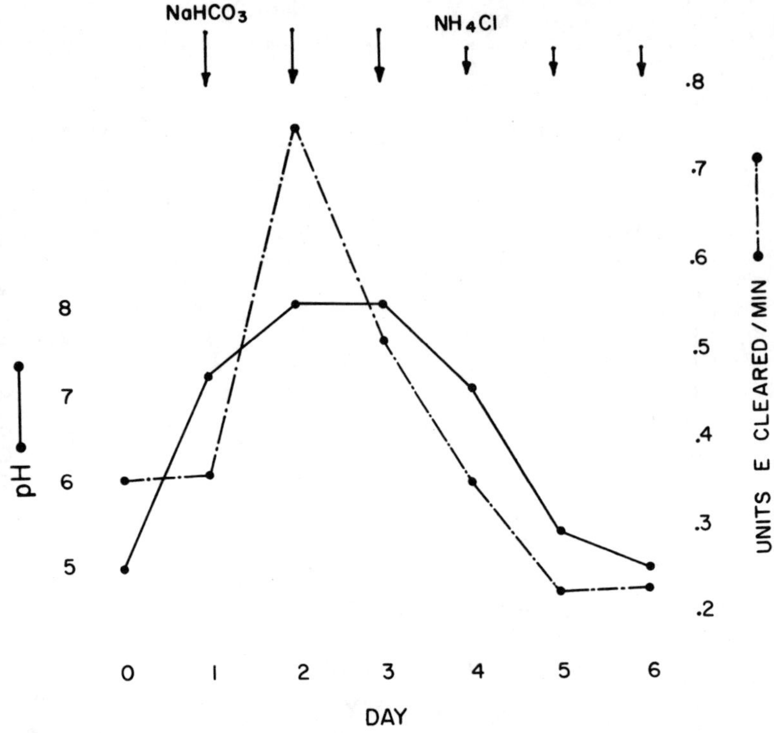

FIGURE 2. Daily change of urine pH (•——•) and approximate "clearance" values (•—•—•—•) in a patient administered $NaHCO_3$ for three days followed by NH_4Cl for three days. Day 0 represents baseline values.

his daily output from about 600 to 2,100 units, as illustrated in FIGURE 3. The approximate clearance per minute is also indicated. When "clearance" $\left(\frac{UV}{P}\right)$ and 24-hour excretion values (UV) are compared, it is apparent that there was little change in plasma concentration, suggesting that the increase seen during alkalosis was not the result of a sudden increase in this parameter. It is also noteworthy that during the second day of alkali consumption, the urinary concentration of erythropoietin slightly exceeded the plasma concentration of 1 unit/ml.

Three possible explanations for the effect observed in these studies, as well as that in one other patient with a refractory anemia subsequently tested, are:

1) Erythropoietin is unstable at acidic pH's, such as those found in urine.
2) Erythropoietin is unstable in the presence of proteolytic enzymes in a bladder containing acidic urine.
3) The excretion of erythropoietin is enhanced at alkaline pH's.

The first hypothesis was ruled out by incubation studies in which Step 1 erythropoietin was diluted to a concentration of 1 unit/ml with 0.05 M phosphate buffers, pH 5.5 to 8.0. Incubation of these solutions at 37° C for one hr in a Dubnoff shaking incubator resulted in no loss of activity. This is in agreement with earlier concepts of erythropoietin's stability, since one method of purifying erythropoietin and maintaining its activity is to acidify plasma to pH 5.5 with hydrochloric acid.[8]

Incubation for one and one-half hr at 37° C of aliquots of urine samples obtained from a patient study dealing with acid and base administration resulted in little of no loss of erythropoietic activity. This suggests that destruction by proteolytic enzymes in the bladder is not the major factor that accounts for the differences seen in this study. These data are consistent with the concept that erythropoietin has acidic glycoprotein properties,[9,10] and Yamashina has found that the alpha-1 acidic glycoproteins are relatively resistant to attack by proteolytic enzymes.[11]

To illustrate further that the differences observed are not wholly due to erythropoietin breakdown in a bladder containing acidic urine, patient H.B. was subjected to water diuresis before and after two days of $NaHCO_3$ administration. On each occasion, the patient emptied his bladder just prior to drinking a one-liter water load. Urine samples obtained during the test periods were immediately frozen until assayed. His initial output during diuresis and before $NaHCO_3$ was 0.09 unit erythropoietin/minute. After two days of $NaHCO_3$ administration, the patient was water-loaded again some 12 hr after taking his last $NaHCO_3$ tablet, at which time the urinary output had increased 19-fold to 1.7 unit/minute. The volumes of urine from both periods were the same, and the pH's were 5.4 and 7.6. Plasma levels obtained from blood samples drawn about half way through

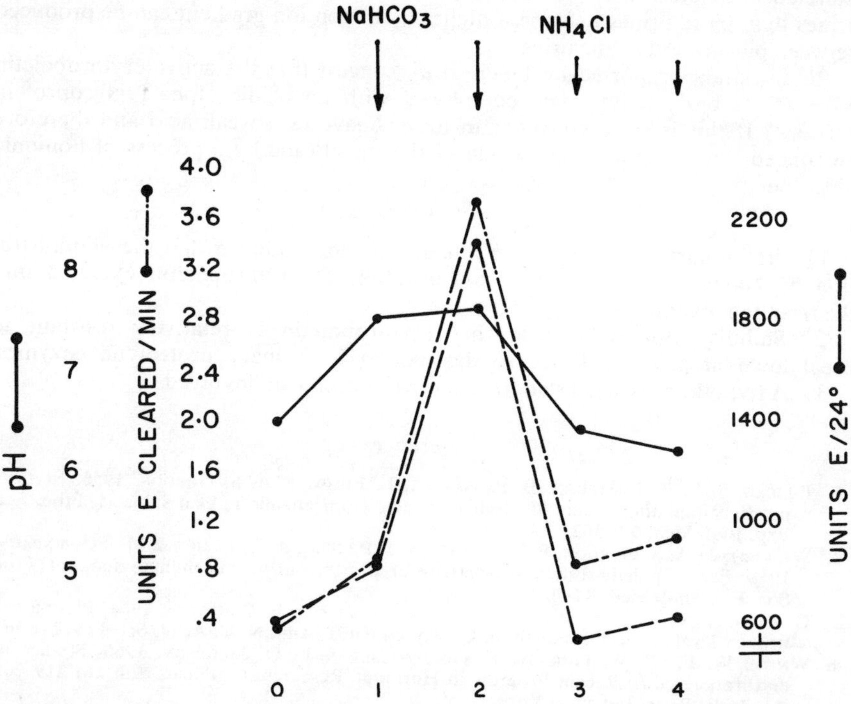

FIGURE 3. Daily change of urine pH (•——•), units of erythropoietin excreted/24 hr (•— — —•) and approximate "clearance" values (•—•—•—•) in a patient administered $NaHCO_3$ for two days followed by NH_4Cl for two days. Day 0 represents baseline values.

each period of diuresis were only slightly elevated during the second test. These studies indicate that even when urine is in the bladder for a short time, there still is a striking effect on erythropoietin excretion during alkalosis.

By exclusion we are left, then, with the suggestion that more erythropoietin is excreted into alkaline urine.

Discussion

The data obtained so far indicate that an alkaline urine enhances the excretion of erythropoietin in the patients tested, although the exact renal mechanism by which this was accomplished is as yet unclear. A few organic compounds, such as aspirin and phenobarbital, have been shown to be preferentially excreted into alkaline urine by a process of 'nonionic diffusion.'[12–14] 'Nonionic diffusion' involves the passive accumulation of a weak base or acid on one side of a membrane. The membrane must be relatively impermeable to the ionized form of the acid or base and highly permeable to the unionized form. A weak base will therefore tend to accumulate on the acidic side of the membrane and a weak acid, on the basic side, provided that there is a pH gradient across the membrane. At basic pH's, studies have indicated that phenobarbital is excreted by a process involving passive diffusion.[15] Salicylate excretion, on the other hand, is somewhat more complicated since it involves decreased tubular reabsorption of free salicylate and may also involve a pH-dependent transport system.[16,17] A great many more compounds, such as the antimalarial drugs, are known to be preferentially excreted in acidic urine;[18] in general, more compounds are excreted into acidic urines than basic urines because a higher hydrogen ion gradient can be produced between plasma and acidic urine.

Recent studies reported by Lewis *et al.* suggest that the active erythropoietin moiety is a basic polypeptide complexed with an acidic alpha-1 glycoprotein carrier.[19] If this is so, erythropoietin may behave as a weak acid and therefore be concentrated on the alkaline side of the membrane by a process of nonionic diffusion.

Summary

1) Preliminary observations in anemic patients indicate that the administration of $NaHCO_3$ increases the concentration of erythropoietin excreted into the resulting alkaline urine.

2) Stability studies indicate that erythropoietin is relatively resistant to breakdown at acidic pH's or to destruction by urinary proteolytic enzymes.

3) A hypothesis is suggested for the renal mechanism involved.

References

1. Piliero, S. J., P. T. Medici, B. Pansky, A. L. Luhby & A. S. Gordon. 1956. Erythropoietic-stimulating effects of plasma extracts from anemic human subjects. Proc. Soc. Exp. Biol. Med. **93:** 302.
2. Winkert, J., A. S. Gordon, P. T. Medici, S. J. Piliero, A. L. Luhby & M. Tannenbaum. 1958. Erythropoietic-stimulating activity of urine from anemic human subjects. Proc. Soc. Exp. Biol. Med. **97:** 191.
3. Gordon, A. S., A. H. Weintraub, J. F. Camiscoli & J. F. Contrera. 1964. Plasma and urinary levels of erythropoietin in Cooley's anemia. Ann. N. Y. Acad. Sci. **119**(2): 561.
4. White, W. F., C. W. Gurney, E. Goldwasser & L. O. Jacobson. 1960. Studies on erythropoietin. *In* Recent Progress in Hormone Research. G. Pincus, Ed. **16:** 219–262. Academic Press, Inc. New York, N. Y.
5. Van Dyke, D. C., M. Layrisse, J. H. Lawrence, J. F. Garcia & M. Pollycove. 1961. Relation between severity of anemia and erythropoietin titer in human beings. Blood **18:** 187.

6. VAN DYKE, D. C. 1960. Sources and properties of human urinary erythropoietin. *In* CIBA Foundation Symposium on Haemopoiesis Cell Production and its Regulation. G. E. W. Wolstenholme & M. O'Connor, Eds. : 397–422. J. A. Churchill, Ltd. London, England.
7. GURNEY, C. W., R. DEGOWIN, D. HOFSTRA & J. BYRON. 1962. Applications of erythropoietin to biological investigations. *In* Erythropoiesis. L. O. Jacobson & M. Doyle, Eds. : 151-161. Grune & Stratton, Inc. New York, N. Y.
8. RAMBACH, W. A., H. L. ALT & J. A. D. COOPER. 1957. The mode of action and nature of a heat-stable plasma erythropoietic factor. Blood **12**: 1101.
9. RAMBACH, W. A., J. A. D. COOPER & H. L. ALT. 1958. Purification of erythropoietin by ion-exchange chromatography. Proc. Soc. Exp. Biol. Med. **98**: 602.
10. GOLDWASSER, E. & W. F. WHITE. 1959. Purification of sheep erythropoietin. Fed. Proc. **18**: 236.
11. YAMASHINA, I. 1956. On the carbohydrate components of the α_1 acid glycoprotein of human plasma. Acta Chem. Scand. **10**: 1666.
12. MILNE, M. D., B. H. SCRIBNER & M. A. CRAWFORD. 1958. Nonionic diffusion and the excretion of weak acids and bases. Amer. J. Med. **24**: 709.
13. WEINER, I. M. & G. H. MUDGE. 1964. Renal tubular mechanisms for excretion of organic acids and bases. Amer. J. Med. **36**: 743.
14. SCRIBNER, B. H., M. A. CRAWFORD & W. J. DEMPSTER. 1959. Urinary excretion by nonionic diffusion. Amer. J. Physiol. **196**(5): 1135.
15. WADDELL, W. J. & T. C. BUTLER. 1957. The distribution and excretion of phenobarbital. J. Clin. Invest. **36**: 1217.
16. GUTMAN, A. B., T. F. YU & J. H. SIROTA. 1955. A study, by simultaneous clearance techniques, of salicylate excretion in man. Effect of alkalinization of the urine by bicarbonate administration; effect of probenecid. J. Clin. Invest. **34**: 711.
17. SCHACHTER, D. & J. G. MANIS. 1958. Salicylate and salicyl conjugates: fluorometric estimation, biosynthesis and renal excretion in man. J. Clin. Invest. **37**: 800.
18. JAILER, J. W., M. ROSENFELD, & J. A. SHANNON. 1947. The influence of orally administered alkali and acid on the renal excretion of quinacrine, chloroquine, and santoquine. J. Clin. Invest. **26**: 1168.
19. LEWIS, J. P., N. I. GALLAGHER, S. E. CARMODY & R. D. LANGE. 1965. Erythropoietin activity and protein-protein interaction in human urine. Biochem. Biophys. Acta. **104**: 218.

ERYTHROPOIETIN PRODUCTION IN THE HUMAN FETUS AND NEWBORN

Sverre Halvorsen and Per Haavardsholm Finne

Pediatric Research Institute, Rikshospitalet, University of Oslo, Norway

The hemolytic disease of the fetus and newborn provides a unique opportunity to study the effect of hypoxia in the fetus with normal oxygenation in the mother. We have used cord blood from normal infants and from erythroblastotic infants to study erythropoietin production in the human fetus.

FIGURE 1 shows the cord blood erythropoietin levels of nonerythroblastic infants plotted against the gestational age of the infant. Premature infants have normal or slightly elevated levels compared with adults. At term there is a wider variation and in postmature infants even higher levels may be found. There may be two explanations for this wide variation in erythropoietin levels at term or after term. Either the ability to produce erythropoietin develops against term, or the elevation in erythropoietin levels is due to fetal hypoxia. The findings of high erythropoietin levels in cord blood from anemic, erythroblastotic infants as early as in the 32nd week of gestation[1] are strong evidence that the human fetus responds to anemic hypoxia with erythropoietin production, and there seems to be no difference in the response to anemia either at this premature stage or at term. High erythropoietin levels in cord blood from cases of severe dysmaturity with high Hb levels[1] indicate that the human fetus also responds to hypoxic hypoxia. The greater variations in the cord blood erythropoietin levels at and after term indicate some degree of hypoxia and not a development of the erythropoiesis-regulating system.

In the first weeks of life no erythropoietic activity was found in the plasma, and the mean of the ^{59}Fe erythrocyte uptake in the recipient polycythemic mice was significantly lower in the mice receiving plasma than in the saline-injected controls.[2] This may have been a methodological error, but may also indicate an inhibitory effect of newborn plasma on erythropoiesis. Preliminary studies in our laboratory support this concept because plasma withdrawn on the fourth and fifth day of life inhibited ^{59}Fe erythrocyte uptake in polycythemic mice given this plasma and control plasma before and after an eight-hour period of hypoxia. However, more data are needed to clarify this point.

Anemic infants and severely cyanotic infants with transposition of the great vessels have elevated levels of erythropoietin in plasma,[2] indicating that newborn infants may produce erythropoietin as a response to anemic and hypoxic hypoxia.

These studies indicate that the erythropoietin production in the human fetus is well established in the 32nd week of gestation. Following birth there is a sudden drop in erythropoietin production and although few, our data suggest that erythropoiesis inhibitors are functioning in the first week of life. Anemic and hypoxic infants may, however, produce erythropoietin in this period. Our general conclusion is, therefore, that in the human the regulation of erythropoiesis through erythropoietin is functioning in the last trimester of pregnancy and in the neonatal period, thus explaining the actual variations in erythropoiesis in the fetus and newborn.

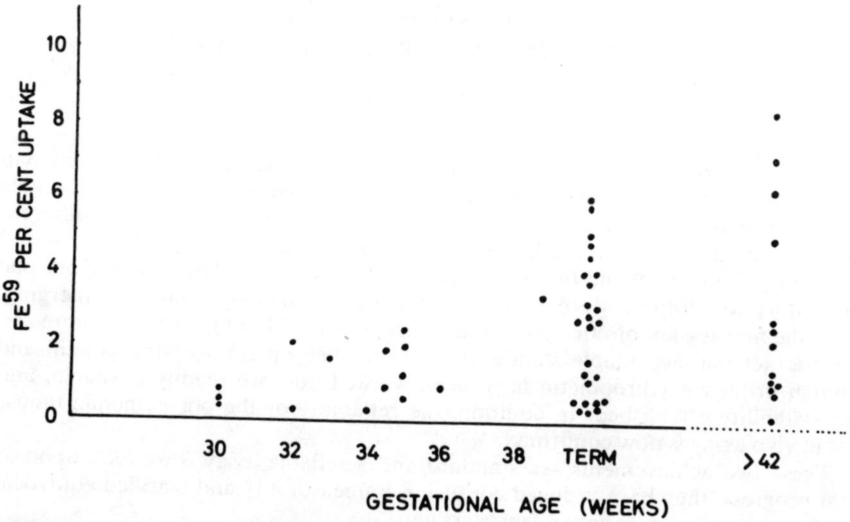

FIGURE 1. Plasma erythropoietin levels in cord blood from nonerythroblastotic infants measured as ^{59}Fe percent erythrocyte uptake in transfusion-induced polycythemic mice plotted against the gestational age at delivery.

References

1. FINNE, P. H. 1966. Erythropoietin production in fetal hypoxia and in anemic, uremic patients. Ann. N. Y. Acad. Sci. This Annal.
2. HALVORSEN, S. 1963. Plasma erythropoietin levels in cord blood and in blood during the first weeks of life. Acta paediat. 52: 425.

SUMMARY OF CONFERENCE ON ERYTHROPOIETIN

Leon O. Jacobson and Sanford B. Krantz

Several years have passed since the Conference on Erythropoiesis in San Francisco. At that conference many questions were unanswered, and considerable confusion existed because erythropoietin was being assayed in several different systems, including the normal rodent, the starved rat, the hypophysectomized rat, and the polycythemic mouse. Thus it was difficult to relate results from one laboratory to another. Moreover, an erythropoietin standard was just emerging.

In the first session of our 1966 Conference, one could not help being impressed by the fact that acceptable standards for both sheep plasma erythropoietin and human urinary erythropoietin have been worked out, are readily available, and their stability established. In addition, the reliability of the polycythemic mouse for in vivo assay is now confirmed.

These two achievements – a standard and a reliable assay – we look upon as real progress; they have reduced confusion immeasurably and clarified equivocal results we puzzled over only a few years ago.

The first session of this Conference was devoted to the assay and standardization of erythropoietin. Papers presented by Doctors Keighley, Linman, McDonald, and Cotes reviewed the in vivo assays now in use and discussed their relative merits and demerits. Dr. Cotes emphasized the importance of selecting a strain of mice which gave reproducible results from week to week, since some strains do not do this, and the importance of using a reference standard with each assay in order to characterize a standard response and avoid confusion with extraneous effects on the marrow. Dr. Cotes and Dr. Keighley showed that plasma erythropoietin could be stored for at least two years without loss of activity if kept under the best conditions, i.e., frozen and dried. The most sensitive in vivo assay still appears to be the mouse that has increased oxygenation in relation to its needs. Several different techniques for preparing such animals were described: The old hypoxic chamber with air evacuation was presented by Dr. Keighley, who finds that ten days in the chamber are sufficient, rather than 16–22 days. The hypoxia caused by silicone rubber membranes was presented by Dr. McDonald. This ingenious device is more permeable to CO_2 than O_2 and causes hypoxia in the chamber as the mice consume the O_2. The silicone membrane chambers are very expensive and may create the additional hazard of different O_2 saturation from group to group unless each chamber is carefully checked for leaks and uniform membranes. When all the hazards of the in vivo mouse assay are controlled, a reasonably useful and sensitive bioassay remains, but one that still needs a reference standard for control so that the pitfalls produced by response variation from day to day may be avoided.

The method of preparing the polycythemic mouse is immaterial. There is no doubt that hypertransfusion, hypoxia, silicone enclosures, or carbon monoxide are all effective. It is therefore largely a matter of using the method that is cheapest and most convenient for a given laboratory. We tend to agree, perhaps mainly from prejudice, that the hypertransfused polycythemic mouse may be physiologically the most satisfactory subject.

The problem of in vitro assay of erythropoietin remains with us. Dr. Goldwasser and we have spent many hours yearning for a rapid, reliable, and simple in vitro method.

The second session concerned the chemistry and purification of erythropoietin. Dr. Goldwasser showed that one of the big problems involved in purification of this material was surface denaturation in dilute solution. This could be corrected by assaying the preparation in a solution with albumin or gelatin. Under these conditions he could purify erythropoietin some 950,000 times to 1600 units per mg, but with only a 2% recovery, which did not provide sufficient material to characterize the final product. Nevertheless, this degree of purification represents a remarkable achievement. Dr. Lowy showed that erythropoietin could also be purified from human urine. The urinary material causes an increase in hematocrit and blood volume and is abolished by antierythropoietin serum, suggesting that it is a similar material to the serum erythropoietin. Purification of this material, however, has proceeded to only 120 units per mg. Dr. Goldwasser commented on the great instability of urinary material, the reason for which is unknown. Dr. Allen reported his ability to purify erythropoietin from mouse plasma by vertical flat bed discontinuous electrophoresis. He reached a purity of 7.9 units per mg of protein by this single procedure. On analysis, this erythropoietin preparation contained six proteins, three of which were esterases; thus further purification is needed for characterization of this molecule. Sedimentation data presented by Dr. Allen and Dr. Goldwasser, and the x-ray inactivation studies of Drs. Hodgson and Rosse indicate a molecular weight in the range of 40,000–60,000.

Having come so very far with the purification of erythropoietin, one would like to know more about this important molecule. Further characterization has been limited by the supply of the material, and thus it was very encouraging to note the report by Dr. Painter of Connaught Laboratories that Step I erythropoietin production and Step III may soon be more readily available. Finally, Dr. Rosse, who has a fondness for Japanese quail, reports that avian erythropoietin is not inactivated by anti-human erythropoietin serum and is not active in mammalian systems, nor does mammalian erythropoietin act on avian marrows. We have come a remarkably long way in the purification of erythropoietin, but much more material and work are still needed to characterize this molecule and perhaps put the finishing touches on purification.

Where is erythropoietin produced? The work of Dr. Jacobson indicating that the kidney is the source of erythropoietin in rats may need certain qualifications on the basis of the work presented at this Conference. Certainly the kidney appears to be a major source of erythropoietin in some species. This is confirmed by Dr. Naets' experiments on dogs; by Dr. Fisher's experiments on the isolated dog kidney perfused with hypoxic blood, and the effect of renal artery constriction; by Dr. Contrera's and Dr. Muirhead's experiments on erythropoietin extraction from kidney section or particulate fractions; and by Dr. Mitus' work on experimental hydronephrosis. In the human, however, and perhaps in rabbits erythropoietin also appears to be produced in an extrarenal site or sites and some control of erythropoiesis persists in addition to and independent of the kidneys, as shown by the work of Dr. Naets and Dr. Nathan. Thus there appear to be species' differences in the site of production, and perhaps other mechanisms of erythropoietic control exist in some species as well.

Associated with increased erythropoietin production is an increase in the granulation of the juxtaglomerular apparatus. However, the conditions that are used to stimulate erythropoietin production also increase renin formation, and although it has been shown that this does not have an erythropoietin-like effect, it indicates the nonspecific nature of the juxtaglomerular apparatus increase. Drs. Halvorsen and Mirand have presented some very interesting observations on hypothalamic stimulation and ablation. The complex ramifications of this work do not provide an easy interpretation. It is still not clear if the plasma erythropoietin (or substance) produced is the same as the erythropoietin produced by reduced tissue O_2 supply, and if so, whether some additional side effects produced by manipulation of the central nervous system, such as an effect on the respiratory center, may reduce tissue oxygenation. Further study of these factors is needed to clarify this matter.

The next question to be taken up was the site of action of erythropoietin. Work with the hypertransfused mouse, in which erythropoietin elicits proerythroblasts where none were present before injection of the hormone, has indicated that the hormone at least works on the primitive stem cell precursor of the erythroblast. Dr. Lajtha has tackled the problem of whether the colony-forming cell is the same as the erythropoietin-responsive cell. By comparing experiments on exocolonization, endocolonization, and erythropoietin response under different conditions, he clearly showed that exocolonization units and erythropoietin-responsive cells respond differently to x-ray. The erythropoietin-responsive cell may be removed from the colony-forming cell, however, by the degree of only one chemical reaction. Is this then a different cell? We may be dealing with the progressive stages of development within one cell, which looks different, but which represents only one unit. At this stage we must agree with Dr. Lajtha that we shall remain in the dark until more of the facts are defined. Dr. Stohlman and Dr. Reissmann have shown that vincristin and Actinomycin D seem to have a far greater effect upon erythropoiesis than upon myelopoiesis or megakaryocytopoiesis. Vincristin delays the usual erythropoietic response but since it has a tendency to hold cells in metaphase, the erythropoietic information may also be held in the stem cell until the latter recovers from the effect of the drug; the cell may then proceed to differentiate. Dr. Yoffey has shown that erythropoietin causes an accelerated reticulocyte discharge from the bone marrow. Dr. Stohlman finds macrocytes after stimulation of normal marrow with erythropoietin, but not after stimulation of hypertransfused marrow. Does this mean that the erythropoietin acts on two cells in normal marrow, the stem cell and the differentiated cell, or can one action on the stem cell account for the macrocytes by promoting premature release of differentiated cells already present? We are still not sure whether erythropoietin also acts at a second site beyond the stem cell.

Dr. Erslev has produced an interesting animal model for the study of the compensated hemolytic state, in which he finds normal erythropoietin levels with increased erythropoiesis. When erythropoietin is given, the response is increased. This may mean, as he suggests, that there are more stem cells present, or that the stem cells are simply in a state of greater receptiveness to erythropoietin. Again, the increased response may be due to the peculiar nature of the dose response curve, which ascends very steeply after a slow plateau where small increments in dose are difficult to measure. Similarly, the work of Jan Fogh showed that a second dose of erythropoietin given up to four days after the first elicited a greater response than the first dose. This may be due to the production of more stem cells, to an increased responsiveness of the stem cells, or to an effect on the increased numbers of differentiated cells. We believe that all these possibilities exist and that further experimentation is necessary to define the exact site of action and kinetics of erythropoietin. Dr. Yoffey has correlated lymphocyte changes with erythropoietic changes and Dr. Orlic has described a primitive cell that takes up tritiated thymidine after erythropoietin administration. Although these conditions may be useful in drawing our attention to certain changes that are occurring, we are still unsure about the appearance of the actual cell upon which erythropoietin exerts its effect. Until we can isolate pure cell populations and show that the hormone acts directly upon these populations, we will still wonder what the stem cell really is.

Finally, Dr. Reissmann and Dr. Takaku reported some experiments on the mechanism of action of erythropoietin. It seems increasingly certain that erythropoietin acts via increased RNA formation, which is followed by increased ALA synthetase that can be detected by eight hr, and then by increased hemoglobin synthesis. Dr. Goldwasser, however, who also likes to think that this is messenger RNA, was quick to point out that it is not proven, and that the increase may be in another species of RNA not yet functionally defined. The sequence of the events that follow RNA stimulation is still not clear. Although there are effects on ALA synthetase, heme, globin, and DNA synthesis, the order of these events has not been determined. There may also be an effect on the production of different hemoglobins in the proerythroblast, as shown by Dr. Borsook, or in mouse marrow, as shown by Dr. Kraus, but further work is needed to characterize these hemoglobin fractions and identify them.

Dr. Matoth explored the generation time of the stem cell and showed that it may be much shorter under certain circumstances than we have expected. It may be as short as 1.75 hours. Dr. Hodgson defined the cell cycle in terms of sensitivity to x-irradiation, and was able to show that there is a well-defined period four hr before erythropoietin acts when the cell is more sensitive to the effect of x-ray and subsequently, will not respond to erythropoietin.

Dr. Schooley has shown clearly that an antibody inhibitory to the function of erythropoietin can be made, and this achievement takes on great significance in view of the recent studies of the Montreal group (Jepson and Lowenstein), which has shown that human anemia can occur in cases of thymus tumors, even in the presence of an erythropoietin inhibitor. The antiserum produces the same effects on the marrow as increased O_2 supply to the whole animal, by reducing the effective circulating erythropoietin. Dr. O'Grady showed that it also affected erythroid colony-forming units by reducing their size and number just as hypertransfusion does. This antibody therefore promises to be a very potent tool for future research on erythropoietin. Finally, the question of its use for an immunoassay of erythropoietin was discussed by Dr. Goudsmit. He correlated an α-2 immunoelectrophoretic preparation band with increased erythropoietic activity in aplastic anemia and reduced activity in human nephritis, and showed by elution that erythropoietic activity was present in this band. However, because of the impure nature of erythropoietin, the antibody must also be impure, and thus, other substances that will not allow complete correlation may well be present. For this we will have to wait and see.

If erythropoiesis is a difficult subject (as is clearly shown above), how much harder must the study of erythropoiesis and sex be! This was plainly demonstrated by the following studies. Dr. Meineke showed that nortestosterone increased erythropoiesis in the hypophysectomized rat, and this was abolished by nephrectomy. Hypertransfusion restricted the marrow response. Dr. Gordon showed increased erythropoiesis after testosterone was injected into the normal rat. Hypoxia increased the marrow response. He also showed that the testosterone had no influence in nephrectomized rats. Perfused kidneys of testosterone-treated rabbits showed erythropoietin levels that were greater than those of perfused kidneys in normal rabbits. Dr. Fried also showed that testosterone-increased serum erythropoietin levels were abolished by nephrectomy. The erythropoietic-stimulating activity was abolished by the antierythropoietin antibody. From all this work it appears that testosterone increases serum erythropoietin levels by acting on the kidney to increase erythropoietin release. This may be a means of reducing anemia where marrow cells show reduced sensitivity to erythropoietin, as in the WW^v mice described by Dr. Fried, but the work of W. Jacobson and Diamond, which shows a direct in vitro effect of testosterone on marrow DNA synthesis, also indicates that other mechanisms of action may exist for the testosterone effects on human aplastic anemias. Of importance for demonstrating testosterone effects was the choice of species and sex of the species, as shown by Dr. Naets. Could the potentiation of the erythropoietin effect, which Dr. Naets and Dr. Meineke suggest for testosterone, be again due to the nature of the dose response curve where there is an initial plateau and then an increased slope of effect? If the androgens increase erythropoietin a little in a state of higher endogenous erythropoietin secretion, then the erythropoietin is clearly easily measured. If they increase it from a state of low endogenous erythropoietin secretion, the effect may not be easily measured because of the plateaued dose response curve. This explanation remains to be clarified but may explain some of the discrepancy.

Dr. Piliero showed that large doses of estrogen exert toxic effects on many organs. It is therefore difficult to conclude that estrogen normally acts to decrease liver production of an erythropoietin precursor. Dr. Medal showed that hemolysates increased erythropoiesis, but he failed to measure endogenous erythropoietin levels. Since hemolysates have great toxic effects on the kidneys, might they not cause increased endogenous elaboration of erythropoietin, rather than a direct effect on erythropoiesis?

The final day of the Conference was mainly devoted to the application of our information concerning erythropoietin to clinical disorders of erythropoiesis. (The in vitro papers have been mainly discussed under mechanism of action of erythropoietin).

As techniques have been perfected, and information about the control mechanism of normal erythropoiesis has increased, we have begun to apply the techniques to clinical diseases. Dr. Russell in her mouse clinic has shown that these techniques can be applied to studies of congenital anemia in two strains of mice. She showed that one of these anemias consisted of reduced sensitivity of the marrow to erythropoietin, and could be alleviated by those conditions that result in increased blood levels of erythropoietin – levels above the normal high for these mice. Another strain, with anemia and increased erythropoietin blood levels, did not respond in the same way unless the marrow was transplanted to another host where it did respond. In this second case, therefore, the primary defect was in a host factor, and not in the marrow cells themselves.

Dr. Adamson reported that by measurement of the daily urinary secretion of erythropoietin and response to phlebotomy, he could distinguish between primary and secondary polycythemias and inappropriate secretion of erythropoietin by tumors. In the latter case the daily urine excretion of erythropoietin was unaffected by phlebotomy. In the secondary polycythemias the erythropoietin secretion was generally high and increased with an exaggerated response after phlebotomy. In the polycythemia veras, virtually no erythropoietin was present in the urine, but it could be elicited after phlebotomy. Dr. Krantz applied in vitro methods to the problem and found reduced sensitivity of the primary polycythemia bone marrow in vitro to the addition of erythropoietin. There was no humoral substance in polycythemia vera plasma which itself stimulated the polycythemia vera marrow, and no inhibitor to the normal action of erythropoietin. Although this work needs further controls, it would seem that polycythemia vera is not caused by erythropoietin.

Dr. Gallagher and Dr. Waldmann reported on many clinical conditions, tumors or cysts, associated with polycythemia, and quite clearly demonstrated increased erythropoietin serum levels under these conditions. Dr. Hoffman reported the phenomenon of polycythemia associated with renal transplantation, thus linking erythropoietin secretion to the state of the kidney. Of interest is the development of increased erythropoiesis even though uremia increased the disassociation between these two functions in the kidney. Dr. Nathan again emphasized the presence of continuing low amounts of erythropoiesis despite nephrectomy, but Dr. Gordon pointed out that nephrectomy might stimulate other organs to take over, to some extent, this single function of the kidney. This point is still not certain and needs further experimentation.

Consideration of the erythropoietin model perhaps led Dr. Hammond to infuse normal plasma into nine children with aplastic anemia and high endogenous levels of erythropoietin, his idea being that their erythropoietin might be abnormal or might need a carrier or cofactor in order to function. In any case, this treatment resulted in four remissions, some of which were permanent. One cannot, however, exclude the possibility that other nonerythropoietin-associated metabolites might have been responsible.

Finally, Dr. Gurney showed that erythropoietin secretion was inhibited by increased CO_2 levels and increased with alkalosis, perhaps because erythropoietin is an acidic molecule. This has important implications for extraction of the hormone from human urine.

Thus we have now progressed to clinical application of the erythropoietin model: We can now classify certain diseases (polycythemias) on the basis of erythropoietin elaboration. As purer and purer preparations of the hormone are produced, we may be able to develop applications for treatment as in uremia. This, however, will have to be reported at some future conference.

Printed in the United States of America